Cecil
Review of
General Internal
Medicine

Cecil
Review of
General Internal
Medicine

8th Edition

J. Allen D. Cooper, Jr., M.D.
Professor of Medicine
Division of Pulmonary, Allergy & Critical Care Medicine
University of Alabama at Birmingham School of Medicine
Chief, Pulmonary Section
Birmingham Veterans Affairs Medical Center
Birmingham, Alabama

Peter G. Pappas, M.D.
Professor of Medicine
Division of Infectious Diseases
University of Alabama at Birmingham School of Medicine
Birmingham, Alabama

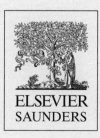

ELSEVIER
SAUNDERS

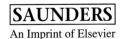

SAUNDERS

An Imprint of Elsevier

The Curtis Center
170 S. Independence Mall W 300 E
Philadelphia, Pennsylvania 19106

NOTICE

Medicine is an ever-changing field. Standard safety precautions must be followed, but as new research and clinical experience broaden our knowledge, changes in treatment and drug therapy may become necessary or appropriate. Readers are advised to check the most current product information provided by the manufacturer of each drug to be administered to verify the recommended dose, the method and duration of administration, and contraindications. It is the responsibility of the treating physician, relying on experience and knowledge of the patient, to determine dosages and the best treatment for each individual patient. Neither the Publisher nor the editor assumes any liability for any injury and/or damage to persons or property arising from this publication.

THE PUBLISHER

Previous editions copyrighted 2001, 1996, 1992, 1989, 1985, 1982, 1980

Library of Congress Control Number: 2004093009

Acquisitions Editor: Kim Murphy
Developmental Editor: Meghan Ziegler
Publishing Services Manager: Frank Polizzano
Project Manager: Jeff Gunning
Design Coordinator: Karen O'Keefe Owens

Printed in the United States of America

Last digit is the print number: 9 8 7 6 5 4 3 2 1

This book is dedicated to our children,
Thomas, Rebecca, Hayden, Cameron, Stavros, and Elias.

CONTRIBUTORS

Eric S. Albright, M.D.
Assistant Professor of Medicine
Department of Medicine, Division of Endocrinology, University of Alabama at Birmingham School of Medicine, Birmingham, Alabama
Endocrinology; Diabetes Mellitus and Metabolism

Vera A. Bittner, M.D., M.S.P.H.
Professor of Medicine
Department of Medicine, Division of Cardiovascular Disease, University of Alabama at Birmingham School of Medicine, Birmingham, Alabama
Cardiology

Joao A. M. de Andrade, M.D.
Assistant Professor of Medicine
Department of Medicine, Division of Pulmonary, Allergy and Critical Care Medicine, University of Alabama at Birmingham School of Medicine
Medical Director, Medical Intensive Care Unit
Birmingham Veterans Affairs Medical Center, Birmingham, Alabama
Pulmonary Diseases

Britt B. Drake, M.D.
Fellow in Gastroenterology and Hepatology
Department of Medicine, Division of Gastrointestinal Disease and Hepatology, University of Alabama at Birmingham School of Medicine, Birmingham, Alabama
Gastrointestinal and Liver Disease

Peter D. Emanuel, M.D.
Professor of Medicine
Associate Director, Division of Hematology/Oncology
Department of Medicine, University of Alabama at Birmingham School of Medicine
Program Director for Hematological Malignancies
Comprehensive Cancer Center, Birmingham, Alabama
Hematology

Stuart J. Frank, M.D.
Professor of Medicine, Cell Biology, and Physiology
Department of Medicine, Division of Endocrinology, Diabetes and Metabolism, University of Alabama at Birmingham School of Medicine
Chief, Endocrinology Section
Medical Service, Birmingham Veterans Affairs Medical Center, Birmingham, Alabama
Endocrinology

Jeffrey R. George, M.D.
Fellow in Hematology/Oncology
University of Alabama at Birmingham School of Medicine and University of Alabama at Birmingham Hospitals, Birmingham, Alabama
Oncology

Ritesh Gupta, M.D., M.P.H.
Fellow in Cardiology
Department of Medicine, Division of Cardiovascular Disease, University of Alabama at Birmingham School of Medicine, Birmingham, Alabama
Cardiology

Julie C. Harper, M.D.
Assistant Professor of Dermatology
Department of Dermatology, University of Alabama at Birmingham School of Medicine, Birmingham, Alabama
Dermatology

Louis W. Heck, Jr., M.D.
Professor of Medicine
Department of Medicine, Division of Rheumatology and Clinical Immunology, University of Alabama at Birmingham School of Medicine, Birmingham, Alabama
Rheumatology and Clinical Immunology

Craig J. Hoesley, M.D.
Assistant Professor of Medicine
Department of Medicine, Division of Infectious Diseases, University of Alabama at Birmingham School of Medicine, Birmingham, Alabama
Infectious Diseases

James E. Johnson, M.D.
Associate Professor of Medicine and Physiology and Biophysics
Department of Medicine, Division of Pulmonary, Allergy and Critical Care Medicine, University of Alabama at Birmingham School of Medicine, Birmingham, Alabama
Critical Care

Lisle M. Nabell, M.D.
Assistant Professor of Medicine
Department of Medicine, Division of Hematology/Oncology, University of Alabama at Birmingham School of Medicine, Birmingham, Alabama
Oncology

Louis Burt Nabors, M.D.

Assistant Professor of Neurology
Department of Neurology, University of Alabama at Birmingham
    School of Medicine, Birmingham, Alabama
Neurology

Fernando Ovalle, M.D.

Associate Professor of Medicine
Director, Clinical Research Unit and Fellowship Training Program
Department of Medicine, Division of Endocrinology, Diabetes and
    Metabolism, University of Alabama at Birmingham School of
    Medicine, Birmingham, Alabama
Diabetes Mellitus and Metabolism

Peter G. Pappas, M.D.

Professor of Medicine
Department of Medicine, Division of Infectious Diseases, University
    of Alabama at Birmingham School of Medicine, Birmingham,
    Alabama
Infectious Diseases

Paul W. Sanders, M.D.

Professor of Medicine and Physiology and Biophysics
Department of Medicine, Division of Nephrology, and Department
    of Physiology and Biophysics, University of Alabama at
    Birmingham School of Medicine, Birmingham, Alabama
Renal Disease

C. Mel Wilcox, M.D.

Professor of Medicine
Department of Medicine, Division of Gastrointestinal Disease and
    Hepatology, University of Alabama at Birmingham School of
    Medicine, Birmingham, Alabama
Gastrointestinal and Liver Disease

PREFACE

The practice of internal medicine presents a formidable and unique challenge to the clinician. The explosion of medical information in the recent past, together with the development of new and innovative therapies and diagnostic techniques, makes the practice of medicine both simpler and more complex than ever before. Thus, the need to remain abreast of current knowledge in internal medicine has never been more important to the physician in training and the practicing clinician—not only to provide the best care for our patients but also to remain well prepared for recertification examinations in our specialties. In an "Information Age," there are several means of acquiring continuing medical education (CME), including traditional board review courses, subspecialty conferences, Internet-based CME activities, and other tools. Fortunately for the physician, access to these various media has never been greater, and access to the Internet has provided physicians, trainees, and patients, even in remote areas, almost limitless access to healthcare-related information. In spite of these significant achievements in alternative methods of CME, we believe that this book continues to play a unique and important role in testing knowledge in the broad discipline of internal medicine. For those individuals who are most comfortable with a readily accessible book of carefully considered questions, clinical scenarios, and detailed answers, this book is ideal in helping to achieve the formidable task of maintaining a current knowledge base in internal medicine.

This is the 8th edition of the *Cecil Review of General Internal Medicine*. It is the companion of the recently published 22nd edition of the *Cecil Textbook of Medicine*. The format of this book is unchanged compared with that in the most recent editions, being composed of questions pertaining to specific areas in internal medicine, divided by major subspecialties. This book represents a significant revision from the 7th edition. All questions have been written by authorities in their field and are presented in a format similar to that used in the American Board of Internal Medicine certification examinations. At the end of each section, detailed explanations and the correct answers are provided for each question. References to the corresponding chapter in *Cecil Textbook of Medicine* are provided for each answer, along with other pertinent references (at the authors' discretion). When used together with *Cecil Textbook of Medicine*, the questions and answers presented herein are both pertinent and sufficiently broad in scope to provide a unique and completely individualized opportunity to review in detail some of the most current information in internal medicine.

Any work of this scope requires the significant input of many contributors. We would like to thank each of the contributors who devoted substantial time and effort to this 8th edition of the *Cecil Review of General Internal Medicine*, for without them, this edition would not have been possible. We sincerely hope that by reviewing the questions and answers along with the *Cecil Textbook of Medicine*, the user will find this to be a useful and enjoyable tutor for maintaining a current fund of knowledge to facilitate the optimal practice of internal medicine.

J. ALLEN D. COOPER, JR., M.D.
PETER G. PAPPAS, M.D.

ACKNOWLEDGMENTS

We would like to thank Ms. Windell Ross, Ms. Cynthia Kirksey, and Ms. Christy Shinn, whose many hours of technical assistance were essential in manuscript preparation.

CONTENTS

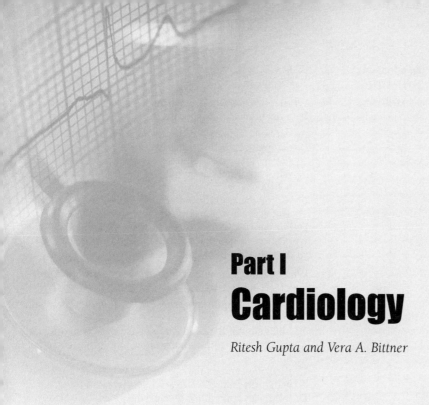

Part I
Cardiology

Ritesh Gupta and Vera A. Bittner

MULTIPLE CHOICE

DIRECTIONS: For questions 1–107, choose the single best answer to each question.

1. Which of the following statements regarding abdominal aortic aneurysms is *not* correct?

    A. Asymptomatic patients with aneurysms less than 5 cm should be monitored with serial imaging.

    B. Asymptomatic patients with aneurysms greater than 5 cm should be referred for elective surgery.

    C. Asymptomatic patients who have aneurysms less than 5 cm but with aortic thrombosis or distal embolization should be anticoagulated with warfarin (Coumadin).

    D. Symptomatic patients should be referred for immediate surgery.

2. Which of the following statements regarding myomectomy for hypertrophic cardiomyopathy is correct?

    A. It reduces the incidence of sudden death.

    B. It has a success rate of 90% for relieving symptoms and reducing outflow tract obstruction.

    C. It is widely applicable in patients with hypertrophic cardiomyopathy.

    D. It may exacerbate the mitral regurgitation associated with hypertrophic cardiomyopathy.

3. Which of the following is *not* associated with a soft S_1?

    A. Wolff-Parkinson-White (WPW) syndrome

    B. First-degree atrioventricular (AV) block

    C. Sinus bradycardia

    D. Severe mitral stenosis

4. Hypertrophic cardiomyopathy (HOCM) is characterized by which of the following echocardiographic findings?

    A. Asymmetrical hypertrophy, most commonly septal hypertrophy

    B. Systolic anterior motion of the anterior mitral valve leaflet

    C. Dynamic systolic gradient in the left ventricular outflow tract

    D. All of the above

5. Hepatojugular (abdominojugular) reflux is found in patients with:

    A. Right ventricular infarction

    B. Superior vena cava syndrome

    C. Left ventricular failure with secondary pulmonary hypertension

    D. Tricuspid regurgitation

6. Paradoxical (reversed) splitting of S_2 is caused by all of the following *except:*

    A. Left bundle branch block

    B. Aortic stenosis

    C. Atrial septal defect

    D. WPW syndrome with a right-sided accessory pathway

7. Which of the following is *not* characteristic of hypertrophic cardiomyopathy?

    A. Hypercontractility of the left ventricular free wall

    B. Hypocontractility of the interventricular septum

    C. Predominant systolic dysfunction

    D. Left ventricular cavity obliteration

8. Which of the following is *not* associated with an increased risk for aortic dissection?

    A. Hemochromatosis

    B. Marfan syndrome

    C. Aortic coarctation

    D. Pregnancy

9. Which of the following statements regarding the effects of physiologic maneuvers on common murmurs is *not* correct?

   A. Handgrip will intensify the systolic murmur of ventricular septal defect.
   B. Handgrip will intensify the systolic murmur of mitral regurgitation.
   C. Valsalva will intensify the systolic murmur of hypertrophic cardiomyopathy.
   D. Squatting will soften the diastolic murmur of aortic insufficiency.

10. Which of the following is *not* a typical symptom in a patient with an expanding thoracic aortic aneurysm?

    A. Hoarseness
    B. Dysphagia
    C. Intrascapular pain
    D. Hemoptysis
    E. All of the above may occur.

11. Kussmaul's sign (an inspiratory increase in the jugular venous pressure) is evident in all of the following *except*:

    A. Right ventricular infarction
    B. Constrictive pericarditis
    C. Pulmonary embolism
    D. Tricuspid regurgitation

12. Acute aortic dissection should be suspected in a patient with:

    A. Anterior chest pain
    B. Intrascapular pain
    C. Diastolic hypertension with an aortic insufficiency murmur
    D. All of the above
    E. None of the above

13. Which of the following is *not* found during orthodromic reciprocating tachycardia, the paroxysmal supraventricular tachycardia (PSVT) seen in patients with WPW syndrome?

    A. A regular, narrow complex tachycardia
    B. Delta waves
    C. Retrograde P waves in the ST segment
    D. Termination with carotid massage or adenosine

14. Which of the following is *not* a typical electrocardiographic (ECG) finding in patients with hypertrophic cardiomyopathy?

    A. Low voltage
    B. Inferior or lateral Q waves mimicking myocardial infarction (pseudoinfarction)
    C. Left atrial enlargement
    D. T wave inversions

15. Which of the following symptoms is *not* typical of claudication?

    A. Intermittent exertional pain in the buttocks, thighs, or calves
    B. A constant amount of exercise required to produce lower extremity pain
    C. Relief of pain with rest
    D. Priapism

16. Which of the following is the most useful way to distinguish ventricular tachycardia (VT) from supraventricular tachycardia (SVT) with aberrancy?

    A. Rate of the tachycardia on the ECG
    B. Stability of the patient (blood pressure [BP], mental status)
    C. AV dissociation on the ECG
    D. Response to adenosine

17. Which of the following statements regarding anticoagulation for atrial fibrillation is *not* correct?

    A. Warfarin (Coumadin) therapy for chronic atrial fibrillation reduces the incidence of stroke.
    B. Anticoagulation is not necessary for patients with paroxysmal atrial fibrillation because the risk of thromboembolism is low.
    C. Aspirin therapy reduces the incidence of stroke but is not as effective as Coumadin.
    D. For patients younger than 65 years with lone atrial fibrillation, aspirin alone is sufficient to prevent stroke because the risk of thromboembolism is low.

18. Which of the following statements regarding cardiac amyloidosis is *not* correct?

    A. Myocardial infiltration results in hypertrophy and restriction.
    B. Infiltration of the conduction system results in arrhythmias, including sinus bradycardia, heart block, and atrial fibrillation.
    C. Digoxin decreases the risk of hospitalization in patients with heart failure due to amyloidosis.
    D. Even with appropriate therapy, the prognosis is poor.

19. Which of the following drugs is *not* useful in the treatment of patients with hypertrophic cardiomyopathy?

    A. Verapamil
    B. Propranolol
    C. Disopyramide
    D. Digoxin

20. Which of the following statements regarding cardioversion of atrial fibrillation is *not* correct?

    A. The absence of thrombus on a transthoracic echocardiogram allows immediate, safe cardioversion.
    B. Patients who have had atrial fibrillation for less than 24 hours do not need anticoagulation before cardioversion.
    C. Patients who have had atrial fibrillation for more than 48 hours should receive Coumadin for 3 weeks before undergoing cardioversion or undergo transesophageal echocardiogram–guided cardioversion.
    D. Maintenance of sinus rhythm with antiarrhythmic drugs does not obviate the need for Coumadin therapy.

21. Which of the following is *not* associated with an increased incidence of sudden cardiac death after a myocardial infarction?

    A. Left ventricular systolic dysfunction
    B. Frequent, multiform premature ventricular contractions
    C. Increased heart rate variability
    D. Late potentials on a signal-averaged ECG

22. A 44-year-old man with a history of sarcoidosis presents with 2 months of dyspnea on exertion and lower leg swelling. ECG reveals low voltages in the precordial and limb leads. He is diagnosed, after a biopsy, with restrictive cardiomyopathy due to sarcoid granulomatous infiltration in the myocardium. His echocardiographic findings are likely to be consistent with:

    A. Bi-atrial enlargement
    B. Restrictive diastolic function and increased wall thickness
    C. Ventricular dilatation

D. Both A and B
E. Both A and C

23. Cardiac MRI has been used in the characterization of which of the following cardiac problems?

    A. Cardiac tumors
    B. Pericardial diseases
    C. Thoracic aorta dissection
    D. Anomalous origin of coronary arteries
    E. All of the above

24. Which of the following statements regarding pharmacologic control of the ventricular response during atrial fibrillation is *not* correct?

    A. Digoxin is useful for sedentary patients.
    B. Digoxin prevents exercise-related increases in the ventricular response during atrial fibrillation.
    C. β-Blockers or calcium-channel blockers are the best agents for young, active patients.
    D. Among the calcium-channel blockers, verapamil and diltiazem, but not amlodipine or nifedipine, are effective in controlling the ventricular response.

25. Which of the following statements regarding acute aortic dissection is *not* correct?

    A. If the ascending aorta or aortic arch is involved, then emergency surgery is indicated.
    B. Patients with dissections involving the proximal aorta should be stabilized with β-blockers and nitroprusside for several hours before proceeding with surgery.
    C. Patients with descending aortic dissections can be managed medically in most cases.
    D. A descending aortic dissection with dissecting hematoma, impending rupture, or uncontrollable pain should be surgically repaired.

26. Which of the following statements regarding radiofrequency catheter ablation is correct?

    A. A permanent pacemaker is implanted after ablation of atrial flutter.
    B. Catheter ablation is extremely painful and requires general anesthesia.
    C. Catheter ablation is curative for most SVTs but is not cost effective compared with medical therapy.
    D. Among patients who have both atrial flutter and atrial fibrillation who undergo ablation of atrial flutter, 50% will have recurrent atrial fibrillation.

27. Which of the following statements about arterial hypertension is *not* correct?

    A. Patients with diabetes have a goal blood pressure of less than 130/80 mm Hg.
    B. Patients with prehypertension have normal blood pressure but multiple lifestyle characteristics that put them at risk for developing hypertension in middle age.
    C. Lifestyle modification is indicated in all stages of hypertension.
    D. Most patients with stage 2 hypertension require multi-drug therapy.

28. In a patient with WPW syndrome who experiences atrial fibrillation with anterograde (AV) conduction over the accessory pathway (pre-excited atrial fibrillation), the drug of choice is:

    A. Verapamil
    B. Digoxin

C. Procainamide
D. Esmolol

29. Which of the following statements regarding doxorubicin cardiotoxicity is *not* correct?

    A. The cardiotoxicity related to doxorubicin is reversible and resolves rapidly after discontinuation of chemotherapy.
    B. Cardiotoxicity is related to peak levels.
    C. Cardiotoxicity is related to cumulative dose.
    D. Cardiotoxicity is uncommonly seen at cumulative doses of less than 500 mg/m^2.

30. Which of the following ECG findings is specific for the diagnosis of pericarditis?

    A. Diffuse ST segment elevation
    B. ST segment elevation that is concave upward
    C. ST segment elevation combined with T wave inversions
    D. PR segment depression

31. A 17-year-old boy experiences lightheadedness and dyspnea, then collapses, and dies during a high school basketball game. Autopsy will likely demonstrate:

    A. Saddle embolism of the main pulmonary artery
    B. Hypertrophic cardiomyopathy
    C. An anomalous coronary artery
    D. Subclinical myocarditis

32. Which of the following statements regarding class Ia antiarrhythmics is *not* correct?

    A. The anticholinergic effects of disopyramide, including urinary retention and dry mouth, limit its use.
    B. Procainamide is associated with a lupus-like reaction and agranulocytosis.
    C. Quinidine results in severe constipation.
    D. Class Ia antiarrhythmics are associated with QT prolongation and torsades de pointes ventricular tachycardia.

33. Which of the following statements regarding peripartum cardiomyopathy is *not* correct?

    A. It usually occurs in the last trimester or first 5 months after delivery.
    B. It usually occurs after a viral illness.
    C. It is reversible in more than half of the patients.
    D. It may occur as a result of an autoimmune mechanism related to release of myocyte antigens from the uterus.

34. Which of the following is *not* a mechanism responsible for cardiac arrhythmias?

    A. Re-entry
    B. Accommodation
    C. Automaticity
    D. Triggered activity

35. Which of the following statements regarding typical atrial flutter is *not* correct?

    A. The re-entry circuit proceeds in a counterclockwise direction around the tricuspid annulus.
    B. Sawtooth flutter waves are best seen in the anterior leads.
    C. The atrial flutter rate is often 250 to 350 beats/minute with a 2:1 ventricular response.
    D. Atrial flutter is amenable to cure with a catheter ablation procedure.

36. Which of the following statements is *not* correct?

    A. Smoking, hyperlipidemia, and diabetes are associated with endothelial dysfunction.
    B. The lipid core of plaques contains tissue factor that promotes lysis of thrombi.
    C. Elevations in high-sensitivity C-reactive protein are associated with greater risk of coronary events.
    D. Family history is an independent risk factor for coronary disease even after adjustment for other known coronary risk factors.

37. Which of the following statements regarding lidocaine is *not* correct?

    A. It is a local anesthetic that causes sodium-channel blockade.
    B. It has activity on both atrial and ventricular myocardium.
    C. The drug mexiletine is an oral drug with properties very similar to those of lidocaine.
    D. Prophylactic administration of lidocaine in the setting of myocardial infarction is not recommended.

38. Which of the following statements regarding paroxysmal supraventricular tachycardia (PSVT) is *not* correct?

    A. Orthodromic reciprocating tachycardia is a narrow complex rhythm using the AV node as the anterograde limb and an accessory pathway as a retrograde limb of the re-entry circuit.
    B. Antidromic reciprocating tachycardia is a narrow complex rhythm using an accessory pathway as the anterograde limb and the AV node as a retrograde limb of the re-entry circuit.
    C. AV nodal re-entrant tachycardia is a narrow complex rhythm using a slow AV nodal pathway as the anterograde limb and a fast AV nodal pathway as the retrograde limb of the re-entry circuit.
    D. Ectopic atrial tachycardia is due to ectopic automaticity or triggered activity in the atrium.

39. Which of the following tissues does *not* normally exhibit automaticity?

    A. Sinus node
    B. Atrial myocardium
    C. AV node
    D. His-Purkinje fibers

40. Which of the following does *not* cause QT prolongation and torsades de pointes ventricular tachycardia?

    A. Hypokalemia and hypomagnesemia
    B. Hypocalcemia
    C. Macrolide antibiotics
    D. Phenothiazines

41. In which of the following patients is an implantable cardioverter-defibrillator not indicated?

    A. A 25-year-old woman with a family history of sudden death, a long QT (550 ms), and syncope
    B. A 75-year-old man with ventricular fibrillation and an acute anterior myocardial infarction
    C. A 55-year-old man with coronary disease, heart failure, and a single episode of resuscitated sudden death
    D. A 65-year-old man with dilated cardiomyopathy and recurrent VT associated with syncope

42. Which of the following statements regarding Marfan syndrome is *not* correct?

    A. Mitral valve prolapse and rupture may occur as a result of elongation of the chordae tendineae.
    B. Aortic regurgitation may occur as a result of aortic dilatation.
    C. Complications of ascending aortic aneurysms account for more than 90% of deaths from Marfan syndrome.
    D. Operation is advisable in symptomatic patients with an ascending aneurysm greater than 6 cm; asymptomatic patients should be followed with serial imaging studies.

43. Which of the following is *not* a known complication of drug therapy with amiodarone?

    A. Hearing loss
    B. Hypothyroidism
    C. Hyperthyroidism
    D. Pulmonary fibrosis

44. Which of the following statements regarding thromboangiitis obliterans is *not* correct?

    A. It occurs more commonly in smokers.
    B. It occurs more commonly in males.
    C. It occurs more commonly in Israel and the Orient.
    D. It occurs more commonly in elderly patients.

45. Which symptom of aortic stenosis is associated with the worst prognosis?

    A. Syncope
    B. Angina
    C. Congestive heart failure
    D. Palpitations

46. What percentage of patients with severe aortic stenosis will have significant coronary artery disease?

    A. 5%
    B. 25%
    C. 33%
    D. 50%

47. Which of the following agents is thought to cause idiopathic dilated cardiomyopathy in the majority of cases?

    A. Alcohol
    B. Iron overload
    C. Subclinical viral infection
    D. Coronary artery disease

QUESTIONS 48–50

A 55-year-old man presents for evaluation of exertional dyspnea and chest pain. His medical history is unremarkable. His carotid pulses are delayed and diminished. His point of maximal intensity is hyperdynamic but not displaced. He has a harsh crescendo-decrescendo murmur along the left sternal border that peaks late in systole. The aortic component of S_2 is not heard. His ECG demonstrates left ventricular hypertrophy with strain pattern. His chest x-ray film shows a normal-sized heart and clear lung fields.

48. The cause of his problem is most likely:

    A. Myxomatous valve degeneration
    B. Bicuspid aortic valve
    C. Rheumatic aortic stenosis
    D. Senile calcific aortic stenosis

49. Which of the following would be most helpful in confirming the diagnosis?

    A. Aortic root angiography
    B. Coronary angiography

C. Echocardiography

D. Pulmonary artery catheterization

50. Appropriate treatment for this patient includes:

A. Digoxin and diuretics

B. Angiotensin-converting enzyme (ACE) inhibitors

C. Nitrates and β-blockers

D. Referral for coronary angiography and cardiac surgery

QUESTIONS 51–53

A 30-year-old woman presents for evaluation of dyspnea and malaise. She has had lower extremity edema, orthopnea, and paroxysmal nocturnal dyspnea. She has had intermittent fevers and chills. BP is 166/56 mm Hg and pulse is 96 beats/minute. The jugular venous pressure is elevated. Her carotid and femoral pulses are bounding with a brisk collapse. She has a II/VI systolic ejection murmur and a III/VI diastolic decrescendo murmur along the left sternal border that is intensified by a handgrip maneuver. An S_3 gallop is present. Bilateral rales and lower extremity edema are present. There are no stigmata of infective endocarditis. ECG is unremarkable. Chest x-ray film shows moderate cardiomegaly and interstitial pulmonary edema.

51. Initial therapy should include:

A. Dopamine and dobutamine

B. Diuretics and ACE inhibitors

C. Nitrates and β-blockers

D. Urgent referral for surgery

52. Initial diagnostic testing should include:

A. Aortic root angiography

B. Coronary angiography

C. Transthoracic echocardiography

D. Pulmonary artery catheterization

53. A fever to 101° F develops, and blood cultures grow gram-positive cocci in clusters. While in the intensive care unit, her dyspnea becomes suddenly worse and she experiences severe respiratory distress. The intensity of her murmur is increased, and rales are heard throughout her chest. The next step in management should be:

A. Sodium nitroprusside

B. Dopamine, dobutamine, and diuretics

C. Transesophageal echocardiography

D. Emergent surgery

QUESTIONS 54–58

A 65-year-old woman presents to the hospital with chest pain. She fell and injured her right hip 3 days ago and has been immobilized because of right hip pain. Yesterday she noticed new pain and swelling of her right leg. She has been previously healthy. Her only medications include hormone replacement therapy with a combination estrogen/progesterone preparation.

54. Which of the following was *not* a primary factor predisposing this patient to her current problem?

A. Immobilization as a result of hip injury

B. Factor V Leiden deficiency

C. Estrogen therapy

D. Traumatic hip injury

55. Which of the following tests, used alone, is *not* useful to make the diagnosis?

A. Impedance plethysmography

B. D-Dimers

C. Ultrasonography

D. Venography

56. Which of the following would *not* be an appropriate treatment regimen for this patient?

A. Fixed-dose unfractionated heparin at 1000 U/hour after a 5000-U bolus

B. Weight-based unfractionated heparin (80 U/kg bolus, followed by 18 U/kg/hour)

C. Low-molecular-weight heparin (LMWH)

D. Combined intravenous heparin and oral warfarin started simultaneously

57. Which of the following statements about LMWH is correct?

A. LMWH affects both antithrombin III and factor Xa.

B. Partial thromboplastin time should be monitored three times daily in patients being treated with LMWH.

C. LMWH results in a slightly greater risk of bleeding than unfractionated heparin.

D. LMWH may be used safely in combination with warfarin.

58. This patient recovers uneventfully after receiving anticoagulation for 6 months. Two years later she undergoes elective hip replacement. Which of the following would *not* be appropriate prophylaxis for DVT?

A. LMWH

B. Unfractionated heparin

C. Warfarin

D. Intermittent pneumatic leg compression

59. A 65-year-old woman presents to the emergency department with a recent history of shortness of breath. She is a current smoker with a 70 pack-year history of smoking. Her blood pressure is 127/80 mm Hg and her heart rate is 90 beats/minute. Oxygen saturation is 80% on room air that increases to 96% with 2 L of oxygen. On examination she has 5 cm JVP, mild basal crackles, and diffuse rhonchi. S_1 and S_2 are normal with a loud P_2, but no S_3 is heard. Her chest x-ray film showed mildly increased vascularity with no obvious infiltrate. The heart size appears mildly increased. Cardiac enzymes and routine laboratory studies are normal. A point of care B-type natriuretic peptide (BNP) level done was measured at 47. Which of the following statements is *true*?

A. Because the BNP level is low, it is highly likely the shortness of breath is due to heart failure.

B. Because the BNP level is low, it is highly likely the shortness of breath is due to respiratory disease.

C. Because the BNP level is low, it is highly likely the shortness of breath is not due to heart failure.

D. Because the BNP level is low, it is highly likely the shortness of breath is not due to respiratory disease.

QUESTIONS 60–64

A 35-year-old man presents for evaluation of worsening dyspnea. He is dyspneic at rest. He smothers if he does not sleep on three pillows. Pitting edema has developed in his legs. He has no history of hypertension or coronary artery disease. He does not drink alcohol. He had a flu-like illness several weeks ago. His BP is 108/84 and pulse is 110 beats/minute. Jugular venous pressure is 14 mm Hg. Rales are present in both lung fields up to the scapulae. He has an S_3 and an S_4 gallop but no murmurs. His liver is mildly enlarged. He has 2++ pitting edema, and his extremities are cool. An ECG shows no acute ST or T wave changes. His chest x-ray film shows bilateral interstitial and alveolar pulmonary edema and cardiomegaly. The creatine kinase and the creatine kinase MB fraction are mildly elevated.

60. The most likely cause of his symptoms is:

    A. Critical aortic stenosis
    B. Severe mitral regurgitation
    C. Idiopathic dilated cardiomyopathy
    D. Coronary artery disease

61. The likelihood of at least partial recovery from his current illness is:

    A. 5%
    B. 15%
    C. 35%
    D. 50%

62. Which of the following would *not* be useful to screen for the cause of his symptoms?

    A. HIV antibody testing
    B. Hepatitis antibody testing
    C. Iron studies
    D. Endomyocardial biopsy

63. Which of the following drugs is *not* indicated in this patient?

    A. ACE inhibitors
    B. Digoxin
    C. Intravenous corticosteroids followed by tapered doses of an oral corticosteroid
    D. Diuretics

64. The patient experiences recurrent VT refractory to all antiarrhythmic drugs except amiodarone shortly after admission to the hospital. Which of the following is now more likely to be the cause of his heart failure?

    A. Lyme carditis
    B. Giant cell myocarditis
    C. Hyperthyroidism
    D. Thiamine deficiency (beriberi)

65. Which of the following is *not* a toxic cause of dilated cardiomyopathy?

    A. Doxorubicin
    B. Cyclophosphamide
    C. Cyclosporine
    D. Ethanol

66. Which of the following statements regarding alcoholic cardiomyopathy is *not* correct?

    A. Ethanol contributes to more than 10% of cases of heart failure in the United States.
    B. The amount of alcohol to produce symptomatic cardiomyopathy is estimated to be six drinks a day for 5 to 10 years.
    C. Binge drinking does not cause alcoholic cardiomyopathy.
    D. Strict abstinence is the most important factor in recovery of systolic function.

QUESTIONS 67 AND 68

A 35-year-old woman presents for evaluation of chest pain. She has had good health except for coryza and cough 1 week ago. Her chest pain is sharp, is worse with deep inspiration, and is better when she leans forward. Her BP is 120/70 mm Hg and pulse is 96 beats/minute. Her cardiac examination is remarkable for a triphasic rub. Her ECG shows diffuse ST segment elevation. The chest x-ray film is normal.

67. The next step in this patient's management should be:

    A. Urgent cardiac catheterization and coronary angiography

    B. Transthoracic echocardiography followed by transesophageal echocardiography if indicated
    C. Immediate admission to an intensive care unit
    D. Outpatient therapy directed at treatment of symptoms

68. Appropriate therapy for this patient includes:

    A. Indomethacin
    B. Tissue plasminogen activator
    C. Immediate surgery
    D. Corticosteroids

QUESTIONS 69–72

A 75-year-old man presents for evaluation of dyspnea. He has smoked since he was a teenager. Except for 20-pound weight loss and a chronic cough that has worsened in the last few months, he states that he has been in good health. His BP is 94/72 mm Hg, and his pulse is 100 beats/minute. His neck veins are distended. His chest is clear except for decreased breath sounds over his right mid-lung field. He has decreased heart sounds. He has no edema in his extremities. The chest x-ray film shows a right hilar mass and an enlarged cardiac silhouette.

69. Which of the following could be performed immediately to help identify the cause of his dyspnea?

    A. Right-sided ECG
    B. Careful auscultation of his BP
    C. Funduscopic examination
    D. Sputum Gram stain and culture

70. Which of the following ECG findings may be seen in this patient?

    A. Diffuse ST segment depression
    B. Sinus bradycardia
    C. Left ventricular hypertrophy
    D. Electrical alternans

71. If a pulmonary artery catheter were inserted, it would demonstrate:

    A. Equalization of right atrial, right ventricular diastolic, pulmonary artery diastolic, and pulmonary artery wedge pressure
    B. Increased cardiac output and reduced systemic vascular resistance
    C. Increased right atrial and right ventricular pressures but normal pulmonary artery wedge pressure and cardiac output
    D. Reduced cardiac output but normal right-sided filling pressures

72. Which of the following tests would be most useful to confirm the diagnosis?

    A. Cardiac catheterization and coronary angiography
    B. Endomyocardial biopsy
    C. Echocardiography
    D. Pulmonary arteriogram

73. Modifiable coronary heart disease (CHD) risk factors include all of the following *except*:

    A. Smoking
    B. Hyperalphalipoproteinemia
    C. Hypertension
    D. Consumption of *trans*-fatty acids
    E. Sedentary lifestyle

74. A patient has a heart rate of 60 beats/minute, an end-diastolic left ventricular volume of 200 mL, and an end-systolic volume of 150 mL. His ejection fraction is:

A. 0.05
B. 3 L/minute
C. 50 mL
D. 0.25
E. 50%

75. All of the following are true *except:*

A. The renin-angiotensin system is activated in heart failure.
B. Renin is produced in the macula densa cells of the juxtaglomerular apparatus.
C. Angiotensin II is a powerful coronary vasoconstrictor.
D. Angiotensin II inhibits release of aldosterone from the adrenal gland.
E. Angiotensin promotes the release of norepinephrine from peripheral sympathetic nervous system sites.

76. On a frontal chest film, the cardiac borders are formed by all of the following structures *except:*

A. Right atrium
B. Superior vena cava
C. Right ventricle
D. Left atrial appendage
E. Main pulmonary artery

77. All of the following medications cause a delay in AV nodal conduction *except:*

A. Diltiazem
B. Dobutamine
C. Adenosine
D. Digoxin
E. Amiodarone

78. Radionuclide perfusion imaging is indicated in all the following settings *except:*

A. Screening of asymptomatic patients for coronary artery disease
B. Risk stratification before noncardiac surgery
C. Assessment of myocardial viability
D. Diagnosis of coronary artery disease in patients with angina who have an abnormal resting ECG
E. Planning of revascularization procedures

79. All of the following conditions are associated with high cardiac output states *except:*

A. Thyrotoxicosis
B. Chronic anemia
C. Hemochromatosis
D. Beriberi
E. Systemic arteriovenous shunting

80. Symptoms of heart failure despite normal left ventricular ejection fraction occur with the following conditions *except:*

A. Amyloidosis
B. Hypertensive heart disease
C. Hemochromatosis
D. Constrictive pericarditis
E. Peripartum cardiomyopathy

81. Factors that may precipitate acute decompensation of chronic heart failure include all of the following *except:*

A. Arrhythmias
B. Infection
C. Poor compliance with medication regimen
D. Transfusion
E. Salt restriction

82. Sympathetic stimulation of the heart results in all of the following *except:*

A. Increased force of contraction of ventricular muscle
B. Increased conduction velocity through the AV node
C. Increased velocity of ventricular muscle relaxation
D. Decreased rate of phase IV depolarization in the sinus node, resulting in increased heart rate
E. Increased velocity of ventricular muscle contraction

83. Which of the following statements regarding the measurement of BP is *not* correct?

A. Mercury manometers are more accurate than aneroid manometers.
B. BP should be measured after the patient has been seated comfortably for at least 5 minutes.
C. Falsely low BP readings occur when the cuff is too narrow or when the bladder is too short to encircle the arm.
D. The BP cuff should be inflated rapidly to 30 mm Hg above the palpated systolic BP to avoid a falsely low reading caused by an auscultatory gap.
E. BP measurements by health care personnel tend to overestimate ambulatory BPs.

84. Which of the following statements regarding hypertension is correct?

A. Secondary hypertension of known cause accounts for approximately 15% of cases of hypertension; the remaining 85% are classified as "essential hypertension".
B. As a result of better and more widely available antihypertensive medications, there has been a decline in the incidence of end-stage renal disease over the past decade.
C. Isolated systolic hypertension is predominantly a disease of advanced age.
D. Whites tend to have more severe and earlier onset of hypertension than blacks.
E. Risk of heart failure is increased in patients with severe hypertension but not in those with milder forms of hypertension.

85. All of the following drugs and chemicals may cause or exacerbate hypertension *except:*

A. Cyclosporine
B. Licorice
C. Calcium supplements
D. Erythropoietin
E. Nonsteroidal anti-inflammatory drugs (NSAIDs)

86. Which of the following medication classes has been shown to decrease stroke mortality among patients with hypertension?

A. ACE inhibitors
B. Calcium-channel blockers
C. Diuretics
D. β-Adrenergic blockers
E. All of the above

87. All of the following lifestyle modifications have been shown to lower BP *except:*

A. Weight reduction
B. Reduction in sodium intake
C. Regular physical exercise
D. Daily intake of 2 ounces of alcohol
E. Increased dietary potassium intake

88. All of the following statements about renovascular hypertension are correct *except:*

    A. Renovascular hypertension is the most common curable cause of hypertension.
    B. Two thirds of patients with renovascular hypertension have atherosclerotic renal artery stenosis.
    C. Patients with fibromuscular dysplasia are less likely to experience cardiovascular complications than those with atherosclerotic disease.
    D. Percutaneous revascularization can often be performed at diagnostic renal arteriography.
    E. Abdominal bruits are present only in a minority of patients with renovascular hypertension.

89. All of the following statements about adverse effects of antihypertensive agents are correct *except:*

    A. When potassium-sparing diuretics are used, hyperkalemia is more likely to occur in patients with diabetes and those with renal insufficiency.
    B. Hyperkalemia is less likely to occur when potassium-sparing diuretics are used in conjunction with ACE inhibitors.
    C. Constipation is a common side effect of verapamil, especially in elderly patients.
    D. Angiotensin II antagonists are contraindicated in pregnancy.
    E. Reserpine is contraindicated in patients with depression.

90. All of the following have been shown to increase pulmonary arterial pressure *except:*

    A. Hypoxia
    B. Increased blood viscosity
    C. Positive end-expiratory pressure in patients who are mechanically ventilated
    D. Elevated endothelin level
    E. Elevated prostacyclin level

91. All of the following are true about primary pulmonary hypertension *except:*

    A. Pulmonary thrombi are often found at autopsy.
    B. Pulmonary scintigraphy may result in hypotension.
    C. Pulmonary vascular endothelial function is abnormal.
    D. Primary pulmonary hypertension is less common in women than men.
    E. Dyspnea on exertion and fatigue are common presenting symptoms.

92. Congenital cardiac defects in which adult survival is expected include all *except:*

    A. Bicuspid aortic valve
    B. Ostium secundum atrial septal defect
    C. Ventricular septal defect
    D. Ebstein's anomaly
    E. Tricuspid atresia

93. All of the following therapies have been associated with improved mortality after myocardial infarction *except:*

    A. ACE inhibitor
    B. β-Blocker
    C. Aspirin
    D. Antiarrhythmics
    E. Thrombolysis

94. Patients with a bicuspid aortic valve often present to the physician with one or more of the following *except:*

    A. Infective endocarditis
    B. Aortic dissection
    C. Papillary muscle rupture
    D. Aortic stenosis
    E. Aortic insufficiency

95. Coarctation of the aorta may be associated with all of the following *except:*

    A. Aneurysm of the circle of Willis
    B. Central cyanosis
    C. Hypertension
    D. Rib notching
    E. Bicuspid aortic valve

96. Cyanosis is a characteristic of which of the following congenital anomalies?

    A. Secundum atrial septal defect
    B. Tetralogy of Fallot
    C. Pulmonary valve stenosis
    D. Coarctation of the aorta
    E. Patent ductus arteriosus

97. Medical complications of cyanotic congenital heart disease include all of the following *except:*

    A. Hyperuricemia
    B. Severe anemia
    C. Cholelithiasis
    D. Abnormal renal function
    E. Abnormal hemostasis

98. All of the following statements about the coronary circulation are true *except:*

    A. Heart rate is the most important determinant of myocardial oxygen consumption.
    B. Coronary perfusion of the left ventricle occurs mainly during diastole.
    C. The subendocardial region of the myocardium is more sensitive to ischemia.
    D. A 50% coronary stenosis on angiography corresponds approximately to a 75% reduction in cross-sectional area.
    E. The abnormal coronary vasodilator response to shear stress and mediators such as acetylcholine is due to deficient prostacyclin production in diseased coronary arteries.

99. All of the following statements about exercise testing are correct *except:*

    A. The deeper the ST segment depression on exercise electrocardiography, the higher is the specificity of the stress test.
    B. The predictive value of the exercise test is influenced by the pretest probability of disease.
    C. Exercise stress testing is contraindicated in severe aortic stenosis.
    D. Exercise stress testing is most useful in patients with a low probability of coronary artery disease.
    E. False-positive ECG responses are more likely in women than in men.

100. All of the following are poor prognostic indicators on exercise testing *except:*

    A. Downsloping ST segment depression of 2 mV or greater
    B. Persistence of ST segment depression for 5 minutes or more into recovery
    C. Exercise-induced hypertension
    D. ST segment depression early during exercise
    E. Poor exercise capacity

101. Which of the following agents have *not* been shown to increase survival in patients with heart failure with left ventricular ejection fraction less than 40%?

    A. β-Blockers
    B. Angiotensin-converting enzyme inhibitors
    C. Spironolactone
    D. Loop diuretics

102. A 56-year-old man is seen in the clinic. He has a history of coronary artery disease with myocardial infarction 1 year ago. A recent echocardiogram demonstrated a left ventricular ejection fraction of 25%. He is currently NYHA class I-II on a medical regimen including acetylsalicylic acid, clopidogrel, β-blockers, and ACE inhibitor. A recent stress myocardial perfusion study showed no evidence of ischemia. Which of the following has the best survival advantage in this patient?

    A. Implantable cardiac defibrillator
    B. Electrophysiologic study
    C. Anticoagulation
    D. Amiodarone therapy

103. Which of the following drugs should be avoided in patients with chronic heart failure?

    A. Nonsteroidal anti-inflammatory drugs
    B. Calcium-channel blockers
    C. Intravenous inotropes
    D. All of the above

104. A 46-year-old woman with a 10-year history of type 2 diabetes mellitus, hypertension, obesity, and hyperlipidemia presents to the emergency department with a recent onset of chest pain. The pain has been worse over the past few hours. ECG in the emergency department showed dynamic ST changes in the lateral leads, and she was admitted to the coronary care unit. A cardiac catheterization demonstrated normal coronary arteries. Which of the following is a possible explanation of her symptoms?

    A. Microvascular angina (syndrome X)
    B. Coronary emboli
    C. Coronary vasculitis
    D. Prinzmetal angina
    E. All of the above

105. A 55-year-old man with a history of diabetes, hypertension, hyperlipidemia, and current smoking presents with a 2-month history of progressively worsening chest pain on exertion. Which of the following diagnostic procedures is most appropriate?

    A. Exercise ECG testing
    B. Adenosine myocardial perfusion scintigraphy
    C. Dobutamine stress echocardiogram
    D. PET scan
    E. Cardiac catheterization

106. A 46-year-old man was treated with thrombolytic therapy and LMWH for anterior ST elevation myocardial infarction. He had complete resolution of chest pain and ST segments came back to baseline. Three days later before discharge he had a sudden onset of severe, sharp persistent chest pain. Which of the following processes could explain the recurrent chest pain?

    A. Post-infarction angina
    B. Infarct expansion
    C. Acute pericarditis
    D. Pulmonary thromboembolism
    E. All of the above

107. A 56-year-old man is status post orthotopic heart transplant 6 years ago for ischemic cardiomyopathy. He has had three episodes of rejection treated successfully by burst doses of intravenous Solu-Medrol. Which of the following is an important concern in this patient?

    A. Allograft rejection
    B. Allograft vasculopathy
    C. Infection
    D. Secondary malignancy
    E. Medication-related side effects including renal and hepatic dysfunction
    F. All of the above

TRUE OR FALSE

DIRECTIONS: For questions 108–140, determine whether *each* choice is true or false. Any combination of answers, from all true to all false, may occur.

108. Which of the following statements are *true* about CHD epidemiology?

    A. By 1990, CHD was the second leading cause of death in developing countries.
    B. Deaths from heart failure in the United States have decreased steadily over the past 10 years as treatment modalities such as ACE inhibitors, digoxin, and β-blockers have been more widely applied.
    C. Women experience myocardial infarction on average 10 to 20 years later than men.
    D. Age-adjusted CHD mortality is higher in blacks than in whites.
    E. CHD mortality has decreased strikingly in eastern European countries over the past decade.

109. Which of the following statements correctly characterize major determinants of cardiac performance?

    A. Stroke volume increases with increasing afterload.
    B. Ventricular preload describes the load against which the ventricle must contract when it ejects blood.
    C. In normal hearts, ventricular inotropic state increases with increasing heart rate because of changes in calcium availability.
    D. Hypoxia, ischemia, and acidosis decrease cardiac contractility.
    E. In failing hearts, right atrial pressure as assessed from the jugular venous pulse is a good indicator of left ventricular filling pressure.

110. Which of the following statements are *true* about echocardiography?

    A. In patients with tricuspid regurgitation, Doppler echocardiography can determine systolic pulmonary arterial pressure.
    B. Echocardiography can distinguish systolic and diastolic dysfunction.
    C. Ejection fraction can be calculated using formulas validated in coronary angiography.
    D. Transthoracic echocardiography is ideally suited to diagnose vegetations on the mitral valve.
    E. Echocardiography is ideally suited for serial noninvasive follow-up of patients with valvular heart disease.

111. Which statements about these cardiac imaging modalities are correct?

    A. Aortic dissection can be assessed by computed tomography, aortography, magnetic resonance imaging, and echocardiography.
    B. Electron beam computed tomography (EBCT) visualizes coronary calcification and has been used to screen asymptomatic individuals for coronary artery disease.
    C. Cardiac catheterization is mandatory in all patients with aortic stenosis who are being considered for aortic valve replacement.
    D. Radionuclide angiography can reliably assess myocardial wall thickness, wall motion, and global left ventricular ejection fraction.
    E. Magnetic resonance imaging can identify cardiomyopathy resulting from hemochromatosis.

112. Which of the following medications have been shown to improve mortality in chronic heart failure?

    A. ACE inhibitors
    B. β-Adrenergic blocking agents
    C. Prazosin
    D. Hydralazine/nitrate combination therapy
    E. Digoxin

113. Which statements about neurohumoral activation in heart failure are *true*?

    A. Circulating norepinephrine levels correlate with survival in heart failure.
    B. Proinflammatory cytokines are elevated in patients with asymptomatic left ventricular dysfunction but diminish as severity of heart failure increases.
    C. Levels of natriuretic peptides are increased in heart failure, but response to these peptides is diminished.
    D. Endothelin levels are increased in heart failure and contribute to peripheral and pulmonary vasoconstriction.
    E. Plasma renin levels are markedly diminished in severe heart failure, resulting in systemic hypotension.

114. Which of the following statements correctly characterize symptoms of heart failure?

    A. Disordered breathing, such as Cheyne-Stokes respiration or nocturnal oxygen desaturation, is common in heart failure.
    B. Nocturnal cough is due to increased pulmonary venous pressure in the recumbent position.
    C. Exercise intolerance occurs only in patients with increased pulmonary venous pressures.
    D. Digestive disturbances are common in heart failure.
    E. Patients with heart failure may present with signs of liver dysfunction.

115. Which of the following statements correctly characterize physical findings in heart failure?

    A. A prominent S_3 gallop is present in the majority of patients with heart failure as a result of systolic dysfunction.
    B. Mitral regurgitation on examination is pathognomonic for heart failure as a result of primary valvular disease.
    C. Jugular venous distention is an early sign of mild left ventricular dysfunction.
    D. The absence of pulmonary rales is very helpful in excluding a diagnosis of heart failure.
    E. A pulsatile liver is a sign of severe tricuspid regurgitation.

116. Which of the following statements are *true* about treatment modalities in heart failure?

    A. Diuretics may increase neurohumoral activation in patients with heart failure.
    B. ACE inhibitors potentiate kinins.
    C. Hypokalemia is a common side effect of ACE inhibitors.
    D. In patients who experience angioedema in response to a short-acting ACE inhibitor, a long-acting ACE inhibitor can be safely substituted.

117. Which of the following statements are *true* about treatment modalities in heart failure?

    A. Aldosterone antagonists increase mortality in heart failure and should be avoided, especially in patients with class IV symptoms.
    B. Digitalis toxicity occurs only when digoxin serum levels exceed 2 ng/mL.
    C. Beneficial effects of digoxin may in part be mediated by diminished activation of the neurohormonal system.
    D. β-Blocker therapy can be administered in most patients with heart failure symptoms.
    E. Premature ventricular contractions, even if asymptomatic, diminish cardiac output in patients with heart failure and should be suppressed pharmacologically.

118. Which of the following statements about heart failure are *true*?

    A. In the United States, heart failure prevalence has increased over the past decade.
    B. The most common cause of heart failure in the current era is valvular heart disease.
    C. Activation of the sympathetic nervous system and the renin-angiotensin system is important in the pathogenesis of heart failure.
    D. Increased BNP levels are seen in elderly patients, women, and those with chronic obstructive pulmonary disease.

119. Which of the following statements about the relationship of BP and lifestyle are *true*?

    A. Weight loss is closely correlated with reductions in BP.
    B. A diet rich in fruits, vegetables, and low-fat dairy products can substantially lower BP in hypertensive patients.
    C. Regular moderate-intensity physical activity can lower BP in normotensive and hypertensive individuals.
    D. Consumption of one to two alcoholic beverages daily has been shown to lower BP in normotensive and hypertensive individuals.
    E. Sodium restriction as a means to lower BP is most effective in populations with high renin hypertension.

120. Which of the following statements are *true* about pharmacologic therapy of hypertension?

    A. Greater than 60% of patients achieve adequate BP control with single-drug therapy.
    B. There are convincing clinical trial data that indicate that initial use of ACE inhibitors and long-acting calcium-channel blockers leads to superior cardiovascular outcomes compared with diuretic and β-blocker therapy.
    C. When choosing an antihypertensive agent, a patient's comorbidities should be carefully considered.
    D. Lack of BP control is often a result of nonadherence.
    E. Volume overload is the most frequent cause of resistant hypertension.

121. Which of the following statements are *true* about co-morbidities in hypertensive patients?

A. Sleep apnea and hypertension often coexist.

B. Hypertension is twice as common in diabetic than non-diabetic patients.

C. Good control of hypertension is less important in older patients compared with younger patients.

D. Tight BP control is contraindicated in patients with renal insufficiency because such therapy often results in worsening renal function (increases in serum creatinine).

E. β-Blockers are contraindicated in patients with a history of asthma.

122. Which of the following statements are *true* about hypertensive crisis?

A. Severe hypertension (BP > 200/120 mm Hg) is an indication for parenteral antihypertensive therapy in an intensive care unit setting.

B. The drug of choice for the treatment of severe hypertension in the setting of aortic dissection is parenteral hydralazine.

C. Eclampsia is best treated with diuretics.

D. Myocardial ischemia and severe hypertension in the setting of a cocaine overdose are best treated by β-adrenergic blocking agents.

E. β-Blockers are contraindicated in hypertensive emergencies complicated by acute left ventricular failure.

123. Which of the following statements are *true* about pulmonary hypertension?

A. Sleep apnea may lead to pulmonary arteriolar vasoconstriction.

B. Bronchiectasis may lead to pulmonary hypertension.

C. Primary pulmonary hypertension is characterized by very high pulmonary venous pressures.

D. Pulmonary hypertension resulting from scleroderma is characterized by increased pulmonary flow with normal pulmonary vascular resistance.

E. Pulmonary hypertension in chronic obstructive pulmonary disease (COPD) is multifactorial in origin.

124. Which of the following abnormalities are seen in patients with abnormalities of the chromosomal band 22q11?

A. Cardiac defects

B. Abnormal facies

C. Thymic hypoplasia

D. Cleft palate

E. Hypocalcemia

125. Which of the following statements are *true* about atrial septal defects?

A. Sinus venosus defects are often accompanied by congenital deformities of the mitral valve.

B. Atrial arrhythmias are common in adults with atrial septal defects.

C. Eisenmenger's syndrome is a frequent complication of uncorrected secundum atrial septal defects.

D. Patients with atrial septal defects are at increased risk of stroke.

E. The systolic murmur typically heard in patients with secundum atrial septal defects is due to shunt flow across the atrial septum.

126. Pregnancy in patients with congenital heart disease warrants special considerations, including:

A. Cesarean section is the preferred mode of delivery.

B. Early ambulation and use of elastic stockings are essential measures to minimize the risk of postpartum thromboembolism.

C. Oxygen administration may predispose to epistaxis.

D. The incidence of congenital heart disease in children born to mothers with congenital heart disease is significantly higher than in the general population.

E. Patients with a secundum atrial septal defect should receive endocarditis prophylaxis.

127. Noncardiac surgery in patients with congenital heart disease warrants special considerations, including:

A. Patients with congenital complete heart block may require temporary pacing.

B. Patients with cyanotic congenital heart disease are at increased risk of paradoxical embolism from peripheral venous catheters.

C. Systemic hypotension increases the right-to-left shunt in cyanotic congenital heart disease.

D. Bleeding risk is increased in cyanotic congenital heart disease.

E. Patients with a bicuspid aortic valve are at increased risk of endocarditis.

128. Which of the following are characteristic of a vulnerable plaque?

A. Thick fibrous cap

B. Large lipid core

C. High content of metalloproteinases

D. Large numbers of inflammatory cells

E. Exposure to repetitive mechanical stress

129. Which of the following are *true* statements about lipoproteins?

A. High-density lipoprotein (HDL) particles have antioxidant properties.

B. Small dense low-density lipoprotein (LDL) particles are believed to be particularly atherogenic.

C. Lipoproteins in diabetic patients may function abnormally because of glycation.

D. Postprandial hyperlipidemia is frequently seen in patients with coronary artery disease.

E. Because LDL cholesterol levels are easily calculated by the Friedewald formula, there is no need for expensive direct measurements of LDL cholesterol.

130. Which statements about angina pectoris are correct?

A. Walk-through angina is defined as angina that occurs with exercise but disappears with continued exertion.

B. Postprandial angina occurs in response to increased oxygen demand in the splanchnic bed after meals.

C. Stable exertional angina is due to intermittent thrombotic occlusion of the culprit vessel.

D. Nocturnal angina is due to increased venous return as the patient assumes a supine position.

E. New-onset angina is a subtype of unstable angina.

131. When evaluating a patient with angina pectoris, which of the following conditions should be considered in the differential diagnosis?

A. Atherosclerotic coronary artery disease

B. Aortic stenosis

C. Aortic insufficiency

D. Hypertrophic cardiomyopathy

E. Syndrome X

132. Which of the following statements are *true* about medical therapy of angina pectoris?

    A. Antiplatelet therapy decreases the risk of myocardial infarction.
    B. Clopidogrel and ticlopidine inhibit the adenosine diphosphate receptors of platelets.
    C. It is important to maintain stable nitrate blood levels throughout the 24-hour period to avoid tachyphylaxis.
    D. β-Blockade is contraindicated in patients with angina pectoris and low ejection fraction.
    E. Angioplasty is preferred over medical therapy in patients with single-vessel coronary artery disease because it lowers mortality and morbidity.

133. Which statements are correct about acute myocardial infarction?

    A. Up to 25% of myocardial infarctions in elderly patients may be silent.
    B. Routine prophylactic use of lidocaine is associated with increased mortality.
    C. Right ventricular myocardial infarction may be associated with cyanosis.
    D. Right bundle branch block is very common in inferior myocardial infarctions because in most patients the right bundle branch is supplied by the right coronary artery.
    E. Complex ventricular ectopy after myocardial infarction is associated with increased mortality; suppression of such ectopy is thus important in improving prognosis.

134. Which statements are correct about coronary artery bypass grafting (CABG)?

    A. CABG prolongs survival in patients with greater than 70% left main stenosis, independent of anginal symptoms.
    B. CABG prolongs survival in patients with three-vessel coronary artery disease and left ventricular systolic dysfunction.
    C. Diabetic patients with multivessel coronary artery disease have a better prognosis with multivessel angioplasty than with CABG.
    D. Women have lower perioperative mortality than men.
    E. Internal mammary grafts remain patent longer than saphenous vein grafts.

135. Which statements are correct about cardiac transplantation?

    A. Contraindications to transplantation include advanced physiologic age, irreversible pulmonary hypertension, irreversible renal dysfunction, diabetes mellitus with significant end-organ involvement, and peripheral vascular disease.
    B. The most common cause of heart failure leading to transplantation is ischemic heart disease.
    C. Only 10 to 20% of suitable harvestable hearts are procured from brain-dead patients.
    D. Some statin drugs have been shown to decrease allograft vasculopathy and the incidence of rejection and may prolong post-transplant survival.
    E. Diltiazem reduces cyclosporine blood levels and should be avoided in transplant patients.

136. Are the following statements true or false?

    A. In a randomized controlled trial with class IV NYHA heart failure patients, LVAD implantation was associated with a better survival compared with medical therapy.
    B. Long QT syndrome has been associated with defects at specific loci on human chromosomes.

    C. Early afterdepolarizations on signal averaged electrocardiograms have been associated with a worse prognosis in patients with heart failure.
    D. Midodrine and fludrocortisone are agents shown to help patients with neurocardiogenic syncope.

137. Which of the following is a contraindication to ibutilide cardioversion of atrial flutter or atrial fibrillation?

    A. Magnesium level less than 2.0 mEq/L
    B. Potassium level less than 4.0 mEq/L
    C. QTc longer than 440 msec
    D. Concurrent use of amiodarone

138. Which of the following statements are *true* about acute coronary syndrome (ACS)?

    A. Acute coronary syndrome is a continuum of ischemia ranging from unstable angina to non–ST elevation myocardial infarction.
    B. ACS is usually precipitated by nonocclusive thrombosis in a coronary vessel.
    C. Negative cardiac enzymes rule out ACS
    D. Elevated troponin enzyme levels are a harbinger of worse prognosis
    E. Plavix reduces the end point of cardiovascular death, nonfatal myocardial infarction, or stroke by a relative 20%. GP IIB/IIIa receptors have been beneficial in all patients with ACS.
    F. Low molecular weight heparin, enoxaparin, is associated with worse outcome in patient with acute coronary syndrome compared to heparin.

139. Which of the following statements are *true* about ST elevation myocardial infarction?

    A. ST elevation myocardial infarction is usually characterized by complete interruption of regional myocardial blood flow.
    B. Positive cardiac enzymes are essential to make a diagnosis of ST elevation myocardial infarction, and treatment decisions should be based on them.
    C. Percutaneous intervention has been shown to have improved survival in randomized clinical trials compared with thrombolytic therapy.
    D. Half-dose thrombolytic therapy with GPIIb/IIIa has been shown to improve survival in patients with ST segment elevation myocardial infarction.
    E. LMWH and tenecteplase are more effective than tenecteplase with standard heparin or GP IIb/IIIa with heparin.

140. Which of the following statements regarding percutaneous intervention (PCI) are *true*?

    A. Diabetics and elderly patients (older than 75 years of age) have a worse prognosis after PCI.
    B. PCI have been shown to reduce angina in patients, compared with medical therapy.
    C. Early aggressive therapy including early PCI in patients with acute coronary syndrome has been shown to reduce death or myocardial infarction.
    D. Patients with diabetes have a better survival after PCI compared with CABG.
    E. In-stent restenosis is a frequent complication of stent placement in the first 6 months after intervention.

MATCHING

DIRECTIONS: Questions 141–207 are matching questions. For each numbered item, choose the most likely associated lettered item from those provided. Each item has *only one* answer.

QUESTIONS 141–144

Match the following conditions with their characteristic chest x-ray film appearance.

    A. Mitral stenosis
    B. Severe aortic insufficiency
    C. Constrictive pericarditis
    D. Angina pectoris
    E. Primary pulmonary hypertension

141. Pulmonary arterial pruning

142. Pericardial calcification

143. Left ventricular enlargement

144. Left atrial enlargement

QUESTIONS 145–148

Select from the list below the cardiac events that correspond most closely to the components of the jugular venous waveform:

    A. Opening of the tricuspid valve and right ventricular relaxation
    B. Right atrial relaxation
    C. Pulmonic valve opening
    D. Right atrial contraction
    E. Passive right atrial filling with a competent tricuspid valve

145. X descent

146. V wave

147. A wave

148. Y descent

QUESTIONS 149–152

Treatments for systolic and diastolic heart failure differ. Match heart failure type with its appropriate treatment(s).

    A. Heart failure resulting from systolic dysfunction
    B. Heart failure resulting from diastolic dysfunction
    C. Both
    D. Neither

149. Digoxin

150. β-Blocker

151. ACE inhibitor

152. Prazosin

QUESTIONS 153–156

For each of the following adverse drug effects, select the most likely causative agent.

    A. Pericardial effusion
    B. Lupus-like syndrome
    C. Coombs' positive hemolytic anemia
    D. Dry cough
    E. Gynecomastia and sexual dysfunction

153. Spironolactone

154. Minoxidil

155. Hydralazine

156. ACE inhibitors

QUESTIONS 157–160

Which mechanisms of pulmonary hypertension best match with these disease entities?

    A. Precapillary pulmonary hypertension
    B. Increased pulmonary venous pressure
    C. Both
    D. Neither

157. Pulmonary embolism

158. Long-standing severe mitral stenosis

159. Acute pulmonary edema resulting from left ventricular dysfunction

160. Pulmonary atresia

QUESTIONS 161–164

Match the following palliative surgical shunts with their anatomic anastomoses.

    A. Superior vena cava to right pulmonary artery
    B. Subclavian artery to pulmonary artery
    C. Ascending aorta to right pulmonary artery
    D. Descending aorta to left pulmonary artery

161. Classic Blalock-Taussig

162. Potts anastomosis

163. Classic Glenn

164. Waterston shunt

QUESTIONS 165–168

Match the following cardiac abnormalities with the disorders listed below.

    A. Floppy mitral valve
    B. Tricuspid atresia
    C. Congenital complete heart block
    D. Ostium primum atrial septal defect
    E. Patent ductus arteriosus

165. Down syndrome

166. Marfan syndrome

167. Maternal systemic lupus erythematosus

168. Congenital rubella

QUESTIONS 169–172

Match the following case scenarios with their probability of coronary artery disease.

    A. A 30-year-old woman with typical angina pectoris
    B. A 49-year-old man with typical angina pectoris
    C. A 49-year-old woman with nonanginal chest pain
    D. A 59-year-old woman with nonanginal chest pain

169. Very low

170. Low

171. Intermediate

172. High

QUESTIONS 173–176

Match the ECG abnormalities with the most likely corresponding coronary artery lesion.

    A. Occlusion of the proximal right coronary artery
    B. Occlusion of the posterior descending coronary artery
    C. Subtotal occlusion of the proximal left anterior descending coronary artery
    D. Occlusion of the left circumflex coronary artery
    E. Occlusion of the mid-left anterior descending coronary artery

173. R/S ratio greater than 1 in leads V_1 and V_2

174. Normal ECG

175. ST segment elevation in V_{4R}

176. T wave inversion in leads V_1 to V_6

QUESTIONS 177–180

Match the following complications of myocardial infarction with their most likely clinical presentation.

    A. Papillary muscle rupture
    B. Ventricular septal rupture
    C. Myocardial free wall rupture
    D. Pericarditis
    E. Right ventricular infarction

177. Hypotension, new systolic murmur, prominent V wave in the pulmonary wedge pressure tracing

178. Hypotension, elevated jugular venous pressure, complete heart block

179. Cardiac arrest 3 days after myocardial infarction; patient has electromechanical dissociation

180. Recurrent chest pain 2 days after myocardial infarction

QUESTIONS 181–184

Match the following valve lesions with their associated murmur.

    A. Decrescendo diastolic blowing murmur heard best along the left sternal border
    B. Holosystolic murmur at the apex radiating to the left axilla
    C. Crescendo-decrescendo systolic murmur along the left sternal border radiating into the carotids
    D. Mid or late systolic murmur at the apex that may be preceded by a click

181. Aortic stenosis

182. Mitral regurgitation

183. Aortic regurgitation

184. Mitral valve prolapse

QUESTIONS 185–188

Match the following physiologic maneuvers with their associated cardiovascular effects.

    A. Increases afterload
    B. Transient increase in preload with a sustained increase in afterload
    C. Reduces preload
    D. Reduces preload and afterload

185. Valsalva maneuver

186. Handgrip

187. Squatting from standing position

188. Standing from a squatting position

QUESTIONS 189–192

Match the following cells with the characteristics of their action potentials.

    A. Sinus node and AV node
    B. Atrial and ventricular myocardium

189. Fast response associated with a rapid inward sodium current

190. Exhibits a slowly rising phase 0

191. Exhibits spontaneous diastolic depolarization

192. Distinct phases 1, 2, and 3

QUESTIONS 193–196

Match the most appropriate diagnostic and/or therapeutic procedure with the patients who would benefit from their use.

    A. Holter monitor
    B. Transtelephonic event recorder
    C. Tilt table testing
    D. Electrophysiologic study and/or radiofrequency catheter ablation

193. A 36-year-old woman with recurrent episodes of PSVT that continue to occur despite therapy with metoprolol and verapamil, singly and in combination

194. A 24-year-old man with sudden episodes of tachypalpitations that occur approximately once per month since he was a teenager

195. A 78-year-old man with episodes of near-syncope occurring several times per day

196. A 55-year-old woman with weekly episodes of syncope preceded by nausea, near-syncope, and flushing

QUESTIONS 197–200

Match the following ECG findings with the appropriate arrhythmia.

    A. Orthodromic reciprocating tachycardia
    B. AV nodal re-entrant tachycardia
    C. Atrial flutter
    D. Ventricular tachycardia

197. Narrow complex tachycardia at 150 beats/minute with regular, sawtooth waves in leads II, III, and aVF

198. Narrow complex tachycardia with no visible P waves

199. Narrow complex tachycardia with P waves superimposed on the ST segment

200. Regular, wide complex tachycardia

QUESTIONS 201–203

Match the following sites of radiofrequency ablation with the appropriate supraventricular arrhythmias.

    A. Low right atrium between the tricuspid valve and inferior vena cava
    B. Mitral or tricuspid valve annulus
    C. Posterior right atrial septum

201. Orthodromic reciprocating tachycardia

202. AV nodal re-entrant tachycardia

203. Atrial flutter

QUESTIONS 204–207

Match the benefits and weaknesses of the common procedures used in the diagnosis of acute aortic dissection.

    A. Portable, relatively noninvasive
    B. Can determine coronary artery involvement, is invasive, and is unable to evaluate the presence of pericardial effusion
    C. The most sensitive and specific but not widely available
    D. Very specific but unable to evaluate for presence of aortic insufficiency or coronary artery involvement

204. Magnetic resonance imaging

205. Aortic angiography

206. Transesophageal echocardiography

207. Computed tomography

Part I
Cardiology
Answers

1. **(C)** *Discussion:* If aortic thrombosis or distal embolization occurs, patients should be referred for surgery. An abdominal aneurysm is a relative contraindication to anticoagulation. (*Cecil, Ch. 75*)

2. **(B)** *Discussion:* There is no evidence that sudden death is reduced after myomectomy. Myomectomy should be reserved for patients who have severe symptoms despite maximal medical therapy. By reducing the Venturi effect on the mitral valves, it reduces the degree of mitral regurgitation. (*Cecil, Ch. 73*)

3. **(A)** *Discussion:* The loudness of S_1 is related to the position of the mitral valve at the onset of ventricular systole. If ventricular systole occurs just as the valve has opened, as occurs with WPW (as a result of the short PR interval), S_1 will be loud. Conversely, if the valve has sufficient time to return to the nearly closed position, the valve closure sounds will be softer. In addition, patients with calcified immobile mitral valves will have a soft S_1. (*Braunwald et al, 2001*)

4. **(D)** *Discussion:* Asymmetrical hypertrophy, commonly seen in the septum, and systolic anterior motion of the anterior mitral valve leaflet are the fundamental features of hypertrophic cardiomyopathy. Contraction of the myocardium is normal, and there is often left ventricular outflow tract obstruction, leading to a dynamic systolic gradient. This can be present at rest and may increase substantially after the Valsalva maneuver or inhalation of amyl nitrate in the echocardiography laboratory. (*Cecil, Ch. 73*)

5. **(C)** *Discussion:* This sign correlates best with elevation of the pulmonary capillary wedge pressure. (*Ewy, 1988*)

6. **(C)** *Discussion:* Any condition that causes electrical or mechanical delay of left ventricular contraction and delayed aortic closure will result in paradoxical splitting of S_2. Atrial septal defect is associated with delayed right ventricular closure and fixed splitting of S_2. (*Cecil, Chs. 46 and 65*)

7. **(C)** *Discussion:* Hypertrophic cardiomyopathy is characterized by severe *diastolic* dysfunction. (*Cecil, Ch. 73*)

8. **(A)** *Discussion:* Hypertension is the most common association with acute aortic dissection. All of the other listed diseases except hemochromatosis are associated with dissection. (*Cecil, Ch. 75*)

9. **(D)** *Discussion:* Squatting increases afterload and intensifies the murmur of aortic regurgitation. (*Cecil, Ch. 46*)

10. **(E)** *Discussion:* Stretching of the recurrent laryngeal nerve can cause hoarseness. Intrascapular pain is the most common site of referred pain, although this is quite variable. Hemoptysis can occur if leakage of blood into the left lung occurs. (*Cecil, Ch. 75*)

11. **(D)** *Discussion:* There is normally an inspiratory decrease in the jugular venous pressure resulting from a reduction in intrathoracic and right-sided heart pressures. In conditions in which right-sided heart pressures are elevated and augmented right ventricular filling is limited, such as right ventricular infarction, constrictive pericarditis, or pulmonary embolism, the increased filling of the right-sided heart chambers that occurs with inspiration is transmitted into the jugular venous pulsation and elevation of the neck veins occurs with inspiration. With tricuspid regurgitation, a prominent V wave in observed but respiratory changes are not affected. (*Cecil, Ch. 46*)

12. **(D)** *Discussion:* If the dissection begins proximally, the pain may be referred anteriorly. As the dissection progresses, posterior chest pain can occur. Unlike other patients with aortic insufficiency, an elevated diastolic pressure is commonly present. (*Cecil, Ch. 75*)

13. **(B)** *Discussion:* Delta waves are caused by simultaneous anterograde conduction over the AV node and accessory pathway *during sinus rhythm*. Orthodromic reciprocating tachycardia (ORT) uses the AV node as the anterograde limb and the accessory pathway as the retrograde limb of the re-entry circuit. For this reason, delta waves are not seen during ORT because conduction occurs retrogradely over the accessory pathway. (*Cecil, Ch. 59*)

14. **(A)** *Discussion:* An ECG from a patient with hypertrophic cardiomyopathy often shows increased voltage suggestive of the marked ventricular hypertrophy seen with this condition. (*Cecil, Ch. 73; Chou, 1991*)

15. **(D)** *Discussion:* Patients with claudication often have impotence because of involvement of pelvic vessels. (*Cecil, Ch. 76*)

16. **(C)** *Discussion:* Rate of the tachycardia or clinical condition of the patient has no use in differentiating the mechanism of a tachycardia. In addition, adenosine is not helpful because some SVTs will not terminate and some VTs will serendipitously stop after intravenous administration of adenosine. The presence of AV dissociation on an ECG is diagnostic of VT. (*Cecil, Ch. 60*)

17. **(B)** *Discussion:* Patients with paroxysmal atrial fibrillation are also at an increased risk of stroke and should be treated with Coumadin. (*Cecil, Ch. 59*)

18. **(C)** *Discussion:* Although a systematic review did not confirm the anecdotal reports of increased digoxin toxicity among patients with cardiac amyloidosis, there are no data to suggest that digoxin favorably alters morbidity and mortality in these patients. (*Cecil, Ch. 73*)

19. **(D)** *Discussion:* Digoxin would worsen the symptoms of hypertrophic cardiomyopathy by increasing contractility and enhancing the diastolic dysfunction and ventricular outflow tract gradient. Negative inotropes such as verapamil, propranolol, and disopyramide are first-line agents for this condition. (*Cecil, Ch. 73*)

20. **(A)** *Discussion:* The left atrial appendage is poorly visualized on a transthoracic echo. The inability to visualize a thrombus does not exclude its presence. (*Braunwald et al, 2001; Cecil, Chs. 51 and 59*)

21. **(C)** *Discussion:* Reduced heart rate variability is associated with an increased incidence of sudden death after a myocardial infarction. Note that these variables have a good negative predictive value but a poor positive predictive value in predicting which patients will die suddenly. (*Cecil, Ch. 60*)

22. **(D)** *Discussion:* Restrictive cardiomyopathy is characterized by generalized wall thickening and impaired diastolic function. There is commonly associated bi-atrial enlargement and modest generalized hypokinesis. Ventricular dilatation is a characteristic of dilated cardiomyopathy and not commonly seen in restrictive cardiomyopathy. Speckling of the myocardium on echocardiography can be noted in certain restrictive disorders classically described in amyloid infiltration of the myocardium (*Cecil, Ch. 51*).

23. **(E)** *Discussion:* Cardiac MRI provides excellent visualization of cardiac tumors, congenital cardiac anomalies, and aortic pathology; it can depict the anomalous origin of coronary arteries and can be helpful in the evaluation of many myocardial and pericardial diseases. Cardiac MRI is still not widely available, remains costly, is not portable, and cannot be used in patients with implanted pacemakers or defibrillators. Although imaging techniques have dramatically improved in recent years and cardiovascular applications have expanded, the role of cardiac MRI relative to other noninvasive imaging modalities such as echocardiography, nuclear imaging, and x-ray computed tomography remains unclear. (*Cecil, Ch. 53*)

24. **(B)** *Discussion:* Digoxin exerts its effects on the AV node by increasing vagal tone, but these effects are abolished by sympathetic stimulation. Thus, digoxin is not useful as sole therapy in patients who are physically active or who have hyperadrenergic states (e.g., fever, thyrotoxicosis). (*Matsuda et al, 1991*)

25. **(B)** *Discussion:* When dissections involve the proximal aorta or arch, emergency surgery is indicated. Morbidity and mortality are directly related to the time between onset of symptoms and surgical treatment. A time lapse of several hours could be potentially fatal. A patient with a descending aortic dissection can be managed medically unless complications develop or symptoms are refractory to medical therapy. (*Cecil, Ch. 75*)

26. **(D)** *Discussion:* Radiofrequency catheter ablation is associated with mild pain and is performed using little or no sedation in many patients. Ablation of atrial flutter restores normal sinus rhythm. Because AV nodal function remains intact, pacemaker implantation is not required. Catheter ablation is cost effective, especially in patients who are young, who have required multiple visits to the emergency department for termination of their tachycardia, or who require chronic drug therapy. (*Cecil, Ch. 61; Philippon et al, 1995*)

27. **(B)** *Discussion:* Patients with diabetes and those with renal insufficiency require intensive treatment of hypertension to prevent progressive end-organ damage. Pre-hypertension is defined as a blood pressure of 120-139/80-89 mm Hg. Patients with pre-hypertension are at increased risk of developing hypertension and should be counseled in appropriate lifestyle modification. Drug therapy is generally not indicated unless there are other compelling reasons. Monotherapy with a single agent is rarely successful in the treatment of severe hypertension. (*Cecil, Ch. 63; JNC VII, 2003*)

28. **(C)** *Discussion:* Any agent that slows conduction through the AV node will increase conduction over the accessory pathway. If the ventricular response is rapid enough, ventricular fibrillation may result. Procainamide prolongs the refractory period of atrial myocardium, slowing conduction over the accessory pathway and reducing the ventricular response. In addition, it may aid conversion to sinus rhythm. (*Cecil, Ch. 59*)

29. **(A)** *Discussion:* Doxorubicin cardiotoxicity is irreversible. The other statements are correct. (*Cecil, Chs. 73 and 191*)

30. **(D)** *Discussion:* PR segment depression is specific for pericarditis and is seen in the early stage of the disease. The other listed ECG findings may be seen with other causes of ST elevation, including acute myocardial injury and early repolarization. (*Cecil, Ch. 74; Chou, 1991*)

31. **(B)** *Discussion:* In seemingly healthy athletes, the most common cause of sudden cardiac death is unrecognized hypertrophic cardiomyopathy. (*Braunwald et al, 2001*)

32. **(C)** *Discussion:* Quinidine commonly causes diarrhea and nausea. (*Cecil, Ch. 62*)

33. **(B)** *Discussion:* Despite a diligent search, no viral cause has been identified. (*Cecil, Chs. 73 and 253*)

34. **(B)** *Discussion:* Accommodation is a normal property of the AV node and does not contribute to the genesis of arrhythmias. (*Cecil, Ch. 57*)

35. **(B)** *Discussion:* Flutter waves are best seen in the inferior leads. (*Cecil, Ch. 59*)

36. **(B)** *Discussion:* Tissue factor is located in the lipid core of plaques and promotes thrombosis when it comes in contact with flowing blood at the time of plaque rupture. Smoking, hyperlipidemia, and diabetes are associated with endothelial dysfunction in coronary and peripheral arteries. C-reactive protein is a marker for inflammation. High levels of C-reactive protein are associated with future coronary events. Family history carries independent prognostic value.

37. **(B)** *Discussion:* Lidocaine has no effect on atrial tissue. (*Cecil, Ch. 62*)

38. **(B)** *Discussion:* Antidromic reciprocating tachycardia is a wide complex rhythm because anterograde AV conduction occurs eccentrically over the accessory pathway. (*Cecil, Ch. 59*)

39. **(B)** *Discussion:* All "pacemaker cells" have diastolic depolarization and are capable of producing spontaneous depolarizations. The rate of the normal sinus node pacemaker is greater than the AV nodal pacemaker, which in turn is greater than the His-Purkinje fibers. (*Cecil, Ch. 57*)

40. **(B)** *Discussion:* Hypocalcemia is not associated with torsades de pointes. (*Cecil, Ch. 60*)

41. **(B)** *Discussion:* Patients with ventricular arrhythmias in the setting of an acute myocardial infarction do not have a worsened prognosis compared with controls. (*Cecil, Chs. 60 and 61*)

42. **(D)** *Discussion:* Because of the unfavorable natural history of patients with Marfan syndrome, prophylactic surgery is recommended in all patients when the ascending aorta is 5 to 5.5 cm or larger. (*Cecil, Ch. 75*)

43. **(A)** *Discussion:* The common adverse effects of amiodarone include pulmonary fibrosis, hypothyroidism or hyperthyroidism, corneal deposits, peripheral neuropathy or myopathy, hepatitis, photosensitivity, and blue-gray skin discoloration. (*Cecil, Ch. 62*)

44. **(D)** *Discussion:* Thromboangiitis obliterans (Buerger's disease) is a disease of young male smokers and has a high prevalence in India, Israel, and the Orient, suggesting a genetic predisposition. (*Cecil, Ch. 77*)

45. **(C)** *Discussion:* Development of congestive heart failure in patients with aortic stenosis is associated with a 50% mortality in 2 years. (*Cecil, Ch. 72*)

46. (D) *Discussion:* Calcific aortic stenosis is a disease of advanced age. Approximately half of all patients will have coronary artery disease even if chest pain is absent. This is the primary reason that patients who have known aortic stenosis undergo left-sided heart catheterization. (*Cecil, Ch. 72*)

47. (C) *Discussion:* Although it is unproven, most cases of idiopathic dilated cardiomyopathy are probably the result of subclinical myocarditis caused by coxsackievirus group B or adenovirus viral infection. (*Cecil, Ch. 73*)

48. (B) *Discussion:* In a 55-year-old man, bicuspid aortic valve is most likely. Senile calcific aortic stenosis develops in the seventh and eighth decades. There was no history of rheumatic fever to suggest rheumatic aortic stenosis. Myxomatous degeneration does not cause aortic stenosis. (*Cecil, Ch. 72*)

49. (C) *Discussion:* Echocardiography can noninvasively evaluate the severity of aortic stenosis with a high degree of certainty. (*Cecil, Ch. 72*)

50. (D) *Discussion:* His symptoms, physical examination, and ECG suggest severe aortic stenosis. After confirmation of this with echocardiography, he should be referred for coronary angiography and then aortic valve replacement. CABG should also be performed if significant coronary obstruction is identified. (*Cecil, Ch. 72*)

51. (B) *Discussion:* She has aortic insufficiency. Diuretics and afterload reduction are of immediate benefit in relieving symptoms until further evaluation can be performed. (*Cecil, Ch. 72*)

52. (C) *Discussion:* Transthoracic echocardiography can evaluate degree of aortic insufficiency, presence of valvular vegetations (although absence of vegetations does not rule out endocarditis), and ventricular function. If endocarditis is strongly suspected, a transesophageal echocardiogram should be performed. (*Cecil, Ch. 72*)

53. (D) *Discussion:* Acute severe aortic insufficiency with left ventricular failure has developed, probably as a result of a ruptured or perforated aortic valve leaflet from staphylococcal endocarditis. Medical stabilization with sodium nitroprusside for afterload reduction and intravenous diuretics to manage the pulmonary edema may be helpful. An intra-aortic balloon pump would be contraindicated because the diastolic flow augmentation would only worsen her aortic insufficiency. Emergency surgery is indicated. (*Cecil, Ch. 72*)

54. (B) *Discussion:* The traumatic hip injury and subsequent immobilization likely caused the venous thrombosis that occurred in this patient. Estrogen therapy may have also contributed to development of venous thrombosis. Factor V Leiden causes activated protein C resistance and predisposes to venous thromboembolic disease. (*Cecil, Ch. 78*)

55. (B) *Discussion:* D-Dimers have good negative predictive value for excluding DVT but should be used with one of the other tests. (*Cecil, Ch. 78*)

56. (A) *Discussion:* Fixed dose unfractionated heparin therapy is not appropriate. Low molecular weight heparins appear to be superior to unfractionated heparin with reduction in major bleeding and lower mortality as documented in clinical trials. Low molecular weight heparins should not be used in patients with renal insufficiency. Warfarin can be started simultaneously with intravenous heparin unless surgical intervention is contemplated. (*Cecil, Ch. 78*)

57. (D) *Discussion:* LMWH does not affect antithrombin III activity, so partial thromboplastin time monitoring is not necessary. The risk of bleeding is less with LMWH and can be used safely during initiation of warfarin. (*Cecil, Ch. 78*)

58. (B) *Discussion:* There is a high risk of DVT after elective hip replacement. Unfractionated heparin is not a recommended prophylaxis regimen for high-risk patients. (*Cecil, Ch. 78*)

59. (C) *Discussion:* B-type natriuretic peptide is released by the left ventricle in response to myocardial stretch and is a relatively sensitive and specific marker of heart failure. It has been shown to have a high negative predictive value; in other words a low BNP level reliably rules out heart failure in a patient with unexplained shortness of breath. A low BNP does not automatically make respiratory disease a cause of this patient's shortness of breath and hence choice B is incorrect. (*Cecil, Ch. 55*)

60. (C) *Discussion:* The viral prodrome and negative medical history suggest viral myocarditis resulting in idiopathic dilated cardiomyopathy. (*Cecil, Ch. 73*)

61. (D) *Discussion:* Up to half of patients with dilated cardiomyopathy presumed secondary to a viral infection will have a major improvement in left ventricular function even in patients in whom an initial biopsy did not show evidence for myocarditis. (*Cecil, Ch. 73*)

62. (D) *Discussion:* Endomyocardial biopsies are not routinely performed in the evaluation of idiopathic cardiomyopathies because they rarely are diagnostic; and treatment with steroids, azathioprine, and cyclosporine in controlled trials has not shown any benefit, even when evidence of myocarditis is demonstrated. (*Cecil, Ch. 73*)

63. (C) *Discussion:* Steroids have not been proven to improve morbidity or mortality for patients with idiopathic dilated cardiomyopathy. (*Cecil, Ch. 73*)

64. (B) *Discussion:* The presence of ventricular tachyarrhythmias raises the possibility of giant cell myocarditis. This is one of the rare instances in which endomyocardial biopsy may be useful because, although unproved, it may respond to immunosuppression. (*Cecil, Ch. 73*)

65. (C) *Discussion:* Doxorubicin, ethanol, and cyclophosphamide have been associated with dilated cardiomyopathy. Cyclosporine does not cause cardiomyopathy. (*Cecil, Ch. 73*)

66. (C) *Discussion:* Frequent binge drinking may also lead to alcoholic cardiomyopathy. (*Cecil, Chs. 17 and 73*)

67. (D) *Discussion:* She has acute viral pericarditis. This is generally a self-limiting disease that can be treated as an outpatient in the majority of patients. (*Cecil, Ch. 74*)

68. (A) *Discussion:* Nonsteroidal anti-inflammatory drugs (NSAIDs) are sufficient for most patients with acute pericarditis. Note that steroids should be reserved for cases that are refractory to NSAIDs because many patients will relapse after withdrawal of steroids. Thrombolytics are not only not helpful but also contraindicated in pericarditis. Anticoagulants should also be avoided, if possible, but may be mandatory in patients with a prosthetic valve or atrial fibrillation. (*Cecil, Ch. 74*)

69. (B) *Discussion:* Careful measurement of his BP to evaluate for pulsus paradoxus is an easy, sensitive, and relatively specific method to diagnose cardiac tamponade. (*Cecil, Ch. 74*)

70. (D) *Discussion:* With large pericardial effusions, electrical alternans, low-voltage QRS complexes, sinus tachycardia, and occasionally diffuse ST elevation secondary to coexistent pericarditis may be seen. (*Cecil, Ch. 74; Chou, 1991*)

71. (A) *Discussion:* Cardiac tamponade results in equalization of diastolic right-sided heart pressures. (*Cecil, Ch. 74*)

72. (C) *Discussion:* Although the diagnosis of cardiac tamponade is primarily made on the basis of clinical findings, the finding of a pericardial effusion on echocardiography would support this diagnosis, especially if right atrial and right ventricular diastolic collapse were also seen. (*Cecil, Chs. 51 and 74*)

73. **(B)** *Discussion:* Hyperalphalipoproteinemia (high HDL cholesterol) is considered a "negative risk factor for CHD" (i.e., it is believed to protect against the development of CHD). Smoking, hypertension, and sedentary lifestyle are potent risk factors for CHD. Recent data show that *trans*-fatty acids contained in many margarines raise serum cholesterol levels. (*Cecil, Ch. 66; ATP III Report, 2002*)

74. **(D)** *Discussion:* Ejection fraction is calculated as stroke volume (volume of blood ejected with each heartbeat) divided by the end-diastolic volume of the left ventricle. In this patient, the stroke volume is 50 mL. The ejection fraction thus is (50 mL/200 mL) = 0.25 or 25%. (*Cecil, Ch. 54*)

75. **(D)** *Discussion:* Renin is produced in the macula densa cells of the juxtaglomerular apparatus. The renin-angiotensin system is activated in heart failure, and the degree of activation correlates with the severity of heart failure and with prognosis. Angiotensin II is a powerful coronary and peripheral arterial vasoconstrictor and stimulates the release of aldosterone from the adrenal gland, leading to avid sodium reabsorption. Angiotensin promotes the release of norepinephrine from peripheral sympathetic nervous system sites. (*Cecil, Chs. 48 and 55*)

76. **(C)** *Discussion:* The right border is formed by the superior vena cava, the right atrium, and sometimes a small portion of the inferior vena cava. The left border is formed by the aortic knob, the main pulmonary artery, the left atrial appendage, and the left ventricle. The right ventricle is located anteriorly and does not reach either heart border. (*Cecil, Ch. 49; Steiner and Levin, 1997*)

77. **(B)** *Discussion:* Dobutamine is a β-adrenergic agonist and enhances AV conduction. All others decrease AV conduction. Adenosine is now frequently used to treat supraventricular re-entrant tachycardias acutely; it is preferred over verapamil in this setting because of its short duration of action. (*Cecil, Chs. 50 and 62*)

78. **(A)** *Discussion:* Perfusion imaging may be useful in very selected asymptomatic patients who are at very high risk for coronary artery disease but is generally not indicated in this setting. Perfusion imaging is critical in the identification of viable myocardium and in the localization of ischemia before revascularization procedures. It has proven useful in risk-stratifying patients before noncardiac surgical procedures, especially peripheral vascular procedures. Exercise stress testing with perfusion imaging has a higher sensitivity and specificity for diagnosis of myocardial ischemia than exercise stress testing with traditional electrocardiographic monitoring. (*Cecil, Ch. 52*)

79. **(C)** *Discussion:* Hemochromatosis is an infiltrative disease that ultimately results in diminished cardiac output. All other conditions are causes of high-output heart failure. (*Cecil, Ch. 55*)

80. **(E)** *Discussion:* Constrictive pericarditis presents as signs of volume overload and diminished exercise tolerance despite normal left ventricular ejection fraction. Because ascites is often a prominent symptom, it is also frequently mistaken for advanced liver disease. Left ventricular hypertrophy and infiltrative diseases such as amyloidosis and storage diseases such as hemochromatosis result in abnormal myocardial compliance and lead to symptoms of heart failure despite preserved left ventricular systolic function. Peripartum cardiomyopathy is a form of dilated cardiomyopathy characterized by global left ventricular systolic dysfunction. (*Cecil, Chs. 55, 73, and 74*)

81. **(E)** *Discussion:* Both bradyarrhythmias and tachyarrhythmias may lead to worsening heart failure symptoms. Decompensation is often precipitated by iatrogenic volume overload such as perioperative volume infusion or transfusion. States of increased metabolic demand such as infection and anemia may lead to increasing heart failure symptoms. Poor compliance with medications, salt, and volume restriction are frequent causes of heart failure decompensation. (*Cecil, Chs. 55 and 56*)

82. **(D)** *Discussion:* Sympathetic stimulation of the heart by sympathetic nerve stimulation or by circulating catecholamines increases heart rate, improves conduction velocity through the AV node, increases force and velocity of ventricular muscle contraction, and enhances ventricular muscle relaxation. Phase IV depolarization in the sinus node is enhanced. (*Cecil, Ch. 48*)

83. **(C)** *Discussion:* Accurately measured blood pressure is paramount in the assessment and treatment of hypertension. Aneroid manometers are less accurate than mercury manometers but are sufficient if frequently standardized against a mercury column. BP should be measured two or three times after the patient has been seated comfortably for at least 5 minutes, and the readings should be averaged. Falsely high BP readings occur when the BP cuff is too narrow or when the bladder is too short to encircle the arm. The auscultatory gap remains unexplained but can cause a significant underestimate of the true pressure unless systolic pressure is first determined by palpation and the BP cuff inflated 30 mm Hg above the palpated pressure. BPs measured in the health care setting tend to be higher than ambulatory readings; the latter correlate better with target organ damage. (*Cecil, Ch. 63; Grim and Grim, 2003*)

84. **(C)** *Discussion:* Secondary causes of hypertension account for only about 5% of cases of hypertension. The incidence of end-stage renal disease has been increasing in the 1990s, and surveys suggest that awareness, treatment, and control rates of hypertension have declined over the same time period. Isolated systolic hypertension increases markedly with age, with an estimated prevalence of 22% among those 80 years and older. Blacks tend to have more severe and earlier onset of hypertension than whites. Data from Framingham indicate an increased risk of heart failure even with moderately elevated blood pressure. (*Cecil, Ch. 63*)

85. **(C)** *Discussion:* Epidemiologic studies and some clinical studies suggest an inverse relationship between calcium intake and BP, and calcium supplementation may be beneficial in the treatment of hypertension. Licorice causes a form of mineralocorticoid hypertension. Cyclosporine, erythropoietin, NSAIDs, and many other drugs may cause or exacerbate hypertension. A careful diet and medication history is an important part of the evaluation of the hypertensive patient. (*Cecil, Ch. 63*)

86. **(E)** *Discussion:* All classes listed have been shown to reduce stroke. Risk of stroke has also been reduced with angiotensin-receptor blocker based regimens. Whether there is a single best class of drugs remains the subject of considerable debate. Most patients will require combination therapy for optimal blood pressure control. (*Cecil, Ch. 63; Blood Pressure Trialists Collaboration, 2003; JNC VII, 2003*)

87. **(D)** *Discussion:* All listed measures with the exception of more than moderate alcohol intake have been shown to reduce BP levels. Intake of alcohol should be limited to 1 oz of ethanol/day in most hypertensive men (24 oz beer, 10 oz wine, or 3 oz of 80-proof whiskey) and to half this amount in hypertensive women or lighter weight individuals. (*Cecil, Ch. 63; JNC VII Report, 2003*)

88. **(E)** *Discussion:* High-pitched, systolic-diastolic, or continuous abdominal bruits are strongly suggestive of renovascular obstruction and are found in one half to two thirds of patients with surgically proven renovascular hypertension. About one third of patients with renovascular hypertension have fibromuscular disease, and two thirds have atherosclerotic disease. Those with

atherosclerotic disease tend to be older, have higher systolic BPs, and have more target organ damage than patients with essential hypertension. Patients with fibromuscular dysplasia are younger and less likely to experience cardiovascular complications. In patients with suitable lesions, percutaneous revascularization can often be performed at the time of diagnostic renal arteriography. (*Cecil, Ch. 63*)

89. **(B)** *Discussion:* Potassium-sparing diuretics are very useful in preventing hypokalemia in patients on thiazide or loop diuretic therapy, but hyperkalemia may occur in the setting of diabetes, renal insufficiency, and concomitant ACE inhibitor therapy. Constipation is a common side effect of verapamil. Both ACE inhibitors and angiotensin II antagonists have teratogenic effects and are contraindicated in pregnant patients. Reserpine is contraindicated in patients with depression. Other side effects include sexual dysfunction, nasal congestion, and lethargy. (*Cecil, Ch. 63*)

90. **(E)** *Discussion:* Hypoxia results in pulmonary arteriolar vasoconstriction. Increased blood viscosity such as that seen in polycythemia vera can increase pulmonary arterial pressures. Increased intrathoracic pressure is transmitted to the pulmonary circulation and causes elevation of pulmonary artery pressures. Endothelin is a powerful vasoconstrictive substance and has been shown to be elevated in some forms of pulmonary hypertension. Prostacyclin is a vasodilatory substance. It causes reduction in pulmonary artery pressure not elevation. (*Cecil, Ch. 64*)

91. **(D)** *Discussion:* Pulmonary thrombi are often found at autopsy and are believed to represent in situ thromboses rather than pulmonary emboli. Pulmonary scintigraphy in patients with severe primary pulmonary hypertension may result in hypotension as a result of obstruction of the pulmonary microvasculature. Pulmonary vascular endothelial function is abnormal in primary pulmonary hypertension. Circulating levels of vasoconstrictors such as endothelin and thromboxane are elevated, whereas vasodilators such as nitric oxide and prostacyclin are diminished. Women outnumber men 3-4:1. Dyspnea and fatigue are common presenting complaints. Because these complaints are fairly nonspecific, the diagnosis of primary pulmonary hypertension is often not made until late in the disease. (*Cecil, Ch. 64; Rich, 1998*)

92. **(E)** *Discussion:* A bicuspid aortic valve is the most common congenital anomaly of the heart. Patients generally come to attention because of progressive stenosis or aortic valve incompetence. Ostium secundum atrial septal defect may not be recognized during childhood. Adults may present with atrial arrhythmias, heart failure, or progressive pulmonary hypertension. Patients with ventricular septal defects generally survive to adulthood, if the ventricular septal defect closes spontaneously or if a nonrestrictive defect is accompanied by elevated pulmonary vascular resistance, thus protecting the left ventricle from chronic volume overload. Ebstein's anomaly is an uncommon congenital defect. Accessory pathways are often present, and patients may present with tachyarrhythmias (WPW syndrome). Uncorrected tricuspid atresia is generally fatal in childhood, although rare instances of survival into adulthood and middle age have been documented. (*Cecil, Ch. 65; Roberts, 1987*)

93. **(D)** *Discussion:* Antiarrhythmic therapies such as prophylactic lidocaine in the hospital and suppression of ventricular ectopy after hospital discharge have been associated with increased mortality after myocardial infarction. All other therapies listed have clear mortality benefits. (*Cecil, Ch. 69*)

94. **(C)** *Discussion:* Patients with a bicuspid aortic valve may experience progressive aortic stenosis or incompetence. They have an increased risk of endocarditis, and thus endocarditis prophylaxis is mandatory. Associated abnormalities of the aortic root may predispose them to aortic dissection. Papillary muscle rupture is not a feature of this anomaly. (*Cecil, Ch. 65; Roberts, 1987*)

95. **(B)** *Discussion:* Cyanosis is not a feature of coarctation of the aorta unless coarctation occurs in association with a cyanotic congenital cardiac anomaly. Adults present with hypertension, and characteristic rib notching may be present on the chest x-ray film. A bicuspid aortic valve is a common associated anomaly. A coexisting aneurysm of the circle of Willis is less common, but a fatal intracranial hemorrhage may be the presenting manifestation in patients in their second or third decade of life. Patients are also at risk of aortic dissection distal to the coarctation site. (*Cecil, Ch. 65; Roberts, 1987*)

96. **(B)** *Discussion:* Only tetralogy of Fallot is an obligatory cyanotic congenital defect. Patients with ostium secundum defect have a left-to-right shunt and are thus characteristically not cyanotic. Neither pulmonary valve stenosis nor coarctation of the aorta is a lesion characterized by shunts. Although usually characterized by a left-to-right shunt, differential cyanosis may occasionally occur in patients who shunt right to left through a patent ductus arteriosus. (*Cecil, Ch. 65; Perloff, 1987*)

97. **(B)** *Discussion:* Patients with cyanotic congenital heart disease have increased red cell mass. High hematocrits may lead to a hyperviscosity syndrome, further worsened by superimposed iron deficiency. Hyperuricemia is believed to be due to increased urate reabsorption as a result of renal hypoperfusion. Renal histology in congenital heart disease is abnormal, and patients are at increased risk of angiographic dye-induced renal failure. The risk of cholelithiasis is increased in cyanotic congenital heart disease (calcium bilirubinate stones). Patients with cyanotic congenital heart disease bruise easily, commonly have gingival bleeding, and may have severe and recurrent epistaxis and hemoptysis. (*Cecil, Ch. 65*)

98. **(E)** *Discussion:* Major determinants of myocardial oxygen consumption include heart rate, afterload, contractility, and preload, in decreasing order of importance. Coronary perfusion in the left ventricle occurs in diastole when wall tension and coronary resistance are low. With increasing severity, ischemia progresses from the most sensitive region in the subendocardium to the subepicardium. Stenoses of 50% or higher on angiography (75% cross-sectional area) can cause angina pectoris during periods of high demand. The vasodilator response is mediated by nitric oxide not prostacyclin. (*Cecil, Ch. 67*)

99. **(D)** *Discussion:* According to Bayes' theorem, the post-test likelihood of coronary disease is influenced by the pretest prevalence of disease. Exercise stress testing is thus most useful in patients with intermediate probability of disease. As ST segment depression increases, specificity of the test increases whereas sensitivity decreases. Women are more likely to have a false-positive ECG response to exercise. Exercise stress testing is contraindicated in severe aortic stenosis and in severe hypertrophic cardiomyopathy. (*Cecil, Ch. 67*)

100. **(C)** Exercise-induced hypotension rather than hypertension is a poor prognostic indicator. Severity of ST segment depression, duration of ST segment depression, early onset of ST segment depression, and poor exercise capacity have been associated with poor prognosis. (*Cecil, Ch. 67*)

101. **(D)** *Discussion:* β-Blockers have been shown to improve survival in class II to class IV heart failure patients in the MERIT-HF, Carvedilol study group trials, COPERNICUS, and other randomized clinical trials. ACE inhibitors have been shown to improve outcomes in patients with symptomatic and asymptomatic left ventricular dysfunction in the SOLVD and CONSENSUS trials. The RALES trial showed a survival benefit of spironolactone in patients with severe heart failure. Diuretics improve patients symptomatically but have never been shown in a randomized clinical trial to improve survival. (*Packer et al, 1996, 2001; MERIT HF*

Study Group, 1999; SOLVD Investigators, 1991; Consensus Trial Study Group, 1987; Pitt et al, 1999)

102. **(A)** *Discussion:* An implantable cardiac defibrillator (ICD) has been shown to improve survival in patients with ischemic cardiomyopathy and left ventricular ejection fraction less than 30% in the randomized clinical trial MADIT-II. These patients did not undergo any electrophysiologic study, unlike in MADIT-I. Anticoagulation is controversial in patients with heart failure and is usually instituted in patients with very low ejection fraction or those with known left ventricular aneurysm or thrombus. Amiodarone therapy is inferior to an ICD in patients with ischemic cardiomyopathy as shown in the AVID trial *(Cecil, Chs. 60 and 61; Moss et al, 1996, 2002; AVID Investigators, 2000)*

103. **(D)** *Discussion:* Prostaglandin inhibitors like aspirin and NSAIDs cause inhibition of the vasodilatory effects of prostaglandins and can impair renal perfusion. Short-acting calcium channel blockers can cause adverse cardiovascular reactions, including hypotension, worsening heart failure, pulmonary edema, and cardiogenic shock. Long-term use of intravenous inotropes is associated with a worsened survival and should only be used as palliative therapy in severely symptomatic heart failure or as a bridge to transplantation. *(Cecil, Ch. 56)*

104. **(E)** *Discussion:* Microvascular angina (syndrome X), coronary emboli, coronary artery vasculitis, and Prinzmetal angina or coronary spasm are all causes of chest pain with ST segment changes. *(Cecil, Ch. 67)*

105. **(E)** *Discussion:* This patient is at high risk for coronary artery disease and describes typical anginal symptoms. Because of the high pre-test likelihood of coronary artery disease, a negative noninvasive study with or without imaging would not help in ruling out the possibility of significant coronary artery disease. In such a patient, coronary angiography is performed with a view toward coronary revascularization. *(Cecil, Ch. 67)*

106. **(E)** *Discussion:* Postinfarction angina, infarct expansion, acute pericarditis, or pulmonary thromboembolism are all causes of post–myocardial infarction pain *(Cecil, Ch. 69)*

107. **(F)** *Discussion:* Allograft rejection requiring augmentation of the immunosuppressive regimen, allograft vasculopathy, infection, secondary malignancy including squamous cell carcinoma of the skin, lymphomas and sarcomas, and medication related side effects are important long-term considerations in patients who receive cardiac transplants. *(Cecil, Ch. 80)*

108. **(A)–True; (B)–False; (C)–True; (D)–True; (E)–False.** *Discussion:* As lifestyles have been westernized, CHD has become an increasingly important cause of death in developing countries and by 1990 had become the second leading cause of mortality. Heart failure hospital discharges and mortality are increasing, at least in part because more patients survive their initial myocardial infarctions. CHD development occurs later in women than men, possibly related to hormonal factors. Blacks have higher CHD mortality rates than their white counterparts. CHD mortality rates are increasing in eastern European countries. *(Cecil, Ch. 47; AHA Statistical Fact Sheet: Populations, 2003; AHA Heart Disease and Stroke Statistics—2003 Update)*

109. **(A)–False; (B)–False; (C)–True; (D)–True; (E)–False.** *Discussion:* Afterload is the load against which the ventricle must contract. Increases in afterload thus tend to decrease stroke volume. Preload describes the loading condition of the heart at the end of diastole. Increases in heart rate enhance the inotropic state of the myocardium via changes in calcium availability, the so-called force-frequency relationship. Hypoxia, ischemia, and acidosis decrease myocardial contractility. Clinically, left ventricular filling pressure is often assessed by measuring pulmonary capillary wedge pressure with a balloon flotation catheter. Right atrial filling pressure is not a reliable estimate of left ventricular loading conditions. *(Cecil, Ch. 55)*

110. **(A)–True; (B)–True; (C)–True; (D)–False; (E)–True.** *Discussion:* Velocities in the regurgitant jet can be measured by Doppler ultrasonography. Using a modification of the Bernoulli equation, a gradient across the tricuspid valve can then be calculated. Right atrial pressure is estimated based on the level of the jugular venous pulsations. Pulmonary arterial systolic pressure can then be estimated as the sum of right atrial pressure and pressure gradient across the tricuspid valve. Distinguishing systolic and diastolic dysfunction is exceedingly important when evaluating patients with symptoms of heart failure. Echocardiography is ideally suited to determine ventricular size, function, and wall motion. Ejection fraction can be determined quantitatively but is often determined by visual estimation. Absence of vegetations does not exclude a diagnosis of endocarditis. Transesophageal echocardiography is better than transthoracic echocardiography in assessing the mitral valve. Patients with valvular heart disease need to be monitored closely clinically. Serial assessment of ventricular function and valve function by echocardiography is helpful in determining progression of disease and timing of surgical intervention. *(Cecil, Ch. 51; ACC/AHA Practice Guideline, 1998)*

111. **(A)–True; (B)–True; (C)–False; (D)–False; (E)–True.** *Discussion:* Aortic dissection can be imaged by a variety of modalities. Use of individual modalities should be guided by local availability and expertise in interpretation and patient characteristics (e.g., claustrophobia, hemodynamic stability, susceptibility to contrast-induced nephropathy). EBCT visualizes coronary calcification and has been used to screen individuals for coronary artery disease. Its precise role in the evaluation of patients at risk for CAD is unclear, however. Quantitation of aortic stenosis can often be accomplished noninvasively with echocardiography, obviating the need for invasive hemodynamic study. Coronary angiography should be performed in patients with aortic stenosis perceived to be at risk for coronary disease. Radionuclide angiography is an excellent method to quantitate ejection fraction and allows assessment of regional wall motion. Quantitation of wall thickness is not feasible, however. MRI has been used to diagnose hemochromatosis, taking advantage of the paramagnetic properties of iron tissue stores. *(Cecil, Chs. 52 to 54)*

112. **(A)–True; (B)–True; (C)–False; (D)–True; (E)–False.** *Discussion:* ACE inhibitors, β-blockers, and hydralazine/nitrate in combination have been shown to improve mortality in heart failure. Hydralazine/nitrate combination therapy is inferior to ACE inhibitors and should be reserved for those individuals who cannot tolerate ACE inhibitors. There was no mortality benefit with prazosin. Digoxin decreases the need for heart failure hospitalization but does not improve CHF mortality. *(Cecil, Ch. 56; ACC/AHA and Heart Failure Society of America Heart Failure Treatment Guidelines)*

113. **(A)–True; (B)–False; (C)–True; (D)–True; (E)–False.** *Discussion:* Circulating levels of neurohumoral mediators, including norepinephrine, correlate with survival in heart failure. Proinflammatory cytokines such as tumor necrosis factor-α are believed to play a role in cardiac cachexia and are seen in severe heart failure. Natriuretic peptides are upregulated in heart failure, but response to these peptides is diminished. Endothelins cause peripheral and pulmonary vasoconstriction and thus contribute to the progression of heart failure. The renin-angiotensin system is upregulated in heart failure; circulating plasma renin levels are thus elevated. *(Cecil, Ch. 56)*

114. **(A)–True; (B)–True; (C)–False; (D)–True; (E)–True.** *Discussion:* Cheyne-Stokes respiration or frank sleep apnea are common in heart failure. As the patient assumes the recumbent

position, venous return increases and pulmonary venous pressure increases. Nocturnal cough, orthopnea, and paroxysmal nocturnal dyspnea may occur as a result of pulmonary venous congestion. Exercise intolerance in heart failure is multifactorial in origin. Pulmonary venous congestion may contribute, but hypoperfusion of skeletal muscles, metabolic abnormalities in skeletal muscle, adverse effects on respiratory muscle function, and deconditioning as a result of inactivity play a role. Bowel wall edema can lead to poor appetite, nausea, abdominal discomfort, and malabsorption. Elevated systemic venous pressures lead to liver congestion and, if severe, to hepatic synthetic dysfunction. Elevated liver function tests and hyperbilirubinemia are not uncommon in advanced heart failure. (*Cecil, Ch. 56*)

115. (A)–False; (B)–False; (C)–False; (D)–False; (E)–True.
Discussion: An S_3 gallop strongly indicates left ventricular dysfunction but is often absent, even in advanced heart failure. Mitral regurgitation often occurs secondary to left ventricular dilatation and is thus not pathognomonic for primary valvular heart disease. Jugular venous distention is a manifestation of high right-sided filling pressures and is thus absent in mild left ventricular dysfunction. Patients with chronic heart failure often have clear lungs to auscultation despite markedly elevated pulmonary wedge pressures. A pulsatile liver is a sign of severe tricuspid regurgitation. (*Cecil, Ch. 56*)

116. (A)–True; (B)–True; (C)–False; (D)–False. *Discussion:* Diuretics are very useful in the treatment of heart failure symptoms but have inherent side effects, including development of electrolyte disturbances, activation of the neurohormonal axis, volume depletion, and azotemia. ACE inhibitors inhibit kininase II and result in kinin potentiation. This potentiation of kinins may be in part responsible for the beneficial hemodynamic effects of ACE inhibitors and is believed to contribute to beneficial effects on ventricular remodeling. ACE inhibitors can cause hyperkalemia. Avoidance of potassium supplements and potassium-sparing diuretics and, if necessary, reduction in ACE inhibitor dose are often sufficient to treat this side effect. Angioedema resulting from ACE inhibitors is a "class effect." Angioedema experienced in response to one ACE inhibitor contraindicates use of any ACE inhibitor. (*Cecil, Ch. 56*)

117. (A)–False; (B)–False; (C)–True; (D)–True; (E)–False.
Discussion: Low doses of spironolactone have been shown to increase survival among patients with advanced symptoms of heart failure. Side effects to digoxin are more common when serum levels are high, but side effects occur frequently at lower levels, especially in elderly patients. Digoxin has been shown to decrease sympathetic outflow from the central nervous system and to suppress renin secretion in the kidney. β-Blockers are beneficial in patients with class II through IV heart failure. Patients with heart failure are at very high risk of proarrhythmia with antiarrhythmic agents. Asymptomatic ventricular ectopy should not be treated with antiarrhythmic agents. (*Cecil, Ch. 56*)

118. (A)–True; (B)–False; (C)–True; (D)–True. *Discussion:* Heart failure is the only cardiovascular disease that is growing in incidence and prevalence over the past few decades. This has been ascribed to an aging population and improved initial management of myocardial infarctions, which reduced mortality but increased heart failure rates. The most common cause of heart failure is ischemic cardiomyopathy; hypertension remains the most common associated factor that is linked to heart failure. Diabetes is a risk factor for heart failure, and its prevalence is also rapidly increasing. Sympathetic activation and activation of the renin-angiotensin system are important in the pathogenesis of heart failure and are the target of therapy with β-blockers and ACE inhibitors, respectively. Other important neurohormones include

tumor necrosis factor-α, interleukin-6, endothelin, and arginine vasopressin. Sleep disorders and nocturnal desaturations are common in patients with heart failure, and supplemental oxygen and nasal oxygen and nasal positive-pressure ventilation may have a beneficial effect on fatigue and other heart failure symptoms. BNP levels are increased in elderly patients, women, and those with chronic obstructive pulmonary disease. (*Cecil, Chs. 55 and 56*)

119. (A)–True; (B)–True; (C)–True; (D)–False; (E)–False.
Discussion: Weight loss appears to be the most efficacious nonpharmacologic means of lowering BP. Dietary content also plays a significant role, as the DASH trial showed. Adequate intake of potassium and calcium seem to be particularly important. At least 30 minutes of moderate intensity physical exercise on most days of the week can lower BP by 4 to 9 mm Hg. Such activity is thus recommended for all hypertensive individuals, although those with manifest cardiovascular disease may require a medical evaluation before initiating such a regimen. Alcohol consumption elevates BP, both acutely and chronically. It is unclear whether the apparent reduction in cardiovascular risk with moderate alcohol consumption in the general population applies to hypertensive individuals. Sodium restriction tends to be most effective in populations with low renin hypertension such as the elderly and black patients. (*Cecil, Ch. 63; JNC VII, 2003*)

120. (A)–False; (B)–False; (C)–True; (D)–True; (E)–True.
Discussion: Monotherapy controls BP in fewer than 50% of hypertensive patients. The comparative efficacy of various antihypertensive agents has been reviewed in a comprehensive meta-analysis, in which it was concluded that larger reductions in blood pressure resulted in greater cardiovascular benefit and that there were no significant differences in total cardiovascular events between agents. JNC VII recommends thiazide-based regimens unless there are compelling indications for use of other drug classes (e.g., ACE inhibitors in impaired left ventricular function). Nonadherence to lifestyle and pharmacologic means of antihypertensive therapy is frequent. Reasons include medication costs, medication side effects, lack of patient education, and complexity of the medication regimen among others. Patients with resistant hypertension often benefit from the addition of a loop diuretic. (*Cecil, Ch. 63; JNC VII, 2003*)

121. (A)–True; (B)–True; (C)–False; (D)–False; (E)–True.
Discussion: It has been estimated that 50% of patients with sleep apnea have hypertension and 30% of hypertensive patients have sleep apnea. It is unclear whether this association is causal or a result of shared risk factors such as age and obesity, but BP often improves with treatment of the sleep apnea. Hypertension and diabetes frequently coexist. Patients with both disorders have a greatly increased cardiovascular risk compared with those who have either hypertension or diabetes. Older patients benefit more from treatment of hypertension than their younger counterparts, at least in the short term. Because older patients are more prone to side effects, BP medications should be started at a lower dose and titrated more slowly than in younger populations. Vigorous control of hypertension is particularly important in patients with renal insufficiency because poor control of BP will accelerate deterioration of renal function. Small rises in creatinine occur frequently as BP is lowered. Large persistent rises in creatinine may be clues to underlying renovascular disease. β-Blockers may precipitate bronchospasm in patients with a history of asthma. (*Cecil, Ch. 63; JNC VII, 2003*)

122. (A)–False; (B)–False; (C)–False; (D)–False; (E)–True.
Discussion: Severe hypertension in the absence of ongoing target organ damage does not require urgent therapy. Patients who have evidence of such target organ damage (funduscopic abnormalities, neurologic and cardiovascular symptoms, and evidence of renal deterioration) should be treated as a medical emergency. In patients with dissection, the goal is to lower BP and heart rate to

minimize shear forces. Hydralazine is contraindicated in this setting. The drugs of choice are β-blockers used in conjunction with sodium nitroprusside or trimethaphan. Intravenous labetalol is another excellent choice because of its combined α- and β-blocking properties. Diuretics are contraindicated in eclampsia. Use of β-blockers as monotherapy in patients with a cocaine overdose leads to unopposed α effects; β-blockers are thus contraindicated as monotherapy in this setting. β-Blockers can be used in conjunction with phentolamine. Labetalol is also a good choice. Although β-blockers have been shown convincingly to improve mortality in mild to severe chronic heart failure, their use is contraindicated in acute left ventricular dysfunction resulting from hypertensive crisis. (*Cecil, Ch. 63; JNC VII, 2003*)

123. (A)–True; (B)–True; (C)–False; (D)–False; (E)–True. *Discussion:* Repeated episodes of hypoxia in patients with sleep apnea may lead to pulmonary arteriolar vasoconstriction and pulmonary hypertension. Bronchiectasis may be associated with systemic-to-pulmonary artery shunts. Such shunts increase pulmonary blood flow and may lead to pulmonary hypertension. Primary pulmonary hypertension is due to pulmonary arteriolar constriction and obliteration. Pulmonary venous pressures are normal in this disease entity. Pulmonary hypertension in scleroderma is due to abnormalities in the pulmonary arteries, not to increased pulmonary blood flow. COPD causes loss of pulmonary parenchyma, hypoxia, and increased intrathoracic pressure, all of which contribute to pulmonary hypertension. (*Cecil, Ch. 64*)

124. A-F: All True. *Discussion:* This constellation of findings is known as the "Catch 22 syndrome." (*Cecil, Ch. 65*)

125. (A)–False; (B)–True; (C)–False; (D)–True; (E)–False. *Discussion:* The sinus venosus defect occurs in 2 to 3% of atrial septal defects and is frequently associated with anomalous pulmonary venous return. Cleft mitral valve is a feature of ostium primum defects. Atrial fibrillation and atrial flutter may be the presenting manifestation of a thus far undiagnosed atrial septal defect. Reverse shunting (Eisenmenger's disease) occurs in 5 to 10% of patients with uncorrected secundum atrial septal defects. Strokes can occur as a result of atrial arrhythmias or paradoxical embolism. The murmur is an ejection type murmur and is due to increased flow across the pulmonic valve. (*Cecil, Ch. 65; Roberts, 1987*)

126. (A)–False; (B)–True; (C)–True; (D)–True; (E)–False. *Discussion:* Vaginal delivery is the preferred mode of delivery in patients with congenital heart disease unless there are clear obstetric indications for cesarean section. Early ambulation and use of elastic stockings are essential measures to minimize the risk of postpartum thromboembolism. This is even more important in patients with a right-to-left shunt who are susceptible to paradoxical embolism. Oxygen administration may predispose to epistaxis as a result of drying of mucous membranes. The incidence of congenital heart disease in children born to mothers with congenital heart disease is significantly higher than in the general population. Patients with a secundum atrial septal defect are not at increased risk of endocarditis; antibiotic prophylaxis is not indicated. (*Cecil, Ch. 65*)

127. A-E: All True. *Discussion:* In patients with congenital complete heart block, vagal stimuli during surgery may significantly decrease heart rate. Those with slow heart rates at baseline, a wide QRS complex, inadequate responses to exercise, and a history of syncope are at increased risk of perioperative complications and should be paced perioperatively. Peripheral intravenous catheters can present a significant hazard in patients with cyanotic congenital heart disease because of the increased risk of paradoxical embolism. Systemic hypotension increases the right-to-left shunt in cyanotic congenital heart disease and may be fatal. Bleeding risk is increased in cyanotic congenital heart disease. Several congenital defects predispose to endocarditis. This consideration is particularly important in patients with a bicuspid aortic valve because this defect is the most common form of congenital heart disease among adults. (*Cecil, Ch. 65; Roberts, 1987*)

128. (A)–False; (B)–True; (C)–True; (D)–True; (E)–True. *Discussion:* Vulnerable plaques tend to be those with thinned fibrous caps, which may be the result of digestion by metalloproteinases. Inflammation, especially in the shoulder regions, is frequently seen. High cholesterol ester content is common. Location and angulation of the plaque as well as hemodynamic factors further determine vulnerability. (*Cecil, Ch. 66*)

129. (A)–True; (B)–True; (C)–True; (D)–True; (E)–False. *Discussion:* HDL promotes cholesterol efflux from atherosclerotic plaques and inhibits the oxidation of LDL particles. Small, dense LDL particles occur often in the setting of hypertriglyceridemia and are associated with increased cardiovascular risk. High-LDL cholesterol levels are not characteristic of the dyslipidemia of diabetes; patients with diabetes tend to have high triglycerides and low-HDL cholesterol. Glycation of lipoproteins may make them more susceptible to oxidation. Postprandial lipoprotein metabolism is often abnormal in patients with obesity, fasting hypertriglyceridemia, diabetes, and coronary artery disease. LDL cholesterol cannot be accurately calculated in patients with hypertriglyceridemia. Direct LDL cholesterol measurements are necessary in this setting. (*Cecil, Ch. 66*)

130. (A)–True; (B)–True; (C)–False; (D)–True; (E)–True. *Discussion:* Unstable angina is often caused by thrombus superimposed on a fixed obstruction. Prinzmetal's angina is due to vasospasm. Other forms of angina in patients with atherosclerotic coronary artery obstruction are due to increased demand, such as occurs with exercise, after meals, or with increased venous return. (*Cecil, Ch. 67*)

131. A-E: All True. *Discussion:* Atherosclerotic coronary artery disease is the most common reason for angina pectoris. Many other disorders can cause angina pectoris resulting from a mismatch of demand and supply, among them severe aortic stenosis, aortic insufficiency, hypertrophic cardiomyopathy, and syndrome X, a disorder of the myocardial resistance vessels. (*Cecil, Ch. 67*)

132. (A)–True; (B)–True; (C)–False; (D)–False; (E)–False. *Discussion:* Antiplatelet therapy decreases the risk of myocardial infarction, stroke, and vascular death. Aspirin irreversibly inhibits platelet cyclooxygenase while clopidogrel and ticlopidine inhibit the adenosine diphosphate receptors of platelets. Continuous nitrate therapy induces tachyphylaxis; a nitrate-free interval is thus recommended. β-Blocker therapy improves survival in patients with heart failure and is not contraindicated in individuals with angina and impaired ejection fraction. Angioplasty in single-vessel coronary disease is indicated for improvement in symptoms but has not been shown to improve mortality. (*Cecil, Ch. 67; Antithrombotic Trialists' Collaboration, 2002*)

133. (A)–True; (B)–True; (C)–True; (D)–False; (E)–False. *Discussion:* Silent myocardial infarction seems to be more common among women and the elderly. Routine prophylactic use of lidocaine has been associated with increased mortality in patients with acute myocardial infarction. In patients with a patent foramen ovale, increased right atrial pressures in the setting of right ventricular infarction may lead to right-to-left shunting and subsequent arterial hypoxemia. The right bundle branch is supplied by the left anterior descending coronary artery. Although complex ventricular ectopy in patients with a recent myocardial infarction is indicative of a poorer prognosis, the CAST trial has convincingly shown that antiarrhythmic therapy in this setting increases mortality. (*Cecil, Ch. 69; Echt et al, 1991*)

134. (A)–True; (B)–True; (C)–False; (D)–False; (E)–True.
Discussion: CABG compared with medical therapy improves survival in symptomatic and asymptomatic severe left main stenosis and in patients with three-vessel coronary artery disease and diminished ejection fraction. The impact of diabetes on the relative benefits of angioplasty and CABG remains controversial. In the BARI study, diabetic patients had a better outcome with CABG than with multivessel PTCA. Women have higher perioperative mortality than men but similar long-term benefit. Internal mammaries are the conduits of choice when available. Free arterial grafts are also increasingly used in preference to saphenous vein grafts. (*Cecil, Chs. 67, 70, and 71; BARI Investigators, 1996; Davis et al, 1995*)

135. (A)–True; (B)–True; (C)–True; (D)–True; (E)–False.
Discussion. All conditions in A are contraindications to transplantation because of limited post-transplant survival. Ischemic heart disease is the most common cause of heart failure in the United States and other developed countries and is thus also the most common reason for cardiac transplantation. Idiopathic dilated cardiomyopathy ranks second in the United States. Organ availability severely limits the number of cardiac transplantations. It is estimated that up to 30% of patients on cardiac transplant lists die before an organ can be procured. Both pravastatin and simvastatin have been shown to decrease cardiac allograft vasculopathy. Diltiazem increases cyclosporine levels and results in significant cost savings because cyclosporine doses can be reduced. (*Cecil, Ch. 80*)

136. (A)–True; (B)–True; (C)–True; (D)–True. *Discussion:* In the REMATCH trial, patients with severe heart failure randomized to a permanent left ventricular assist device (LVAD) had a 48% lower risk of death than those treated medically. Six different subtypes of long QT syndrome have been described; gene mutations responsible for subtypes 1 through 5 have been characterized. The mutations affect the sodium and potassium channels involved in repolarization. Signal averaged electrocardiogram abnormalities predict arrhythmic, cardiac, and total mortality in patients with coronary artery disease, left ventricular dysfunction, and nonsustained ventricular tachycardia. Fludrocortisone acts by expanding the total blood volume, and midodrine is a pure α-agonist that serves as a vasoconstrictor; both these agents are useful in patients with neurocardiogenic syncope. (*Cecil, Chs. 56, 59, and 60; Rose et al, 2001*)

137. (A)–True; (B)–True; (C)–True; (D)–False. *Discussion:* Ibutilide is a class III agent that is only available in intravenous form and is used for chemical cardioversion of atrial fibrillation and atrial flutter. It is associated with QTc prolongation, and its use is contraindicated in patients with baseline QTc longer than 440 msec. Hypokalemia and hypomagnesemia are associated with increased incidence of torsades, and, ideally, potassium concentration should be greater than 4.0 mEq/L and magnesium level greater than 2.0 mEq/L before ibutilide administration. Pretreatment with amiodarone may increase the conversion rate to sinus rhythm and is not a contraindication to ibutilide administration if the QTc interval is less than 440 msec. (*Cecil, Ch. 59*)

138. (A)–True; (B)–True; (C)–False; (D)–True; (E)–False; (F) False. *Discussion:* Acute coronary syndrome is characterized by nonocclusive thrombus in a coronary artery causing a continuum of ischemia ranging from unstable angina to non–ST segment elevation myocardial infarction. Unstable angina is described as new-onset, worsening angina or post–myocardial infarction angina and does not have to include a rise in cardiac markers. Elevated troponins lead to a diagnosis of non–ST segment elevation myocardial infarction and is a harbinger for worse short- and long-term prognosis. The CURE study showed a 20% reduction in the combined end point of cardiovascular death, nonfatal myocardial infarction, or stroke in ACS patients treated with clopidogrel in addition to standard therapy. GP IIb/IIIa inhibitors have been

shown to decrease mortality in patients who subsequently undergo percutaneous intervention and also in subgroups with elevated troponins or dynamic ST segment changes. Enoxaparin is superior to unfractionated heparin. (*Cecil, Ch. 68; Yusuf et al, 2003; Boersma et al, 2002*).

139. (A)–True; (B)–False; (C)–False; (D)–False; (E)–True.
Discussion: ST segment elevation myocardial infarction (STEMI) is caused by complete occlusion of blood flow to a particular area of the myocardium causing profound ischemia and eventually cell death. Cardiac enzymes are usually elevated in patients with STEMI, but at the initial presentation may be negative. A characteristic presentation with a supporting ECG is adequate to make the diagnosis because the enzymes do not rise for a few hours after myocardial infarction. Percutaneous intervention has been shown to be superior to thrombolytic therapy based on moderate-sized comparative studies, registry data, and indirect evidence. It has now become the standard of care in appropriately equipped hospitals. Half-dose thrombolytic therapy with GP IIb/IIIa inhibitors did not improve survival, although there was a reduction in the recurrent events at 6 months' duration. Low-molecular-weight heparin in combination with tenecteplase was more effective than tenecteplase combined with standard heparin or with a GP IIb/IIIa inhibitor plus heparin in STEMI. (*Keeley et al, 2003; Topol, 2001; ASSENT 3, 2001; Cecil, Ch. 69*).

140. (A)–True; (B)–True; (C)–True; (D)–False; (E)–True.
Discussion: Patients who are older than 75 years of age, diabetics and those with renal insufficiency have a worse prognosis compared with others. PTCA has not been shown to reduce death or myocardial infarction although there is a significant reduction in angina. For high-risk patients with acute coronary syndrome, early referral for cardiac catheterization and percutaneous angioplasty or CABG is recommended. Diabetics had a worse prognosis with PTCA compared with CABG in the BARI trial. In-stent restenosis is now the most significant long-term limitation of coronary angioplasty. Drug-eluting stents are associated with significantly lower restenosis rates. (*Cecil, Ch. 70*)

141. (E); 142. (C); 143. (B); 144. (A). *Discussion:* In primary pulmonary hypertension there is enlargement of the central pulmonary arteries with sudden tapering in the periphery, giving the appearance of a pruned tree. Pericardial calcification is sometimes seen in constrictive pericarditis and should be distinguished from intramyocardial calcification, which sometimes occurs in old myocardial infarcts. In severe aortic insufficiency, the left ventricle is dilated as a result of chronic volume overload. In contrast, in mitral stenosis, the left ventricle is small but there is marked enlargement of the left atrium and left atrial appendage. (*Cecil, Ch. 49; Steiner, 2001*)

145. (B); 146. (E); 147. (D); 148. (A). *Discussion:* The jugular venous pulse is best observed when the patient is positioned to allow observation of the venous column throughout the cardiac cycle. The A wave reflects right atrial contraction. The X descent reflects right atrial relaxation and continues with early right ventricular contraction. The V wave represents passive right atrial filling while the tricuspid valve is closed. The Y descent reflects tricuspid valve opening and right ventricular relaxation. Pulmonic valve opening is not reflected in the jugular venous pulsation. (*Cecil, Ch. 46; Bates, 1994*)

149. (A); 150. (C); 151. (C); 152. (D). *Discussion.* Digoxin diminishes the need for hospitalization in patients with heart failure resulting from systolic dysfunction but is not useful and may be detrimental in patients with diastolic dysfunction. β-Blockers improve survival in patients with systolic dysfunction and help control symptoms in patients with diastolic dysfunction by lowering BP and decreasing heart rate. The latter prolongs diastole and may improve left ventricular filling. ACE inhibitors improve survival in patients with symptomatic systolic left ventricular dysfunction and prevent progression to overt heart failure among patients with impaired left ventricular systolic function but minimal or no symptoms of heart failure. Their role in diastolic dysfunction is less well defined, but patients with hypertensive heart disease may benefit. Prazosin is not useful in either condition. (*Cecil, Ch. 56*)

153. (E); 154. (A); 155. (B); 156. (D). *Discussion:* Spironolactone may cause mastodynia, gynecomastia, and sexual dysfunction. Minoxidil may cause both pleural and pericardial effusions. Hydralazine frequently causes a positive antinuclear antibody test but only rarely causes a lupus-like syndrome at commonly used antihypertensive doses. Methyldopa may cause liver toxicity and rarely causes a Coombs-positive hemolytic anemia. Dry cough is a common side effect of ACE inhibitors. (*Cecil, Ch. 56*)

157. (A); 158. (C); 159. (B); 160. (D). *Discussion:* Pulmonary embolism is a form of precapillary pulmonary hypertension. Pulmonary venous pressure is normal in this entity. Mitral stenosis initially results in elevation of pulmonary venous pressure but when of long standing is often associated with pulmonary arteriolar vasoconstriction. Pulmonary hypertension resulting from pulmonary arteriolar vasoconstriction in mitral stenosis may not improve after mitral commissurotomy or mitral valve replacement. Acute pulmonary edema is due to acute increases in pulmonary venous pressure. Pulmonary atresia is characterized by diminished pulmonary blood flow and is thus not associated with pulmonary hypertension. (*Cecil, Chs. 64, 65, and 72*)

161. (B); 162. (D); 163. (A); 164. (C). *Discussion:* In the current era, many patients with cyanotic congenital heart disease undergo complete repair. In the past, patients with cyanotic congenital heart disease were treated with palliative shunts. A proportion has survived to adulthood and may present to general internists and adult cardiologists for ongoing care. Familiarity with the most commonly performed shunts is thus important for any internist. (*Cecil, Ch. 65; Roberts, 1987*)

165. (D); 166. (A); 167. (C); 168. (E). *Discussion:* Down syndrome is frequently associated with congenital cardiac anomalies. Endocardial cushion defects are most common. Marfan syndrome is a disorder of connective tissue and may be manifested by fusiform aortic aneurysms, aortic regurgitation, aortic dissection, or a floppy mitral valve. Maternal systemic lupus erythematosus is associated with complete heart block in the offspring. At times, the maternal lupus may not become symptomatic until years after the birth of an infant with congenital complete heart block. When mothers are infected with rubella during the first trimester, infants may be born with the congenital rubella syndrome. Patent ductus arteriosus is a characteristic congenital cardiac anomaly in this syndrome. (*Cecil, Ch. 65; Perloff, 1987*)

169. (C); 170. (D); 171. (A); 172. (B). *Discussion:* Based on age, gender, and presenting symptoms, the probability of coronary artery disease can be estimated. Such an estimate is very useful in determining further work-up and therapy. (*Cecil, Ch. 67; ACC/AHA Guidelines for Exercise Testing*)

173. (B); 174. (D); 175. (A); 176. (C). *Discussion:* An R/S ratio greater than 1 in V_1 and V_2 is indicative of a true posterior myocardial infarction. Occlusion of the left circumflex coronary artery is often electrocardiographically silent. ST segment elevation in V_{4R} is indicative of right ventricular myocardial infarction and suggests an occlusion proximal to the right ventricular branches of the right coronary artery. T wave inversion throughout the precordium should raise suspicion for a subtotal occlusion in the proximal left anterior descending coronary artery. (*Cecil, Ch. 69; Chou, 1991*)

177. (A); 178. (E); 179. (C); 180. (D). *Discussion:* Papillary muscle rupture causes acute mitral regurgitation with hypotension, elevated pulmonary capillary wedge pressure with a prominent V wave, and a new systolic murmur. The murmur may be very soft and difficult to appreciate, especially because most patients are quite tachycardic as well. Clinically, ventricular septal rupture and papillary muscle rupture are difficult to distinguish. Doppler echocardiography documenting the shunt or mitral regurgitation, respectively, or right-sided heart catheterization documenting oxygen step-up in the right ventricle or prominent V waves on the pulmonary capillary wedge pressure tracing are helpful in distinguishing the two diagnoses. Inferior myocardial infarctions with right ventricular involvement often present as significant hemodynamic compromise and AV conduction disturbances. Myocardial free wall rupture generally presents as cardiac arrest from which the patient cannot be resuscitated. Recurrent chest pain after myocardial infarction could be due to recurrent ischemia or pericarditis. (*Cecil, Ch. 69*)

181. (C); 182. (B); 183. (A); 184. (D). *Discussion:* Aortic stenosis produces a harsh crescendo-decrescendo systolic murmur along the left sternal border that radiates into the carotid arteries. Severe aortic stenosis is characterized by a late-peaking murmur and a soft aortic component of the second heart sound (A_2). Mitral regurgitation produces an apical blowing holosystolic murmur that radiates into the left axilla. Of the choices listed, aortic insufficiency is the only one that is associated with a diastolic murmur. It is blowing and heard best along the left sternal border. This murmur is often missed if the patient is examined only in the supine position. It can be heard best with the patient leaning forward at end expiration. This positions the aortic valve closer to the chest wall. Mitral valve prolapse produces a characteristic mid or late systolic murmur that is often preceded by a click. Although similar in quality to mitral regurgitation, it is not holosystolic because the valves are not regurgitant in early systole. (*Cecil, Chs. 46 and 72*)

185. (C); 186. (A); 187. (B); 188. (D). *Discussion:* The Valsalva maneuver increases intrathoracic pressure and reduces venous return to the heart. This produces a reduction in cardiac preload. The handgrip maneuver produces an increase in systolic BP, left ventricular end-systolic pressure, and end-diastolic pressure. It is important to instruct the patient not to perform the Valsalva maneuver while performing the handgrip maneuver because this can confuse the response of the murmur to the maneuver. Squatting from a standing position produces transient increases in venous return as a result of compression of lower extremity musculature. An increase in systemic vascular resistance and afterload is then produced by compression of the leg arteries. Standing from a squatting position produces a reduction in venous return as a result of venous pooling in the legs and in systemic vascular resistance. (*Cecil, Ch. 46*)

189. (B); 190. (A); 191. (A); 192. (B). *Discussion:* Working cells of the atria and ventricles have a fast response action potential with a rapidly rising phase 0 mediated by an inward sodium current. Phases 1, 2, and 3 are distinctly seen. Pacemaker cells of the sinus and AV node exhibit a slow response and are mediated by an inward calcium current. Unlike myocardial cells that have a stable resting membrane potential, pacemaker cells exhibit spontaneous diastolic depolarization. (*Cecil, Ch. 57*)

193. (D); 194. (B); 195. (A); 196. (B). *Discussion:* Patients with PSVT refractory to medical therapy should be referred for a catheter ablation procedure. The second patient most likely has PSVT. A transtelephonic event recorder that is worn for 30 days is the most effective method of demonstrating the presence of an arrhythmia. Because his symptoms occur infrequently, a Holter monitor would not be likely to demonstrate the cause. In the third patient, a

bradyarrhythmia is the most likely cause. Because symptoms occur several times per day, a Holter monitor would be useful to rule out an arrhythmia as the cause of symptoms. The last patient's symptoms are compatible with vasovagal syncope. A tilt table test is appropriate in the initial diagnostic evaluation. (*Cecil, Chs. 58 and 61*)

197. **(C)**; 198. **(B)**; 199. **(A)**; 200. **(D)**. *Discussion:* Typical atrial flutter is characterized by the absence of an isoelectric interval in the inferior leads and a sawtooth appearance of the flutter waves. The atrial flutter cycle length is typically 200 msec or 300 beats/minute. Because 2:1 conduction commonly occurs at this rate, this tachycardia is usually 150 beats/minute. Because atrial and ventricular activation are simultaneous, P waves are rarely seen during atrioventricular nodal re-entrant tachycardia. Retrograde atrial activation over the accessory pathway is slightly delayed, so that it appears 40 to 80 msec after the QRS complex, usually within the ST segment. A regular, wide complex tachycardia is ventricular tachycardia in the vast majority of cases and should be treated as such until proven otherwise. (*Cecil, Chs. 50 and 59*)

201. **(B)**; 202. **(C)**; 203. **(A)**. *Discussion:* Accessory pathways are myocardial bridges from the atrium to the ventricle. They are ablated along the annulus of the mitral or tricuspid valve. The slow pathway is ablated in the posterior right atrial septum at the base of Koch's triangle, which is formed by the tendon of Todaro, the septal insertion of the tricuspid valve, and the coronary sinus. The atrial flutter circuit revolves around the tricuspid annulus and is ablated in its narrowest portion between the inferior vena cava and the tricuspid annulus. (*Cecil, Ch. 61*)

204. **(C)**; 205. **(B)**; 206. **(A)**; 207. **(D)**. *Discussion:* Cardiac magnetic resonance imaging is very sensitive and specific for the diagnosis of acute aortic dissection but is not widely available. In addition, it may not be the optimal imaging modality for patients who are unstable and need close hemodynamic monitoring. Aortic angiography is invasive and cannot determine the presence of a pericardial effusion. It is useful in determining whether the dissection involves the coronary arteries or whether concomitant coronary artery disease is present. Transesophageal echocardiography may be the most widely used modality for the diagnosis of dissection because it is noninvasive and can be performed at the bedside in the intensive care unit. In addition, valvular and pericardial involvement can be readily determined. Computed tomography is also widely available and very specific but cannot determine whether valvular insufficiency is present or whether the coronary arteries are involved. (*Cecil, Chs. 51, 53, 54, and 75*)

BIBLIOGRAPHY

Practice guidelines and position statements on cardiovascular disease topics can be accessed at American College of Cardiology: http://www.acc.org/clinical/statements.htm
American Heart Association: http://americanheart.org/presenter.jhtml?identifier=2158
Heart Failure Society of America: http://www.hfsa.org/hf_guidelines.asp

American Heart Association Statistical Fact Sheet: Populations. Dallas, TX, American Heart Association, 2003.

American Heart Association: Heart Disease and Stroke Statistics—2003 Update. Dallas, TX, American Heart Association, 2002.

Anti-thrombotic Trialists' Collaboration: Collaborative meta-analysis of randomised trials of antiplatelet therapy for prevention of death, myocardial infarction, and stroke in high risk patients. BMJ 2002;324:71-86. Erratum in BMJ 2002;324:141.

Antiarrhythmics versus Implantable Defibrillators (AVID) Investigators: A comparison of antiarrhythmic-drug therapy with implantable defibrillators in patient resuscitated from near fatal arrhythmias. N Engl J Med 2000;337:1576.

ASSENT-3: Efficacy and safety of tenecteplase in combination with enoxaparin, abciximab, or unfractionated heparin: The ASSENT 3 randomised trial in acute myocardial infarction. Lancet 2001;358:605-613.

Bates B: The cardiovascular system. In A Guide to Physical Examination and History Taking, 6th ed. Philadelphia, JB Lippincott, 1994.

Blood Pressure Lowering Treatment Trialists' Collaboration: Effects of different blood-pressure-lowering regimens on major cardiovascular events: Results of prospectively-designed overviews of randomized trials. Lancet 2003;362:1527-1535.

Boersma E, Harrington RA, Moliterno DJ, et al: Platelet glycoprotein IIb/IIIa inhibitors in acute coronary syndromes: A meta-analysis of all major randomized clinical trials. Lancet 2002;359:189-198.

Braunwald E, Zipes D, Libby P (eds.): Heart Disease, A Textbook of Cardiovascular Medicine, 6th ed. Philadelphia, WB Saunders, 2001.

Chou TC: Electrocardiography in Clinical Practice, 3rd ed. Philadelphia, WB Saunders, 1991.

Comparison of coronary bypass surgery with angioplasty in patients with multivessel disease. The Bypass Angioplasty Revascularization Investigation (BARI) investigators. N Engl J Med 1996;335:217.

CONSENSUS Trial Study Group: Effects of enalapril on mortality in severe congestive heart failure. Results of the Cooperative North Scandinavian Enalapril Survival Study (CONSENSUS). N Engl J Med 1987;316:1429-1435.

Davis KB, Chatiman B, Ryan T, et al: Comparison of 15-year survival for men and women after initial medical or surgical treatment for coronary artery disease: A CASS Registry Study. J Am Coll Cardiol 1995;25:1000.

Echt DS, Kiebson PR, Mitchell LB, et al: Mortality and morbidity in patients receiving encainide, flecainide, or placebo. The Cardiac Arrhythmia Suppression Trial. N Engl J Med 1991;324:781.

Ewy GA: The abdominojugular test: Technique and hemodynamic correlates. Ann Intern Med 1988;109:456.

Goldman L, Ausiello D (eds): Cecil Textbook of Medicine, 22nd ed. Philadelphia, WB Saunders, 2004.

Grim CM, Grim CE: Blood pressure measurement. In Izzo JL, Black HR (eds): Hypertension Primer, 3rd ed. Dallas, TX, American Heart Association, 2003.

Keeley EC, Boura JA, Grines CL: Primary angioplasty versus intravenous thrombolytic therapy for acute myocardial infarction: A quantitative review of 23 randomised trials. Lancet 2003;361:13-20.

Matsuda M, Matsuda Y, Yamagishi T, et al: Effects of digoxin, propranolol, and verapamil on exercise in patients with chronic isolated atrial fibrillation. Cardiovasc Res 1991;25:453.

MERIT-HF Study Group: Effect of metoprolol CR/XL in chronic heart failure: Metoprolol CR/XL Randomized Intervention Trial in Congestive Heart Failure (MERIT-HF). Lancet 1999;353:2001-2007.

Moss AJ, Hall WJ, Cannon DS, et al: Improved survival with an implantable defibrillator in patients with coronary artery disease at high risk for ventricular arrhythmia. N Engl J Med 1996;335:1933.

Moss AJ, Zareba W, Hall WJ, et al: Prophylactic implantation of a defibrillator in patients with myocardial infarction and reduced ejection fraction. N Engl J Med 2002;346:877.

National Cholesterol Education Program: Third Report of the Expert Panel on Detection, Evaluation, and Treatment of High Blood Cholesterol in Adults (Adult Treatment Panel III) (NIH publication No. 02-5215). Washington, DC, National Institutes of Health, 2002.

Packer M, Bristow MR, Cohn JN, et al: The effect of carvedilol on morbidity and mortality in patients with chronic heart failure. N Engl J Med 1996;334:1349-1355.

Packer M, Coats AJ, Fowler MB, et al: Effect of carvedilol on survival in severe chronic heart failure. N Engl J Med 2001;344:1651-1658.

Perloff JK: The Clinical Recognition of Congenital Heart Disease, 3rd ed. Philadelphia, WB Saunders, 1987.

Philippon F, Plumb VJ, Epstein AE, Kay GN: The risk of atrial fibrillation following radiofrequency catheter ablation of atrial flutter. Circulation 1995;92:430.

Pitt B, Zannad F, Remme WJ, et al: The effect of spironolactone on morbidity and mortality in patients with severe heart failure. Randomized Aldactone Evaluation Study Investigators. N Engl J Med 1999;341:709-717.

Rich S: Clinical insights into the pathogenesis of primary pulmonary hypertension. Chest 1998;114(3, Suppl.):237S.

Roberts WC: Adult Congenital Heart Disease. Philadelphia, FA Davis, 1987.

Rose EA, Gelijins AC, Moskowitz AJ, et al: Randomized Evaluation of Mechanical Assistance for the Treatment of Congestive Heart Failure (REMATCH) Study Group. Long-term mechanical left ventricular assistance for end-stage heart failure. N Engl J Med 2001;345: 1435-1443.

SOLVD Investigators: Effect of enalapril on mortality and the development of heart failure in asymptomatic patients with reduced left ventricular ejection fractions. N Engl J Med 1992;327:685.

SOLVD Investigators: Effect on enalapril on survival in patients with reduced left ventricular ejection fractions and congestive heart failure. N Engl J Med 1991;325:293.

Steiner RM: Radiology of the heart. *In* Braunwald E (ed): Heart Disease. A Textbook of Cardiovascular Medicine. Philadelphia, WB Saunders, 2001.

The 7th Report of the Joint National Committee on Prevention, Detection, and Treatment of High Blood Pressure (JNC VII). NIH publication 03-5233. Bethesda, MD, National Institutes of Health, 2003.

Topol EJ: Reperfusion therapy for acute myocardial infarction with fibrinolytic therapy or combination reduced fibrinolytic therapy and platelet glycoprotein IIb/IIIa inhibition: The GUSTO V randomized trial. Lancet 2001;357:1905-1914.

Yusuf S, Mehta SR, Zhao F, et al. on behalf of the CURE (Clopidogrel in Unstable angina to prevent Recurrent Events) Trial Investigators: Early and late effects of clopidogrel in patients with acute coronary syndromes. Circulation 2003;107:966-972.

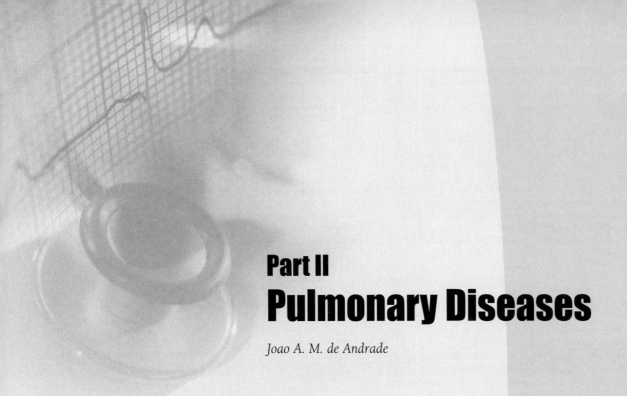

Part II
Pulmonary Diseases

Joao A. M. de Andrade

MULTIPLE CHOICE

DIRECTIONS: For questions 1–70, choose the single best answer to each question.

1. A 32-year-old patient was found to have a large, free-layering, transudative pleural effusion at the right hemithorax. All of the following are expected findings on physical examination *except:*

   A. Absent or decreased breath sounds at the right hemithorax
   B. Increased vocal fremitus at the right hemithorax
   C. Lag on chest wall motion at right hemithorax
   D. Normal percussion at left hemithorax
   E. Normal breath sounds at left hemithorax

2. A 19-year-old patient with known diagnosis of asthma presents to your office complaining of more frequent episodes of wheezing and shortness of breath. He is experiencing symptoms about three times per week and during the last month woke up three nights with dyspnea, which improved after using a short-acting inhaled β2-agonist. Which of the following is the best approach to this patient's therapy?

   A. Increase frequency of β2-agonist inhalation
   B. Start theophylline, combined with nedocromil
   C. Start low-dose inhaled corticosteroid
   D. Start combination of cromolyn and leukotriene receptor antagonist
   E. Start long-acting β2-agonist

3. The following are expected physiologic changes that may occur in the airways during an acute asthma exacerbation *except:*

   A. Tachypnea is present and is the result of stimulation of intrapulmonary receptors.
   B. Hypoxemia occurs due to shift to lower $\dot{V}/\dot{Q}$ ratio at a larger number of alveolar capillary units.
   C. Work load of ventilatory muscles is increased.
   D. The pleural pressure at inspiration becomes more positive.
   E. Resistance to airflow is increased.

4. A 24-year-old white male with a history of recurrent respiratory tract infections and infertility presented complaining of chronic productive cough. A high resolution CT of the chest showed widespread bronchiectasis, with pulmonary function tests showing airflow obstruction. Considering the most likely diagnosis, the following statements about this condition are correct *except:*

   A. Meconium ileus suggests the diagnosis in a newborn.
   B. It is an autosomal recessive genetic disease and the most common mutation is a 3 base-pair deletion that causes the loss of a phenylalanine at position 508.
   C. A sweat chloride level more than 60 mEq/L associated with typical clinical manifestations suggests the diagnosis.
   D. Pancreatic insufficiency and progressive malnutrition accounts for over 90% of the mortality related to this disease.
   E. Colonization and severe infection with *Pseudomonas aeruginosa* are very frequent in more advanced stages.

5. A 65-year-old man who was a former foundry worker presented with progressive dyspnea and chronic cough. Pulmonary function testing shows a restrictive pattern and the chest x-ray film showed bi-apical micronodular infiltrates with calcified hilar adenopathy. Considering the most likely diagnosis, the following statements about this condition are correct *except:*

A. It is a granulomatous disease that results from inhaling silica particles and susceptibility to it may be linked to the HLA-DP B1.

B. Patient is at increased risk of mycobacterial infections and should receive yearly tuberculin skin testing.

C. Supportive therapy, oxygen, and rehabilitation are the main forms of therapy.

D. Massive inhalation may cause acute form characterized by alveolar filling with proteinaceous material.

E. The risk of developing disease increases with the level and duration of exposure.

6. Which of the following treatments has been shown to alter the course of chronic obstructive pulmonary disease (COPD)?

A. Long-acting inhaled β_2-agonists

B. Theophylline

C. Pulmonary rehabilitation program

D. Smoking cessation

E. Pneumococcal vaccine

7. A 75-year-old man with a history of severe COPD on home oxygen presents to the emergency department with a 3-day history of worsening dyspnea and productive cough with purulent sputum. He has never required admission to an intensive care due to COPD before. Initial evaluation reveals an elderly gentleman in moderate to severe respiratory distress not able to speak in full sentences and slightly obtunded. Lungs had decreased breath sounds with occasional expiratory wheezing. Initial arterial blood gas analysis is as follows: pH, 7.25; $PaCO_2$, 70; and PaO_2, 50. Chest radiograph shows hyperinflation without infiltrates or pneumothorax. Treatment with oxygen (Venturi mask with FIO_2 of 0.50), bronchodilators, antibiotics, and corticosteroids is started. After 1 hour, on follow up, he is more obtunded and the arterial blood gas now shows a pH of 7.15, $PaCO_2$ of 100, and PaO_2 of 70. Which of the following is the *best* course of action at this time?

A. Increase frequency of nebulized β_2-agonists and increase dose of intravenous corticosteroids

B. Decrease FIO_2 because of worsening CO_2 retention

C. Intubation and mechanical ventilation

D. Obtain a spiral CT angiography to rule out pulmonary embolism

E. Obtain an echocardiogram and serum levels of B-type natriuretic pepetide (BNP) because the patient may have concomitant congestive heart failure

8. All of the following tests may be indicated in the investigation of a patient presenting with diffuse bronchiectasis *except:*

A. High resolution CT of chest

B. Swallowing study by speech pathologist to rule out aspiration

C. Serum precipitating antibodies

D. Serum quantitative immunoglobulins

E. Sweat chloride concentration

9. The following interstitial lung diseases may present as preserved lung volumes or even hyperinflation on chest radiograph and a pattern of airflow obstruction on pulmonary function test *except:*

A. Idiopathic pulmonary fibrosis

B. Sarcoidosis

C. Histiocytosis X

D. Lymphangioleiomyomatosis

E. Tuberous sclerosis

10. The following statements about amiodarone-induced pulmonary toxicity are correct *except:*

A. The most common presentation includes development of insidious dyspnea, cough, fever, and malaise, along with weight loss.

B. Doses greater than 400 mg/day increase the risk of pulmonary toxicity, which may respond to corticosteroids.

C. The majority of patients will have a reduction in the diffusion capacity (DLCO) of over 15%.

D. Pleuritic chest pain occurs in a minority of patients.

E. The presence of phospholipid-laden inclusions within lung parenchymal cells and alveolar macrophages are diagnostic findings of pulmonary toxicity in a lung biopsy specimen.

11. The following statements about carbon monoxide poisoning are correct *except:*

A. Nonsmoking individuals will usually present symptoms with carboxyhemoglobin (HbCO) levels above 10%.

B. Loss of consciousness may be a risk factor for prolonged neurologic problems such as memory loss and difficulty concentrating.

C. Use of hyperbaric oxygen is recommended whenever the HbCO level is above 15%.

D. Hyperbaric oxygen therapy may avoid neurologic symptoms in more severe cases if started within 6 hours of the intoxication.

E. The severity of the clinical illness usually correlates better with the duration of exposure than with the HbCO level.

12. A 35-year-old man with known HIV infection presents with induration of 7 mm to a tuberculin skin test using 5 tuberculin units of PPD. Chest radiograph is normal. Patient is on HAART (antiretroviral therapy) and is asymptomatic. Which of the options below describe what you should do next?

A. No therapy is warranted at this time because PPD induration is less than 10 mm.

B. Check three samples of sputum for acid-fast bacilli and, until cultures are available, start anti-tuberculosis therapy.

C. Start isoniazid for 12 months.

D. Start isoniazid and rifampin for 9 months.

E. Repeat PPD test in 2 weeks and start prophylactic therapy if induration is more than 15 mm.

13. The following statements about bronchogenic carcinoma are correct *except:*

A. It is the leading cause of death from cancer in the United States in both men and women.

B. Cigarette smokers have a 10- to 25-fold increased risk of developing lung cancer.

C. The preferred therapy for stage I non–small cell bronchogenic carcinoma is combination chemotherapy.

D. The syndrome of inappropriate secretion of ADH may complicate cases of small cell bronchogenic carcinoma.

E. Adenocarcinoma is the most prevalent histologic type and tends to be located in the periphery of the lung.

14. A 35-year-old white woman presents with recurrent low-grade fever and diffuse arthralgias. On physical examination, raised, red, tender and nodular subcutaneous lesions are noted in the anterior surface of her legs. A chest x-ray film showed bilateral adenopathy. There were no infiltrates. Considering the most likely diagnosis, the following statements about this condition are correct *except:*

    A. It is a form of granulomatous inflammation and usually the skin biopsy of the nodular lesions described will yield the diagnosis in the majority of cases.
    B. The constellation of symptoms or signs described is usually associated with good prognosis and spontaneous resolution.
    C. In the United States it is a condition that affects predominantly people of African background.
    D. The presence of persistent hypercalcemia is an indication for treatment with corticosteroids.
    E. In the presence of lung parenchymal involvement, pulmonary function tests often will have a restrictive pattern.

15. The following conditions are associated with increased risk for lung abscess *except:*

    A. Cerebrovascular accident complicated by dysphagia
    B. Seizure disorder
    C. Binge drinking
    D. Use of inhaled corticosteroids
    E. General anesthesia

16. The following pulmonary manifestations may be seen associated with rheumatoid arthritis *except:*

    A. Interstitial lung disease
    B. Diaphragmatic dysfunction
    C. Pleural effusion
    D. Bronchiolitis obliterans with organizing pneumonia (BOOP)
    E. Cricoarytenoid dysfunction with airway obstruction

17. A 70-year-old gentleman presents with sudden onset of dyspnea and tachycardia. He just came back from a trip to Europe the day before starting with symptoms, and he was on an airplane for about 12 hours. On physical examination, he is somewhat anxious and in mild respiratory distress; his blood pressure is 145/84 mm Hg. The electrocardiogram shows sinus tachycardia and signs of right ventricle strain. Chest radiograph was unremarkable. ABG analysis showed mild hypoxemia and respiratory alkalosis. A ventilation/perfusion scan of his lungs showed large, unmatched perfusion defect in the right lower lobe. All of the following would be appropriate therapies for this patient *except:*

    A. Oxygen therapy to maintain hemoglobin saturation above 90%
    B. Unfractionated heparin, IV bolus of 5000 units followed by maintenance dose to maintain aPTT of 1.5 to 2.0 times control values
    C. Placement of inferior vena cava filter if patient has recurrent episode while appropriately anticoagulated
    D. Tissue-type plasminogen activator, 100 mg IV over 2 hours, followed by maintenance dose of intravenous unfractionated heparin
    E. Enoxaparin, 1.0 mg/kg subcutaneously every 12 hours

18. The following diseases typically will present as pleural effusion with low glucose levels (<60 mg/dL) *except:*

    A. Empyema secondary to *Streptococcus pneumoniae* infection
    B. Rheumatoid arthritis pleurisy
    C. Esophageal rupture

    D. Systemic lupus erythematosus effusion
    E. Chylothorax secondary to non-Hodgkin's lymphoma

19. The following statements about idiopathic pulmonary fibrosis (IPF) are correct *except:*

    A. A surgical lung biopsy will show a pattern of "usual interstitial pneumonia."
    B. The majority of cases will have a favorable response to corticosteroids and azathioprine.
    C. Mortality is about 50% within 3 to 5 years of diagnosis.
    D. Chest radiograph will have reticular infiltrates that predominate at the bases.
    E. Pulmonary function tests will typically show a restrictive pattern.

20. The following are causes of posterior mediastinal masses *except:*

    A. Bochdalek hernia of diaphragm
    B. Enteric cysts
    C. Esophageal cancer
    D. Thymoma
    E. Neurogenic tumors

21. All of the following conditions or drugs decrease theophylline clearance, resulting in increased serum levels of this drug *except:*

    A. Cimetidine
    B. Cirrhosis
    C. Allopurinol
    D. Rifampin
    E. Erythromycin

22. All of the following are risk factors for the development of asthma *except:*

    A. Birth prematurity
    B. Lower socioeconomic status
    C. Maternal cigarette smoking
    D. Females older than age 40 years
    E. Child born to mother older than age 40 years

23. All of the following diseases are associated with cigarette abuse *except:*

    A. Lung cancer
    B. Goodpasture's syndrome
    C. Emphysema
    D. Sarcoidosis
    E. Eosinophilic granuloma of the lung

24. All of the following conditions generally occur only after a latent period of more than 15 years after asbestos exposure *except:*

    A. Benign pleural effusion
    B. Pulmonary fibrosis
    C. Pleural plaques
    D. Mesothelioma
    E. Bronchogenic carcinoma

25. The following statements are true about pulmonary thromboembolism or deep vein thrombosis (DVT) *except:*

    A. Ventilation-perfusion lung scan showing two or more segmental perfusion defects without corresponding ventilation defect is more than 90% specific for the diagnosis of pulmonary embolism.
    B. Left ventricular dysfunction predisposes to pulmonary infarction.
    C. Massive pulmonary embolism with hemodynamic alterations is an indication for fibrinolytic agents.

D. Nephrotic syndrome is a risk factor for DVT and pulmonary thromboembolism.

E. Hemoptysis is a contraindication to heparin anticoagulation of patients with pulmonary embolism.

26. All of the following are proteinase inhibitors present in the lung parenchyma *except:*

A. Glutathione
B. α_1-Antiprotease inhibitor (α_1-antitrypsin)
C. Secretory leukoprotease inhibitor (SLPI)
D. α_2-Macroglobulin
E. Cystatin C

27. Use of carbon monoxide to measure lung diffusion is optimal because of all of the following characteristics of this gas *except:*

A. Carbon monoxide is diffusion limited.
B. Carbon monoxide distribution is not affected by lung volume.
C. Hemoglobin avidly binds carbon monoxide.
D. There is little capillary blood partial pressure for carbon monoxide in normal individuals.
E. Carbon monoxide can be easily produced and is stable for use.

28. All of the following contribute to the diagnosis of allergic bronchopulmonary aspergillosis *except:*

A. Elevated serum immunoglobulin E level
B. Underlying asthma
C. Positive serum precipitins for *Aspergillus*
D. Positive delayed hypersensitivity skin tests to *Aspergillus* antigens
E. Central bronchiectasis

29. All of the following systemic disorders are associated with pulmonary fibrosis *except:*

A. Diabetes mellitus
B. Scleroderma
C. Ankylosing spondylitis
D. Hermansky-Pudlak syndrome
E. Neurofibromatosis

30. Characteristics of patients with rheumatoid arthritis that increase risk for pulmonary disease include all of the following *except:*

A. High rheumatoid factor titer
B. Subcutaneous nodules
C. Male gender
D. Severe erosive arthritis
E. History of tobacco abuse

31. All of the following have been associated with occupational asthma *except:*

A. Rat urinary protein
B. Latex
C. Aluminum fluxes
D. Flour dust
E. Asbestos

32. All of the following symptoms are associated with obstructive sleep apnea *except:*

A. Loud snoring
B. Nocturia
C. Morning headaches
D. Dyspepsia
E. Tinnitus

33. All of the following molecules are secreted by T helper type 1 (Th1) lymphocytes *except:*

A. Interleukin-5
B. Interleukin-2
C. Interferon
D. Transforming growth factor-β_1 (TGF-β_1)
E. Granulocyte-macrophage colony-stimulating factor (GM-CSF)

34. A 24-year-old man presents with symptoms of cough and intermittent shortness of breath. He works as a spray painter and has had no significant prior illnesses. He does not smoke. Chest radiograph is normal. Spirogram shows normal FEV_1 and forced vital capacity. Which one of the following tests would most likely demonstrate a reason for his symptoms?

A. High-resolution CT scan
B. Methacholine challenge test
C. Persantine-thallium scan
D. Echocardiogram
E. Ventilation-perfusion lung scan

35. A 54-year-old woman presents with symptoms of intermittent shortness of breath and wheezing. Examination reveals inspiratory and expiratory wheezes primarily auscultated over the neck. Which one of the following tests or procedures should be performed *first* in the evaluation of the patient?

A. Spirogram with flow-volume loop
B. Bronchoscopy
C. CT of the neck
D. Transtracheal aspiration
E. Ventilation-perfusion lung scan

36. Which one of the following organisms most commonly causes postinfluenza bacterial pneumonia?

A. *Streptococcus pneumoniae*
B. *Staphylococcus aureus*
C. *Pseudomonas aeruginosa*
D. *Haemophilus influenzae*
E. *Pneumocystis carinii*

37. Which one of the following pulmonary conditions is associated with pulmonary lymphangioleiomyomatosis?

A. Chylous pleural effusion
B. Bronchogenic carcinoma
C. Diaphragmatic paralysis
D. Bronchial hyperreactivity to methacholine
E. Mesothelioma

38. Which one of the following medications should be initial therapy for a symptomatic patient with COPD resulting from tobacco abuse?

A. Theophylline
B. Ipratropium by inhalation
C. Prednisone
D. Salmeterol by inhalation
E. Spironolactone (Aldactone)

39. Which one of the following statements is *true* regarding exercise-induced asthma?

A. Bronchodilation often occurs at the start of exercise.
B. Mast cell–originating mediators are not involved in the process.
C. High humidity exacerbates the syndrome.
D. Inhaled lidocaine is the most effective treatment.
E. Approximately 10% of asthmatics have increased bronchospasm with exercise.

40. What is the *most* appropriate treatment for pulmonary alveolar proteinosis?

    A. Cyclophosphamide
    B. Prednisone
    C. Trimethoprim-sulfamethoxazole
    D. Lung lavage
    E. Lung resection

41. Which one of the following patients with DVT should have an inferior vena caval filter placed?

    A. A 76-year-old man with severe obstructive pulmonary disease, requiring home oxygen, and a large pelvic vein thrombus
    B. A 45-year-old man in whom recurrent pulmonary thromboemboli (PTEs) develop while he is treated with warfarin (Coumadin) (international normalized ratio [INR] on admission, 1.3)
    C. A 27-year-old 28-week pregnant woman with a femoral vein thrombus
    D. A patient on Coumadin for DVT with pulmonary embolus who has guaiac-positive stools
    E. A patient with a large pelvic vein thrombus and pulmonary embolism who has blood-streaked sputum

42. All of the following factors are associated with increased risk of pulmonary damage resulting from bleomycin administration *except:*

    A. Age of patient
    B. Cumulative dose of drug
    C. History of tobacco abuse
    D. Concurrent radiation therapy to the lung
    E. Administration of bleomycin with other chemotherapeutic agents

43. Which one of the following is the most definitive therapy for obstructive sleep apnea?

    A. Tracheostomy
    B. Nasal continuous positive airway pressure (CPAP)
    C. Weight reduction
    D. Uvulopalatopharyngoplasty (UPPP)
    E. Tricyclic antidepressants

44. Which one of the following serum enzymes may be elevated in pneumonia caused by *Pneumocystis carinii?*

    A. γ-Glutamyltransferase
    B. Alkaline phosphatase
    C. Lactate dehydrogenase (LDH)
    D. Amylase
    E. Elastase

45. A 48-year-old woman presents with a history of nonproductive cough that has been present for 3 months. Which one of the following elements of the patient's history would be important to determine?

    A. The patient often awakens with a bitter taste in her mouth.
    B. The patient is taking nifedipine for treatment of hypertension.
    C. The patient works as a secretary.
    D. The patient has no dyspnea at rest.
    E. The patient has had a similar cough in the past.

46. All of the following syndromes can be a manifestation of methotrexate pulmonary toxicity *except:*

    A. Noncardiogenic pulmonary edema
    B. Pulmonary fibrosis
    C. Pleural effusion
    D. Bronchospasm
    E. Hypersensitivity pneumonitis

47. A 70-year-old man presents with a lobar pneumonia on chest radiograph. Sputum Gram stain shows kidney-shaped gram-negative diplococci. What is the *most* likely pathogen?

    A. *Moraxella catarrhalis*
    B. *Neisseria gonorrhoeae*
    C. *Haemophilus influenzae*
    D. *Yersinia enterocolitica*
    E. *Streptococcus pneumoniae*

48. Which one of the following cytokines is a powerful eosinophil chemoattractant that is *most* likely involved in the pathogenesis of asthma?

    A. Interleukin-6
    B. Tumor necrosis factor-α
    C. Transforming growth factor-β
    D. Interleukin-5
    E. Interferon-α

49. All of the following are causes of hemoptysis *except:*

    A. Bronchitis resulting from tobacco abuse
    B. Asthma
    C. Pulmonary tuberculosis
    D. Mitral stenosis
    E. Bronchiectasis

50. All of the following cause digital clubbing *except:*

    A. Idiopathic pulmonary fibrosis
    B. Bronchiectasis
    C. Wegener's granulomatosis
    D. Crohn's disease
    E. Bronchogenic carcinoma

51. All of the following statements are true about community-acquired pneumonia (CAP) *except:*

    A. Most cases of CAP result from aspiration of oropharyngeal secretions.
    B. Influenza virus infection predisposes to CAP partially through effects on respiratory epithelium.
    C. The presence of hemolytic anemia and pneumonia in a young person suggests *Mycoplasma pneumoniae* is the causative agent.
    D. Proven methods for reducing CAP occurrence are immunization with pneumococcal and influenza vaccines.
    E. CAP resulting from *S. pneumoniae* is associated with a positive sputum culture for the organism in more than 50% of cases.

52. All of the following can cause a reduction in diffusing capacity (DLco) without other pulmonary function abnormality *except:*

    A. Chronic PTE
    B. Primary pulmonary hypertension
    C. Scleroderma
    D. Bleomycin administration
    E. Lobectomy

53. All of the following are manifestations of fat embolism syndrome *except:*

    A. Pleural effusion
    B. Diffuse alveolar infiltrates on chest radiograph
    C. Petechiae over upper half of body
    D. Retinal blood vessels showing fatty droplets
    E. Confusion

54. All of the following physical findings have been associated with sarcoidosis *except:*

    A. Cranial nerve palsy
    B. Angina
    C. Erythema nodosum
    D. Uveitis
    E. Digital clubbing

55. Each of the following has been associated with an increased risk of bronchogenic carcinoma *except:*

    A. Passive smoke exposure
    B. Asbestos exposure
    C. Chronic obstructive pulmonary disease
    D. Diet low in vitamin A
    E. Air pollution

56. Which of the following are *true* about patients with obstructive sleep apnea?

    A. Female patients outnumber male patients.
    B. Patients with the problem commonly awaken at night and have difficulty returning to sleep.
    C. Mean age at onset is 40 to 50 years.
    D. The majority of patients will improve with weight reduction.
    E. All of the above

57. Which of the following disorders are associated with obstructive sleep apnea?

    A. Hypothyroidism
    B. Acromegaly
    C. Down syndrome
    D. Chronic obstructive pulmonary disease
    E. All of the above

58. Nocturnal symptoms of obstructive sleep apnea include which of the following?

    A. Snoring
    B. Somnambulism
    C. Gastroesophageal reflux
    D. Enuresis
    E. All of the above

59. Which of the following manifestations are contraindications to resection of a bronchogenic carcinoma?

    A. Hypercalcemia
    B. Pleural effusion
    C. Mediastinal adenopathy on CT scan
    D. Histologically documented hepatic metastases
    E. All of the above

60. Which of the following is an indication for chest tube placement and drainage of a parapneumonic pleural effusion?

    A. pH < 7.10
    B. Positive pleural fluid Gram's stain
    C. Lactate dehydrogenase (LDH) level >1000 units/mL
    D. Glucose ratio < 0.5
    E. All of the above

61. Which of the following factors help define asthma?

    A. Low diffusing capacity for carbon monoxide
    B. Airway hyperreactivity to methacholine
    C. Proximal bronchiectasis
    D. Eosinophilia
    E. All of the above

62. Which of the following chest radiographic abnormalities can be caused by rheumatoid arthritis?

    A. Pleural effusion
    B. Hyperexpansion
    C. Multiple nodules
    D. Reticulonodular infiltrates
    E. All of the above

63. A 30-year-old man presents with symptoms of shortness of breath and nonproductive cough. Pulmonary function tests are shown in the following table. Which other tests might be helpful in the diagnosis of his pulmonary disease?

Test	% Predicted
FVC	45
FEV_1	51
FEV_1/FVC	.85
TLC	40
RV	50
DL_{CO}	40

    A. Serum immunoglobulin precipitins to thermophilic fungi
    B. Antinuclear antibody (ANA)
    C. Gallium scan of the lungs
    D. Open lung biopsy
    E. All of the above

64. Which of the following collagen vascular diseases can cause pleural effusions?

    A. Rheumatoid arthritis
    B. Scleroderma
    C. Polymyositis/dermatomyositis
    D. Fibromyalgia
    E. All of the above

65. Which of the following can predispose to clot formation and subsequent pulmonary thromboembolism?

    A. Immobilization
    B. Obesity
    C. Trauma
    D. Malignancy
    E. All of the above

66. Which of the following are side effects of isoniazid therapy?

    A. Decreased visual acuity
    B. Orange discoloration of secretions
    C. Thrombocytopenia
    D. Peripheral neuropathy
    E. All of the above

67. A 65-year-old patient presents to the emergency department and a chest radiograph shows a right lower lobe posterior infiltrate. All of the following are important in the history for determining appropriate initial coverage *except:*

    A. The patient drinks 1 gallon of vodka per day.
    B. The patient is a member of the American Legion.
    C. The patient had an illness consistent with influenza infection starting 1 week ago.
    D. The patient recently excavated a building site.
    E. The patient uses prednisone chronically

68. Which of the following are associated with *Mycoplasma pneumoniae* infection?

    A. Erythema multiforme
    B. Raynaud's phenomenon
    C. Hemolytic anemia
    D. Bullous myringitis
    E. All of the above

69. Which of the following pathogens more frequently cause nosocomial pneumonia than community-acquired pneumonia?
    A. Influenzavirus
    B. *Streptococcus pneumoniae*
    C. *Haemophilus influenzae*
    D. *Pseudomonas aeruginosa*
    E. All of the above

70. A 65-year-old woman presents with a chronic cough. Which of the following problems might be contributing to this symptom?
    A. Gastroesophageal reflux
    B. Congestive heart failure
    C. Asthma
    D. Postnasal drip
    E. All of the above

MATCHING
QUESTIONS 71–78

Match each of the following bronchogenic carcinomas with the most appropriate clinical presentation. Each tissue cell type can be used as an answer once or more than once.

   A. Bronchoalveolar carcinoma
   B. Adenocarcinoma
   C. Squamous cell carcinoma
   D. Small cell carcinoma
   E. Bronchial carcinoid

71. A 65-year-old male smoker with new-onset seizures and a chest radiograph that shows a peripheral, noncalcified lung nodule

72. A 35-year-old nonsmoker with a history of pulmonary sequestration and a nonresolving pulmonary infiltrate with air bronchograms on chest radiograph

73. A 74-year-old nonsmoker with a history of IPF and a new ill-defined nodule on a chest radiograph

74. A 59-year-old smoker with a large central lung mass on a chest radiograph and hypercalcemia

75. A 64-year-old smoker with a central lung mass on a chest radiograph, proximal muscle weakness, and peripheral paresthesias

76. A 60-year-old smoker with a large central lung mass on a chest radiograph, hepatomegaly, and lymphadenopathy.

77. A 45-year-old nonsmoker with a right lower lobe atelectasis on a chest radiograph and a hypervascular pedunculated mass seen at the takeoff of the right lower lobe on bronchoscopy.

78. A 55-year-old nonsmoker with a lung nodule on a chest radiograph, liver nodules on abdominal chest tomography, and intermittent episodes of wheezing and flushing.

QUESTIONS 79–83

Match the following interstitial lung diseases with the associated clinical presentation.

   A. Idiopathic pulmonary fibrosis
   B. Sarcoidosis
   C. Eosinophilic granuloma of the lung

   D. Hypersensitivity pneumonitis
   E. Lymphangioleiomyomatosis

79. A 68-year-old man with digital clubbing, pulmonary crackles, an antinuclear antibody titer of 1:80, and restrictive lung disease on pulmonary function testing

80. A 34-year-old woman with recurrent chylous pleural effusions and restrictive lung disease on pulmonary function testing

81. A 45-year-old smoker with restrictive lung disease on pulmonary function testing, a lytic rib lesion, and recent history of pneumothorax

82. A 55-year-old woman who has noted low-grade fevers, cough, and shortness of breath since using a humidifier at home

83. A 24-year-old with painful red areas on the anterior aspect of the lower extremities and hilar adenopathy on a chest radiograph

QUESTIONS 84–90

Match the following clinical pulmonary syndromes with the causative environmental exposure. Each clinical syndrome may be used more than once.

   A. Pulmonary fibrosis
   B. Bronchitis
   C. Asthma
   D. Pleural effusion
   E. Progressive massive fibrosis
   F. Hypersensitivity pneumonitis

84. Asbestos

85. Silica

86. Cotton dust

87. Grain dust

88. Isocyanates

89. Flour dust

90. Moldy hay

QUESTIONS 91–95

Match the following characteristics noted in pleural effusions with the associated disorders.

   A. Fluid LDH level of 120 IU/L; fluid protein/serum protein ratio of 0.4
   B. Fluid values: pH 6.8, glucose level of 10 mg/dL, amylase level of 500 U/L
   C. Fluid values: pH 7.25, glucose level of 10 mg/dL, amylase level of 50 U/L
   D. Fluid values: LDH level of 120 IU/L; creatinine level of 10 mg/dL
   E. Fluid values: pH 7.3, glucose level of 30 mg/dL; amylase level of 500 U/L
   F. Fluid values: LDH level of 250 IU/L; triglyceride level of 200 mg/dL
   G. Fluid value: ANA titer of 1:256 (peripheral 1:64)

91. Bronchogenic carcinoma

92. Esophageal perforation

93. Rheumatoid arthritis

94. Urinary obstruction

95. Cirrhosis

QUESTIONS 96–100

Match the following initial therapies with the most appropriate pulmonary pathogen.

 A. Oseltamivir
 B. Doxycycline
 C. Erythromycin
 D. Cefotaxime
 E. Ciprofloxacin
 F. Piperacillin
 G. None of the above

96. *Mycoplasma pneumoniae*

97. Influenzavirus A

98. *Chlamydia psittaci*

99. *Legionella pneumophila*

100. *Pseudomonas aeruginosa*

Part II
Pulmonary Diseases
Answers

1. **(C)** *Discussion:* Large pleural effusions will increase the distance between the lung and the chest wall; furthermore, typically, the vocal fremitus will be decreased as the fluid will absorb the sounds coming from the lung. The same mechanism explains why the breath sounds will be diminished in the affected hemithorax. The physical examination of the contralateral hemithorax should be normal. (*Cecil, Ch. 81*)

2. **(C)** *Discussion:* The patient has mild persistent asthma, which is defined as symptoms more than twice a week but less than daily and/or more than two nights per month. The preferred therapy for patients presenting with this degree of severity is low-dose inhaled corticosteroids. Alternatively, one can consider use of cromolyn and its derivatives or sustained-release theophylline, keeping serum concentration at 5-15 μg/mL. (*Cecil, Ch. 84 and National Asthma Expert Panel Report—Guidelines for the Diagnosis and Management of Asthma 1997, updated in 2002*)

3. **(D)** *Discussion:* During an acute asthma exacerbation, resistance to airflow is increased. On inspiration, the pleural pressure becomes more negative. The peak pleural pressure during expiration may be increased as the expiratory phase becomes active and the patient struggles to force air out of the lungs. Tachypnea is secondary to stimulation of central respiratory centers by intrapulmonary receptors. Asthma is a patchy disease, so airways narrowing results in imbalance between ventilation ($\dot{V}$) relative to perfusion ($\dot{Q}$). (*Lumb, 2000*)

4. **(D)** *Discussion:* The patient likely has cystic fibrosis (CF). It is an autosomal recessive genetic disease in which the most common mutation is ΔF508, which causes a 3 base-pair deletion and loss of a phenylalanine at position 508. The presence of meconium ileus in a newborn strongly suggests the diagnosis, and the diagnosis can be corroborated by a sweat chloride concentration more than 60 mEq/L. In later stages, chronic infection with *Pseudomonas* is very common and the most frequent cause of mortality is respiratory failure. (*Cecil, Ch. 86*)

5. **(A)** *Discussion:* The patient has silicosis, which is a form of interstitial lung disease associated with crystalline silica exposure. It has three forms of presentation: acute, accelerated, and chronic. The risk of developing the disease, like in other pneumoconiosis, increases with the level and duration of exposure. Pathologic evaluation may show dust-laden macrophages, silicotic nodules, or massive fibrosis, which indicates accelerated silicosis. Polarized light microscopy may show the presence of birefringent material, indicating silica particles. Acute silicosis is a cause of secondary alveolar proteinosis. In chronic or classic silicosis, the chest radiograph shows small nodularities that predominate in the upper lobes. Patients with silicosis are at increased risk of *Mycobacterium* infections and should have yearly tuberculin skin testing. There are no data to support use of corticosteroids, and therapy is largely supportive. Beryllium disease is characterized by the presence of noncaseating granulomas in a pattern similar to sarcoidosis, and a genetic marker (HLA-DP B1 Gluc 69) has been linked to increased susceptibility to it. (*Cecil, Chs. 89 and 91*)

6. **(D)** *Discussion:* The only treatment ever shown to alter the progression of COPD is smoking cessation. Patients with hypoxemia will have mortality benefit from home oxygen therapy. Pulmonary rehabilitation programs have been shown to increase quality of life and exercise capacity but will not reduce mortality or alter the rate of disease progression. Pneumococcal and influenza vaccines should be given to all patients with COPD to prevent exacerbations and avoid the devastating effects of such infections. Theophylline and bronchodilators provide symptomatic relief only. (*Cecil, Ch. 85*)

7. **(C)** *Discussion:* The patient has COPD exacerbation, probably from purulent bronchitis, and has developed respiratory failure. Provided the patient and/or his family agree, intubation and mechanical ventilation is the best course of action at this point. Most patients who develop respiratory failure from COPD and who are started on mechanical ventilation will eventually be liberated from it. About half of those patients, however, will die within the next year. Increased frequency of nebulized β_2-agonists will probably be helpful, but it is unlikely that it will resolve his respiratory failure. Although higher concentrations of oxygen can cause worsening CO_2 retention, persistent hypoxemia has much more daring consequences and must be avoided. Oxygen therapy should be titrated so arterial saturation of oxygen is maintained at about 90%. Obtaining spiral CT angiogram, performing echocardiography, and testing for BNP may become necessary subsequently but at the present time would delay the appropriate therapy. (*Cecil, Ch. 85*)

8. **(C)** *Discussion:* Serum precipitating antibodies are related to hypersensitivity pneumonitis (allergic extrinsic alveolitis), which does not cause bronchiectasis. High-resolution CT of the chest is the test of choice for diagnosis and characterization. Patients with humoral immunodeficiency may present later in life, after repeated sinopulmonary infections, with bronchiectasis, hence the need for serum levels of immunoglobulins. Chronic aspiration is a common cause of bronchiectasis, especially in patients with a history of altered state of consciousness due to stroke, seizures and alcohol intoxication. Patients with cystic fibrosis usually present with repetitive respiratory infections and upper lobe bronchiectasis and frequently become infected with *Pseudomonas aeruginosa*. (*Cecil, Ch. 88*)

9. **(A)** *Discussion:* The majority of interstitial lung diseases will present with decreased lung volumes on chest radiograph and a restrictive pattern on pulmonary function test. Idiopathic pulmonary fibrosis follows that rule. Bronchiolitis obliterans organizing pneumonia (BOOP), chronic hypersensitivity pneumonitis, histiocytosis X, lymphangioleiomyomatosis, neurofibromatosis, sarcoidosis, and tuberous sclerosis often present as formation of cysts and/or significant airflow obstruction and consequent hyperinflation. (*Cecil, Ch. 88*)

10. **(E)** *Discussion:* Amiodarone may cause lung toxicity in up to 10% of patients. Doses above 400 mg/day, previous pulmonary disease, and concomitant use of general anesthesia, cardiopulmonary bypass, or pulmonary angiography are risk factors for lung injury. The most common clinical presentation consists of very nonspecific complaints, but a minority can have an acute course similar to pneumonia or even acute respiratory distress syndrome. Pleuritic chest pain is reported by less than 20% of patients. Most patients will show impairment of the diffusion capacity. If the drug cannot be withdrawn, corticosteroids might be of benefit. The findings of the so-called foamy macrophages and cells with lamellar inclusions are present in a lung biopsy specimen of any patient using amiodarone and are not specific for toxicity. *(Cecil, Ch. 88)*

11. **(C)** *Discussion:* Carbon monoxide poisoning is caused by tissue hypoxia due to its greater affinity for hemoglobin, which displaces oxygen from it. Hyperbaric oxygen therapy is recommended in cases of more severe carbon monoxide poisoning defined by the presence of loss of consciousness or seizures as well as evidence of cardiac disease or HbCO level above 20-25%. Patients with more severe poisoning are at risk for the development of delayed neurologic impairment, which may include memory loss, decreased concentration capacity, as well as personality changes. Hyperbaric oxygen therapy may avoid neurologic impairment if started within 6 hours of exposure. Risk factors for the development of prolonged neurologic problems include older age, prolonged exposure, and loss of consciousness. The diagnosis of carbon monoxide poisoning is made by the finding of elevated HbCO level, and the severity of the clinical illness tends to correlate better with the duration and intensity of exposure. *(Cecil, Ch. 90)*

12. **(C)** *Discussion:* The criteria to define a PPD test as positive depend on the probability with which one is infected with *Mycobacterium tuberculosis.* Patients with known or suspected HIV infection are considered to have a positive PPD if the induration is ≥ 5 mm. Patients with HIV infection should receive preventive therapy for tuberculosis, preferably with isoniazid for at least 12 months. *(Schlossberg, 1999; American Thoracic Society, 1990)*

13. **(C)** *Discussion:* Bronchogenic carcinoma is now the leading cause of death from cancer in the United States in both men and women. Cigarette smoking increases the risk of it by at least 10-fold. Adenocarcinoma is the most prevalent cell type and tends to present as peripheral nodules/masses. Small cell lung cancers arise from neuroendocrine cells located in the respiratory tree and often are complicated by SIADH and other endocrine syndromes. The only modality of therapy that can cure non–small cell bronchogenic carcinoma is surgical resection; therefore, if no contraindication is present, it will always be the preferred treatment for stage I non–small cell bronchogenic carcinoma. Small cell bronchogenic carcinomas are a more aggressive histologic type and tend to be a "systemic" disease with early metastatic lesions, so combination chemotherapy is the preferred therapy for such cases. *(Cecil, Ch. 198)*

14. **(A)** *Discussion:* Sarcoidosis is a multisystemic granulomatous inflammatory condition that affects predominantly people of African background. Pulmonary disease can range from bilateral mediastinal lymphadenopathy to diffuse parenchymal scarring and usually the pulmonary function test will have a restrictive pattern. The presence of erythema nodosum combined with bilateral mediastinal lymphadenopathy as well as low-grade fever and arthralgias is called Lofgren's syndrome, which is more common in whites and is associated with better prognosis. The nodular lesions of erythema nodosum are not caused by granulomas; therefore, skin biopsy will have a very low yield. Hypercalcemia is a relatively common complication of more severe cases and tends to respond to corticosteroids. *(Cecil, Ch. 91)*

15. **(D)** *Discussion:* Any condition that causes aspiration of oropharyngeal or gastric contents with or without reduced airway ciliary's action will predispose to lung abscess, especially if there is concomitant periodontal disease or gingivitis. Use of inhaled corticosteroids is associated with increased incidence of oral candidiasis and may also be complicated by hoarseness but it is not associated with lung abscess. *(Cecil, Ch. 92)*

16. **(B)** *Discussion:* Rheumatoid arthritis is the collagen vascular disease that most commonly affects the lung. Pleural disease is relatively common and effusions with very low glucose levels may be present. Interstitial lung disease with a pattern indistinguishable from idiopathic pulmonary fibrosis is frequently reported and may actually precede joint manifestations in about 20% of the cases. BOOP manifested by subacute onset of respiratory symptoms, associated patchy infiltrates on a chest radiograph, and airflow obstruction has been described and may carry a poor prognosis. The small cartilages of the larynx can be affected, producing airflow obstruction. Diaphragmatic dysfunction is part of the so-called shrinking lung syndrome, which has been described in cases of systemic lupus erythematosus. *(Cecil, Ch. 88)*

17. **(D)** *Discussion:* The use of thrombolytic therapy for pulmonary thromboembolism is still a matter of great controversy. It is recommended only in patients with hemodynamic instability defined by hypotension as well as severe hypoxemia in the midst of an acute event. There are no data favoring one or another thrombolytic regimen. All other options are established therapies for acute pulmonary thromboembolism. *(Cecil, Ch. 94)*

18. **(E)** *Discussion:* Chylothorax is defined by a concentration of triglycerides greater than 110 mg/dL in a pleural fluid. Most common causes are tuberculosis, trauma to the thoracic duct, or invasion of it from malignancy. Glucose levels will be normal or elevated. The other options are conditions that can present as low levels of glucose in a pleural fluid. *(Cecil, Ch. 95; Sahn, 1988)*

19. **(B)** *Discussion:* Idiopathic pulmonary fibrosis (IPF) is a clinical syndrome characterized by progressive dyspnea and nonproductive cough with a restrictive pattern on pulmonary function tests and hypoxemia that usually appears first during exercise. Chest radiograph and high-resolution CT of the chest shows reticular infiltrates associated with honeycombing that predominate at the bases and are usually pleural based. A surgical lung biopsy will show a pattern of usual interstitial pneumonia, and 50% of patients will die within 3 to 5 years from the time of diagnosis. There is no approved therapy for IPF, and only a small number of patients will respond to immunosuppressant therapy. *(Cecil, Ch. 88; Schwartz and King, 1998)*

20. **(D)** *Discussion:* Thymomas are neoplasms that arise from the thymus and are located in the anterior mediastinum. The other options will typically be found in the posterior mediastinum. *(Cecil, Ch. 95)*

21. **(D)** *Discussion:* Theophylline is a methylxanthine that is a second-line agent in the management of asthma and COPD resulting from tobacco abuse. Although this drug was initially believed to have bronchodilating effects primarily through generation of increased levels of cyclic adenosine monophosphate, which relaxes bronchial smooth muscle, studies suggested that this agent may have other effects as well. Unfortunately, the use of theophylline is somewhat limited by the potential for toxicity. Drugs or conditions that affect hepatic clearance of this drug can potentiate or diminish toxicity by modulating serum theophylline levels. Cigarette smoking, rifampin, phenytoin, and barbiturates can reduce serum levels by increasing hepatic clearance of theophylline. In contrast, cimetidine, cirrhosis, allopurinol, erythromycin, congestive heart failure, febrile viral illness, ciprofloxacin, troleandomycin, oral contraceptives, propranolol, and clarithromycin can increase

theophylline levels by reducing hepatic clearance. (*Fishman, 1998; Cecil, Ch. 85*)

22. **(E)** *Discussion:* Asthma affects more than 10 million Americans, and the incidence of this disorder appears to be increasing. More than two thirds of people affected by asthma are younger than 18 years. Although all of the risk factors for asthma are not understood, some have been delineated. Premature infants are four times as likely to acquire asthma. Low birth weight may also predispose to asthma independent from prematurity. Race, gender, and socioeconomic status also appear to be associated with development of asthma. Blacks have a higher prevalence of asthma than whites. Males are most commonly affected in childhood, but following puberty there is a higher incidence of the disorder in females than males. Lower socioeconomic status also appears to be associated with a higher prevalence of asthma, possibly because of exposure to more indoor pollution, allergens, or passive cigarette smoke. Maternal factors also affect the incidence of asthma. Younger mothers, particularly those younger than age 20 years, bear infants who more commonly acquire asthma. This association is not related to the common association of younger maternal age and premature birth or socioeconomic status. Maternal cigarette smoking is also a clear risk factor for development of asthma in the first year of life. Respiratory infections early in life also appear to cause asthma. (*Fishman, 1998; Cecil, Ch. 84*)

23. **(D)** *Discussion:* Tobacco abuse is the number one preventable cause of health problems in the world today. Although the prevalence of smoking has decreased since the first surgeon general's report in 1964 demonstrated a link between smoking and ill health, the overall incidence of smoking in the general population has remained 25% over the past few years. There are also subgroups of the general population who have shown a recent upswing in prevalence, including white adolescents. The effects of tobacco smoke on health are wide and varied. Virtually all organ systems, including the lung, can be involved with benign and malignant processes induced by tobacco smoke. The best studied associations have been between cigarette smoking and COPD or lung cancer. Approximately 15% of smokers acquire symptomatic COPD. The other 85% probably do not become symptomatic because large pulmonary reserve is not diminished enough to cause symptoms. However, the great majority of smokers do have at least subclinical pulmonary dysfunction, as evidenced by a more rapid decline in pulmonary flow rates with age. Smokers are also more prone to lung cancer. Statistics suggest there is a 20-fold increase in risk of developing lung cancer in smokers compared with nonsmokers. Malignancies of other organ systems are also increased with smoking, suggesting that carcinogens absorbed from the smoke may be important. The risk of developing COPD or lung cancer is dose related; the amount smoked and the duration of smoking both correlate independently with the chance of developing these problems. Although the reason for the association is unclear, almost 100% of patients with eosinophilic granuloma of the lung are current or previous smokers. Smoking also appears to be a risk factor for developing pulmonary hemorrhage and glomerulonephritis (Goodpasture's syndrome), although nonsmokers may also experience this problem. (*Fishman, 1998*)

24. **(A)** *Discussion:* Asbestos is a fibrous material that has been used for insulation because of its fire resistance and durability for almost 2000 years. Inhalation of this material was first noted to cause pulmonary alterations in 1924. Since that time significant safeguards have been put in place to reduce the complications of exposure to this material. However, because of the long lag period between exposure and development of certain clinical syndromes, there continue to be a significant number of patients suffering from asbestos-related disorders. Pleural plaques are the most common complication of asbestos exposure. Development of pleural

plaques is related to the intensity of exposure and the time since exposure. In one study, pleural plaques developed in 17% of shipyard workers 10 years after initial exposure whereas 70% of workers acquired plaques after 30 years. Development of pulmonary fibrosis also appears to be time dependent. Ten percent of insulation workers have evidence of pulmonary fibrosis after 10 to 19 years of exposure, whereas 73% experience the problem after 20 to 29 years of exposure. In contrast, bloody effusions resulting from asbestos exposure may occur closer to the initial exposure. Generally, these benign pleural effusions develop 12 to 15 years after initial exposure. The risks of mesothelioma and bronchogenic carcinoma also increase with time of exposure. In general, these malignancies only develop 20 to 40 years after initial exposure. Although asbestos exposure and cigarette smoking are synergistic for increased risk of bronchogenic carcinoma, smoking does not appear to be a risk factor for the development of mesothelioma. (*Fishman, 1998; Cecil, Ch. 89*)

25. **(E)** *Discussion:* Pulmonary thromboembolism occurs in more than 500,000 Americans per year. The majority of emboli originate from deep veins in the legs. When pulmonary thromboembolism goes undiagnosed, the mortality approaches 30%, whereas diagnosed thromboembolism carries a 10% mortality, primarily in the first hour of the process. Factors that predispose to pulmonary thromboembolism are those proposed by Virchow: stasis, hypercoagulability, and endothelial injury. Nephrotic syndrome results in loss of natural anticoagulant factors causing hypercoagulability. When a clot travels to the pulmonary circulation, a number of consequences may occur, including pulmonary ventilation-perfusion imbalances, acute massive vascular occlusion with hemodynamic compromise, and pulmonary infarction. Distal emboli more commonly cause infarction as a result of loss of bronchial collateral circulation. Chronic left ventricular dysfunction also predisposes to infarction, possibly through alterations in bronchial venous return. The clinical diagnosis of pulmonary thromboembolism can be difficult. Although pulmonary angiography is the gold standard for diagnosis of the problem, it carries significant risk. Ventilation-perfusion lung scans can be very useful in the diagnosis of pulmonary thromboembolism if limitations are recognized. A normal perfusion scan virtually rules out pulmonary thromboembolism. Two or more segmental or lobar perfusion defects have a 97% specificity and 88% positive predictive value for pulmonary thromboembolism. Any other pattern detected on ventilation-perfusion scanning has less than 50% positive predictive value. Treatment of most patients with pulmonary thromboembolism involves administration of heparin to prevent further clot formation and prevent platelet activation with consequent release of mediators that impair gas exchange in this situation. Hemoptysis after pulmonary embolism is related to decreased blood flow to the affected area of lung and is not a contraindication for heparin therapy unless it is massive. In fact, massive hemoptysis resulting from pulmonary thromboembolism is uncommon; and if it is present, other diagnoses should be considered. The role of fibrinolytic agents in the treatment of pulmonary thromboembolism is controversial. The one situation in which it appears there is a definite indication is in the patient with hemodynamic compromise resulting from massive central embolism. In this setting, thrombolytic agents have essentially replaced pulmonary embolectomy. (*Cecil, Ch. 94; American College of Chest Physicians, 2001*)

26. **(A)** *Discussion:* Extracellular proteinases degrade cellular matrix to allow normal lung remodeling. Antiproteinase molecules modulate this process by preventing overdigestion of matrix. When there is an excess of proteinase activity or a deficiency of antiproteinase activity, matrix degradation results in pulmonary dysfunction manifesting as bronchitis, emphysema, or pulmonary fibrosis. α_1-Antiprotease inhibitor is a 52-kD glycoprotein secreted

by hepatocytes and macrophages. This glycoprotein inhibits the action of elastase and other serine proteinases. Genetic deficiency of this antiproteinase results in a number of syndromes, including emphysema. α_2-Macroglobulin is a 725-kD protein that inhibits several classes of proteinases by adhering to them after it has been digested. SLPI is a 12-kD protein that is produced by airway cells and inhibits a number of serine proteinases. Cystatins are a family of cysteine proteinase inhibitors. Cystatin C is a ubiquitous secreted molecule that competes with substrates of a number of proteinases, sparing them from destruction. Glutathione, a major antioxidant molecule that is also involved in arachidonic acid metabolism, does not have antiproteinase activity. (*Fishman, 1998*)

27. **(B)** *Discussion:* Gas diffusion is dependent on a number of factors, most importantly the area of interface between alveoli and capillaries. Carbon monoxide, an easily produced gas, is an ideal gas for measurement of this surface area because factors other than alveolocapillary surface area do not play a major role in diffusion of carbon monoxide from alveolus to capillary. This is because (1) the gas is diffusion limited and (2) there is virtually no partial pressure of carbon monoxide in capillary blood, resulting in a steep concentration gradient for this gas driving it from the alveolus to the capillary. Avid binding of carbon monoxide to hemoglobin helps to maintain this concentration gradient. Unfortunately, there are some conditions that may nonspecifically affect the measurement of diffusing capacity with this gas. If overall lung volume is reduced, the diffusing capacity for carbon monoxide will be proportionately reduced. This effect can be estimated by comparing the apparent reduction in diffusing capacity with the degree of reduced lung volume. The concentration of hemoglobin in capillary blood can also affect the diffusing capacity for carbon monoxide and lower the value in the absence of an alteration in diffusion membrane surface area. The effect of low hemoglobin concentration can be estimated by comparing the degree of apparent impairment in diffusing capacity with the severity of hemoglobin reduction. Polycythemia can also increase the diffusing capacity as a result of elevated hemoglobin in the capillary blood. (*Cecil, Ch. 82*)

28. **(D)** *Discussion:* Allergic bronchopulmonary aspergillosis is a disorder that occurs in asthmatics who have colonization of bronchi with *Aspergillus* or, rarely, with other fungi. This colonization stimulates an immediate hypersensitivity reaction, resulting in increased serum IgE concentrations and peripheral eosinophilia. Pulmonary infiltrates can also develop. Asthmatics in whom this condition develops demonstrate serum IgE antibodies that are specific for *Aspergillus* and may acquire specific precipitating IgG antibodies to the fungus (serum precipitins). Although patients with allergic bronchopulmonary aspergillosis can exhibit skin test reactivity to *Aspergillus* preparations, the response is an immediate reaction rather than a delayed response. (*Fishman, 1998*)

29. **(A)** *Discussion:* A number of collagen vascular diseases can cause pulmonary fibrosis, including rheumatoid arthritis, scleroderma, and SLE. Subclinical pulmonary fibrosis is probably very prevalent in scleroderma patients. In addition to pulmonary fibrosis, pulmonary hypertension, pleural effusions, aspiration resulting from esophageal dysfunction, and obstructive lung disease are also associated with scleroderma. Ankylosing spondylitis is a common inflammatory disorder of the musculoskeletal system, which occurs most frequently in young men. In addition to multiple skeletal abnormalities, patients with ankylosing spondylitis can acquire pulmonary fibrosis, primarily in the lung apices. Hermansky-Pudlak syndrome is an inherited lysosomal storage disease with associated oculocutaneous albinism in which affected individuals can acquire pulmonary fibrosis. Neurofibromatosis is also an inherited disorder, characterized by neurofibromas in the skin and other sites, cafe au lait spots, and axillary freckles, in

which patients can develop pulmonary fibrosis, usually noted first between the ages of 35 and 60 years. (*Cecil, Ch. 88*)

30. **(E)** *Discussion:* Rheumatoid arthritis is associated with a number of pleuropulmonary manifestations, including pleural fibrosis/effusion, pulmonary nodules, bronchiolitis, and pulmonary fibrosis. All of these manifestations are increased in patients with more severe underlying disease as manifested by high rheumatoid titers, subcutaneous nodules, and more erosive arthritis. In contrast to the overall population of patients with rheumatoid arthritis, in which females outnumber males, patients with pulmonary disease resulting from rheumatoid arthritis are more likely to be male. Although tobacco abuse is certainly associated with other pulmonary diseases, it does not raise the risk of pulmonary fibrosis resulting from rheumatoid arthritis. (*Fishman, 1998; Cecil, Ch. 88*)

31. **(E)** *Discussion:* Asthma caused by the workplace environment can be the result of exposure to more than 200 different materials generally classified as high- or low-molecular-weight substances. Animal handlers are prone to asthma because of exposure to a number of allergens at the workplace. More than 50% of animal handlers will experience respiratory symptoms after 3 months of employment. A history of atopy and elevated serum IgE levels are risk factors for development of asthma in animal handlers. One allergen to which animal handlers experience sensitivity is a protein found in rat urine. Measures to prevent aerosolization of this protein such as utilization of adsorbent bedding can reduce the incidence of asthma in these workers. Risk factors for asthma caused by latex include (1) frequent use of disposable latex gloves, (2) presence of atopic disease, and (3) prior or current evidence of hand dermatitis. A large percentage of patients in whom latex-related asthma develops also report rhinitis and conjunctivitis on exposure to latex. Skin testing with latex can identify affected individuals. One study has shown that 20% of bakers' apprentices have positive skin tests to flour extracts after 5 years of work. Overall, 7 to 20% of bakers experience some allergic symptoms, including asthma, that worsen at the workplace. Using properly fitting occlusive masks can minimize these symptoms. Although asbestos exposure can cause a respiratory bronchiolitis, asthma has not been associated with exposure to this fiber. (*Fishman, 1998; Cecil, Ch. 89*)

32. **(E)** *Discussion:* Although all snorers do not have obstructive sleep apnea, it is generally present in those who are affected. Nocturia is also a common symptom in patients with this disorder and, although not as common as snoring, is probably due to release of atrial natriuretic factor at night because of right atrial stretch. Morning headaches are also common in patients with obstructive sleep apnea; they commonly quickly remit after the patient is awake for a short period of time. Dyspepsia occurs more frequently in these patients, probably because of increased gastroesophageal reflux occurring as a result of increased intrathoracic negative pressures generated at night. Tinnitus is not a symptom of obstructive sleep apnea. (*Cecil, Ch. 96; Pack, 1994*)

33. **(A)** *Discussion:* Accumulating evidence suggests subtypes of pulmonary lymphocytes are involved in different disease processes that involve the lung. B cells are important for clearance of antibody-sensitive invading pathogens such as *S. pneumoniae*. Natural killer cells are important for lysis of tumor cells. Two subsets of T helper cells initially were thought to act primarily by enhancing B-cell activity but subsequently have been shown to secrete a number of inflammatory mediators. Th1 lymphocytes are involved in antiviral and antifungal defense, cell-mediated immunity, granuloma formation, and graft rejection. In addition to interleukin-2, interferon, and TGF-β_1, Th1 cells also secrete interleukin-3, -6, -12, and -16 as well as GM-CSF. In contrast, Th2 lymphocytes are involved primarily in processes of immediate hypersensitivity, such

as allergic inflammation and antiparasitic defense. Interleukin-5 is a cytokine that stimulates proliferation and attracts eosinophils. This cytokine is a major secretory product of Th2 cells. Other cytokines secreted by Th2 cells include interleukin-2, -3, -4, -9, -10, -13, and -16 as well as GM-CSF and TGF-β_1. (*Mossman and Sad, 1996*)

34. **(B)** *Discussion:* The patient most likely has hyperreactive airway syndrome because of exposure to isocyanates contained in the spray paint. Isocyanates are highly reactive chemicals that are found in paints, varnishes, flexible foams, and adhesives. Overall, 5 to 30% of exposed individuals experience respiratory symptoms. After an individual is sensitized, very low concentrations of isocyanates can trigger bronchospasm. Isocyanate-induced asthma may be intermittent and associated with normal pulmonary function tests, as in this case, when the individual is away from the exposure. However, airway hyperreactivity, manifested by a drop in flow rates with low doses of inhaled methacholine, is present even in the absence of concurrent isocyanate exposure. Exposure to the suspected isocyanate can also induce a reduction in flow rates, but this can be dangerous even in a controlled setting. Although isocyanates contained in spray paint can also cause hypersensitivity pneumonitis, which may be distinguishable on high-resolution CT scan of the lungs, this is much less common than airway hyperreactivity caused by these chemicals. Although ventilation-perfusion scan would be useful in eliminating PTEs as a cause of the dyspnea in this patient, there are no clues in the history to suggest this diagnosis. Performance of the other tests mentioned is also not supported by the clinical presentation. (*Cecil, Ch. 89*)

35. **(A)** *Discussion:* Stridor (inspiratory wheezing) is suggestive of upper airway obstruction at an extrathoracic site. This may be associated with flattening of the inspiratory flow-volume loop. Alternatively, upper airway obstruction occurring at an intrathoracic site (vocal cords or below) can cause flattening of the expiratory flow-volume loop. Visualization of the upper airway by CT may be useful in this setting, but it is relatively insensitive. Examination of the upper airway through bronchoscopy or laryngoscopy should be performed in these patients, but, because of the invasive nature of these procedures, the degree of impairment and site of obstruction should first be evaluated by spirometry. Although emergent tracheostomy may be occasionally required in patients with upper airway obstruction, there is no role for transtracheal aspiration. (*Fishman, 1998*)

36. **(A)** *Discussion:* Influenza infection puts the affected patient at risk for superimposed bacterial pneumonia. This is probably due to deactivating effects of this virus on polymorphonuclear leukocytes as well as effects on pulmonary epithelium. Although the incidence of pneumonia resulting from *S. aureus* is increased after influenza infection, this organism is not the most common pathogen in this setting. Instead, *S. pneumoniae* is the most common bacterial pathogen involved in postinfluenza pneumonia. *P. aeruginosa* and *H. influenzae* can also cause postinfluenza pneumonia. In fact, *H. influenzae* received its name because it was initially isolated from a patient with clinical influenza. The risk for pneumonia resulting from *P. carinii* is not increased with influenza infection. Influenza can also directly cause pneumonia. This should be considered in a patient in whom infiltrates develop in this setting. (*Cecil, Ch. 92; American Thoracic Society, 2001; Bartlett et al, 1998*)

37. **(A)** *Discussion:* Lymphangioleiomyomatosis is a disorder affecting women of childbearing age that is characterized by proliferation of smooth muscle in the lung, resulting in cystic changes and lymphatic obstruction. Cyst formation can subsequently cause pneumothorax, whereas lymphatic obstruction causes recurrent pleural effusions that are chylous in nature. Patients with this disorder have decreased lung volumes on pulmonary function testing, but a chest radiograph may suggest hyperexpansion as a result of

the cyst formation. High-resolution CT scan is useful and may be diagnostic. Other disorders listed in the question have not been associated with this disorder. (*Taylor et al, 1990*)

38. **(B)** *Discussion:* Emerging data suggest that ipratropium bromide treatment improves prognosis in patients with COPD. Patients with this disorder commonly respond to ipratropium more favorably than asthmatics. Although some patients with mild COPD may be managed with an albuterol inhaler alone, they are the minority. Theophylline may be useful in patients with COPD but only after treatment with inhaled bronchodilators has failed. Prednisone is effective in acute exacerbations of COPD and may be used chronically in stable COPD but only after all other treatments have proven ineffective and only with objective verification of treatment efficacy using pulmonary function testing. Salmeterol, a long-acting β-agonist inhaled bronchodilator, is useful in the chronic treatment of COPD if short-acting bronchodilators are not sufficient to control symptoms. Aldactone may be useful in treating edema related to cor pulmonale caused by end-stage COPD, but it is generally not required early in the treatment of COPD. (*Cecil, Ch. 85*)

39. **(A)** *Discussion:* Normal individuals as well as asthmatics manifest bronchodilation at early stages of exercise because of release of catecholamines. In normal individuals this is followed by a return to normal baseline airway tone, whereas asthmatics with exercise-induced bronchospasm experience a reduction in airway diameter coincidental with symptoms of wheezing and coughing. Although mechanisms of these exercise-induced changes are not totally clear, it appears that mast cell activation is involved as a result of airway heat loss during exercise. Airway water loss also appears to occur during exercise, and this may also be a cause of bronchospasm in asthmatic airways in this setting. In this regard, dry air worsens exercise-induced bronchospasm in affected asthmatics. In contrast, humid air, such as that present in indoor swimming pools, can improve symptoms. A number of treatments can prevent exercise-induced asthma, including inhaled cromolyn sodium or β-adrenergic agonists used 10 to 20 minutes before exercise. Various studies suggested that exercise-induced asthma is very common, occurring in 50 to 90% of asthmatics. (*Cecil, Ch. 84*)

40. **(D)** *Discussion:* Pulmonary alveolar proteinosis is a disease characterized by accumulation in alveoli of phospholipid-rich periodic acid–Schiff (PAS)-positive proteinaceous material. This disorder can occur as a result of no definable cause or after a number of associated pathologic processes, including hematologic malignancies, exposure to silica, and *P. carinii* infection in HIV-infected individuals. If pulmonary alveolar proteinosis is due to an underlying process, treatment of that process is indicated. However, the only currently effective therapy of primary pulmonary alveolar proteinosis is whole-lung lavage. Most patients require multiple lavage procedures to maintain adequate gas exchange. (*Cecil, Ch. 88*)

41. **(A)** *Discussion:* Indications for inferior vena caval filter placement are (1) a contraindication to anticoagulation in a patient with documented DVT or PTE, (2) a complication of current anticoagulation, (3) failure of adequate anticoagulation as reflected by recurrent DVT or PTE, and (4) a patient with low pulmonary reserve who is at high risk for death with PTE. Poor compliance with anticoagulation regimens or difficulty in anticoagulation may also be indications, but these are far less proven. The patient described in answer A has severe pulmonary disease and thus would have high mortality with PTE. (*Cecil, Ch. 94; American College of Chest Physicians, 2001; Moser, 1990*)

42. **(C)** *Discussion:* Overall, 4% of patients who receive bleomycin will acquire pulmonary fibrosis from this drug. However, certain risk factors markedly increase the chance of pulmonary side effects from this drug. In addition to the elements listed in the question, oxygen therapy can increase the risk of bleomycin pul-

monary toxicity. Although the use of colony-stimulating factors to improve neutropenia has been associated with enhanced bleomycin pulmonary toxicity, this relationship needs further study. Tobacco abuse has not been associated with a higher risk for bleomycin pulmonary toxicity. (*Cecil, Ch. 88; Cooper et al, 1986*)

43. **(A)** *Discussion:* Although other forms of therapy are less invasive, tracheostomy is the most effective therapy for obstructive sleep apnea. Uvulopalatopharyngoplasty will be successful in approximately 45% overall and 75 to 80% successful if the level of obstruction is documented to be at the soft palate. Weight reduction should be encouraged if the patient is overweight, but improvement in apnea only occurs in approximately 20% of patients with this intervention. Nasal CPAP is the preferred therapy for the majority of patients because of its noninvasive nature and proven efficacy. Tricyclic antidepressants can improve apnea if it occurs primarily during rapid-eye-movement sleep. (*Cecil, Ch. 96; Kales et al, 1987; Pack, 1994*)

44. **(C)** *Discussion:* Although serum LDH may rise in several pulmonary disorders and thus is nonspecific for diagnosis, this enzyme may be useful for following the course of pneumonia from *P. carinii* in HIV-infected patients. Increased LDH levels (>300 IU/mL) are present in the majority of patients with this disorder. Levels greater than 600 IU/mL are predictors of poor prognosis. Another serum enzyme that can be elevated with *P. carinii* pneumonia is angiotensin-converting enzyme. (*Cecil, Ch. 92; Bartlett et al, 1998*)

45. **(A)** *Discussion:* Chronic cough may be due to a variety of mechanisms. When the cause of chronic cough goes undiagnosed for several months, certain specific problems should be considered. Occult asthma with normal pulmonary tests or only mild reductions in flow rates is a common cause of this problem. Because inhaled β-adrenergic agonists can sometimes precipitate the cough in this setting, oral forms may be more effective. Chronic esophageal reflux is also a common cause of cough from either aspiration of refluxed material or a reflex triggered by acid reflux into the lower esophagus. Patients with this problem may awaken with a bitter taste as a result of refluxed material. Alternatively, patients may commonly awaken with a sore throat. Postnasal drip can be difficult to control and may cause chronic cough that does not diminish until sinus drainage is controlled. If cough persists despite efforts at treatment of any of these disorders, bronchoscopy should be considered to rule out an endobronchial lesion as the cause of the cough. (*Fishman, 1998*)

46. **(D)** *Discussion:* Methotrexate can cause pulmonary side effects when it is used for the treatment of benign or malignant processes. Although the most common pulmonary process associated with methotrexate therapy is a subacute syndrome most consistent with hypersensitivity pneumonitis, this drug can also cause noncardiogenic pulmonary edema, particularly when given intrathecally. Pulmonary fibrosis or an isolated pleural effusion can also be caused by methotrexate. One study demonstrated that pleural fluid associated with methotrexate contains high concentrations of the drug, suggesting a possible direct toxic effect. (*Cooper et al, 1986*)

47. **(A)** *Discussion:* Organisms that commonly cause CAP include *M. pneumoniae, S. pneumoniae,* and *H. influenzae,* in that order. *Chlamydia* species are also probably a major cause of this problem, but the relative importance of these organisms is uncertain. *M. catarrhalis, S. aureus,* and *P. aeruginosa* are relatively uncommon causes of CAP except in the presence of other complicating factors such as COPD. *M. catarrhalis* is a gram-negative diplococcus that causes sinusitis and otitis media as well as pneumonia. Most isolates are β-lactamase positive, which should guide therapy. (*American Thoracic Society, 2001; Bartlett et al, 1998*)

48. **(D)** *Discussion:* Knowledge of the role of cytokines in pulmonary disease is becoming increasingly important because of the development of therapeutic agents that specifically inhibit production or actions of these molecules. Interleukin-5 is a cytokine that selectively supports the differentiation of progenitor cells into mature eosinophils. In addition, interleukin-5 is a specific chemotaxin for eosinophils. Studies suggested that this cytokine is important in the pathogenesis of immediate hypersensitivity reactions that are involved in allergic phenomena such as asthma and rhinitis. Inhibitors of interleukin-5 are under investigation for the treatment of patients with these disorders. (*Cecil, Ch. 84*)

49. **(B)** *Discussion:* Bronchitis secondary to infection or environmental exposures such as tobacco smoke is the most common cause of hemoptysis. However, other causes need to be considered when a patient presents with this symptom. Bronchiectasis is a potential cause of massive hemoptysis; occasionally, vascular embolization or lung resection is needed to control hemorrhage in this setting. Aspergilloma within cavities can also cause massive hemoptysis. The diagnosis is suggested by a rounded opacity within the cavity that changes in location with position of the patient. Pulmonary embolism can cause hemoptysis, although this is rarely massive and is usually associated with an infiltrate/density on chest radiograph. Mitral stenosis was a major cause of hemoptysis resulting from pulmonary venous hypertension when this was a more prevalent cardiac problem, but this has diminished as more effective therapy for the valvular disease has been developed. Although asthma is a form of bronchitis, it does not cause hemoptysis. (*Cecil, Ch. 81; Winter and Ingbar, 1988*)

50. **(C)** *Discussion:* Clubbing of the fingers or toes is defined by a bulbous enlargement of the distal digit resulting from an increase in soft tissue. Pulmonary syndromes that are associated with digital clubbing are (1) primary and metastatic pulmonary malignancies; (2) bronchiectasis, including cystic fibrosis; (3) lung abscess and empyema; (4) mesothelioma; (5) pulmonary fibrosis; and (6) neurogenic diaphragmatic tumors. Cardiac and gastrointestinal disorders that cause this finding include (1) congenital heart defects, (2) bacterial endocarditis, (3) cirrhosis, and (4) inflammatory bowel diseases. Hemiplegia can also cause clubbing, and it may be hereditary and not related to any pathologic process. (*Fishman, 1998*)

51. **(E)** *Discussion:* Pneumonia is the sixth leading cause of death in the United States. Overall there are 2 to 3 million new cases of CAP annually in the United States. CAP probably occurs as a result of aspiration of normal pharyngeal secretion because the majority of organisms that cause CAP are normal inhabitants of the pharynx, and studies demonstrated that normal individuals regularly aspirate upper airway secretions, especially at night. Influenza infection predisposes to CAP, probably through several effects of the virus on epithelial and inflammatory cells. Because of this association, influenza immunization reduces the incidence of CAP. Pneumococcal vaccine is also important because this organism is the most common cause of CAP. Because *S. pneumoniae* is a fastidious organism, expectorated sputum culture will only be positive in 40 to 50% of cases; this percentage decreases if the patient is receiving antibiotics. (*American Thoracic Society, 2001; Bartlett et al, 1998*)

52. **(E)** *Discussion:* The diffusing capacity for carbon monoxide (DLco) attempts to measure the area of alveolocapillary membrane by determining the amount of hemoglobin in the thorax using the avid hemoglobin-binding properties of carbon monoxide. An isolated reduction in DLco suggests obliteration of capillary bed volume, which can occur secondary to pulmonary hypertension (as occurs in scleroderma and primary pulmonary hypertension), embolic phenomenon, or toxic effects of drugs such as bleomycin on endothelium. Lobectomy should not alter DLco disproportional to the degree of lung volume loss. (*Cecil, Ch. 82*)

53. (A) *Discussion:* Fat embolism results in a clinical syndrome of neurologic and pulmonary abnormalities occurring within 12 to 24 hours after skeletal trauma. Overall, 5% of patients who sustain severe, multiple orthopedic injuries experience this syndrome. Signs and symptoms of the syndrome include fever, respiratory failure, mental confusion, a petechial rash predominantly over the upper torso, and retinal vessel fat globules. Fat in the urine may also be present, and the chest radiograph commonly shows evidence of noncardiogenic pulmonary edema. In general, a pleural effusion is not part of the syndrome. (*Fishman, 1998*)

54. (E) *Discussion:* Sarcoidosis is a multisystem disorder that is characterized by granulomatous inflammation in a number of organ systems; the lung and intrathoracic lymph nodes are involved most frequently. Four complications of sarcoidosis that warrant corticosteroid therapy are (1) hypercalcemia, (2) uveitis, (3) cardiac involvement, including heart block, and (4) neurologic involvement, including cranial nerve alterations. Sarcoidosis can cause angina by involving the coronary arteries, although this is very rare. Chronic uveitis in combination with sarcoidosis is relatively common, occurring in approximately 20% of patients. Erythema nodosum also occurs in conjunction with sarcoidosis, usually in association with bilateral hilar adenopathy, fevers, polyarthritis, and uveitis (Lofgren's syndrome). Clubbing is not associated with sarcoidosis. (*Cecil, Ch. 91*)

55. (D) *Discussion:* Chronic inhalation of passive second-hand tobacco smoke has been associated with increased risk of bronchogenic carcinoma. Because second-hand smoke does not pass through cigarette filters, the level of carcinogens is actually higher than that of direct smoke. Other air pollutants can also increase the risk for bronchogenic carcinoma. There is a higher incidence of lung cancer in workers who are chronically exposed to fossil fuel fires, and roofers who are exposed to coal-tar fumes also have significantly increased risk after 20 years of exposure. Patients who smoke and acquire COPD also are at increased risk for bronchogenic carcinoma compared with those who do not acquire airway obstruction. Asbestos exposure alone increases the risk of bronchogenic carcinoma, and exposure to this mineral markedly increases the risk in the setting of tobacco smoke exposure. Although there is increasing evidence that diet, particularly vitamin intake, may place a patient at risk for a number of malignancies, the association of low vitamin A intake and bronchogenic carcinoma has not been established. (*Cecil, Ch. 198*)

56. (C) *Discussion:* The majority of patients with obstructive sleep apnea are men, by a 7:1 to 20:1 ratio. In general, patients with sleep apnea are not aware of arousal after episodes of apnea. Although sleep apnea can occur at any age, the usual age at onset is 40 to 50 years, and the incidence increases with age from that point. Weight loss can improve symptoms of apnea, but the majority of affected patients need some other form of therapy. (*Kales et al, 1987*)

57. (E) *Discussion:* Patients with hypothyroidism have blunted respiratory drive responses to hypercapnia and hypoxia. In addition, goiters associated with this problem can add to upper airway obstruction. The association of acromegaly and Down syndrome is probably due to redundant upper airway tissue that results in obstruction at night. Normal individuals demonstrate some evidence of mild airway obstruction at night; this is amplified by the presence of COPD. Although the most common apnea associated with COPD is hypopnea, intermittent upper airway obstruction with apnea also occurs. (*Kales et al, 1987*)

58. (E) *Discussion:* Virtually 100% of patients with obstructive sleep apnea are noted to snore. However, snoring does not necessarily imply the presence of apnea, and relief of snoring with upper airway surgery does not necessarily mean apnea has been adequately treated. Somnambulism occurs to a greater degree in patients with obstructive sleep apnea than in unaffected patients, but it is still relatively uncommon. Increased gastroesophageal reflux occurs, probably as a result of a marked decline in intrathoracic pressures during airway obstruction. Enuresis occurs in approximately 5% of patients affected with obstructive sleep apnea. (*Kales et al, 1987*)

59. (D) *Discussion:* Resection of bronchogenic carcinoma is the best hope for cure of a patient. Therefore, thorough examination is needed to establish that a particular finding is definitely a contraindication to resection. Paraneoplastic hypercalcemia can be due to release of a parathyroid-like hormone that is not indicative of metastases; thus an elevated serum calcium level in the setting of bronchogenic carcinoma is not necessarily a contraindication to surgery. Pleural effusion can be caused by proximal obstruction resulting from the carcinoma and does not necessarily indicate pleural metastases. Mediastinal adenopathy on CT scan also does not necessarily indicate tumor involvement; tissue sampling by mediastinoscopy or thoracotomy is indicated before rejecting the patient for surgery. Documented hepatic metastases suggest metastatic disease and are a contraindication for resection. (*Cecil, Ch. 198*)

60. (E) *Discussion:* Although the clinical situation must dictate the need for chest tube drainage in a particular patient, certain fluid characteristics suggest it may be necessary. All of the findings noted in the question suggest the fluid is an empyema, with large numbers of inflammatory cells metabolizing glucose, resulting in a low pleural fluid glucose level, and producing carbon dioxide, resulting in a low pleural fluid pH. The markedly elevated pleural fluid LDH level suggests the normal filtration barrier has been markedly disrupted by the process. Although pleural effusions with some of these parameters might respond to conservative measures, a pleural effusion with a positive Gram stain virtually never responds to anything less than chest tube drainage and antibiotic therapy. (*Sahn, 1988*)

61. (B) *Discussion:* Asthma is a disease associated with bronchial edema, increased mucus production, and heightened bronchial reactivity to nonspecific agents such as histamine or methacholine. In general, tissue destruction does not occur in this syndrome until very late in its course, when subepithelial fibrosis may develop. Therefore, unlike emphysema, the diffusing capacity for carbon monoxide is normal in asthmatics and the airway obstruction is reversible to a variable degree. Proximal bronchiectasis can occur in the setting of allergic bronchopulmonary aspergillosis in the setting of asthma but does not occur in asthmatics without this syndrome. Peripheral eosinophilia may not be present in all cases of asthma. (*Cecil, Ch. 84*)

62. (E) *Discussion:* Rheumatoid arthritis can cause a variety of thoracic abnormalities. Risk factors for developing these abnormalities are the presence of (1) severe articular disease, (2) high rheumatoid factor titers, (3) subcutaneous nodules, and (4) systemic manifestations such as Felty's syndrome or myopericarditis. The most common thoracic abnormality associated with this disease is pleural effusion. Pulmonary nodules caused by rheumatoid arthritis are usually multiple and may cavitate. They usually are present in patients with concomitant subcutaneous nodules and are histologically indistinguishable. Hyperexpansion on chest radiograph may occur secondary to bronchiolitis obliterans associated with rheumatoid arthritis. In general, this problem is resistant to therapy. Reticulonodular infiltrates occur in conjunction with pulmonary fibrosis caused by rheumatoid arthritis as well as other collagen vascular diseases. (*Cecil, Ch. 88; Hunninghake and Fauci, 1979*)

63. (D) *Discussion:* The pulmonary function tests demonstrate a restrictive ventilatory defect with reduced lung volumes and increased FEV_1/FVC ratio. In addition, the diffusing capacity is decreased, suggesting a tissue-damaging process rather than simple respiratory muscle weakness. A number of diseases can cause this pulmonary function abnormality, which is indicative of an interstitial pulmonary process. These include hypersensitivity pneumonitis, collagen vascular diseases such as SLE, idiopathic pulmonary fibrosis, and sarcoidosis. Although serum precipitins are commonly elevated in patients with hypersensitivity pneumonitis, they are not diagnostic of this disorder because they may be elevated in subjects who have been exposed to thermophilic fungi but have no pulmonary disease. In addition, an elevated ANA titer is not diagnostic of a particular pulmonary process because it may be positive at low titer in patients with idiopathic pulmonary fibrosis as well as patients with SLE. Gallium scanning of the lungs is also nonspecific because it will be positive in lungs with virtually any type of inflammation from infectious or noninfectious causes. Of all the possible answers to this question, open lung biopsy is the only test that will commonly differentiate among all of the causes of restrictive ventilatory defects. (*Cecil, Ch. 88*)

64. (A) *Discussion:* Although pleural fibrosis is common in patients with scleroderma, pleural effusion is uncommon. Any form of pleural disease is uncommon in patients with polymyositis or dermatomyositis. Pleural effusion caused by rheumatoid arthritis is exudative, with low pH and low glucose level. A rheumatoid factor titer greater than 1:320 is suggestive that a pleural effusion is due to rheumatoid arthritis. Pleural effusion in SLE is commonly associated with pleuritic pain. A pleural fluid ANA titer greater than 1:160 is suggestive that the effusion is due to SLE. Fibromyalgia does not present as pleural disease. (*Cecil, Ch. 88; Hunninghake and Fauci, 1979*)

65. (E) *Discussion:* The three general factors that contribute to clot formation are stasis, trauma to blood vessels, and clotting abnormalities. Immobilization and obesity probably predispose to clot formation through venous stasis. Malignancy may predispose to clot formation through stasis resulting from obstruction by the malignancy or through paraneoplastic clotting abnormalities. Body trauma results in damage to blood vessels, with subsequent changes in endothelium that makes it more susceptible to clot formation. In addition to the factors listed, other factors that predispose to clot formation include surgery, particularly of the pelvis or hip area; excess estrogen states; advanced age; and primary hypercoagulable states. (*Cecil, Ch. 94; Moser, 1990*)

66. (D) *Discussion:* A number of antituberculosis medications are hepatotoxic, including rifampin, pyrazinamide, and isoniazid. In general, hepatitis induced by isoniazid is reversible unless there is underlying liver disease. Peripheral neuropathy induced by isoniazid is commonly responsive to thiamine; other antituberculosis medications do not cause a peripheral neuropathy. Orange discoloration of secretions is a complication of rifampin therapy; the discoloration is harmless. Thrombocytopenia is also a significant side effect of rifampin only. Ethambutol may cause retrobulbar neuritis that is manifested by decreased visual acuity, central scotomas, and red/green color blindness. (*American Thoracic Society/Centers for Disease Control/IDSA, 2003*)

67. (B) *Discussion:* The most common location for aspiration pneumonia to occur is the lower lobe superior segment, followed by the lower lobe posterior basal segment. Aspiration pneumonias such as those that occur after passing out as a result of drinking alcohol or during a seizure are due commonly to anaerobic organisms. Therefore, an elicited history of excessive alcohol consumption would be important. Influenza infection also results in a shift in the type of organisms that cause pneumonia. Influenza predisposes an individual to bacterial pneumonias and, with *S. aureus*, plays a greater role than in community-acquired pneumonias in

the absence of previous influenza infection. Building excavation sites are a common source of certain pathologic fungi, particularly *Histoplasma capsulatum*. Therefore, although a localized lobar pneumonia would be atypical for this organism, this part of the history would be important. Conversely, although pneumonia caused by *Legionella pneumophila* was first reported at a convention for legionnaires, it has been shown to be a major cause of pneumonia in all patient groups. Use of corticosteroids increases the risk of infections with encapsulated organisms and fungi as well as reactivation of mycobacterial infections. (*Cecil, Ch. 92; American Thoracic Society, 2001*)

68. (E) *Discussion: Mycoplasma pneumoniae* only exists in a human reservoir. Only 3 to 10% of infections result in pneumonia; the rest result in an upper respiratory tract illness. Bullous myringitis, when seen, should strongly suggest *Mycoplasma* infection. However, this manifestation, although relatively specific for the organism, is relatively rare. All of the other manifestations listed can be associated with *Mycoplasma* infection. The finding of cold agglutinin hemolytic anemia in a patient with pneumonia should strongly suggest *Mycoplasma* infection. (*Cecil, Ch. 92; American Thoracic Society, 2001*)

69. (D) *Discussion:* The most common causes of community-acquired pneumonia are *Mycoplasma pneumoniae, Streptococcus pneumoniae,* and *Haemophilus influenzae,* in that order. *Staphylococcus aureus* and *Pseudomonas aeruginosa* are relatively uncommon causes of community-acquired pneumonia except in the presence of other complicating factors such as COPD. In contrast, patients who are hospitalized more commonly develop pneumonias caused by other staphylococci or *Pseudomonas*, possibly because of the change in flora secondary to antibiotic therapy. (*Cecil, Ch. 92; American Thoracic Society, 2001*)

70. (E) *Discussion:* Chronic cough may be due to a variety of mechanisms. In cases in which the cause of chronic cough goes undiagnosed for several months, certain specific problems should be considered. Occult asthma with only mild reductions in flow rates is a common cause of this problem. Because inhaled β-adrenergic agonists can sometimes precipitate the cough, the oral forms may be more effective. Chronic esophageal reflux is also a common cause of cough as a result of either aspiration of refluxed material or a reflex triggered by acid reflux into the lower esophagus. Patients with left ventricular dysfunction can also present with cough. This group of patients is hypersensitive to inhalation of methacholine, suggesting they have hyperactive airways similarly to patients with traditional asthma. Postnasal drip can be difficult to control and may cause chronic cough that does not diminish until sinus drainage is controlled. If cough persists despite efforts at treatment, bronchoscopy should be considered to rule out an endobronchial lesion as the cause of the cough. (*Fishman, 1998*)

71. (B); 72. (A); 73. (A or B); 74. (C); 75. (D); 76. (D); 77. (E); 78. (E). *Discussion:* Clinical presentation can be very helpful in the initial assessment of bronchogenic carcinoma cell type because certain tumors tend to present in relatively distinct patterns. However, there is overlap in presentation, so that definitive histologic typing only occurs with biopsy. Small cell carcinoma usually originates centrally, in larger airways, and metastasizes early. In addition, small cell carcinoma is known to be associated with a number of paraneoplastic syndromes, including Eaton-Lambert syndrome, in which involved patients manifest muscle weakness and electromyography shows a characteristic increased action potential with repeat stimulation. Squamous cell carcinoma of the lung also usually presents as a central lung mass. In addition, squamous cell carcinoma is the primary lung malignancy associated with hypercalcemia, usually resulting from secretion of a parathyroid-like peptide by this malignancy. Bronchoalveolar carcinoma is a malignancy consisting of cells resembling airway lining cells. The chest radiograph manifestation of bronchoalveolar cell carcinoma is commonly an alveolar-like infiltrate that may contain air bronchograms. Adenocarcinoma of the lung is the bronchogenic carcinoma that is most likely to cause a single metastasis to the brain. In contrast, squamous cell carcinoma usually invades locally and small cell carcinoma metastasizes distally, but usually in multiple sites. The carcinoid syndrome, characterized by flushing, diarrhea, and bronchospasm, is due to release of a number of mediators by carcinoid tumors or, more rarely, small cell carcinomas. This syndrome generally only occurs with the tumor in a position where venous drainage does not pass through the liver before entering the systemic circulation. Carcinoid tumors are generally hypervascular on direct visualization. (*Cecil, Ch. 198*)

79. **(A)**; 80. **(E)**; 81. **(C)**; 82. **(D)**; 83. **(B)**. *Discussion:* Interstitial lung disease results from a number of processes with distinct histopathologic manifestations. IPF, a disorder that generally starts in the fifth or sixth decade, is manifested by insidious onset of exertional dyspnea with or without digital clubbing. Physical examination demonstrates lung crackles, and serum may show low-titer positive antinuclear antibody. Biopsy of the lung shows usual interstitial pneumonitis. Sarcoidosis is a multisystem disorder that is characterized by granulomatous inflammation in a number of organ systems; the lung and intrathoracic lymph nodes are involved most frequently. The syndrome of hilar adenopathy, erythema nodosum, and uveitis (Lofgren's syndrome) is almost always due to sarcoidosis and carries a favorable prognosis. Eosinophilic granuloma of the lung is a disease affecting smokers in which interstitial inflammation contains Langerhans' cells. Immunohistochemical stains that specifically detect these cells can be useful for the diagnosis of this disorder. Hypersensitivity pneumonitis (extrinsic allergic alveolitis) is a disorder associated with exposure to thermophilic fungi or other allergens that induce a delayed-type hypersensitivity reaction in the lung of the affected individual. Biopsy of the lung in this disorder demonstrates interstitial inflammation containing lymphocytes and monocytes as well as loosely formed noncaseating granulomas. Serum precipitins (precipitating antibodies) are generally positive in these patients, although these antibodies may be detected in patients who have been exposed to these allergens but do not have pulmonary disease. (*Cecil, Ch. 88*)

84. **(A or D)**; 85. **(A or E)**; 86. **(B)**; 87. **(B)**; 88. **(C or F)**; 89. **(C)**; 90. **(F)**. *Discussion:* Occupational exposures can result in a variety of pulmonary disorders. Pulmonary fibrosis can result from chronic exposure to minerals such as asbestos or silica. Asbestosis (pulmonary fibrosis secondary to asbestos exposure) occurs after a lag time of 10 to 20 years of exposure and can result in severe disability and widespread fibrosis. Silicosis (pulmonary disease caused by silica exposure) also occurs after a lag period, but the initial pulmonary lesion shows small, rounded opacities that consist of collagen fibrils histopathologically. With progressive disease, silicosis results in progressive fibrosis when the small nodules coalesce into larger opacities and symptoms can be more pronounced than in the early stages of the disorder. Diffuse alveolar damage and pulmonary alveolar proteinosis have also been described after short exposure periods to silica. Cotton dust and grain dust exposures cause occupational bronchitis. Endotoxins within these dusts are probably the inciting components for this syndrome. Both of these dusts can also cause fever in the absence of pulmonary symptoms, also probably resulting from endotoxin inhalation. Bronchitis secondary to cotton dust exposure tends to improve with continued exposure during the work week but worsen once again after returning to work from a period off the job. Many agents found in the workplace can cause asthma, manifested by variable bronchospasm and airway hyperreactivity. Isocyanates, chemicals used in spray paints and other industrial products, are an example of low-molecular-weight substances that cause asthma. Flour dust contains high-molecular-weight components, specifically proteins that induce antibody formation in some individuals and asthma in a subgroup of those individuals. In contrast, thermophilic fungi found in moldy hay can also induce production of antibodies by certain exposed individuals but a subgroup of these individuals experience interstitial inflammation containing lymphocytes and macrophages with loosely formed granulomas rather than asthma. The difference in disease manifestation between these two exposures probably relates to the type of subclass of antibody stimulated. (*Cecil, Ch. 89*)

91. **(E)**; 92. **(B)**; 93. **(C)**; 94. **(D)**; 95. **(A)**. *Discussion:* Pleural fluid exists in a balanced state between formation and absorption of fluid at the parietal surface. Excessive formation of pleural fluid results from an alteration in this balance. Increased formation may occur as a result of a reduction in plasma oncotic pressure (as in cirrhosis) or increased hydrostatic pressure (as in urinary obstruction or congestive heart failure), resulting in a transudation of plasma that is filtered through a relatively normal pleura, making the resultant transudate low in protein. Increased fluid formation can also occur as a result of involvement of the pleural surface with a process that alters the normal filtering process, and thus the resultant pleural fluid is relatively high in protein. One protein, LDH, is used to determine the amount of protein exudation into the pleural fluid. A value greater than 200 IU/L or a ratio of pleural fluid LDH to serum LDH of greater than 0.6 is strongly suggestive of an exudative pleural effusion. A ratio of total protein in the pleural fluid to serum total protein of greater than 0.5 is also suggestive of an exudative pleural effusion. Low glucose level or pH in pleural fluid is suggestive of an inflammatory process that results from metabolism of glucose, with formation of CO_2 and subsequent lowering of pH. A reduction in glucose can also occur as a result of impaired glucose transport into the pleural space, as in the case of pleural effusion caused by rheumatoid arthritis. Amylase may be elevated in pleural fluid for a variety of reasons, including carcinomatosis and pancreatitis. (*Cecil, Ch. 198; Sahn, 1988*)

96. **(C)**; 97. **(A)**; 98. **(B)**; 99. **(C)**; 100. **(F)**. *Discussion:* "Atypical pneumonias" (i.e., pneumonias with no culturable organism) are commonly caused by *Mycoplasma* or *Legionella* infection. Both of these organisms are susceptible to erythromycin therapy. *Chlamydia psittaci* can also cause an atypical pneumonia. Although this organism may be partially responsive to erythromycin, doxycycline is currently the drug of choice. *Pseudomonas aeruginosa*, a major cause of nosocomial pneumonia, has developed resistance patterns over the years, making use of certain agents, such as ampicillin, ineffective against this organism. In addition, although ciprofloxacin is an effective antibiotic against *Pseudomonas*, the development of resistance can be rapid, so ciprofloxacin is indicated only in infections caused by strains of *Pseudomonas* that are documented to be resistant to other agents. Both zanamivir and oseltamivir are effective against influenza A and will reduce symptoms if given within 30 to 36 hours after onset of symptoms. (*Cecil, Ch. 92; American Thoracic Society/CDC/IDSA, 2003*)

BIBLIOGRAPHY

American College of Chest Physicians: Sixth ACCP Consensus Conference on Antithrombotic Therapy. Chest 2001;119(Suppl.).

American Thoracic Society: Guidelines for the initial management of adults with community acquired pneumonia. Am Rev Respir Dis 2001;163:1730.

American Thoracic Society: Targeted tuberculin testing and treatment of latent tuberculosis infection. Am Rev Respir Dis 1999;161:5221.

American Thoracic Society/Centers for Disease Control: Diagnostic standards and classification of tuberculosis. Am Rev Respir Dis 1990;142:725.

American Thoracic Society/CDC/IDSA: Treatment of tuberculosis. Am Rev Respir Dis 2003;167:603.

Bartlett JG, Breiman RF, Mandell LA, File TM Jr: Community-acquired pneumonia in adults: Guidelines for management. Clin Infect Dis 1998;26:811.

Cooper JAD Jr, White DA, Matthay RA: State of the art: Drug-induced pulmonary disease. Am Rev Respir Dis 1986;133:321, 488.

Crystal RG: α_1-Antitrypsin deficiency, emphysema, and liver disease: Genetic basis and strategies for therapy. J Clin Invest 1990;85:1343.

Ferrer J: Pleural tuberculosis. Eur Respir J 1997;10:942.

Fishman AP (ed): Fishman's Pulmonary Diseases and Disorders, 3rd ed. New York, McGraw-Hill, 1998.

Goldhaber SZ: Pulmonary embolism. N Engl J Med 1998;339:93.

Goldman L, Ausiello D (eds): Cecil Textbook of Medicine, 22nd ed. Philadelphia, WB Saunders, 2004.

Hunninghake GW, Fauci AS: State of the art: Pulmonary involvement in the collagen vascular diseases. Am Rev Respir Dis 1979;119:471.

Kales A, Vela-Bueno A, Kales JD: Sleep disorders: Sleep apnea and narcolepsy. Ann Intern Med 1987;106:434.

Lumb A (ed): Nunn's Applied Respiratory Physiology, 5th ed. Woburn, MA, Butterworth-Heinemann, 2000

Metlay JP, Kapoor WN, Fine MJ: Does this patient have community-acquired pneumonia? Diagnosing pneumonia by history and physical examination. JAMA 1997;278:1440.

Moser KM: Venous thromboembolism. Am Rev Respir Dis 1990;141:2.

Mossman TR, Sad S: The expanding universe of T cell subsets: Th1, Th2 and more. Immunol Today 1996;17:138.

National Asthma Expert Panel Report—Guidelines for the Diagnosis and Management of Asthma. National Heart Lung and Blood Institutes, National Institutes of Health, 1997, updated in 2002.

Pack AI: Obstructive sleep apnea. Ann Intern Med 1994;39:517.

Sahn SA: State of the art: The pleura. Am Rev Respir Dis 1988;138:184.

Schlossberg D (ed): Tuberculosis and Nontuberculosis Mycobacterial Infections, 4th ed. Philadelphia, WB Saunders, 1999.

Schwarz MI, King TE (ed): Interstitial Lung Disease, 3rd ed. Hamilton, Ontario, BC Decker, 1998.

Taylor JR, Ryu J, Colby TV, Raffin TA: Lymphangioleiomyomatosis: Clinical course of 32 patients. N Engl J Med 1990;323:1254.

Winter SM, Ingbar DH: Massive hemoptysis: Pathogenesis and management. J Intensive Care Med 1988;3:171.

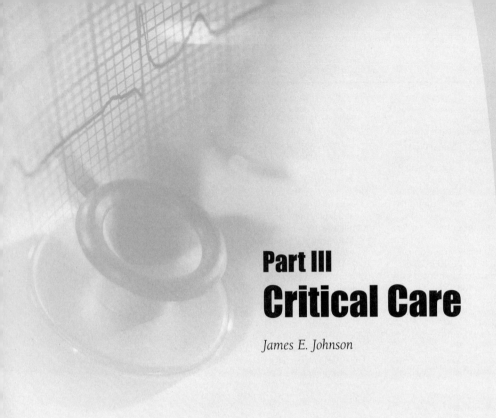

Part III
Critical Care

James E. Johnson

ABBREVIATIONS

ARDS—Acute respiratory distress syndrome
COPD—Chronic obstructive pulmonary disease
CVP—Central venous pressure
FIO_2—Fraction of inspired gas that is oxygen
J—Joules
PCO_2—Partial pressure of carbon dioxide
$PaCO_2$—Partial pressure of carbon dioxide in arterial blood
PEEP—Positive end-expiratory pressure
PO_2—Partial pressure of oxygen
PaO_2—Partial pressure of oxygen in arterial blood
SIMV—Synchronized intermittent mandatory ventilation
SVR—Systemic vascular resistance

MULTIPLE CHOICE

DIRECTIONS: For questions 1–30, choose the single best answer.

1. A 24-year-old man is seen in the emergency department for a severe asthma attack that does not respond to initial treatment. He is sedated, paralyzed, and intubated. The initial ventilator settings are as follows: assist control, volume control; rate 16; tidal volume, 700 mL; FIO_2, 100%; PEEP, 5 cm H_2O. The patient is not making any spontaneous ventilatory efforts. His peak pressure is 48 cm H_2O and plateau pressure is 28 cm H_2O. An arterial blood gas drawn after 20 minutes on these settings shows a pH of 7.24, $PaCO_2$ of 53 mm Hg, and PaO_2 of 342 mm Hg. Which of the following ventilator adjustments would be best?

   A. Reduce the FIO_2 to 80%
   B. Reduce the FIO_2 to 80% and increase the tidal volume to 800 mL
   C. Reduce the FIO_2 to 80% and increase the set rate to 20 per minute
   D. Reduce the FIO_2 to 80% and increase the PEEP to 10 cm H_2O
   E. Make no changes

2. A 75-year-old man develops diffuse bilateral infiltrates after an episode of bacteremia related to a urinary tract infection. He is intubated and placed on a mechanical ventilator. The application of positive end-expiratory pressure would be expected to do all of the following *except* which one?

   A. Increase the PaO_2/FIO_2 ratio
   B. Increase lung compliance
   C. Reduce intrapulmonary shunting
   D. Reduce lung water
   E. Increase end-expiratory lung volume

3. A 25-year-old 80-kg man has a motorcycle accident with a right midshaft femur fracture and develops diffuse bilateral infiltrates on the following day. The patient was wearing a helmet, and there was no significant head trauma or loss of consciousness. The most likely cause of the patient's lung condition is which of the following?

   A. Aspiration of gastric contents
   B. Nosocomial pneumonia due to gram-negative organisms
   C. Fat embolization syndrome
   D. Pulmonary thromboemboli
   E. Community-acquired pneumonia

4. The patient in Question 3 is intubated and placed on mechanical ventilation. After about 12 hours his settings and results of arterial blood gas analysis are as follows: assist control, volume control; set rate 18 (actual rate 18); tidal volume, 700 mL; FIO_2, 50%; PEEP, 10 cm H_2O; pH, 7.43; $PaCO_2$, 38 mm Hg; and PaO_2, 74 mm Hg. The peak and plateau pressures are 42 and 38 cm H_2O, respectively. What ventilator setting changes should be made at this point?

   A. Reduce the FIO_2 to 40%
   B. Reduce the rate to 14
   C. Reduce the tidal volume to 500 mL and increase the rate to 25 per minute
   D. Reduce the PEEP to 7.5 cm H_2O
   E. Make no changes

5. A 63-year-old 60-kg woman was intubated and ventilated with assist control, volume control for hypercapnic respiratory failure due to COPD and right lower lobe pneumonia. After 48 hours of treatment with antibiotics, bronchodilators, and corticosteroids, a spontaneous breathing trial is performed on the ventilator at a pressure support of 5 cm H_2O, FIO_2 of 30%, and PEEP of 0 cm H_2O. After 30 minutes on these settings, the monitoring equipment shows a tidal volume of 250 mL, a respiratory rate of 34 breaths per minute, and an oxygen saturation of 95%. What would you do at this point?

A. Extubate the patient
B. Resume mechanical ventilation at previous assist control settings
C. Resume mechanical ventilation using pressure control ventilation
D. Sedate and paralyze the patient and switch to SIMV

6. A patient is being mechanically ventilated with 100% oxygen and has the following arterial blood gas: pH 7.40; $PaCO_2$, 39 mm Hg; PaO_2, 63 mm Hg. What is the most likely mechanism of the hypoxemia?

A. Ventilation-perfusion mismatch
B. Intrapulmonary shunting
C. Pulmonary diffusion abnormalities
D. Hypoventilation
E. Low inhaled oxygen partial pressure

7. A 21-year-old man is found unconscious by his roommate and brought by ambulance to the emergency department. His vital signs are as follows: pulse, 90 beats/minute; blood pressure (BP), 120/70 mm Hg; temperature, 97.2° F; respirations, 12 breaths/minute. He is unresponsive to verbal or painful stimuli. His pupils are 2 mm and reactive, and his examination is otherwise unrevealing. An arterial blood gas analysis on room air shows a pH of 7.18; $PaCO_2$, 63 mm Hg; PaO_2, 75 mm Hg. His hypoxemia is most likely due to which of the following?

A. Hypoventilation only
B. Hypoventilation and aspiration pneumonia
C. Pulmonary thromboemboli
D. Neurogenic pulmonary edema
E. ARDS

8. All of the following are diagnostic criteria for ARDS except which one?

A. PaO_2/FIO_2 ratio of 200 or less
B. Bilateral pulmonary infiltrates
C. Increased respiratory compliance
D. No evidence of left atrial hypertension
E. Acute onset with appropriate clinical setting

9. A 21-year-old asthmatic man is brought to the emergency department for severe dyspnea that came on while mowing his grass. He is intubated for respiratory distress and is treated overnight with nebulized albuterol, intravenous steroids, and synchronized intermittent mandatory ventilation (SIMV). In the morning, he is agitated and requiring restraints. He is given a spontaneous breathing trial with pressure support of 5 cm H_2O, PEEP of 0 cm H_2O, and an FIO_2 of 30%; and after 30 minutes his tidal volume is 550 mL, his respiratory rate is 24 breaths/minute, and his oxygen saturation is 98%. What should be done at this point?

A. Sedate with lorazepam and resume SIMV
B. Sedate with lorazepam and paralyze with vecuronium and resume SIMV

C. Sedate with lorazepam and increase pressure support to 15 cm H_2O
D. Sedate with lorazepam and switch to assist control
E. Extubate the patient

10. A 16-year-old girl develops weakness in her lower extremities that progresses over a 3-day period to inability to walk unassisted. She then develops weakness in both of her arms. Physical examination on admission is normal with the exception of severe bilateral lower extremity weakness with inability to overcome gravity and less pronounced bilateral arm weakness. The best test to monitor this patient for the onset of life-threatening respiratory muscle weakness is which of the following?

A. Vital capacity
B. FEV_1
C. Peak flow
D. Negative inspiratory force
E. Arterial blood gases

11. Noninvasive ventilation by means of a face mask can be used at times to avoid endotracheal intubation. Which of the following clinical findings would indicate a need to proceed directly to endotracheal intubation without a trial of noninvasive ventilation?

A. Bronchospasm
B. Unresponsiveness
C. Pulmonary edema
D. Bilateral pneumonia
E. Neuromuscular weakness

12. Which one of the following vasopressors has the *least* direct effect on the heart?

A. Dopamine
B. Vasopressin
C. Dobutamine
D. Norepinephrine
E. Epinephrine

13. With hypovolemic shock, all of the following are reduced *except* which one?

A. Central venous pressure
B. Mean arterial pressure
C. Systemic vascular resistance
D. Cardiac output
E. Pulmonary capillary wedge pressure

14. A 75-year-old woman presents with pyuria and a temperature of 38.5° C (101.3° F), BP of 110/70 mm Hg, pulse of 115 beats/minute, respiratory rate of 22 breaths/minute, and a white blood cell count of 14,500/mm³. Which of the following does she have?

A. Systemic inflammatory response syndrome (SIRS)
B. Severe sepsis
C. Septic shock
D. Multiple organ dysfunction syndrome (MODS)
E. Bacteremia

15. A 68-year-old white woman presents with multilobar pneumonia, hypotension, and acute renal failure and is treated initially with broad-spectrum antibiotics, mechanical ventilation, vasopressors, and fluids. In addition to these measures, which of the following should also be given?

A. Methylprednisolone, 1g intravenously
B. Ibuprofen, 800 mg per nasogastric tube
C. Activated protein C intravenously
D. Monoclonal antibodies to tumor necrosis factor (TNF) intravenously

16. Severe hypothermia is sometimes missed on initial evaluation. The temperature may be reported as the lower limit of the thermometer, which may be only a few degrees below normal. Which of the following tests has findings that are characteristic enough to indicate the diagnosis?

    A. Serum electrolytes
    B. Electrocardiogram
    C. Arterial blood gases
    D. Serum thyroid-stimulating hormone (TSH) level
    E. Chest radiograph

17. A 19-year-old man collapses while training for a marathon and is brought to the emergency department. His temperature is measured to be 41.6° C (106.8° F). Which of the following should be the initial treatment?

    A. Cold intravenous fluids
    B. Iced saline gastric lavage
    C. Peritoneal lavage
    D. Wetting and fanning of the skin
    E. Intubation and muscular paralysis with vecuronium

18. A black widow spider bite is most likely to be associated with which of the following?

    A. Disseminated intravascular coagulation
    B. Painful muscle spasm
    C. Coma
    D. Local tissue necrosis
    E. Bradyarrhythmias

19. The initial decision about the dose of antivenin for a patient with a rattlesnake bite should be made based on the local reaction at the bite, systemic signs and symptoms, and which of the following?

    A. Coagulation parameters
    B. Serum BUN and creatinine
    C. Serum creatine phosphokinase
    D. Hematocrit
    E. White count

20. A patient who presents with botulism from eating home-processed food is most likely to have which of the following?

    A. Tetany
    B. Diplopia
    C. Fever
    D. Acute renal failure
    E. Rhabdomyolysis

21. A 24-year-old woman with long-standing type I diabetes presents with a 5-day history of severe nausea and vomiting with coffee-ground emesis for the past 12 hours. The pulse rate is 134 beats/minute; BP, 95/50 mm Hg; temperature, 36.5° C; and respiratory rate, 22 breaths/minute. Selected laboratory tests are as follows: pH, 7.40; $Paco_2$, 39 mm Hg; Pao_2, 164 mm Hg (breathing oxygen at 3 L/minute); sodium, 141 mEq/L; potassium, 4.1 mEq/L; chloride, 83 mEq/L; bicarbonate, 22 mEq/L; BUN, 89 mg/dL; creatinine, 3.6 mg/dL; glucose, 909 mg/dL. Which of the following best describes the patient's acid-base status?

    A. No acid-base disturbance
    B. Primary metabolic alkalosis
    C. Primary metabolic acidosis
    D. Primary metabolic acidosis and primary metabolic alkalosis
    E. Triple primary disturbance—metabolic acidosis, respiratory acidosis, and metabolic alkalosis

22. A 63-year-old man presents to the emergency department with sudden severe chest pain radiating through to his back.

He has a long history of hypertension and a remote smoking history. His pulse is 108 beats/minute and BP is 160/100 mm Hg in both arms. He has a left femoral bruit, but otherwise his cardiovascular examination is unremarkable. His electrocardiogram shows left ventricular hypertrophy, and his portable chest x-ray film is normal. A CT scan with contrast medium enhancement shows an aortic dissection beginning just distal to the left subclavian artery and extending to the diaphragm. Which of the following should be done?

    A. Aortography
    B. Coronary angiography
    C. Surgical repair
    D. Intra-aortic balloon counter-pulsation
    E. Intravenous labetalol

23. A 62-year-old man with chronic alcoholism is admitted for nausea, vomiting, and abdominal pain. His clinical findings and laboratory tests are consistent with pancreatitis, and he is treated with intravenous dextrose 5% in 0.5 normal saline with 20 mEq/L of potassium and multivitamins at a rate of 125 mL/hour. After 48 hours, he develops rising creatine phosphokinase levels along with myoglobinuria. An abnormal level of which of the following is the probable cause for this?

    A. Potassium
    B. Sodium
    C. Bicarbonate
    D. Phosphorus
    E. Calcium

24. A 32-year-old male body builder is brought to the emergency department after being found unresponsive in the locker room of the gym. On arrival he is apneic and is immediately intubated. He is agitated and combative when stimulated but quickly becomes lethargic and apneic when he is not stimulated. BP is 136/68 mm Hg; pulse is 96 beats/minute; and he is afebrile. The remainder of his examination is unrevealing. He does not respond to administration of naloxone, flumazenil, or D_5W. Specimens drawn for arterial blood gas analysis after intubation show pH of 7.32, $Paco_2$ of 51 mm Hg, and Pao_2 of 479 mm Hg while he is receiving 100% oxygen via mechanical ventilator. Initial electrolytes, CBC, liver enzymes, and coagulation studies were normal. ECG shows sinus rhythm at 92 beats/minute and normal QRS and QT intervals. Urine drug screen was negative for opiates, benzodiazepines, tricyclics, cocaine, or cannabinoids. Blood ethanol level was 0. Which of the following statements best describes the expected outcome?

    A. He becomes progressively more alert, responsive, and appropriate over the next 3-5 hours. He is extubated 6 hours after admission with no sequelae.
    B. Oxalate crystals are found in the urine. He develops progressive acidosis and shock requiring pressor support. Fomepizole is given along with hemodialysis with gradual improvement over 36 hours.
    C. Two hours after admission, he develops ventricular tachycardia. A bicarbonate infusion is begun, but he develops seizures and refractory ventricular tachycardia and dies.
    D. Cardiac enzymes reveal evidence of myocardial necrosis. A subsequent ECG shows ST segment elevation in V_1 to V_3. He improves over 24 hours, and a cardiac catheterization shows normal coronary arteries.

25. A 35-year-old multiparous woman in her 37th week of pregnancy is referred because of suspected hepatitis. She

presented to a walk-in clinic 1 week ago with malaise and nausea and was treated symptomatically. She now reports continued malaise, nausea, and right upper quadrant abdominal pain. She reports no fever or chills. BP is 160/100 mm Hg, pulse is 104 beats/minute, respiratory rate is 22 breaths/minute, and temperature is 37.1° C. There is mild scleral icterus. The lungs are clear. A grade 2/6 systolic murmur is present at the upper left sternal border. The abdomen is nontender. The uterus is gravid, and fetal heart tones are normal. There is pitting edema of the lower extremities. Neurologic examination is normal. Laboratory tests are notable for hematocrit of 30%, WBC count of 7,800/μL, and platelet count of 65,000/μL, INR is 1.2, creatinine is 1.6 mg/dL, and electrolytes are normal. Urinalysis shows 1+ protein with a normal sediment. Serum glutamic oxaloacetic transaminase (alanine transaminase) is 140 U/L (normal 0-31), and lactate dehydrogenase is 1020 U/L (normal 120-240). Total bilirubin is 3.4 mg/dL (normal 0-1.0). All of the following statements are true *except* which one?

A. She is at increased risk for seizures, renal failure, and/or hepatic rupture
B. The peripheral blood smear is likely to show schistocytes.
C. Immediate delivery is the most appropriate therapy.
D. Platelet transfusion is indicated because of the increased risk of maternal bleeding.

26. All of the following decrease delivery and uptake of oxygen to peripheral tissues *except* which one?

A. Decreased cardiac output
B. Increased carboxyhemoglobin concentration
C. Alkalosis
D. Fever
E. Decreased 2,3-diphosphoglycerate (2,3-DPG)

27. A 24-year-old woman is being mechanically ventilated for ARDS. On the fifth hospital day, subcutaneous air is noted in her neck along with what sounds like a pericardial rub. Chest radiograph shows pneumopericardium, pneumomediastinum and a small amount of subcutaneous air in the neck. The patient's status is otherwise unchanged from the day before. Which one of the following is true?

A. Placement of bilateral chest tubes is indicated.
B. Mediastinal drainage should be performed.
C. A pericardial catheter should be inserted.
D. A needle drainage catheter should be placed in the neck.
E. The patient is at increased risk of pneumothorax and should be monitored.

28. A 22-year-old man with known human immunodeficiency virus infection is admitted to the hospital with progressive dyspnea and fever. He has been on dapsone for prophylaxis against *Pneumocystis*. The chest radiograph reveals right lower lobe pneumonia, and a cephalosporin is administered. A pulse oximeter shows an adequate waveform with a saturation of 85% on 6 L/minute of oxygen by nasal cannula. However, an arterial blood gas sample drawn simultaneously reveals a PaO_2 of 150 mm Hg. What is the most likely diagnosis?

A. Elevated methemoglobin
B. Elevated carboxyhemoglobin
C. A congenital hemoglobinopathy with left shift of the oxygen-hemoglobin dissociation curve
D. Shock with digital hypoperfusion

29. The antidote for digitalis intoxication works by which of the following mechanisms?

A. Altering tissue binding by increasing plasma pH
B. Increasing clearance by reducing urinary pH
C. Reducing metabolism to a toxic metabolite by inhibiting an enzyme
D. Binding to the molecule, thereby reducing its effect and increasing clearance
E. Raising intracellular cyclic adenosine monophosphate by stimulating an alternate cell membrane receptor

30. A 53-year-old man is admitted to the intensive care unit (ICU) with a history of increasing angina. Nitroglycerin and heparin infusions are started. Two hours later he develops severe chest pain and diaphoresis. During examination, he suddenly becomes unresponsive and no pulse can be obtained. The monitor shows coarse ventricular fibrillation. Which of the following is the best initial intervention?

A. Unsynchronized countershock, 200 J
B. Synchonized countershock, 100 J
C. Lidocaine, 100 mg intravenous bolus
D. Intubation and bag ventilation
E. Epinephrine, 1 mg intravenous bolus

MATCHING

DIRECTIONS: Please match the following questions with the most appropriate answer. Each answer may be used only once.

Four clinical scenarios are followed by four sets of ventilator settings. Please match the scenario with the most appropriate ventilator settings. All of the patients are on assist control, volume control.

31. A 40-year-old 60-kg woman with ARDS due to alcoholic pancreatitis

32. A 21-year-old 60-kg woman with severe diabetic ketoacidosis and urosepsis with a normal chest radiograph (pH, 6.92; Pco_2, 12 mm Hg; Po_2, 110 mm Hg on room air before intubation)

33. A 68-year-old, 60-kg woman with an exacerbation of COPD due to lobar pneumonia

34. A 56-year-old 60-kg woman with bullous emphysema and wedge resection of right upper lobe nodular lesion now with large air leak and a chest tube

	Tidal Volume (mL)	Machine Resp Rate (per min)	Fio_2 (%)	PEEP (cm H_2O)
A.	550	14	35	0
B.	550	28	28	0
C.	550	14	35	5
D.	360	32	50	14

The following are four clinical settings. Please match them to the hemodynamic parameters obtained from pulmonary artery catheterization that follow. Pressures are given in mm Hg and systemic vascular resistance (SVR) is in dyne sec/cm⁵.

35. A 57-year-old man presents with dizziness, fatigue, and weight loss. He had a stage II lung cancer resected a year ago. Examination reveals a pulse rate of 125 beats/minute and a BP of 78/40 mm Hg. Chest x-ray film shows an enlarged cardiac silhouette.

36. A 63-year-old man presents with severe substernal chest pain and diaphoresis. Examination reveals a pulse rate of 110 beats/minute and a BP of 85/42 mm Hg. The electrocardiogram shows ST segment elevation in V_1 through V_4.

37. A 73-year-old woman presents with fever and flank pain. Examination reveals a temperature of 103.2° F, a pulse of 122 beats/minute, and BP of 80/48 mm Hg. Urinalysis documents pyuria.

38. A 60-year-old man has chest pain and dyspnea 4 days after a hip replacement. His pulse is 110 beats/minute and BP is 90/50 mm Hg.

	Mean Arterial Pressure	Central Venous Pressure	Pulmonary Artery Pressure	Wedge Pressure	Cardiac Output (L/min)	SVR
A.	56	12	38/28	26	2.3	1530
B.	60	15	48/30	9	2.6	1380
C.	53	2	22/8	4	9.8	420
D.	55	18	30/18	19	3.1	950

Please match the drug with the most appropriate treatment for overdose/intoxication.

39. Acetaminophen

40. Metoprolol

41. Organophosphate insecticide

42. Ethylene glycol

43. Cyclic antidepressant

    A. Fomepizole
    B. Glucagon
    C. Pralidoxime
    D. *N*-Acetylcysteine
    E. Alkalinization of the blood

Match the following types of respiratory failures to the most appropriate causative disease.

44. Hypercapnic respiratory failure

45. Hypoxemic respiratory failure

46. Failure of oxygen extraction

47. Reduced arterial oxygen content

48. Normal arterial oxygen content with reduced delivery

    A. Carbon monoxide poisoning
    B. Cardiac tamponade
    C. Acute respiratory distress syndrome
    D. Amyotrophic lateral sclerosis
    E. Cyanide poisoning

Match the following clinical syndrome of toxicity to the appropriate agent.

49. Delirium, dry mucous membranes, urinary retention

50. Abdominal pain, fasciculations, paralysis

51. Abdominal pain, blurred vision, altered mental status, anion-gap acidosis

52. Cardiac arrhythmias, vomiting, seizures

53. Seizures, hypotension, prolonged QT interval

54. Hypotension, bradycardia, coma

    A. Theophylline
    B. Verapamil
    C. Scopolamine
    D. Amitriptyline
    E. Insecticide
    F. Wood alcohol

Please match the following nutrient with the clinical finding associated with its deficiency.

55. Thiamine

56. Vitamin C

57. Zinc

58. Vitamin K

    A. Coagulopathy and bleeding
    B. Ophthalmoplegia
    C. Capillary fragility
    D. Diarrhea

TRUE OR FALSE

DIRECTIONS: Please answer true or false for the following questions.

Figures III-1 and III-2 are plots of airway pressure vs. time for a patient who is heavily sedated and making no effort to breathe as she is given

Airway Pressure vs. Time

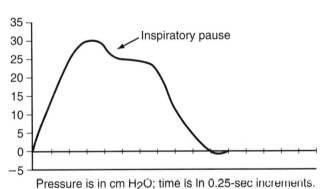

Pressure is in cm H_2O; time is in 0.25-sec increments.

FIGURE III-1

Airway Pressure vs. Time

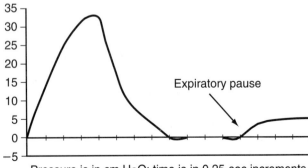

Pressure is in cm H_2O; time is in 0.25-sec increments.

FIGURE III-2

500 mL tidal volumes. Expiratory and inspiratory pauses are done at separate times. Please answer the following questions true or false.

59. The peak pressure is 30 cm H_2O

60. The inspiratory plateau pressure is 15 cm H_2O

61. The patient has no intrinsic PEEP (auto-PEEP)

Which of the following are true regarding arterial P_{CO_2} (Pa_{CO_2}) in patients who are intubated and mechanically ventilated?

62. A patient with normal lungs with a minute ventilation of 7 L/minute and a Pa_{CO_2} of 40 mm Hg would be expected to have a Pa_{CO_2} of about 20 mm Hg if the minute ventilation is doubled.

63. A patient with normal lungs and a Pa_{CO_2} of 40 mm Hg would be expected to have an end-tidal P_{CO_2} of 38 to 40 mm Hg.

64. A patient with severe COPD and a Pa_{CO_2} of 40 mm Hg would be expected to have an end-tidal P_{CO_2} of about 45 to 50 mm Hg.

65. At a constant minute ventilation and calorie intake, a high fat feeding formula would be expected to increase Pa_{CO_2} as compared with a high carbohydrate formula.

Which of the following are true in regard to various modalities for mechanically ventilating patients?

66. Two patients are on mechanical ventilators, each receiving a tidal volume of 500 mL at a machine set rate of 12 breaths/minute. Both are breathing faster than the set rate such that the total respiratory rate is about 20 breaths/minute. The one on synchronized intermittent mechanical ventilation (SIMV) is more likely than the one on assist control to get 500 mL of gas with every breath.

67. A patient on pressure support ventilation can vary the tidal volume delivered by increasing or decreasing his own respiratory effort.

68. Pressure control ventilation cycles (goes from inhalation to exhalation) based on gas flow.

69. Pressure support is a better modality than pressure control for a patient who may not initiate breaths.

All of the following modalities have been shown to improve arterial oxygenation in patients with ARDS. Please mark true for the ones that have also been shown conclusively in randomized clinical trials to reduce mortality in this patient group.

70. Inhaled nitric oxide

71. Prone positioning

72. Positive end-expiratory pressure (PEEP)

73. Extracorporeal membrane oxygenation

Which of the following are true regarding cardiogenic shock in patients with acute myocardial infarction?

74. It is more likely in patients with myocardial infarctions with ST segment elevation as compared with those without ST segment elevation.

75. Mixed venous saturation levels are reduced.

76. Intra-aortic balloon counter-pulsation is contraindicated in the presence of acute mitral regurgitation.

77. Acute coronary revascularization improves survival in this setting.

QUESTIONS 78–82

A 19-year-old male diabetic is admitted for diabetic ketoacidosis brought on by a gastrointestinal infection. He initially has a serum glucose of 645 mg/dL, a serum bicarbonate of 8 mEq/L, and an arterial pH of 7.22. Over the first 8 hours he is given 2 L of saline and an insulin infusion at 7 units/hour. At the end of 8 hours he feels better and his pulse is 105 beats/minute, BP 115/60 mm Hg, temperature is 36.8° C, and respirations are 18 breaths/minute and unlabored. His laboratory tests are as follows: sodium, 136 mEq/L; potassium, 3.2 mEq/L; chloride, 98 mEq/L; bicarbonate, 14 mEq/L; BUN, 22 mg/dL; creatinine, 1.3 mg/dL, and glucose, 164 mg/dL. Please mark true for the things that should be done at this point.

78. Discontinue the insulin drip and give regular insulin subcutaneously

79. Discontinue intravenous fluids

80. Give intravenous bicarbonate

81. Begin 5% dextrose in normal saline by constant IV infusion

82. Add potassium to intravenous fluids

QUESTIONS 83–87

A 22-year-old woman with advanced cystic fibrosis is admitted to the ICU after coughing up about 700 mL of blood over a 12-hour period. The patient had an FEV_1 measured 3 months ago at 24% of predicted. Chest radiograph shows increased interstitial markings with preserved lung volumes and extensive cystic appearing changes consistent with diffuse bronchiectasis. There is a new infiltrate in the right upper lobe. Bronchoscopy confirms the right upper lobe as the bleeding site. Which of the following are true?

83. Lung cancer due to chronic inflammation is the probable cause of the bleeding.

84. Surgical lobectomy should be recommended.

85. Antibiotic therapy is likely to be sufficient treatment for the hemoptysis.

86. If bronchial artery embolization is attempted, the patient should be counseled about paraplegia as a possible complication.

87. The patient should have the left lung down during active bleeding.

QUESTIONS 88–92

A 72-year-old woman is hospitalized with urosepsis. Acute respiratory distress syndrome (ARDS) subsequently develops, prompting transfer to the ICU. Because of high peak pressures, the patient is switched from assist control, volume control to assist control, pressure control with a driving pressure of 24 cm H_2O, inspiratory time of 0.75 second, set rate of 20/minute, PEEP of 10 cm H_2O, and F_{IO_2} of 60%. Delivered tidal volumes are initially 420 mL and total minute ventilation is 8.4 L/minute. When you examine the patient the next morning the tidal volume has dropped to 300 mL. Please indicate as true the possible explanations for the reduction in tidal volume.

88. The patient's lung inflammation and pulmonary edema are improving.

89. The patient is making less respiratory effort.

90. The patient is breathing faster than the set rate of the ventilator and has developed auto-PEEP.

91. The patient has retained secretions in her endotracheal tube.

92. The patient has developed a pneumothorax.

QUESTIONS 93–97

A 76-year-old man with severe COPD is admitted to the ICU with influenza complicated by right lower lobe pneumonia and respiratory failure. Other than COPD, his medical problems are minor. By the fourth hospital day, his fever has gone but he remains unable to breathe on his own. He is being treated with amantidine, ceftriaxone (Rocephin), azithromycin, and methylprednisolone as well as inhaled albuterol and ipratropium. Indicate as true those things that are likely to reduce his overall complication rate or his chance of dying in the ICU.

93. Changing his ventilator circuitry every 24 hours.

94. Transfusing packed red blood cells whenever his hemoglobin drops below 9 g/dL

95. Beginning an insulin infusion to maintain tight control of his blood sugar for persistent elevations of the glucose in the 160- to 220-mg/dL range.

96. Giving heparin, 5000 units, subcutaneously twice or three times per day

97. Giving ranitidine, 50 mg, intravenously every 8 hours

QUESTIONS 98–100

Which of the following are benefits of tracheostomy over continued endotracheal intubation for a patient who has already been mechanically ventilated with an endotracheal tube for two weeks and who is not likely to be extubated within the immediately foreseeable future?

98. Patient comfort is increased

99. The risk of laryngeal trauma is reduced.

100. The risk of tracheal stenosis is substantially reduced

Part III
Critical Care
Answers

1. **(A)** *Discussion:* The patient has a very high PaO_2, so the FIO_2 can be reduced. Answer B is incorrect because peak airway pressure is already high and increasing tidal volume will raise it farther. Answer C is incorrect because high respiratory rates produce auto-PEEP in patients with severe airflow obstruction. The patient likely already has substantial amounts of auto-PEEP contributing to his high airway pressures. Both B and C are tempting answers in that increasing ventilation usually improves respiratory acidosis. In this case, allowing some degree of respiratory acidosis (permissive hypercapnia) is preferable to increasing airway pressures farther. Answer D is incorrect because external PEEP is of little benefit to obstructed patients. If the patient is spontaneously breathing on the ventilator and has substantial auto-PEEP, applied PEEP at less than 80% of the auto-PEEP level can lower the threshold to trigger the breath. We are not told the amount of auto-PEEP in this case, and the patient is not spontaneously breathing. *(Cecil, Ch. 99)*

2. **(D)** *Discussion:* In patients with ARDS, PEEP works by recruiting alveoli that contain fluid. Ventilation of these alveoli reduces the amount of blood that is shunted through the lungs without ever coming into close proximity with air. This increases PaO_2 at any given inhaled oxygen percentage. Also, ventilation of these additional alveoli increases lung compliance by allowing the tidal volume to be distributed through more lung tissue. The lungs are more inflated at end-exhalation owing to the additional pressure. PEEP does not actually remove fluid from the lungs. Also, using PEEP prophylactically in situations with high risk of developing ARDS does not prevent the development of ARDS. *(Cecil, Chs. 99 and 101)*

3. **(C)** *Discussion:* Patients with long bone fractures are at risk for embolization of bone marrow contents. Fatty acids are toxic to the lung when arriving in this fashion. The result is an acute lung injury with all the clinical features of ARDS. In the absence of head trauma or loss of consciousness, aspiration of gastric contents is unlikely but could produce the same picture. There is no reason to think the patient would have a community-acquired pneumonia, and it is too early for nosocomial pneumonia. Pulmonary thromboemboli are not associated with diffuse infiltrates. *(Cecil, Ch. 99)*

4. **(C)** *Discussion:* Patients with ARDS have improved survival with lower tidal volume ventilation, as demonstrated by the ARDSnet trial comparing 6 mL/kg to 12 mL/kg in a randomized study. Reducing the patient's tidal volume to 500 mL comes close to that goal for this 80-kg patient. This should reduce the plateau pressure as well. A plateau pressure of 30 cm H_2O or less is a secondary goal in ventilating these patients. Reducing the tidal volume without increasing the rate is likely to lead to CO_2 retention if the rate is not increased. The overall minute ventilation will be about the same if the rate is increased to 25 from 18 at the same time the tidal volume is reduced. A follow-up arterial blood gas analysis should be obtained in 20 to 30 minutes. *(Cecil, Ch. 99)*

5. **(B)** *Discussion:* Patients with respiratory failure must be assessed for evidence that they have improved enough to be extubated. The best single indicator is the rapid shallow breathing index calculated as the respiratory frequency divided by the tidal volume (in liters) during a spontaneous breathing trial. In this case the F/TV ratio is 34/0.25 = 136. The cutoff value predicting successful extubation is a value less than 105. The original study was done with the patient taken transiently off the ventilator and allowed to breathe through a handheld spirometer, but spontaneous breathing trials done on low levels of pressure support work just about as well. The ratio at 30 to 60 minutes is more predictive than the ratio immediately after initiation of spontaneous breathing. Conditions that produce respiratory failure tend to cause the patient to breathe in a rapid shallow manner (high ratio). Improvement in the patient's condition tends to produce a reduction in the ratio. This patient should not be extubated yet but should be put back on mechanical ventilation. Pressure control has little advantage in obstructed patients over volume control. Paralysis should be avoided if at all possible especially in patients who are on steroids. *(Cecil, Ch. 101)*

6. **(B)** *Discussion:* Hypoxemia that is refractory to 100% oxygen is essentially always due to shunting of blood from the right- to left-sided circulation in either the lungs (ARDS with blood traversing alveoli filled with fluid) or in the heart (right to left intracardiac shunt such as an atrial septal defect with reversed flow). Hypoventilation as a cause of hypoxemia is associated with an elevated $PaCO_2$. Ventilation-perfusion mismatch, diffusion abnormalities, and hypoventilation all have substantial increases in PaO_2 with breathing 100% oxygen. Low inhaled PO_2 is by definition not present when breathing 100% oxygen at any barometric pressure present in the lower levels of the Earth's atmosphere. However, with acute unexplained hypoxemia, the possibility that the gas administered is not actually 100% oxygen should be entertained. Giving compressed air instead of oxygen happens occasionally, and there has been at least one instance of a hospital oxygen system being filled with the wrong gas (argon). *(Cecil, Ch. 99)*

7. **(A)** *Discussion:* The case description is that of a sedative overdose vs. an intracranial catastrophe such as a subarachnoid hemorrhage. Such patients are at risk for respiratory failure due to lack of respiratory effort from brain stem suppression or damage. They are also at risk for neurogenic pulmonary edema or aspiration due to lack of airway protective reflexes. In this case the problem appears to be hypoventilation alone, based on the result of blood gas analysis. One could do a formal alveolar gas equation calculation assuming a barometric pressure of about 760 mm Hg or just recognize that when breathing room air at any barometric pressure the PaO_2 drops about 1 mm Hg for every 1 mm Hg the $PaCO_2$ rises (the exact relationship is 1/R, where R is the respiratory quotient—about 0.8 for most people). Given that the $PaCO_2$ has risen 23 mm Hg above normal, the PaO_2 would be expected to drop about the same amount. Hence, the entire drop to 75 mm Hg can be explained by

hypoventilation (assuming a starting Pa_{O_2} in the 90s) without invoking a process such as pneumonia, neurogenic pulmonary edema, or ARDS. Pulmonary thromboemboli usually are associated with a low Pa_{CO_2}. Also, one would have to invoke two unrelated processes to account for the patient's findings because pulmonary thromboemboli would not explain the unresponsiveness. (*Cecil, Ch. 99*)

8. **(C)** *Discussion:* Based on the American European Consensus Conference definition, acute respiratory distress syndrome is a condition characterized by bilateral infiltrates with poor oxygenation ($Pa_{O_2}/F_{IO_2} < 200$). Because a similar picture could occur owing to left-sided heart failure, the patient should have no evidence of elevated left atrial pressure (this can be determined either clinically or by invasive testing by pulmonary artery catheterization). Because chronic conditions such as advanced diffuse infiltrative lung diseases can meet these criteria, the diagnosis should only be made when the infiltrates come on acutely (hours to days) in a proper clinical setting known to be associated with lung injury. Lung compliance is usually reduced, not increased, with ARDS although this is not part of the formal definition. (*Cecil, Ch. 99*)

9. **(E)** *Discussion:* This patient has a rapid shallow breathing index (see discussion for question 5) of 24/0.55 = 44, well below the cutoff value of 105. His agitation is probably due to the endotracheal tube rather than to his underlying respiratory problems. Although he almost certainly has some ongoing bronchospasm, he will probably do well with removal from assisted ventilation at this point. If he is kept on the machine, he should be sedated. Benzodiazepams such as lorazepam are effective, and often narcotics such as morphine are needed as well to reduce the cough reflex and relieve discomfort associated with intubation. Paralyzing agents should be avoided or minimized especially with concomitant treatment with steroids because the combination increases neuromuscular complications. (*Cecil, Ch. 101*)

10. **(A)** *Discussion:* This patient almost certainly has Guillain-Barré syndrome with ascending symmetrical weakness. Many of these patients go on to develop respiratory failure due to involvement of phrenic and intercostal nerves. Changes in arterial blood gases occur late in the course and should not be used as the primary means of following them. Traditionally, the vital capacity has been measured at the bedside with a simple handheld spirometer. The measurement can be repeated every few hours by respiratory therapists or nursing personnel. The normal value is about 70 mL/kg, and as respiratory muscle dysfunction progresses this declines. Values at or below 10 mL/kg are associated with respiratory failure. Timed volumes like the FEV_1 require more sophisticated equipment. FEV_1, peak flow, and respiratory pressures will also decline with worsening respiratory muscle function but have not been as well studied as means of following such patients. (*Cecil, Ch. 100*)

11. **(B)** *Discussion:* Noninvasive ventilation can be delivered via tight-fitting nose/mouth or nose-only masks with less expensive machines that typically use pressure assistance for the patient's own spontaneous breaths. This can reduce the need for intubation in a variety of clinical settings as the patient's problem is treated. It works best with an awake, cooperative patient. Unresponsiveness may be associated with a lack of airway protective reflexes. Also, obstructive sleep apnea (OSA) is fairly common in the general population. Upper airway obstruction due to OSA whether previously diagnosed or not is more of a problem when the patient is unconscious. Finally, such a patient is at greater risk of becoming apneic due to the underlying central nervous system dysfunction. Whereas noninvasive ventilation can be set up to have mandatory timed triggering, it usually does not work well for providing full ventilatory support for a completely apneic person. (*Cecil, Ch. 101*)

12. **(B)** *Discussion:* Vasopressin has essentially no direct effects on the heart. It is the only one of the pressors listed that is not chemically related to epinephrine. All of the others stimulate heart rate, contractility, or both, with norepinephrine having the least direct cardiac effect. Vasopressin, once used mainly for variceal bleeding, is now being used as a pure vasoconstricting pressor. It is typically added at a fixed intravenous constant infusion dose as a second or third pressor for patients with severe shock. (*Cecil, Ch. 103*)

13. **(C)** *Discussion:* Hypovolemic shock occurs due to blood or fluid volume loss. As a result, cardiac filling pressures such as central venous pressure and left atrial pressure (and hence pulmonary capillary wedge pressure) are reduced. Cardiac output is therefore reduced because of the low preload. Systemic vascular resistance is high as compensatory measures such as increased sympathetic autonomic activity attempt to maintain systemic BP. As compensatory measures fail, mean arterial pressure falls as well. (*Cecil, Ch. 102*)

14. **(A)** *Discussion:* The patient meets the definition of SIRS, which requires at least two of the following four criteria: temperature $> 38°$ or $< 36°$ C; heart rate > 90 beats/minute; respiratory rate > 20 breaths/minute or $Pa_{CO_2} < 32$ mm Hg; and WBC > 12,000 or $< 4,000/\mu L$, or > 10% immature forms. She also meets the definition of sepsis (which was not one of the choices) because she meets the SIRS definition in the presence of evidence of infection. The question does not give enough information to decide whether she has severe sepsis or MODS because there is no information about organ function. Both of these definitions require the presence of organ dysfunction. The patient does not meet the definition of septic shock because this requires hypotension or vasopressor use despite adequate fluid repletion in addition to organ dysfunction. She may have bacteremia, but this will not be known until blood culture results are available. (*Cecil, Ch. 104*)

15. **(C)** *Discussion:* Activated protein C (drotrecogin alfa), given in addition to standard therapy, has been shown to reduce mortality. In the study, patients received the medication by continuous intravenous infusion for 96 hours. The drug has effects on the inflammatory cascade as well as inhibiting coagulation. High doses of steroids do not improve survival, but evidence suggests that aggressively searching for relative adrenal insufficiency in these patients and treating with replacement corticosteroids may improve the outcome. Evidence also supports that aggressively repleting fluid volume early (in the first 6 hours) and using vasopressors and inotropic agents to reach specific circulatory goals improves mortality. Ibuprofen and monoclonal anti-TNF antibodies have not been shown to help. (*Cecil, Ch. 104*)

16. **(B)** *Discussion:* Hypothermia must be considered in patients who present with mental status changes. If mildly reduced temperature values are recorded for such a patient (94° to 95° F), measurement with a device with a broader range should be undertaken. The diagnosis is sometimes first considered after the electrocardiogram is examined. At about 32° C (90° F), the J wave of Osborne appears on the ECG. This is an extra hump on the end of the R wave. Typically, the electrocardiogram also shows bradycardia, slowing of AV conduction, widening of the QRS and QT intervals, and T wave inversion, but these findings are less specific. The TSH may be elevated if hypothyroidism is a contributing factor to the hypothermia, but most of these patients are not hypothyroid. Neither serum electrolytes nor the chest radiograph have specific abnormalities, but they help screen for comorbidities. Hypothermia affects arterial blood gases because the blood gas machine microprocessor is programmed to assume that the blood was drawn from a person with normal body temperature. Because of the effect of temperature on solubility of the gases and on the interaction with hemoglobin, the measured values will have a higher

Pa_{O_2} and Pa_{CO_2} and lower pH than are actually present in vivo. While these effects may be important in proper interpretation of the blood gas report, they do not help with making the diagnosis of hypothermia. (*Cecil, Ch. 105*)

17. **(D)** *Discussion:* This patient has hyperthermia due to environmental exposure and exertion. Neuromuscular paralysis is not going to help substantially with cooling at this point. The key intervention for such patients is to immediately begin external cooling by wetting the patient and fanning him. This takes advantage of the heat of vaporization of water, which can remove a considerable amount of heat quickly. It is also easy to start this in the prehospital phase, and many athletic and military personnel are acquainted with this approach. Intravenous fluids should be room temperature. Iced saline gastric lavage can be used as can peritoneal lavage, but these are more invasive and take longer to initiate. (*Cecil, Ch. 105*)

18. **(B)** *Discussion:* A black widow spider bite often goes unnoticed and begins producing symptoms in as little as 10 minutes or up to 2 hours later. The bite site itself is unremarkable with little tissue reaction. The venom has neuromuscular effects first in the local area and then more generally with dull pain and then painful muscle spasms. The patient may have a boardlike abdomen and may have enough muscle rigidity to have some respiratory difficulties. Cardiac dysrhythmias sometimes occur but usually are tachyarrhythmias. (*Irwin and Rippe, 2003*)

19. **(A)** *Discussion:* Pit viper envenomations can produce severe local reactions to include compartment syndromes and local tissue necrosis. A variety of systemic effects can occur, and these are typically accompanied by coagulation abnormalities. The decision to give antivenin is based on a constellation of findings, including the severity of the local reaction, the degree of systemic symptoms, and the degree of abnormality of these laboratory tests. The presence of even mild systemic symptoms or coagulopathy should prompt antivenin therapy, particularly if these findings appear to be progressing. (*Irwin and Rippe, 2003*)

20. **(B)** *Discussion:* Botulism is a disease due to exposure to a toxin produced by *C. botulinum*. This usually occurs as a result of ingesting the preformed toxin in improperly home canned foods. The syndrome is mainly that of a descending paralysis with prominent cranial nerve features (diplopia, dysphagia, dysarthria). The differential diagnosis includes other paralyzing syndromes such as organophosphate poisoning, myasthenia, or the Miller-Fisher variant of Guillain-Barré syndrome. Gastrointestinal symptoms may also be seen, but fever is not a feature. Tetany is a feature of another clostridial toxin (from *C. tetani*) but not botulism. (*Irwin and Rippe, 2003*)

21. **(D)** *Discussion:* This patient has two primary acid-base disturbances that offset each other in terms of the serum bicarbonate and pH values. Calculation of the anion gap (141 − 83 − 22 = 36 mEq/L) demonstrates a marked elevation. Nothing causes this degree of elevation of the anion gap other than an anion gap metabolic acidosis. The list of disorders causing this is short, and in this patient diabetic ketoacidosis is most likely. Lactic acidosis and various ingestions can be ruled out by laboratory testing and history. This degree of an anion gap can be present in the face of a normal (as opposed to reduced) bicarbonate level, if a primary process tending to elevate the bicarbonate is also present. In this case, acid loss through vomiting is probably the mechanism. One way to quantify this is with the concept of the "starting bicarbonate" concentration. In other words, what would the bicarbonate concentration be if the metabolic acidosis were not there or before the metabolic acidosis "started" (realizing that the metabolic acidosis and alkalosis may develop concurrently as they probably did in this case)? The starting bicarbonate is calculated

by subtracting the normal anion gap (10 mEq/L) from the patient's anion gap and adding the result to the patient's serum bicarbonate level. In this case, the answer is (36 − 10) + 22 = 48 mEq/L. This high value confirms a process that would be forcing the bicarbonate level up above normal if it were not for the acidosis. So, the patient has a primary anion gap metabolic acidosis based on measuring the anion gap and has a primary metabolic alkalosis based on calculating the starting bicarbonate. She does not have a primary respiratory acidosis because the Pa_{CO_2} is actually slightly below normal. It is close enough to normal that it does not represent a respiratory alkalosis either. (*Andreoli, Ch. 26*)

22. **(E)** *Discussion:* This patient has an aortic dissection beginning distal to the left subclavian (type B by the Stanford classification). Physical examination shows no evidence of organ ischemia and distal pulses are normal with the exception of a bruit, which is probably due to atherosclerotic disease and not directly related to the dissection. Treatment of this type of dissection is medical with outcomes that are as good or better than surgical treatment. Type A dissections (beginning more proximally than the left subclavian) have a better outcome with surgery. Institution of intravenous medication to control heart rate and BP and thus reduce the rate of change of pressure over time (dP/dT) is done to reduce the chance of further extension or rupture. Labetalol has both α- and β-blocking properties and is a reasonable choice in this setting. Aortography and coronary angiography will add little information that will change the acute management and will add a second contrast load to what has already been given for the CT scan. Intra-aortic balloon counter-pulsation would serve no purpose and would be likely to worsen the dissection or rupture the aorta. (*Irwin and Rippe, 2003*)

23. **(D)** *Discussion:* Patients with chronic alcoholism have substantial complications after admission to the hospital. They can have a variety of withdrawal syndromes from alcohol. Often they have gastrointestinal problems that limit oral intake and place them at risk for metabolic disturbances due to partial refeeding with intravenous fluids and nutrients. Acute thiamine deficiency is well known and avoided by giving supplemental multivitamins. These patients also can develop reductions in serum levels of potassium, magnesium, and phosphorus as intravenous dextrose and fluids are given. Severe hypophosphatemia with a level less than 1 mg/dL can be associated with rhabdomyolysis, with resulting renal failure in this setting. (*Irwin and Rippe, 2003*)

24. **(A)** *Discussion:* The scenario described is typical for an overdose of γ-hydroxybutyrate (GHB). This is a drug used in a variety of settings. It is alleged to enhance sexual desire and performance. This assertion with its sedative properties has led to its use as a "date-rape" drug. The use of this drug at parties by large numbers of people has become an increasingly common phenomenon. It has also been used by some body-builders because of claims that it can enhance the increase in muscle mass. Respiratory depression is the most serious side effect, and this can be enhanced by the presence of other sedatives. Flumazenil does not reverse its effects, which will eventually abate as the drug is eliminated. Oxylate crystals may be seen with ingestion of ethylene glycol. The absence of an increased anion gap acidosis makes this unlikely. Ventricular arrhythmias are among the most serious complications of tricyclic antidepressant overdose. Widening of the QRS complex would be the most likely clue to this ingestion. The negative urine drug screen also makes this less likely. Cocaine ingestion is common and can be associated with chest pain and myocardial injury, even in persons with normal coronary anatomy. The absence of initial hypertension, tachycardia, or other signs of increased adrenergic activity make this ingestion unlikely. (*Irwin and Rippe, 2003; Chin et al, 1998; Li et al, 1998*)

25. **(D)** *Discussion:* The patient described exhibits typical symptoms and findings of the HELLP (hemolysis, elevated liver enzymes, low platelets) syndrome. This typically develops in the third trimester in patients with preeclampsia or eclampsia and is more common in multiparous women. Abdominal pain, especially right upper quadrant pain, is a common presenting feature. Microangiopathic hemolytic anemia is a cardinal finding. Seizures, renal failure, ARDS, and hepatic subcapsular hematoma with rupture are all potential complications. If the fetus is viable, immediate delivery is the treatment of choice. In women with HELLP who have a platelet count greater than 40,000/μL, postpartum bleeding is unlikely and platelet transfusion is usually not required. (*Irwin and Rippe, 2003; Geary, 1997; Stone, 1998*)

26. **(D)** *Discussion:* Delivery of oxygen to peripheral tissues is directly related to the cardiac output and arterial oxygen content. Uptake by the tissues occurs as oxygen diffuses down a concentration gradient created by ongoing O_2 consumption by the mitochondria. This process is influenced by the affinity of the hemoglobin for the oxygen, with factors that decrease hemoglobin affinity tending to favor oxygen movement into tissue. A reduction in cardiac output directly reduces bulk oxygen delivery. The presence of carboxyhemoglobin also reduces bulk transport because the carbon monoxide (CO) occupies oxygen-binding sites. The presence of CO has another deleterious effect in that it causes left shifting of the oxygen hemoglobin dissociation curve so that what oxygen that is bound to hemoglobin adheres more tightly. Of the other three choices only fever causes right shifting of the dissociation curve (meaning hemoglobin binds less avidly to oxygen). A reduction in 2,3-DPG (as happens with prolonged banking of blood) and alkalosis both left shift the curve. (*Levitzky, 2003*)

27. **(E)** *Discussion:* Pneumothorax follows the development of mediastinal emphysema in 40 to 50% of ventilated patients. Because the patient can be watched closely in the ICU, the usual practice is to withhold chest tube placement until it is actually needed to avoid placing a large number of unnecessary tubes. Drainage procedures for air in the pericardium, mediastinum, or subcutaneous tissue are of no value. (*Marcy, 1993*)

28. **(A)** *Discussion:* This patient is taking a drug that can induce methemoglobin. The actual percentage of hemoglobin that is methemoglobin can be measured in arterial blood with a co-oximeter that uses absorption of multiple frequencies of light to quantitate the percentage of oxyhemoglobin, deoxyhemoglobin, carboxyhemoglobin, and methemoglobin. This test is automatically done with arterial blood gas analysis in many hospitals. When it is not done, the percentage of oxyhemoglobin (percent saturation) reported is a calculated quantity that the machine determines based on the shape of the normal oxygen hemoglobin dissociation curve corrected for the $Paco_2$ and pH because these shift the curve. Routine arterial blood gas analysis done in this fashion will miss the presence of methemoglobin or carboxyhemoglobin. Also, pulse oximeters used at the bedside are designed only to determine the percentage of oxyhemoglobin, with the assumption that all hemoglobin is either the oxy or deoxy form. The color alteration due to methemoglobin tends to lower the oxyhemoglobin percentage measured by the machine, although the measured percentage is unlikely to be accurate. This patient has a low oxygen saturation by pulse oximetry, with a high Pao_2 most consistent with the presence of methemoglobin. Carboxyhemoglobin does not lower the measured saturation by pulse oximetry. If the patient had poor digital perfusion, the pulse oximeter would not pick up an adequate waveform. A congenital hemoglobinopathy would not produce this degree of discrepancy between saturation and Pao_2. Also, a left shift would result in the Pao_2 at a given saturation being lower, not higher, than expected. (*Irwin and Rippe, 2003*)

29. **(D)** *Discussion:* Digoxin-specific antibody Fab fragments are the treatment of choice for severe digitalis toxicity. They are sheep anticardiac glycoside IgG antibodies cleaved to isolate the Fab fragments. These bind to digoxin or other cardiac glycosides. Response is rapid, with complete or partial response occurring within about 1 hour of infusion. (*Irwin and Rippe, 2003*)

30. **(A)** *Discussion:* Early defibrillation is critical in patients with ventricular fibrillation and should be the initial intervention. The initial countershock should be 200 J. This should be followed with shocks at 300 and then 360 J each if the rhythm is not corrected. Epinephrine, airway control, and antiarrhythmic agents are important for patients who do not respond to defibrillation. Synchronized cardioversion has no role in the resuscitation of ventricular fibrillation. (*Irwin and Rippe, 2003*)

31. **(D)**; 32. **(B)**; 33. **(C)**; 34. **(A)**. *Discussion:* Ventilator settings can vary widely depending on the clinical setting. Two of the patients have obstructive lung disease. In such patients, the general strategy is to try to avoid high respiratory rates to minimize auto-PEEP. Auto-PEEP increases peak and plateau pressures because it elevates the starting point for alveolar pressure as a breath is pushed in. It also creates a threshold effect, making it more difficult for patients to initiate breaths on their own because the inspiratory muscles must first activate sufficiently to overcome the positive pressure in the alveolus before subatmospheric alveolar and airway pressures can be generated and sensed by the machine to trigger a breath. Adding some PEEP can raise machine pressure up closer to the auto-PEEP level, reducing this threshold. Hence, the COPD patient has 5 cm H_2O of applied PEEP. Even if the patient has no auto-PEEP, this low level of PEEP is unlikely to have any harmful effects. The bullous emphysema patient with the large air leak has no PEEP in order to make every effort to reduce airway pressure and reduce the leak. The patient with the metabolic acidosis has normal lungs and needs a very high minute ventilation and hence a high rate. Oxygenation is not a problem, so the Fio_2 is low and PEEP is not necessary. The patient with ARDS is the most challenging. She needs a reduced tidal volume (about 6 mL/kg ideal weight) because this has been shown to improve mortality. The rate therefore needs to be faster and often has to be quite fast because of increased dead space ventilation due to the disease. PEEP is necessary to improve oxygenation (see also the discussions for questions 2, 4, and 8). These lower tidal volumes can be somewhat problematic. In clinical settings other than ARDS, there is no evidence that they offer an advantage and usually 8 to 10 mL/kg ideal weight tidal volumes are used initially and adjusted downward if peak and plateau pressures are excessive. (*Cecil, Ch. 101*)

35. **(D)**; 36. **(A)**; 37. **(C)**; 38. **(B)**. *Discussion:* Pulmonary artery catheterization has been used less commonly in the ICU in recent years owing to emerging evidence that it does not alter clinical outcome. However, it clearly provides information that helps to understand the pathophysiology of some disease states, particularly those associated with shock and/or pulmonary infiltrates. Why this does not clearly translate into improved clinical outcome parameters has been the subject of a good deal of speculation. Possible reasons include adverse events from the catheter itself and treatment decisions based on data that may be incorrectly measured, misinterpreted, or inadequately correlated with the patient's clinical status. Still, most intensivists believe information from these catheters can be helpful in making proper treatment decisions in selected patients. The clinical scenario in question 35 is that of a patient with a malignant pericardial effusion due to lung cancer. With hypotension in this setting, one typically sees equalization in diastolic pressures in the heart. Answer D has CVP, wedge, and pulmonary artery diastolic pressures all in the 18- to 19-mm Hg range associated with a low cardiac output. Question 36 is a patient with a large anterior myocardial infarction. BP is low

due to poor cardiac output and there is a reactive rise in SVR. Wedge pressure is high due to the low output and possibly also from worsening ventricular compliance. Question 37 is a patient with urosepsis. Shock is distributive in this case with inappropriate vasodilatation due to endotoxin and cytokines. SVR and filling pressures are low and cardiac output is high. Later in the course of septic shock, the cardiac output may also drop due to myocardial depression. Question 38 is a patient with a pulmonary thromboembolus. His pulmonary artery and pressures are high. BP is low because of poor cardiac output due to the pulmonary vascular occlusion. (*Cecil, Chs. 102-104*)

39. (D) *Discussion:* Acetaminophen in large doses exceeds the capability of the liver to metabolize it by the usual pathway, and a hepatotoxic metabolite is produced that requires glutathione for detoxification. Fulminate hepatic failure may occur without prompt treatment. If *N*-acetylcysteine treatment is instituted early, patients very seldom die of this overdose. This agent probably acts by increasing glutathione levels. (*Cecil, Ch. 106; Irwin and Rippe, 2003*)

40. (B) *Discussion:* β-Blocker overdoses mainly cause bradyarrhythmias and myocardial depression. Glucagon probably acts by activating the adenyl cyclase system independent of the β-receptors. It has a short half-life so it must be given by infusion. Glucagon has also been used to treat calcium channel blocker intoxication, although calcium is the first line of treatment for those agents. (*Cecil, Ch. 106*)

41. (C) *Discussion:* Organophosphate insecticides act by inhibiting cholinesterase. Cholinergic nerve endings are then flooded with acetylcholine, causing parasympathetic effects at muscarinic endings and depolarizing paralysis at nicotinic neuromuscular junctions. Atropine will counter the muscarinic effects but not the nicotinic effects. Pralidoxime reverses the binding of the organophosphate to the enzyme and rapidly reverses the paralysis. Pralidoxime has been issued to soldiers who may be exposed to chemical weapons because nerve agents work by the same mechanism. (*Cecil, Ch. 106*)

42. (A) *Discussion:* Ethylene glycol and methanol are both toxic alcohols whose main effects are exerted by their metabolites. Fomepizole inhibits alcohol dehydrogenase, thereby blocking the formation of the toxins. Hemodialysis may be used to remove both of these agents. (*Cecil, Ch. 106*)

43. (E) *Discussion:* Cyclic antidepressants cause ventricular arrhythmias, coma, and seizures. The tissue binding of the drugs is very dependent on pH, with an alkaline pH favoring removal from the tissue to the soluble phase. While alkalinization of the urine is easily accomplished with bicarbonate, it is more difficult to do in the blood because the extra bicarbonate is filtered by the kidney. Still, a bicarbonate infusion may help somewhat. Alkalinization of the blood is more rapidly and reliably accomplished by intubation and hyperventilation. Severely intoxicated patients can have resolution of wide complex tachycardia simply by increasing minute ventilation by increasing respiratory rate on the ventilator. (*Cecil, Ch. 106*)

44. (D); 45. (C); 46. (E); 47. (A); 48. (B). *Discussion:* Hypercapnic respiratory failure, characterized by inability to achieve adequate CO_2 removal, is common in obstructive airway diseases and neuromuscular diseases, in this case amyotrophic lateral sclerosis. ARDS is the prototype of hypoxemic respiratory failure, with shunt physiology and the requirement for a high concentration of inspired oxygen. Although hypercapnic and hypoxemic respiratory failure are the classic forms, the term *respiratory failure* also is used loosely to describe any process that interferes with tissue oxygen delivery or utilization. In cyanide poisoning, adequate oxygen is delivered to the tissues but cannot

be used because of blockade of mitochondrial cytochrome oxidase. Carbon monoxide binds to hemoglobin with a much greater affinity than oxygen, leading to a reduced arterial oxygen content despite a normal PaO_2. The low output state of cardiac tamponade leads to reduced tissue oxygen delivery in the presence of normal arterial oxygen content. (*Cecil, Ch. 99*)

49. (C); 50. (E); 51. (F); 52. (A); 53. (D); 54. (B). *Discussion:* The primary manifestations of scopolamine toxicity relate to anticholinergic properties, leading to altered mental status, dry mucous membranes, and urinary retention. Organophosphates, common components of insecticides, irreversibly inhibit acetylcholinesterase, leading to cholinergic manifestations with abdominal pain, vomiting, tachycardia, salivation, lacrimation (all muscarinic), as well as depolarizing neuromuscular blockade (nicotinic). The latter produces fasciculations and eventual paralysis. Methanol (wood alcohol) is converted to formic acid in the body, with classic symptoms including blurred vision and anion-gap acidosis. Permanent blindness may result. Theophylline toxicity causes nausea and vomiting early, which can be followed by cardiac arrhythmias and seizures. Severe tricyclic overdose (amitriptyline being one of them) causes prolongation of the QT interval, ventricular arrhythmias, seizures, and hypotension. Calcium-channel blocker overdoses cause bradycardia, hypotension, and coma; intravenous calcium may be life saving in such instances. (*Cecil, Ch. 106*)

55. (B) *Discussion:* Nutrition is a major issue in the ICU because deficiencies often contribute to the patient's disease process and because intravenous nutritional replacement can produce clinical syndromes by repleting some but not all the patient's deficits. Thiamine is a classic example of this. Alcoholics are often very malnourished but need glucose-containing fluids to treat such conditions as alcoholic ketoacidosis. Glucose repletion can rapidly deplete the minimal tissue thiamine stores, causing neurologic findings (i.e. Wernicke-Korsakoff syndrome characterized by mental status changes, vomiting, nystagmus, and ophthalmoplegia). (*Cecil, Ch. 257, 258, 259*)

56. (C) *Discussion:* Scurvy is very uncommon in western society but can occasionally be seen in patients who adopt fad diets or who have food intolerances from prior intestinal manipulation (surgery and/or radiation therapy). Vitamin C is involved in collagen metabolism, and one of the findings of deficiency is capillary fragility and bleeding. Hemorrhage around hair follicles is a feature of advanced disease. Chronic intermittent bleeding into soft tissues can produce chronic anemia and necessitate transfusion. Joint and bone pain due to subperiosteal hemorrhage may occur. The finding of petechiae on the arm after use of a sphygmomanometer is referred to as a positive Rumpel-Leed test. (*Cecil, Ch. 257, 258, 259*)

57. (D) *Discussion:* Acute zinc deficiency has been described in patients receiving parenteral nutrition. The clinical features include diarrhea, mental status changes, and skin lesions. (*Cecil, Ch. 257, 258, 259*)

58. (A) *Discussion:* Vitamin K is a well-known cofactor for a number of coagulation factors produced by the liver. Elevation of the prothrombin time is typically seen with deficiency. (*Cecil, Ch. 257, 258, 259*)

59. (True); 60. (False); 61. (False). *Discussion:* Review of airway pressure and airflow graphics can help with understanding pathophysiology in patients with respiratory failure. This patient has a peak pressure on inspiration of 30 cm H_2O and a plateau pressure of about 25 cm H_2O (airway pressures are given in cm H_2O and vascular pressures as mm Hg; 1 cm H_2O = 1.36 mm Hg). The inspiratory pause button causes a delay in exhalation after the breath is given, allowing an assessment of elastic recoil/compliance properties of the respiratory system after flow resistive forces have dissipated. This patient does have auto-PEEP given that the pressure rises when the expiratory pause button is pushed. This button closes the exhalation valve near the end of expiration. If there is continued flow of gas near end-expiration, stopping the flow by closing the exhalation valve will result in the pressure sensor in the machine circuit registering the alveolar pressure. When this valve is open, the reading from this sensor does not reflect alveolar pressure because flow is occurring down a pressure gradient. Accurate measurement of auto-PEEP by this method depends on the patient being relaxed or paralyzed. Attempts by the patient to initiate a breath or actively exhale will result in pressure fluctuations being transmitted to the pressure sensor. (*Cecil, Ch. 100*)

62. (True); 63. (True); 64. (False); 65. (False). *Discussion:* The numerical value of $PaCO_2$ is proportional to CO_2 production divided by alveolar ventilation. In a normal person, doubling total ventilation would be expected to approximately double alveolar ventilation and hence reduce the $PaCO_2$ value to one half of the original value. Measuring $PaCO_2$ requires arterial puncture, so noninvasive methods of determining $PaCO_2$ have been sought. One method that has been extensively studied is capnography of exhaled gas (measurement and graphing of PCO_2 during each tidal volume). With normal lungs, alveolar PCO_2 is equal to $PaCO_2$ due to equilibrium achieved between blood and gas at the alveolar membrane. Gas exhaled late in the tidal volume (end-tidal PCO_2) is mainly alveolar gas. Measuring PCO_2 continuously throughout the tidal volume will show the level rising as dead space gas is cleared and reaching a plateau at or slightly below the $PaCO_2$ level. In patients with lung disease, the relationship is not so simple. These patients have ventilation-perfusion mismatching such that some of the gas throughout exhalation is coming from areas with poor gas exchange and hence low PCO_2 values. Therefore, PCO_2 levels do not plateau near end exhalation but are still rising and remain less than $PaCO_2$, sometimes considerably less. High fat formulas produce less CO_2 than high carbohydrate formulas. Because fat contains less oxygen than carbohydrate, more oxygen is required for each molecule of CO_2 produced as it is metabolized. Said another way, less CO_2 is produced compared with oxygen consumed when metabolizing fat as compared with carbohydrate. CO_2 production divided by O_2 consumption is referred to as the respiratory quotient (RQ or just R). It is about 0.7 for fat and 1.0 for carbohydrate. A high fat formula would be expected to decrease $PaCO_2$ at a constant minute ventilation compared with a high carbohydrate formula. (*Cecil, Ch. 100*)

66. (False); 67. (True); 68. (False); 69. (False). *Discussion:* SIMV and assist control (AC) set at the same rate and tidal volume behave identically for apneic patients. Both modalities will deliver the set tidal volume at the set rate. They vary in how they handle spontaneous breaths. AC gives a full tidal volume any time the machine senses that the patient is initiating a breath (usually by sensing subatmospheric pressure as the patient tries to inhale). The timer for the next breath then resets. In this sense, the machine behaves like a demand pacemaker. As long as the patient breathes faster than the set rate, all of the breaths will be patient initiated and all will be the set tidal volume, in this case 500 mL. With SIMV, for most of the time between breaths, the patient gets whatever amount of air he or she can pull without any help from the ventilator. The timer for the next machine breath does not reset (hence the name intermittent *mandatory* ventilation). Therefore, spontaneous breaths can be of any tidal volume with SIMV but will be at the set tidal volume with AC. Pressure support is a modality designed to assist patients with spontaneous breaths. There is no set rate, so it is a poor modality for a patient who may become apneic. When the patient attempts to inhale, the machine senses subatmospheric pressure and responds by opening an inspiratory valve, allowing gas flow and pressurization of the machine circuit to the desired level. This assists the patient in taking the breath, and the actual tidal volume will depend on the magnitude and

duration of the patient's own inspiratory effort. The machine closes the inspiratory valve and opens the expiratory valve when flow drops off to some percentage of the initial flow. Pressure control uses similar technology, but typically a rate is specified and the pressure is held for a specified time. Hence pressure control is time cycled whereas pressure support is flow cycled (cycling refers to what makes the machine stop inhalation and begin exhalation). (*Cecil, Ch. 101*)

70-73. (All False). *Discussion:* Prone positioning, inhaled nitric oxide, and extracorporeal ventilation have all been studied looking for a mortality benefit with no improvement identified despite favorable effects on gas exchange. The effect of PEEP on mortality in ARDS has never been studied in a randomized trial including a subgroup ventilated without PEEP. Its use rapidly became standard of care after it was found to improve oxygenation in these patients in the late 1960s. It seems likely that it reduces mortality in at least a subgroup of more severe patients who would die of complications of severe hypoxemia without it. In the ARDSnet trial, which showed reduced mortality with lower tidal volumes, both groups got PEEP, as have patients in all ARDS trials in the past few decades. Theoretically, PEEP may improve clinical outcome for reasons other than its effect on oxygenation. It is known to keep alveoli open throughout the respiratory cycle. By avoiding opening and closing of these alveoli, PEEP may reduce ventilator-induced lung injury, but this has not been proven conclusively. (*Cecil, Ch. 101; Irwin and Rippe, 2003*)

74. (True); 75. (True); 76. (False); 77. (True). *Discussion:* Cardiogenic shock occurs in 5 to 19% of acute myocardial infarctions and is about twice as common in ST segment elevation vs. non–ST segment elevation events. Because cardiac output is low, mixed venous saturation tends to be low because peripheral tissues have to extract more oxygen per deciliter of blood to meet metabolic needs. Intra-aortic balloon counter-pulsation (IABP) increases diastolic coronary artery perfusion pressure, increases cardiac output, decreases left ventricular afterload, and decreases cardiac oxygen demand. It has been shown to improve hemodynamics and survival at both 30 days and 1 year. It provides a valuable bridge to revascularization procedures, which have been shown to reduce 6-month mortality. IABP can be used in the presence of mitral regurgitation but not aortic regurgitation. (*Cecil, Ch. 103; Irwin and Rippe, 2003*)

78. (False); 79. (False); 80. (False); 81. (True); 82. (True). *Discussion:* In diabetic ketoacidosis (DKA), serum glucose levels are high but the cells are deficient in glucose because the lack of insulin impairs uptake. As insulin levels are restored with intravenous insulin, serum glucose levels often decline more rapidly than the acidosis clears. Once the glucose level is near normal (< 200 mg/dL), continued insulin infusion will produce hypoglycemia if the patient is not given glucose. The insulin infusion must be maintained in this case because the patient still has evidence of ongoing acidosis based on the continued elevation of the anion gap. Continued insulin infusion will inhibit the breakdown of stored fat and therefore stop the production of ketoacids. So, the end point for insulin infusion is not just control of the blood glucose concentration but also normalization of the anion gap. The patient also needs more fluid. Two liters is not enough, given that most of these patients are depleted by 5 to 10 L. The patient's tachycardia in the absence of fever is probably due to continued fluid volume depletion. He also needs potassium, given that his serum level is low and ongoing insulin and glucose infusion will shift more of it into the cells. Intravenous bicarbonate is definitely not indicated at this point, and it is controversial whether it should ever be used in DKA. (*Irwin and Rippe, 2003*)

83. (False); 84. (False); 85. (False); 86. (True); 87. (False). *Discussion:* This patient has massive hemoptysis because she has more than 500 mL in a 24-hour period. Cystic fibrosis patients have extensive bronchiectasis owing to their chronic mucous clearance problems and infections. Minor hemoptysis may clear with antibiotic therapy alone, but this degree of bleeding is much more ominous. The blood is almost certainly coming from the bronchial circulation feeding the inflamed bronchiectatic tissue. Lobectomy is an effective treatment for massive hemoptysis if the site of origin can be determined. Unfortunately, this patient has poor lung function and chronic infection and is therefore a very poor operative candidate. A much better option for her is bronchial artery embolization. The bronchial arteries arise from the aorta and become hypertrophied in such patients, making them easier to cannulate than they are in normal persons. They can both be embolized without any pulmonary ischemic complications, probably owing to collaterals with the pulmonary circulation (in fact, bronchial arteries are not reconnected during lung transplantation). Embolization removes the high pressure blood supply to the bronchiectatic airway and often stops the bleeding. Bronchial artery embolization has been complicated by paraplegia due to accidental embolization of penetrating spinal arteries, although this is rare. During active hemoptysis, the bleeding lung should be positioned downward to limit blood entering the good lung. (*Irwin and Rippe, 2003*)

88. (False); 89. (True); 90. (True); 91. (True); 92. (True).
Discussion: Pressure control is a specialized tool that should mainly be reserved for patients with diffuse alveolar filling and ARDS pathophysiology. This is because changes in the patient's status produce more complicated effects than are seen with volume-targeted modalities. With pressure control, pressure is the independent variable and volume is the dependent variable. Anything that reduces lung compliance or increases airway or endotracheal resistance will reduce tidal volume. Also, the patient may alter the tidal volume by altering the amount of effort that he or she makes. More vigorous activation of the diaphragm will increase the pressure gradient from the machine to the alveolus, pushing more gas in; and less effort will have the opposite effect. Also, auto-PEEP can have a major effect on tidal volume with pressure control. If a patient has no auto-PEEP at a rate of 20/minute, but has 5 cm H_2O of auto-PEEP at a rate of 25, the effective driving pressure for the tidal volume will be eroded by 5 cm H_2O. This is a major limiting factor when increasing the rate in patients with ARDS on pressure control. With the very high rates used, even patients without airflow obstruction develop auto-PEEP. One must look at the effect a change has on total minute ventilation and not just tidal volume when making adjustments with pressure control. Number 88 is false because an improvement in lung inflammation and edema would be expected to increase lung compliance and increase tidal volume. The rest are true for the reasons just given. The pneumothorax will increase pressure in the chest and erode the inspiratory pressure gradient. In all of these circumstances, a volume-targeted modality will continue to give the same tidal volume but airway pressures will change as the patient's status changes. (*Cecil, Ch. 101*)

93. (False); 94. (False); 95. (True); 96. (True); 97. (True).
Discussion: The care of an ICU patient is not confined to addressing the primary disease process. The science behind proper supportive care is expanding rapidly and should be incorporated to improve patient outcome. Nothing is accomplished if a patient survives respiratory failure from pneumonia only to die of pulmonary thromboemboli or gastric stress ulceration. A number of studies have shown that frequent ventilator circuit changes are detrimental. Nosocomial pneumonia incidence is actually reduced and costs are lower with circuit changes once per week as compared with once per day. Bacterial colonization of the circuit comes from the endotracheal tube and is not reduced by frequent changes (*Irwin and Rippe, 2003*). Anemia is very common in the ICU. A large study comparing a transfusion at a threshold of 9 g/dL vs. 7 g/dL in 838 ICU patients demonstrated no difference in survival in the groups. The less ill patients appeared to do better with the 7 g/dL strategy unless they had ischemic cardiac disease (*Hebert et al, 1999*). Hyperglycemia is also very common in the ICU whether the patient has diagnosed diabetes or not. This is because of stress and treatments such as steroids and intravenous fluids containing glucose. A recent study of 1548 ICU patients randomized to intensive control of blood sugar with a goal of 110 mg/dL or less vs. loose control at 180 mg/dL or less showed reduced mortality with tight control (*Van Den Berghe et al, 2001*). Immobilized patients are at a substantially increased risk of deep venous thrombosis (DVT). For medically ill patients such as this one, low-dose subcutaneous heparin can decrease the risk from about 30% to about 10%. The dose is 5000 units, and studies have used it both twice and three times per day (*Irwin and Rippe, 2003*). ICU patients are at increased risk of stress ulcers and gastrointestinal bleeding. Not all ICU patients are at increased risk, but the list of risk factors for this is long and essentially everyone admitted to the ICU who is likely to be there for more than 48 hours should be considered for stress ulcer prophylaxis. Specifically, mechanical ventilation for more than 48 hours, as in this case, is a risk factor. H_2 blockers, proton pump inhibitors, and sucralfate are all effective in reducing the rate of this complication. (*Irwin and Rippe, 2003*)

98. (True); 99. (True); 100. (False). *Discussion:* Tracheostomy is typically recommended at between 2 and 3 weeks of mechanical ventilation if extubation is unlikely within the immediately foreseeable future. Definite advantages include improved patient comfort and improved secretion control. Also, tracheostomy eliminates further tube trauma to the larynx. The incidence of tracheal stenosis is not definitely reduced, although the currently available data are inadequate to come to a firm conclusion about this. (*Irwin and Rippe, 2003*)

BIBLIOGRAPHY

Andreoli TE, Bennett JC, Carpenter CC, Plum F (eds.): Cecil Essentials of Medicine, 4th ed. Philadelphia, WB Saunders, 1997.

Chin RL, Sporer KA, Cullison B, et al: Clinical course of gamma hydroxy butyrate use—New York and Texas, 1995-1996. JAMA 1997;277:1511.

Geary M: The HELLP syndrome. Br J Obstet Gynaecol 1997;104:887.

Goldman L, Ausiello D (eds): Cecil Textbook of Medicine, 22nd ed. Philadelphia, WB Saunders, 2004.

Herbert PC, Wells G, Blajchman MA, et al: A multicenter, randomized, controlled clinical trial of transfusion requirements in critical care. N Engl J Med 1999;340:409.

Irwin RS, Rippe JM (eds): Intensive Care Medicine, 5th ed. Philadelphia, Lippincott Williams & Wilkins, 2003.

Levitzky MG (ed): Pulmonary Physiology, 6th ed. New York, McGraw-Hill, 2003.

Li J, Stokes SA, Woeckener A: A tale of novel intoxication: Seven cases of gamma-hydroxybutyric acid overdose. Ann Emerg Med 1998;31:723.

Marcy TW: Barotrauma: Detection, recognition, and management. Chest 1993;104:578.

Stone JH: HELLP syndrome: Hemolysis, elevated liver enzymes, and low platelets [clinical conference]. JAMA 1998;280:559.

Van Den Berghe G, Wouter P, Weekers F, et al: Intensive insulin therapy in critically ill patients. N Engl J Med 2001;345:1359.

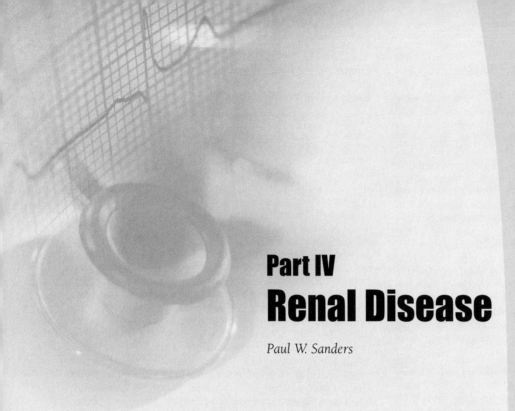

Part IV
Renal Disease

Paul W. Sanders

TRUE OR FALSE

DIRECTIONS: For questions 1–35, decide whether *each* choice is true or false. Any combination of answers, from all true to all false, may occur.

1. In obstructive uropathy:

   A. The presence of polyuria rules out obstruction.
   B. The absence of hydronephrosis on ultrasound examination rules out urinary tract obstruction.
   C. Infection is a frequent complication.
   D. Hypertension is uncommon.
   E. Renal tubular acidosis (RTA), type IV, can occur.

2. Membranous nephropathy:

   A. May occur as a result of a systemic illness or be a primary (intrinsic) disorder
   B. Merits an evaluation for malignancy when found in a patient older than age 50 years
   C. Infrequently improves without treatment
   D. Does not recur in the transplanted kidney
   E. Is the most common cause of idiopathic nephrotic syndrome in adults

3. Features of magnesium depletion include:

   A. Hypokalemia
   B. High serum parathyroid hormone levels
   C. Prolongation of the PR and QT intervals
   D. Amelioration of cardiac toxicity of cardiac glycosides
   E. Can occur with aminoglycoside administration

4. Which of the following statement(s) is/are true about the renal hypoperfusion syndromes?

   A. Salt avidity and hyperreninemia are usually observed.
   B. Effective circulating volume has a greater effect on systemic blood pressure than does renin secretion in the setting of renal hypoperfusion.
   C. Occlusive arterial disease causes renal hypoperfusion, elevated renin secretion, and hypertension in the setting of a normal effective circulating volume.
   D. Unilateral renal arterial occlusive disease is not associated with azotemia if the contralateral kidney maintains normal function.
   E. Nonsteroidal anti-inflammatory agents can exacerbate renal hypoperfusion in predisposed individuals.

5. Normal pregnancy is associated with:

   A. Increased glomerular filtration rate (GFR) and renal blood flow
   B. Respiratory alkalosis
   C. Hypouricemia
   D. Mild non–anion-gap type metabolic acidosis
   E. Slight increase in blood pressure

6. Which of the following statement(s) is/are *true* concerning creatinine clearance?

   A. Creatinine clearance normally exceeds "true" measurements of GFR.
   B. Cimetidine and trimethoprim can block the secretory component of creatinine clearance.
   C. Urinary creatinine excretion is primarily influenced by the muscle mass in the steady state.
   D. The secretory component of creatinine excretion may become more apparent when serum creatinine concentrations are elevated.
   E. Creatinine clearance is directly related to the serum creatinine concentration.

7. Which of the following statement(s) is/are *true* concerning urinary chloride excretion rates?

   A. Urinary chloride excretion provides an index of extracellular fluid volume.
   B. Urinary chloride excretion is increased in metabolic alkalosis caused by excessive use of furosemide or thiazides.
   C. Laxative abuse is associated with increased urinary chloride excretion.

D. Increase adrenocortical hormone activity increases urinary chloride excretion.

E. Vomiting is associated with increased urinary chloride excretion.

8. Which of the following statement(s) is/are *true* concerning calcium/phosphate balance in chronic renal failure?

   A. Increased circulating level of parathyroid hormone (PTH) is uncommon in chronic kidney disease.
   B. Hyperphosphatemia is related to reduced renal excretion and reduces PTH secretion.
   C. Extrarenal production of 25-hydroxyvitamin D is increased in chronic renal failure.
   D. 1,25(OH)$_2$ Vitamin D (calcitriol) increases gut absorption of calcium and phosphorus.
   E. A normal calcemic response to PTH is not observed in chronic renal failure with 1,25(OH)$_2$ vitamin D (calcitriol) deficiency.

9. Which of the following statement(s) is/are *true* concerning "uremic" pericarditis?

   A. A friction rub, pleuritic chest pain, and enlarged cardiac size are typical findings in uremic pericarditis.
   B. Hypotension, tachycardia, and raised jugular venous pressures are hallmarks of cardiac tamponade.
   C. Intensive dialysis can worsen "uremic" pericarditis.
   D. Volume overload can be improved by ultrafiltration in the setting of tamponade.
   E. Emergent surgical intervention is indicated if the pericardial effusion causes hemodynamic compromise.

10. Which of the following statement(s) is/are *true* concerning the anemia of end-stage renal disease (ESRD)?

    A. Erythropoietin deficiency is primarily related to the loss of renal mass.
    B. Iron deficiency and hyperparathyroidism are important causes of resistance to erythropoietin response.
    C. Normalizing the hematocrit can increase mortality in this population of patients.
    D. Increased release of oxygen from hemoglobin is an important factor in the adaptation to anemia in chronic renal failure.
    E. Erythropoietin reduces blood transfusion requirements and the incidence of iron overload and transfusion-related infections in the ESRD population.

11. Which of the following statement(s) is/are *true* concerning chronic ambulatory peritoneal dialysis?

    A. Relatively reduced peritoneal surface limits the usefulness of this approach in children.
    B. Insulin-dependent diabetics have severe problems with glycemic control because of the large amounts of dextrose absorbed from the peritoneal dialysate.
    C. The dialysis prescription is tailored to the characteristics of the patient's peritoneal membrane.
    D. Fluid removal is adjusted by changing the concentration of dextrose in the dialysate.
    E. Peritonitis is a common problem with CAPD and is usually caused by gram-negative organisms.

12. Which of the following statement(s) is/are *true* concerning tissue typing and renal transplantation?

    A. Siblings with the same biologic parents have a 25% chance of being HLA incompatible.
    B. By definition, a biological parent shares one HLA haplotype with each child.
    C. In vitro cytotoxicity tests do not predict rejection in the transplant setting.

D. MHC class II antigens, expressed on B lymphocytes and vascular endothelial cells, are pivotal in the rejection process.

E. Mandatory sharing of 6-antigen matched cadaver kidneys with the best-matched recipient will dramatically improve graft survival for nearly all transplant recipients.

13. Which of the following statement(s) is/are *true* concerning cyclosporine?

    A. This agent has dramatically improved renal allograft survival.
    B. The use of more specific, targeted immunosuppressants (cyclosporine, OKT3) has reduced the incidence of opportunistic infections.
    C. Cyclosporine markedly slows the recovery from acute tubular necrosis (ATN) and potentiates the adverse effects of other nephrotoxic agents.
    D. Side effects of cyclosporine include nephrotoxicity, tremor, hyperglycemia, hypertension, and hyperkalemia.
    E. Calcium-channel blockers that include verapamil and diltiazem increase serum concentrations of cyclosporine.

14. Which of the following statements about membranoproliferative glomerulonephritis (MPGN) is/are *true*?

    A. MPGN does not recur after renal transplantation.
    B. This clinicopathologic entity occurs primarily in young adults.
    C. Hypocomplementemia may be severe.
    D. MPGN may be a primary (intrinsic) renal lesion or may occur in systemic illnesses, including hepatitis B antigenemia and other infections and systemic lupus erythematosus.
    E. The incidence of primary (intrinsic) MPGN is increasing.

15. Which of the following statements about hemolytic-uremic syndrome (HUS) is/are *true*?

    A. HUS may occur after gastroenteritis, especially verotoxin-producing *Escherichia coli* infections.
    B. HUS has a particularly poor renal prognosis in children.
    C. An HUS syndrome may occur with pregnancy or the use of oral contraceptive agents.
    D. Important features of HUS include microangiopathic hemolytic anemia, thrombocytopenia, reduced haptoglobin levels, and minimal evidence of disseminated intravascular coagulation.
    E. Relapse of HUS does not occur.

16. Which of the following is/are *true* of the nephrotic syndrome?

    A. Plasma volume is usually increased.
    B. It is usually associated with renal sodium wasting.
    C. It occurs with diffuse and focal forms of glomerulonephritis.
    D. The incidence of infection is increased.
    E. Albumin infusions are of significant benefit for treatment of hypoalbuminemia and edema.

17. Which of the following is/are the direct results of chronic, but rarely acute, renal failure?

    A. Elevated alkaline phosphatase from bone
    B. Radiographic signs of renal osteodystrophy
    C. Bilaterally small kidneys
    D. Hyposthenuria
    E. Hypertension

18. Which of the following is/are features of analgesic-associated nephropathy?

    A. Equal gender distribution
    B. Normal-sized kidneys
    C. Anemia out of proportion to azotemia
    D. Sterile pyuria
    E. Papillary necrosis

19. A 47-year-old man has an excretory urogram for investigation of microscopic hematuria discovered on a routine urinalysis. He is apparently healthy and entirely without complaints. Kidneys are of normal size, with calcification of and collection of dye in dilated medullary structures. Serum electrolytes, blood urea nitrogen (BUN), creatinine, calcium, phosphorus, and uric acid are normal. Creatinine clearance is 103 mL/minute. Urinalysis reveals rare red blood cells and no protein. Which of the following is/are *true* of this patient?

    A. There is a significant chance that he will develop symptomatic renal stones.
    B. There is a significant chance that he has hypercalciuria.
    C. He is likely to have impaired urine-concentrating ability.
    D. His condition is likely to progress gradually to ESRD.
    E. His children each have a 1-in-2 chance of developing the same condition.

20. A 32-year-old man has a 15-year history of diabetes mellitus. His serum creatinine concentration is 2.3 mg/dL. A diagnosis of diabetic nephropathy is established by renal biopsy. Which of the following is/are *true* of this patient?

    A. Angiotensin-converting enzyme (ACE) inhibitors are unlikely to help this condition at this time.
    B. He has a less than 30% chance of having hypertension at this time.
    C. He has a 50% chance of having the nephrotic syndrome at this time.
    D. Because of his age, nephropathy is likely to be his only major organ system diabetic complication to date.
    E. He is likely to develop ESRD requiring dialysis within the next 4 years.

QUESTIONS 21–22

A 57-year old woman presents for evaluation of malaise and edema. She has been previously healthy and takes no medicines. A comprehensive physical examination, including routine laboratory tests, was performed 3 months ago and was entirely normal. The patient reports these symptoms for a few weeks. She has noted no change in her urine volume but does report nocturia. Physical examination shows a mildly ill woman with hypertension and pedal edema. No other remarkable physical findings were noted. Laboratory studies show:

Serum electrolytes	
Sodium	138 mEq/L
Potassium	5.3 mEq/L
Chloride	100 mEq/L
Bicarbonate	18 mEq/L
BUN	62 mg/dL
Serum creatinine	4.8 mg/dL
Hematocrit	31%
White blood cell count	9700/mm^3
Erythrocyte sedimentation rate	40 mm/hr

Urinalysis shows a pH of 5.5, 2+ protein, 10 to 20 RBCs per high-power field, and rare red blood cell casts.

Antinuclear antibodies, total hemolytic complement (CH50), anti-streptolysin-O (ASO) titer, and rheumatoid antibodies were normal.

A percutaneous renal biopsy is performed. Light microscopy reveals that about 80% of the glomeruli seen are affected with proliferating epithelial crescents. Immunofluorescence shows absence of IgG, IgA, and complement in the kidney.

21. Which of the following renal syndromes is/are likely to have this clinical and histologic picture?

    A. IgA nephropathy
    B. Polyarteritis nodosa
    C. Wegener's granulomatosis
    D. Post-streptococcal glomerulonephritis
    E. Primary (idiopathic) crescentic glomerulonephritis

22. Which of the following therapy is/are appropriate at this time?

    A. Hemodialysis
    B. Plasmapheresis
    C. Observation
    D. Intravenous methylprednisolone
    E. Warfarin and dipyridamole

23. Which of the following is/are *true* of uremic acidosis?

    A. Urine pH is usually greater than 6.0.
    B. Hyperkalemia worsens acidosis by suppressing ammonia production.
    C. Anion gap acidosis develops only when the GFR falls below 20 mL/minute.
    D. Renal ammonia production and excretion are low, considering the degree of acidosis.
    E. Bicarbonate wasting is observed when isotonic bicarbonate is infused to restore the serum bicarbonate to normal levels.

24. Which of the following statements about aminoglycoside-induced tubule damage is/are *true*?

    A. Functional tubular abnormalities may cause hypokalemia and hypomagnesemia.
    B. Oliguric acute renal failure is the rule.
    C. Toxicity is related to the dose of aminoglycoside and the duration of therapy.
    D. Risk factors include the age of the patient, the baseline serum creatinine concentration, and extracellular fluid volume depletion.
    E. All aminoglycosides are equally nephrotoxic.

25. Which of the following statements about pregnancy-induced hypertension (preeclampsia) is/are *true*?

    A. Onset is associated with elevation of the serum uric acid level.
    B. Nephrotic-range (> 3.5 g/day) proteinuria can occur.
    C. This syndrome typically occurs at between 12 and 24 weeks of gestation.
    D. GFR and renal blood flow are usually unchanged in preeclampsia.
    E. Clinical manifestations of preeclampsia generally resolve within 6 weeks after delivery.

26. Which of the following statements about renal calculi is/are *true*?

    A. Crystals seen on urinalysis confirm their formation in the kidney.
    B. Treatment of all patients with renal calculi should include a high fluid intake (minimum 2 L) if tolerated.
    C. Hexagonal-shaped crystals in the urine are always pathologic.

D. Magnesium ammonium phosphate crystals (struvite) are associated with urinary tract infections with urea-splitting organisms.
E. Alkalinization of the urine with potassium citrate may be effective in preventing the formation of both uric acid and calcium stones.

27. Which of the following statements about autosomal-dominant polycystic kidney disease (ADPKD) is/are *true*?

   A. ADPKD is the most common hereditary disease in the United States.
   B. Hepatic cysts support the diagnosis of ADPKD.
   C. Although half of the offspring of one affected parent will inherit the gene that produces ADPKD, expression of the disease is variable.
   D. Renal calculi are uncommon in ADPKD.
   E. Microscopic and macroscopic hematuria can occur.
   F. The incidence of intracranial aneurysms is higher in patients with ADPKD than the general population.

28. Episodic gross hematuria may be associated with which of the following:

   A. IgA nephropathy
   B. Cyclophosphamide therapy
   C. Analgesic nephropathy
   D. Sickle cell disease
   E. Schönlein-Henoch purpura

29. Clinical features of the syndrome of acute glomerulonephritis include:

   A. Hypertension
   B. Hypercholerolemia
   C. Red blood cell casts in the urinary sediment
   D. Edema
   E. Hypoalbuminemia

30. Causes of the syndrome of acute glomerulonephritis associated with hypocomplementemia include:

   A. Systemic lupus erythematosus
   B. Membranoproliferative glomerulonephritis
   C. Wegener's granulomatosis
   D. Infective endocarditis
   E. Hemolytic-uremic syndrome

31. Disease states associated with profound salt retention along with low fractional sodium excretion include:

   A. Acute glomerulonephritis
   B. ATN
   C. Acute interstitial nephritis
   D. Hepatorenal syndrome
   E. Hypovolemic shock

32. Common causes of ATN include:

   A. β-Lactam antibiotics
   B. Aminoglycoside antibiotics
   C. Cholesterol embolic disease
   D. Radiocontrast media
   E. Vancomycin

33. Risk factors for radiocontrast agent-induced acute renal failure include:

   A. Volume depletion
   B. Multiple myeloma
   C. Hypercalcemia
   D. Diabetes mellitus
   E. Chronic renal insufficiency

34. Effective strategies for minimizing the risk of radiocontrast nephropathy in diabetic patients with renal insufficiency include:

   A. Low-dose dopamine infusion
   B. Atrial natriuretic peptide infusion
   C. Volume expansion with 0.45% saline solution
   D. Intravenous furosemide
   E. Intravenous mannitol

35. In the treatment of the nephrotic syndrome, interventions that decrease urinary protein excretion include:

   A. Diltiazem
   B. ACE inhibitors
   C. Nonsteroidal anti-inflammatory agents
   D. α-Adrenergic receptor antagonists
   E. Low protein diet

MULTIPLE CHOICE

DIRECTIONS: For questions 36–107, choose the *single best* answer for each question.

QUESTIONS 36 AND 37

A 43-year-old man developed cellulitis of his left lower extremity but resisted medical evaluation for 2 weeks. When it did not improve, he saw his physician, who admitted him to the hospital. His admission serum creatinine concentration was 1.2 mg/dL. He was treated with a 2-week course of intravenous antibiotics that consisted of nafcillin, clindamycin, and gentamicin. Ten days into this treatment, a serum creatinine concentration is obtained and is 3.5 mg/dL. Renal ultrasound showed normal-sized kidneys without hydronephrosis.

36. Possible causes of this patient's acute renal failure include:

   A. ATN
   B. Acute glomerulonephritis
   C. Allergic interstitial nephritis
   D. A, B, and C are correct.
   E. Only A and C are correct.

37. On further evaluation, he was found to have a blood pressure of 160/95 mm Hg, a decrease in urine output to less than 30 mL/hour, and a urinalysis that showed 2+ protein, 2+ hemoglobin, red blood cells, and red blood cell and tubule epithelial cell casts. Based on these findings, the *most* likely diagnosis is:

   A. Gentamicin nephrotoxicity
   B. Postinfectious acute glomerulonephritis
   C. Hypersensitivity reaction to a β-lactam antibiotic
   D. Cannot determine from information available
   E. None of the above

38. *True* statements regarding poststreptococcal glomerulonephritis include:

   A. Serum complement, C3, and total hemolytic complement are usually low.
   B. Poststreptococcal acute glomerulonephritis has an excellent prognosis for recovery.
   C. Glomerulonephritis can develop after either skin or pharyngeal streptococcal infections.
   D. A, B, and C are correct.
   E. Only A and C are correct.

39. The *most* common intrinsic (primary) glomerular lesion is:

    A. Anti–glomerular basement membrane (GBM) glomeru-
       lonephritis
    B. Membranoproliferative glomerulonephritis
    C. Amyloidosis
    D. IgA nephropathy
    E. Focal and segmental glomerulosclerosis

40. A 45-year-old black man presents with hilar adenopathy,
    pulmonary infiltrates, and erythema nodosum. On trans-
    bronchial biopsy, he is found to have noncaseating granulo-
    mas. Special stains of the tissue reveal no organisms.
    Potential clinical renal manifestations in this patient may
    include:

    A. Hypercalcemic nephropathy
    B. Hyposthenuria
    C. Granulomatous infiltration of the renal interstitium
    D. Immune complex–mediated glomerulonephritis
    E. A, B, C, and D are correct.
    F. None of the above is correct.

41. The hypercalcemia of sarcoidosis:

    A. Reflects extrarenal 1α–hydroxylation of 25(OH) vitamin
       D3
    B. Rarely produces nephrocalcinosis
    C. Responds well to prednisone
    D. Only A and C are correct.
    E. A, B, and C are correct.

QUESTIONS 42–44

*A 60-year-old man with end-stage renal failure from chronic glomeru-
lonephritis presents with acute onset of gross hematuria and mild flank
pain. He has been on dialysis for 4 years, and his course has otherwise
been uneventful. He was afebrile and the hematuria resolved without
intervention.*

42. Which of the following is most appropriate now?

    A. Renal ultrasound
    B. Computed tomography
    C. Angiography
    D. Intravenous pyelography
    E. None of the above

43. True statements about acquired cystic kidney disease
    (ACKD) include all of the following *except:*

    A. ACKD occurs exclusively in hemodialysis patients and
       not in patients receiving peritoneal dialysis.
    B. ACKD is rare in patients without renal failure.
    C. ACKD is frequently asymptomatic but can produce pain,
       fever, and hematuria.
    D. ACKD is associated with renal cell carcinoma.
    E. ACKD has a male predominance.

44. Renal cell carcinoma in dialysis patients:

    A. Responds well to chemotherapy
    B. Is rarely bilateral
    C. Does not occur in native kidneys in renal transplant
       recipients
    D. Infrequently metastasizes unless the tumor size is larger
       than 3 cm
    E. None of the above is correct.

QUESTIONS 45–47

*A 67-year-old white male is referred for evaluation of renal failure.
Evaluation includes the following laboratory values:*

Serum Studies

Sodium	135 mEq/L
Potassium	4.2 mEq/L
Chloride	109 mEq/L
Bicarbonate	24 mEq/L
Glucose	101 mg/dL
Calcium	10.9 mg/dL
Phosphorus	4.3 mg/dL
Albumin	4.0 g/dL

Urine Studies

Creatinine clearance	55 mL/minute
Urine protein	6.2 g/day
Hematocrit	29%

45. Based on the data presented, the patient appears to have:

    A. Acute glomerulonephritis
    B. Acute vasculitic lesion
    C. Reflux nephropathy
    D. Atheroembolic renal disease
    E. Nephrotic syndrome
    F. None of the above

46. Tests to perform at this point to make a diagnosis might
    include:

    A. Urine immunofixation electrophoresis
    B. Bone marrow aspiration and biopsy
    C. Serum immunofixation electrophoresis
    D. Urine protein electrophoresis
    E. A, B, and C are correct.
    F. A, B, C, and D are correct.

47. The low anion gap in this patient most likely reflects:

    A. The presence of lithium
    B. Acidosis
    C. A low serum albumin
    D. A high circulating level of IgG
    E. None of the above

48. Deposition of monoclonal immunoglobulin light chains in
    the kidney can produce all of the following *except:*

    A. Casts in the lumen of the tubules
    B. Amyloidosis, type AL
    C. Granular deposits with glomerular injury
    D. Vasculitis
    E. ATN

QUESTIONS 49–51

*A 50-year-old woman presents with an abrupt decline in urine output
and renal failure. Her only past medical history is significant for hysterectomy 1 month earlier and chronic migraine headaches controlled
with methysergide. She takes no other medications. The following data
were obtained:*

Serum Studies

Sodium	130 mEq/L
Potassium	6.2 mEq/L
Chloride	99 mEq/L
Bicarbonate	16 mEq/L
Glucose	101 mg/dL
Calcium	7.9 mg/dL
Phosphorus	6.3 mg/dL
Albumin	4.0 g/dL
Creatinine	3.2 mg/dL

Urine Studies

pH	1.010
Protein	Trace
Hb	Trace
Sediment	Unremarkable

Urine output over the past 12 hours was 60 mL.

49. Which study do you perform now to assist with the diagnosis?

    A. Renal ultrasound
    B. Kidney biopsy
    C. Selective renal arteriogram
    D. 24-Hour urine for protein and immunofixation electrophoresis
    E. None of the above is appropriate

The patient receives treatment for the hyperkalemia. The fractional excretion of sodium was 1.3%. Repeat urinalysis was unchanged, and renal function did not improve with gentle hydration. A renal ultrasound demonstrated echogenic, normal-sized kidneys with minimal hydronephrosis bilaterally. No stones were evident.

50. Possible causes of the renal failure include:

    A. ATN
    B. Urinary tract obstruction
    C. Acute glomerulonephritis
    D. Allergic interstitial nephritis
    E. Cannot determine from the data given

51. A computer tomogram of the abdomen demonstrated mild hydronephrosis of both kidneys with mildly dilated proximal ureters that were deviated medially and appeared to be extrinsically compressed at the level of the mid to lower ureter. The *most* likely diagnosis is:

    A. Obstruction related to kidney stones bilaterally
    B. Obstruction secondary to retroperitoneal adenopathy
    C. Retroperitoneal fibrosis
    D. Obstruction secondary to adenocarcinoma
    E. ATN
    F. Cannot determine from the data given

QUESTIONS 52–54

A 25-year-old man presents with a history of upper respiratory symptoms followed by streaky hemoptysis and malaise. His blood pressure is 140/90 mm Hg, and he has trace lower extremity edema. Pertinent laboratory include a serum urea nitrogen of 86 mg/dL and creatinine of 3.5 mg/dL. Urinalysis shows 2+ protein, 3+ blood, 5 to 10 RBCs per high-power field, and rare red cell casts. Chest radiograph demonstrates opacities in both lung fields.

52. The most likely diagnosis at this point is:

    A. Wegener's granulomatosis
    B. Anti–glomerular basement membrane (anti-GBM) disease
    C. Postinfectious glomerulonephritis
    D. Allergic interstitial nephritis
    E. None of the above

53. The most appropriate initial diagnostic study should be:

    A. Bronchoscopy with biopsy
    B. Open lung biopsy
    C. Biopsy of the nasal mucosa
    D. CT of the chest and abdomen
    E. Percutaneous renal biopsy with immunofluorescence microscopic examination

54. The clinical course of this lesion:

    A. Depends on how rapidly treatment is initiated
    B. Can be predicted by the amount of urine output
    C. Can be predicted by the serum creatinine concentration at presentation
    D. Only A and C are correct.
    E. All are correct.

QUESTIONS 55–58

A 50-year-old woman with a 10-year history of non–insulin-dependent diabetes mellitus complains of low back pain and is prescribed indomethacin, 25 mg, three times a day. She returns for evaluation 4 weeks later with the following laboratory abnormalities:

Serum electrolytes	
Sodium	136 mEq/L
Potassium	6.2 mEq/L
Chloride	106 mEq/L
Bicarbonate	18 mEq/L
Serum urea nitrogen	55 mg/dL
Serum creatinine	5.3 mg/dL

Her serum creatinine was 2.2 mg/dL when checked 1 and 6 months previously.

55. Potential causes of the deterioration in this patient's renal function include:

    A. Renal ischemia secondary to reduced renal blood flow from prostaglandin inhibition
    B. Urinary tract obstruction
    C. Allergic interstitial nephritis
    D. A, B, and C are correct.
    E. Only A and C are correct.

56. *True* statements about allergic interstitial nephritis secondary to nonsteroidal anti-inflammatory agents include:

    A. Hematuria is frequently present.
    B. Eosinophilia is frequently present.
    C. The presence of eosinophils in the urine supports the diagnosis.
    D. A, B, and C are correct.
    E. Only A and C are correct.

57. Further review of the patient's record revealed a history of use of acetaminophen and aspirin over the past 20 years for low back pain and headache. Urinalysis showed 1+ protein, 10 to 20 WBCs per low power field and 4 to 6 WBC casts per low power field. Renal ultrasound demonstrated small kidneys with hydronephrosis bilaterally. On the second hospital day, small fragments of tissue were identified in the urine. Given this information, the *most* likely diagnoses should now include:

    A. Chronic interstitial nephropathy
    B. Allergic interstitial nephritis
    C. Papillary necrosis
    D. A, B, and C are correct.
    E. Only A and C are correct.

58. Potential causes of this patient's hyperkalemia include:

    A. Hyporeninemia from prostacyclin inhibition
    B. Renal tubular acidosis from urinary tract obstruction
    C. Renal failure
    D. A, B, and C are correct.
    E. Only A and C are correct.

QUESTIONS 59–62

A 39-year-old, 50-kg man presents to the emergency department with a history of alcoholism and recent onset of obtundation. He lives alone and can provide no other information. On presentation, he has a grand mal seizure that lasts for 2 minutes. Findings after a routine physical examination include a blood pressure of 120/70 mm Hg; heart rate of 110/minute, and no evidence of head trauma, papilledema, or focal neurologic findings. His mental status does not change with intravenous injections of thiamine and 50% dextrose. Laboratory evaluation includes:

Serum electrolytes
    Sodium   136 mEq/L
    Potassium   5.0 mEq/L
    Chloride   100 mEq/L
    Bicarbonate   12 mmol/L
Serum urea nitrogen   42 mg/dL
Serum creatinine   4.2 mg/dL
Arterial pH   7.10
Arterial P_{CO_2} 40 mm Hg
Arterial P_{O_2} 85 mm Hg

59. This patient has the following acid-base disorder(s):

    A. Simple metabolic acidosis
    B. Simple respiratory acidosis
    C. Mixed metabolic and respiratory acidosis
    D. Combined metabolic acidosis, respiratory acidosis, and metabolic alkalosis
    E. None of the above

60. Potential causes of this patient's problem might include:

    A. Methanol ingestion
    B. Uremia
    C. Ethylene glycol ingestion
    D. A, B, and C are possible.
    E. A and C are possible.

61. Ethylene glycol overdose:

    A. Produces an anion-gap metabolic acidosis
    B. Is associated with the presence of octahedral crystals typical of calcium oxalate in the urine
    C. Can cause oliguric acute renal failure
    D. A, B, and C are correct.
    E. A and C are correct.

62. Initial emergency management of ethylene glycol overdose can include:

    A. Creation of an osmotic diuresis
    B. Intravenous infusion of ethyl alcohol
    C. Hemodialysis
    D. A, B, and C are correct.
    E. Only A and C are correct.

63. In acute alcohol poisoning:

    A. The difference between observed and calculated serum osmolality is a rapid way to determine the degree of intoxication.
    B. The arterial pH correlates with the production of metabolites from alcohol dehydrogenase.
    C. Infusion of inhibitors of alcohol dehydrogenase is efficacious.
    D. A and C are correct.
    E. A, B and C are correct.

64. True statements about type IV renal tubular acidosis include all of the following *except:*

    A. Hyperkalemia is common.
    B. Renal ammoniagenesis is impaired.
    C. Urine pH is never below 5.5.
    D. It can occur during treatment with nonsteroidal anti-inflammatory agents.
    E. It can develop from urinary tract obstruction.

QUESTIONS 65–68

A 56-year-old white man with a history of symptomatic coronary artery disease and mild hypertension presents to his physician with complaints of headache and fatigue. He reportedly had a blood pressure of 196/115 mm Hg and a "normal" laboratory evaluation. His physician prescribed an ACE inhibitor and instructed the patient to return in 2 weeks. The patient is brought into the emergency department 5 days later with severe proximal muscle weakness to the point where he cannot rise from a chair, extreme fatigue, nausea, and vomiting.

65. Without other information available, which of the following is/are possible?

    A. The patient has symptomatic renal failure related to ACE-II inhibition.
    B. Life-threatening hyperkalemia is present.
    C. This patient probably has renovascular hypertension.
    D. A, B, and C are correct.
    E. Only A and C are correct.

66. If the serum potassium concentration was 7.2 mEq/L and his electrocardiogram revealed absent P waves and markedly prolonged QRS duration suggestive of a "sine-wave" pattern, appropriate initial management could include:

    A. Calcium gluconate, 10%, 10 mL administered intravenously
    B. Albuterol, 20 mg, via nebulized inhaler
    C. Intravenous regular insulin, 5 units, plus 50 mL of 50% dextrose
    D. A, B, and C are correct.
    E. Only A and C are correct.

67. The patient's serum creatinine concentration was 6.7 mg/dL. After stopping the ACE inhibitor, his creatinine value fell to 1.5 mg/dL. Which of the following is/are correct?

    A. The patient probably had hemodynamically significant bilateral renal artery stenosis.
    B. This patient probably had a glomerulonephritis related to the captopril therapy.
    C. If a selective ACE II receptor antagonist was used, this complication should not recur.
    D. A, B, and C are correct.
    E. Only A and C are correct.

68. Potential complications of ACE inhibitors include:

    A. Acute renal failure
    B. Persistent cough
    C. Acute severe hypotension
    D. Hyperkalemia
    E. A, B, C, and D are correct.
    F. Only A and C are correct.

QUESTIONS 69–72

An 18-year-old man presents to the emergency department with dysuria and fever. On further questioning, he relates two prior episodes of a urinary tract infection successfully treated with oral antibiotics. His evaluation is unremarkable except for a blood pressure of 160/105 mm Hg. Urinalysis revealed 3+ protein, a specific gravity of 1.012, pH of 5.5, and a microscopic examination showing 2 to 5 RBCs and 5-10 WBCs per high-power field. The serum creatinine concentration was 4.9 mg/dL. He was referred to a urologist, who performed a voiding cystourethrogram, which demonstrated vesicoureteral reflux bilaterally.

69. Which of the following is the most likely cause of this clinical syndrome?

    A. Obstructive uropathy at the level of the prostate
    B. Chronic tubulointerstitial nephritis
    C. Chronic glomerulonephritis

D. Reflux nephropathy
E. Acute glomerulonephritis

70. The cause of this patient's renal failure:

A. Will likely progress to ESRD
B. Will stabilize and cause no further problems
C. Is producing the hypertension
D. Only A and C are correct.
E. None of the above

71. A 24-hour urine protein excretion rate was 2.9 g/24 hours. This suggests:

A. The patient has focal segmental glomerulosclerosis.
B. The patient has membranoproliferative glomerulonephritis.
C. The patient will eventually progress to end-stage renal failure.
D. Only A and C are correct.
E. None of the above

72. The initial renal lesion in this patient:

A. Could be prevented by surgical intervention now
B. Is most likely associated with a renal cortical scar
C. Is an uncommon cause of end-stage renal failure
D. Only A and C are correct.
E. None of the above

QUESTIONS 73–76

A 24-year-old woman is admitted for abnormal uterine bleeding and a uterine mass. A preoperative ultrasound demonstrated mild bilateral hydronephrosis and normal-sized kidneys. She undergoes general anesthesia with resection of a large uterine leiomyoma. Her postoperative course was complicated with confusion, followed by obtundation. Her blood pressure is 120/80 mm Hg supine and upright, and her resting heart rate is 90 beats/minute. Her weight is now 55 kg. These laboratory studies were obtained the morning after the operation:

Serum electrolytes	
Sodium	170 mEq/L
Potassium	4.0 mEq/L
Chloride	136 mEq/L
Bicarbonate	22 mmol/L
Serum urea nitrogen	24 mg/dL
Serum creatinine	0.9 mg/dL
Serum glucose	90 mg/dL
Urine osmolality	80 mOsm/kg
Urine sodium	25 mEq/L

73. The most appropriate initial choice of intravenous fluids is:

A. 5% Dextrose in water
B. 5% Dextrose in 0.25% sodium chloride
C. 5% Dextrose in 0.45% sodium chloride
D. 5% Dextrose in 0.9% sodium chloride
E. None of the above is appropriate.

74. If one assumes no loss of solute, what is the calculated water deficit?

A. 3 L
B. 5 L
C. 7 L
D. 9 L
E. 11 L

75. Factors that control serum osmolality include:

A. Thirst

B. Atrial natriuretic hormone
C. Antidiuretic hormone (ADH)
D. A, B, and C are correct.
E. Only A and C are correct.

76. The patient is given aqueous vasopressin, 10 mU/kg intravenously, and her urine osmolality 2 hours later is 520 mOsm/kg. The most likely diagnosis of this patient's hypernatremia is:

A. Nephrogenic diabetes insipidus secondary to relief of urinary tract obstruction
B. Central diabetes insipidus
C. Osmotic diuresis secondary to retention of nitrogenous waste products
D. Sodium chloride retention
E. None of the above

QUESTIONS 77 AND 78

A 67-year-old man is brought to the emergency department with fever, nausea, and vomiting. For the past 10 days he has taken ampicillin for a urinary tract infection. Temperature is 100.6° F. Blood pressure is 125/70 mm Hg (supine) and 90/56 mm Hg (standing). Pulse rate is 92 beats/minute (supine) and 122 beats/minute (standing). Physical findings include rare basilar rales and wheezes, a faint macular rash on the trunk and legs, and a moderately enlarged prostate. Urinalysis shows 1+ proteinuria, 10-20 WBCs per high-power field, 20-30 RBCs per high-power field, and several white cell casts. A Wright stain of spun urinary sediment reveals many eosinophils. Other laboratory data include:

Serum electrolytes	
Sodium	134 mEq/L
Potassium	5.8 mEq/L
Chloride	110 mEq/L
Bicarbonate	14 mEq/L
BUN	88 mg/dL
Serum creatinine	2.8 mg/dL
WBC count	13,200/μL
Eosinophils	12%
Polymorphonuclear leukocytes (PMNs)	68%
Lymphocytes	12%
Monocytes	8%
Arterial pH	7.24
Urine studies	
Sodium	58 mEq/L
Chloride	34 mEq/L
Potassium	17 mEq/L
pH	5.7

77. Which of the following is the most likely cause of this clinical syndrome?

A. Obstructive uropathy at the level of the prostate
B. Acute glomerulonephritis
C. Tubulointerstitial nephritis
D. Volume depletion
E. Mild chronic renal insufficiency

78. Which of the following is least likely to contribute to hypotension in this patient?

A. Vomiting
B. Decreased GFR
C. Salt-losing nephropathy
D. Nausea and vomiting
E. Fever

QUESTIONS 79 AND 80

A 59-year-old male truck driver comes to the emergency department because of lethargy, nausea, and vomiting over the preceding 5 days and markedly decreased urinary volume. He has a history of mild hypertension treated with dietary salt restriction. For the past several months he has had urinary hesitancy and nocturia. Blood pressure is 105/60 mm Hg; pulse rate is 125 beats/minute. There is a 20-mm Hg orthostatic drop in blood pressure. Physical examination shows prostatic enlargement. The patient is unable to produce a urine specimen. The bladder is not distended by percussion. Plain film of the abdomen shows two renal outlines of normal size. Ultrasound examination of the kidneys shows normal renal size; there is no dilatation of the renal pelvis or ureters. Laboratory studies show:

Serum electrolytes	
Sodium	132 mEq/L
Potassium	5.2 mEq/L
Chloride	110 mEq/L
Bicarbonate	22 mEq/L
BUN	110 mg/dL
Serum creatinine	13 mg/dL
Calcium	8.1 mg/dL
Phosphate	6.2 mg/dL
Hemoglobin	13.5 g/dL

After rehydration with 5 L of normal saline, the patient remains anuric. The next morning, repeat ultrasound examination of the kidneys shows bilateral distention of the renal pelvis. Placement of a bladder catheter yields 2000 mL of clear urine, and urine production continues at 1000 mL/hour over the next 5 hours.

79. Which of the following is the most likely explanation of the abnormalities of renal function seen in this patient?

   A. Chronic renal failure
   B. High circulating levels of vasopressin
   C. Obstructive uropathy at the level of the prostate
   D. Renal artery stenosis
   E. A toxic nephropathy

80. Which of the following best explains the initially normal ultrasound examination?

   A. Improper interpretation of the examination
   B. Extracellular fluid volume depletion
   C. Acute glomerulonephritis
   D. Bilateral ureteral obstruction
   E. Uric acid nephropathy

QUESTIONS 81 AND 82

A 66-year-old man with recently diagnosed small cell carcinoma of the lung, without apparent central nervous system metastases, comes to the hospital with confusion. There is no history of vomiting and he takes no medicine. Physical examination reveals a blood pressure of 116/80 mm Hg, jugular vein pressure of 6 cm H_2O, and obtundation without any localizing findings. There is no clinical evidence of extracellular fluid (ECF) depletion. Laboratory tests include:

Serum electrolytes	
Sodium	108 mEq/L
Potassium	4.4 mEq/L
Chloride	82 mEq/L
Bicarbonate	20 mEq/L
BUN	6 mg/dL
Serum creatinine	0.7 mg/dL
Serum uric acid	3.8 mg/dL
Serum osmolality	222 mOsm/kg

Urine studies	
Sodium	50 mEq/L
Potassium	12 mEq/L
pH	5.0
Osmolality	860 mOsm/kg

81. What is the major mechanism contributing to this patient's hyponatremia?

   A. Osmotic diuresis
   B. Impaired free water clearance
   C. Laboratory artifact in the measurement of serum sodium
   D. ADH effect based on a physiologic nonosmotic stimulus
   E. Decreased total body water with a larger decrease in total body sodium

82. Which mechanism explains the measured level of urine sodium?

   A. Osmotic diuresis
   B. Salt-losing nephropathy
   C. Impaired free water clearance
   D. Increased distal delivery of an impermeant anion
   E. The patient is in sodium balance and the extracellular fluid compartment is not depleted

QUESTIONS 83 AND 84

A 68-year-old man has increasing hypertension 3 weeks after an aortic angiogram and subsequent repair of an abdominal aortic aneurysm. In the hospital he received brief courses of several drugs, including a cephalosporin, cimetidine, and heparin. He is currently receiving aspirin and dipyridamole. Physical examination now shows a blood pressure of 170/110 mm Hg. Bruits are heard in both femoral arteries. Mottling of the lower extremities and subungual petechiae on a lower extremity nail bed are present. Laboratory data include:

Serum electrolytes	
Sodium	140 mEq/L
Potassium	5.1 mEq/L
Chloride	104 mEq/L
Bicarbonate	20 mEq/L
BUN	60 mg/dL
Serum creatinine	3.2 mg/dL
Complete blood cell count	
Hematocrit	35%
White blood cell count	10,500 /mm³
Polymorphonuclear leukocytes	80%
Lymphocytes	12%
Eosinophils	8%

Urinalysis shows a pH of 5.0, 2+ protein, 1 to 3 WBCs per high-power field, and 10 to 15 RBCs per high-power field.

Wright's stain of the urine is positive for eosinophils.

83. Choose the diagnosis most likely to explain the azotemia and hypertension in this patient.

   A. Nephrosclerosis
   B. Atheroembolic renal disease
   C. Drug-induced interstitial nephritis
   D. Radiocontrast-induced renal disease
   E. Postoperative ATN

84. Which is the most likely prognosis for the renal disease?

   A. Complete recovery in 2 to 3 days
   B. Complete recovery in 10 to 14 days
   C. Stabilization of the renal function at the current level
   D. Progressive deterioration of renal function over months
   E. The disorder has no characteristic course.

QUESTIONS 85 AND 86

A 49-year-old woman with known polycystic kidney disease and a serum creatinine concentration of 3.0 mg/dL comes to the emergency department because of abdominal and flank pain. She states that she noted some blood-tinged urine the preceding day. Physical examination showed blood pressure of 180/105 mm Hg, pulse of 92 beats/minute, and temperature of 38°C. There is no orthostasis. Large bilateral upper quadrant masses are palpated; the right is somewhat tender. Bowel sounds are normal. A plain film of the abdomen reveals large upper quadrant masses bilaterally. An abdominal sonogram shows large polycystic kidneys with multiple overlapping echoes. A few areas in the upper pole of the right kidney have complex echoes. No solid masses are seen. Urinalysis shows 1+ protein, RBCs >100 per high-power field, and WBCs of 5 to 10 per high-power field.

85. Which of the following is the most likely cause of the patient's condition?

    A. Renal infarction
    B. Urinary tract infection
    C. Renal cell carcinoma
    D. Hemorrhage into a renal cyst
    E. Arteriovenous malformation of the kidney

86. Which procedure is most reasonably indicated at this time?

    A. Observation and bed rest
    B. Surgical exploration
    C. Renal angiography
    D. Intravenous pyelogram
    E. CT scan of the abdomen

QUESTIONS 87 AND 88

A 40-year-old woman was evaluated for edema of some months' duration and was found to have the nephrotic syndrome. The 24-hour urinary protein excretion was 11 g. Serum creatinine was 0.9 mg/dL, and creatinine clearance was 88 mL/minute. A percutaneous renal biopsy obtained a small piece of cortex that revealed only four glomeruli with a normal light microscopic pattern. Immunofluorescence was negative, and electron microscopy revealed fusion of the glomerular foot processes without evidence of immune deposits. She has no other clinical findings.

After a 16-week course of prednisone, 60 mg daily, the edema was slightly improved, although the patient noted a cushingoid appearance. The 24-hour urinary protein excretion was 5 g. Prednisone was discontinued, and she was managed with diuretics and sodium restriction with an improvement of the edema.

Two years later, the patient is found to have persistent edema and a serum creatinine value of 3.7 mg/dL, with 14 g of protein in a 24-hour collection of urine.

87. If a renal biopsy were to be performed now, the most likely histologic diagnosis would be

    A. IgA nephropathy
    B. Minimal change glomerulopathy
    C. Membranous glomerulonephritis
    D. Focal segmental glomerulosclerosis
    E. Membranoproliferative glomerulonephritis

88. Which of the following should be used to treat the persistent nephrotic syndrome in this patient?

    A. Aspirin plus dipyridamole
    B. Prednisone, 60 mg orally daily
    C. Prednisone plus cyclophosphamide

D. Methylprednisolone, 1 g daily for 3 days
E. None of the above

QUESTIONS 89 AND 90

A 78-year-old man is brought to the emergency department by a neighbor who was alarmed after not hearing from him for 3 days. The patient is barely conscious and has an obvious left hemiparesis. Blood pressure is 90/60 mm Hg with a pulse rate of 120 beats/minute. He is afebrile. The mucous membranes are dry, and there is tenting of the skin over the forehead. There is early skin breakdown on the left hip. The remainder of the physical examination is consistent with a cerebrovascular accident. There is no sign of heart failure or pulmonary infiltrates. Weight is 70 kg. Laboratory studies show:

Serum electrolytes	
Sodium	162 mEq/L
Potassium	5.0 mEq/L
Chloride	120 mEq/L
Bicarbonate	24 mEq/L
Serum glucose	181 mg/dL

89. This patient's total body sodium content is

    A. High because the serum sodium concentration is high
    B. Low
    C. Normal
    D. Cannot determine from the information given

90. In planning fluid therapy, which of the following is appropriate?

    A. Half of the calculated water deficit should be administered as hypotonic fluid immediately and the remainder over 8 to 12 hours.
    B. Initial extracellular volume (ECV) repletion should be made with isotonic saline, followed by correction of the free water deficit with hypotonic fluids over 48 hours.
    C. Furosemide should be administered and the measured urinary sodium loss should be replaced with hypotonic saline.
    D. The calculated free water deficit should be administered as half-normal saline over the next 24 hours.
    E. The calculated free water deficit should be administered as half-normal saline over the next 48 hours.

QUESTIONS 91 AND 92

A 78-year-old woman is evaluated in the emergency department because of a 4-day history of vomiting, muscle cramps, and low-grade fever. She has been unable to eat anything and has drunk only tea, water, and carbonated drinks. The previous history is unremarkable.

91. Which of the following would be the most likely electrolyte disturbance?

    A. Hyponatremia
    B. Hyperkalemia
    C. Hypokalemia
    D. Anion gap acidosis
    E. Hyperchloremic metabolic acidosis

92. The most likely urinary electrolyte findings would be

    A. Urine sodium = 30 mEq/L; urine potassium = 60 mEq/L
    B. Urine sodium = 30 mEq/L; urine chloride = 90 mEq/L
    C. Urine sodium = 30 mEq/L; urine chloride = 30 mEq/L
    D. Urine sodium = 3 mEq/L; urine potassium = 20 mEq/L
    E. Urine sodium = 3 mEq/L; urine chloride = 50 mEq/L

QUESTIONS 93 AND 94

A 60-year-old man is seen in the emergency department because of muscle cramps and paresthesias. He has a history of recurrent squamous cell carcinoma of the head and neck and finished a course of cisplatin 3 weeks before admission. Local radiation therapy is planned for the immediate future. He has also noted frequent watery diarrhea over the past month and has not been able to eat or drink well. Physical examination does not show significant volume depletion. There is a positive Chvostek sign, serum calcium concentration of 5.8 mg/dL, and serum magnesium level of 0.7 mEq/L. The urinary magnesium concentration on a random urine sample is 20 mEq/L.

93. Which factor is *least* likely to have contributed to the hypomagnesemia in this patient?

    A. Diarrhea
    B. Hypocalcemia
    C. Poor oral intake
    D. Cisplatin therapy
    E. A paraneoplastic syndrome from a squamous cell carcinoma

94. Which factor is most likely to have contributed to the hypocalcemia?

    A. Diarrhea
    B. Hypomagnesemia
    C. Poor oral intake
    D. Cisplatin therapy
    E. A paraneoplastic syndrome from a squamous cell carcinoma

QUESTIONS 95–98

A 70-year-old white man presented to the emergency department with several months of dyspnea, fatigue, and weight loss culminating in the recent onset of hemoptysis. Initial physical examination demonstrates euvolemia and normotension. Initial laboratory examination showed the following:

Serum electrolytes	
Sodium	136 mEq/L
Potassium	4.9 mEq/L
Chloride	101 mEq/L
Bicarbonate	21 mEq/L
BUN	46 mg/dL
Serum creatinine	4.3 mg/dL
Hematocrit	31%
Platelets	475,000/µL
Urinalysis	2+ protein, 3+ Hb

Urine sediment showed numerous granular casts and RBCs with occasional RBC casts.

Chest radiograph demonstrates patchy infiltrates in both lung fields.

95. Possible diagnoses include all of the following *except:*

    A. Wegener's granulomatosis
    B. Microscopic polyarteritis nodosa
    C. Anti–glomerular basement membrane disease (Goodpasture's syndrome)
    D. Post-streptococcal acute glomerulonephritis
    E. All of the above

Renal biopsy demonstrated crescent formation in 80% of the glomeruli, and immunofluorescent microscopy reveals a "pauci-immune" pattern (C_3 and IgM only).

96. Appropriate therapies for the constellation of findings include:

    A. Cyclophosphamide
    B. Interferon-α
    C. Methylprednisolone
    D. A and C are correct.
    E. All of the above are correct.

97. Antineutrophil cytoplasmic antibodies (ANCA) would be expected to be positive in all of the following *except:*

    A. Cryoglobulinemia
    B. Wegener's granulomatosis
    C. Microscopic polyarteritis nodosa
    D. Churg-Strauss syndrome
    E. All of the above are correct.

98. All of the following are true of Wegener's granulomatosis *except:*

    A. Without treatment, 1-year survival is < 20%.
    B. Oliguria and serum creatinine > 4 are indicators of a poor renal prognosis.
    C. Once requiring dialysis, patients do not recover renal function.
    D. Remissions of up to 4 years can be achieved with appropriate therapy.
    E. Patients with limited sinus disease may benefit from chronic therapy with trimethoprim/sulfamethoxazole.

QUESTIONS 99–101

A 45-year-old white man with ethanol-related cirrhosis presents to the emergency department with nausea, vomiting, and oliguria 5 days after undergoing a large-volume paracentesis (10 L). He is taking furosemide, spironolactone, and isosorbide dinitrate. Laboratory investigation demonstrates:

Serum electrolytes	
Sodium	125 mEq/L
Potassium	3.3 mEq/L
Chloride	84 mEq/L
Bicarbonate	28 mEq/L
BUN	34 mg/dL
Serum creatinine	3.7 mg/dL
Urine studies	
Sodium	7 mEq/L
Creatinine	74 mg/dL

99. Likely causes for acute azotemia include:

    A. Prerenal azotemia (volume depletion)
    B. ATN
    C. Hepatorenal syndrome (HRS)
    D. A and C are correct.
    E. All of the above are correct.

100. Features of the hepatorenal syndrome include:

    A. It may be precipitated by volume depletion.
    B. It is caused by a renal tubular defect.
    C. It is associated with a 50% mortality rate.
    D. It has no known cure.
    E. Moderate proteinuria is usually present.

101. Hyponatremia is common in cirrhotic patients. This finding can be attributed to:

    A. Increased renal sodium losses
    B. Increased renal free water retention
    C. Effective circulatory volume expansion

D. Decreased adrenal aldosterone production

E. None of the above

QUESTIONS 102–104

A 67-year-old black man had a recent episode of acute renal failure caused by prostatic hypertrophy and urethral obstruction. His renal function has stabilized and a typical set of blood chemistries is presented:

Serum electrolytes	
Sodium	138 mEq/L
Potassium	5.8 mEq/L
Chloride	108 mEq/L
Bicarbonate	18 mEq/L
BUN	28 mg/dL
Serum creatinine	2.3 mg/dL
Arterial blood gases	
pH	7.33
$Paco_2$	35 mm Hg
Pao_2	82 mm Hg

102. Regarding the above electrolyte abnormalities, which of the following would be *true* of this patient?

A. He would be unable to raise his urinary pH in response to an oral bicarbonate load.

B. Given his hyperkalemia, the metabolic acidosis likely represents nonrenal bicarbonate loss.

C. These abnormalities represent a decrease in production or effect of aldosterone.

D. Increased distal sodium delivery would be unlikely to improve either the acidosis or the hyperkalemia.

E. Oral bicarbonate administration is the treatment of choice.

103. Recovery of renal function after urinary obstruction:

A. Is inversely proportional to the duration of obstruction

B. Is inversely proportional to the degree of obstruction

C. Is proportional to renal cortical thickness

D. A and C are correct.

E. All of the above are correct.

104. Postobstructive diuresis is caused by:

A. Loss of the medullary salt/urea gradient

B. Decreased sensitivity to ADH

C. Salt retention and volume expansion

D. Accumulation of solutes (osmotic diuresis)

E. All of the above are correct

QUESTIONS 105–107

A 47-year-old white man underwent an abdominal ultrasound to evaluate gallstones. A complicated cyst was incidentally noted on the right kidney. A CT scan of the abdomen confirmed a 3-cm cystic mass "highly suspicious for renal cell carcinoma" in the right kidney but discovered no adenopathy, metastases, or intravascular involvement.

105. The most appropriate initial intervention is:

A. A combination of external-beam radiation and vinblastine-based chemotherapy

B. Radical nephrectomy with regional lymph node dissection

C. Serial CT scans every 3 months

D. Fine-needle aspiration and biopsy

E. Excisional biopsy

106. Which of these are risk factors for renal cell carcinoma?

A. Acquired cystic kidney disease

B. Autosomal-dominant polycystic kidney disease

C. von Hippel-Lindau syndrome

D. A and C are correct.

E. All of the above are correct.

107. Which of the following syndromes have been associated with renal cell carcinoma?

A. Polycythemia

B. Anemia

C. Hypercalcemia

D. Myopathy/neuropathy

E. All of the above are correct.

MATCHING

DIRECTIONS: Questions 108–125 are matching questions. For each numbered item, choose the *most* likely associated lettered item from those provided. Each numbered item has *only one* answer. Within each set of questions, each lettered item may be the answer to one, more than one, or none of the numbered items.

QUESTIONS 108–115

For each of the therapeutic agents listed below, select the most likely associated complication.

A. Impaired free water excretion

B. Nephrogenic diabetes insipidus

C. Secondary nephrotic syndrome

D. Hypokalemia

E. Hyperkalemia

108. Gold

109. Chlorpropamide

110. Lithium

111. Cyclosporine

112. Succinylcholine

113. D-Penicillamine

114. Spironolactone

115. Trimethoprim

QUESTIONS 116–120

For each of the following clinical diagnoses, select the most appropriate serum electrolyte determinations. Each answer can only be used once.

	A.	B.	C.	D.	E.
Sodium	142	138	138	138	122
Potassium	5.7	2.2	3.4	5.7	5.7
Chloride	100	112	112	112	76
Bicarbonate	16	16	16	16	16

116. Diabetic ketoacidosis

117. Type IV renal tubular acidosis (RTA)

118. Distal (type I) RTA

119. Proximal (type II) RTA

120. Uremic acidosis

QUESTIONS 121–125

For each of the following immunosuppressant medications, select the most appropriate mechanism of action.

A. Inhibits T cell function by binding to the CD3 complex on the surface of the T cell
B. Inhibits T cell activation by inhibiting cytokine production by antigen-presenting cells
C. Inhibits T cell activation by preventing interleukin (IL)-2 production
D. Inhibits cytokine-stimulated T cell proliferation by binding to mammalian target of rapamycin (mTOR) in the T cell cytoplasm

121. OKT3

122. Cyclosporine

123. Corticosteroids

124. Tacrolimus

125. Sirolimus

Part IV
Renal Disease
Answers

1. (A)–False; (B)–False; (C)–True; (D)–False; (E)–True.
Discussion: Obstruction should always be considered in patients who present with renal failure. Whereas anuria occurs when obstruction is complete, in partial obstruction, polyuria may be seen. Although ultrasound is an excellent screening tool, obstruction may occur without hydronephrosis. Complications of obstruction include frequent urinary tract infections, hypertension, and type IV renal tubular acidosis (RTA). *(Cecil, Ch. 121)*

2. (A)–True; (B)–True; (C)–False; (D)–False; (E)–False.
Discussion: Membranous nephropathy, diagnosed with renal biopsy, warrants an investigation for systemic diseases that include systemic lupus erythematosus, infections, and malignancy. Up to 25% of patients older than age 50 years have an associated malignancy, especially of the stomach, colon, and lung. Membranous nephropathy has in recent years been replaced by focal and segmental glomerulosclerosis as the most common cause of idiopathic nephrotic syndrome in adults. The variable course of membranous nephropathy makes the assessment of therapy difficult. Membranous nephropathy can recur in the transplanted kidney. *(Haas et al., 1997; Cecil, Ch. 119)*

3. (A)–True; (B)–False; (C)–True; (D)–True; (E)–True.
Discussion: Magnesium depletion can be difficult to diagnose, but persistent hypomagnesemia suggests the diagnosis. Drugs that can produce magnesium depletion from renal magnesium wasting include loop diuretics, aminoglycosides, and cisplatin. Magnesium depletion causes hypokalemia from renal potassium wasting and hypocalcemia by preventing parathyroid hormone secretion. Cardiac effects of magnesium depletion include prolongation of the PR and QT intervals and ventricular arrhythmias. Cardiac toxicity of digitalis is enhanced by magnesium depletion. *(Cecil, Ch. 115)*

4. (A)–True; (B)–True; (C)–True; (D)–True; (E)–True.
Discussion: Renal hypoperfusion can be caused by a primary reduction in effective circulating volume, unilateral renal occlusive disease, or bilateral acute renal vasoconstriction. Increased renal salt avidity and renin secretion are constant findings. Azotemia and hypertension depend on the volume status and whether the hypoperfusion is a unilateral (i.e., occlusion) or bilateral (i.e., vasoconstriction, hypovolemia) process. The nonsteroidal anti-inflammatory agents can produce a hemodynamically mediated acute renal failure in predisposed individuals, such as those with severe liver disease or congestive heart failure. *(Cecil, Chs. 116 and 124)*

5. (A)–True; (B)–True; (C)–True; (D)–False; (E)–False.
Discussion: Renal hemodynamics change dramatically with normal pregnancy. Both GFR and renal blood flow increase by up to 150% during the course of pregnancy, starting as early as the fourth week of gestation. Renal clearance of urate increases, producing hypouricemia. An increase in uric levels coincides with development of preeclampsia. Respiratory alkalosis is also common. Metabolic acidosis does not develop during normal pregnancy, and blood pressure typically decreases in early gestation. *(Brenner and Rector's The Kidney)*

6. (A)–True; (B)–True; (C)–True; (D)–True; (E)–False.
Discussion: Creatinine is an end product of muscle creatine metabolism. The creatinine production rate correlates with muscle rather than whole body mass and is reasonably constant from day to day in the same individual. Urinary creatinine excretion is the sum of filtration and secretion. Creatinine secretion normally accounts for only 20% of creatinine excretion but can increase if glomerular filtration is impaired out of proportion to impairments of renal plasma flow. Organic bases such as cimetidine can block creatinine secretion but do not affect the filtration component of creatinine excretion. Thus, cimetidine can increase serum creatinine and decrease creatinine clearance rate but in the steady state will not change the absolute excretion of creatinine. Because of the nonlinear relationship between creatinine clearance and the serum creatinine concentration, changes in serum creatinine concentration can be an insensitive indicator of reductions in the GFR in the 60 to 100 mL/minute range. *(Cecil, Ch. 110)*

7. (A)–True; (B)–True; (C)–False; (D)–True; (E)–False.
Discussion: Urinary chloride excretion provides important information about the status of whole body fluid balance and the pathogenesis of metabolic alkalosis. Extrarenal losses of fluid can cause chloride depletion and low urinary chloride concentrations (e.g., vomiting, laxative abuse). Diuretics can cause metabolic alkalosis and renal losses of NaCl, whereas adrenocortical hormones cause metabolic alkalosis with NaCl retention. Although urinary chloride concentration will be elevated in both conditions, saline administration will improve the metabolic alkalosis in the first instance but not in the latter ("saline-resistant" metabolic alkalosis). *(Cecil, Ch. 110)*

8. (A)–False; (B)–False; (C)–False; (D)–True; (E)–True.
Discussion: Secondary hyperparathyroidism is a common complication of chronic kidney disease and is related to several pathophysiologic events. Obligatory phosphate retention occurs when the GFR approaches 20 to 25 mL/minute. The kidney is the principal site of enzymatic conversion of 25(OH) vitamin D to the highly active metabolite 1,25(OH)$_2$ vitamin D (calcitriol). Renal production of calcitriol is impaired very early in the course of chronic renal failure. As a primary consequence of reduced gut calcium absorption, hypocalcemia ensues, which stimulates PTH secretion. In this setting of secondary hyperparathyroidism and reduced calcium absorption, the development of renal osteodystrophy is a near certainty. *(Brenner and Rector's The Kidney)*

9. (A)–True; (B)–True; (C)–False; (D)–False; (E)–True.
Discussion: Inadequate dialysis is the most common cause of uremic pericarditis. Because of the development of extensive pericardial capillaries and the bleeding tendency in uremia, the pericardial fluid is usually hemorrhagic and may accumulate quite rapidly. Any evidence of hemodynamic compromise becomes a surgical emergency. Right-sided filling pressures are critical in maintaining cardiac output in the setting of pericarditis, so volume depletion should be avoided. *(Cecil, Ch. 117)*

10. **(A)–True; (B)–True; (C)–True; (D)–True; (E)–True.**
Discussion: The availability of erythropoietin has changed the clinical features of ESRD. Cardiac performance, appetite, and general sense of well being are augmented by maintenance of the hematocrit in a reasonable range (33-36%). However, completely correcting the hematocrit with erythropoietin does not provide additional benefit and, for unclear reasons, in one study, appeared to increase mortality in patients on dialysis. *(Cecil, Ch. 117)*

11. **(A)–False; (B)–False; (C)–True; (D)–True; (E)–False.**
Discussion: Children do quite well with peritoneal dialysis because of a relative increase in peritoneal surface area. Diabetics generally do well and have minimal hemodynamic instability on peritoneal dialysis. Adding insulin to the dialysate typically controls hyperglycemia. Permeability characteristics of the peritoneal membrane vary from one person to the next and can even change in the same individual over time. The dialysis prescription is therefore adjusted according to the peritoneal equilibration test (PET), which is obtained in every patient on peritoneal dialysis. Ultrafiltration is achieved by changing the concentration of dextrose in the dialysate. Peritonitis is a major complication of peritoneal dialysis and is most often caused by gram-positive organisms from the skin. *(Cecil, Ch. 118)*

12. **(A)–True; (B)–True; (C)–False; (D)–True; (E)–False.**
Discussion: Tissue typing and proper matching have a beneficial effect on graft survival. In vitro cytotoxicity testing between donor cells and recipient serum has nearly eliminated "hyperacute" rejection. Despite these advances, it is unusual to find the "perfect" 6-antigen match for a cadaver kidney because of the high frequency of polymorphisms of the HLA system. In the meantime, advances in immunotherapy have dramatically improved graft survival in the usual setting when the HLA matching is less than perfect. *(Cecil, Ch. 118)*

13. **(A)–True; (B)–True; (C)–True; (D)–True; (E)–True.**
Discussion: Cyclosporine has revolutionized organ transplantation and represents the first generation of targeted immunosuppressants. It is currently being used in combination with conventional immunosuppressants (glucocorticoids, azathioprine) and other targeted immunosuppressants like OKT3 and antilymphocyte globulin. Cyclosporine toxicity remains a constant problem, despite careful monitoring of blood levels. The drug is metabolized through the hepatic cytochrome P-450 enzyme system. Drugs that alter this system can affect serum concentrations of cyclosporine. *(Cecil, Ch. 118)*

14. **(A)–False; (B)–True; (C)–True; (D)–True; (E)–False.**
Discussion: Membranoproliferative glomerulonephritis (MPGN) refers to a clinicopathologic entity that occurs primarily in young adults. Interestingly, the incidence of idiopathic MPGN is declining. Activation of the complement pathway is a typical feature of this lesion, and hypocomplementemia may be severe, especially in type II MPGN. Most of these patients have a circulating IgG autoantibody (termed *C3 nephritic factor*) that binds to C3 convertase of the alternative complement pathway, protecting it from inactivation. About 70% of patients will have a depressed serum C3. MPGN may occur in association in several infective conditions (e.g., hepatitis B or infective endocarditis), systemic lupus erythematosus, mixed essential cryoglobulinemia, sickle cell disease, scleroderma, and α_1-antitrypsin deficiency. MPGN can recur after renal transplantation. *(Cecil, Ch. 119)*

15. **(A)–True; (B)–False; (C)–True; (D)–True; (E)–False.**
Discussion: Hemolytic-uremic syndrome (HUS) is a form of thrombotic microangiopathy characterized clinically by microangiopathic hemolytic anemia, thrombocytopenia, reduced haptoglobin levels, and minimal evidence of disseminated intravascular coagulation. HUS may occur in children 3 to 10 days after a bout of gas-troenteritis, particularly with verotoxin-producing *Escherichia coli* infections. HUS occurs less frequently in adults, often in association with pregnancy or oral contraceptives. The renal prognosis in children is good: although renal failure may occur in 60% of children, it usually resolves spontaneously within about 2 weeks. However, about 14% will develop chronic renal failure. Those patients who present with a diarrheal prodrome tend to have the most favorable outcome. *(Cecil, Ch. 124)*

16. **(A)–False; (B)–False; (C)–True; (D)–True; (E)–False.**
Discussion: The nephrotic syndrome—heavy proteinuria, edema, and hypoalbuminemia—is a common consequence of a variety of glomerular diseases of both focal and diffuse pathology. It is characterized by an often-decreased plasma volume and avid sodium retention. Management of nephrotic edema includes salt restriction and diuretics. Although albumin infusions are of transient benefit, the added albumin is rapidly lost from the circulation. There is an increased infection rate in the nephrotic syndrome, a finding attributed to loss of circulating immunoglobulins. *(Cecil, Ch. 119)*

17. **(A)–True; (B)–True; (C)–True; (D)–False; (E)–False.**
Discussion: Although hypocalcemia, hyperphosphatemia, and disorders of parathyroid hormone are present in both acute and chronic renal failure, elevation of bone alkaline phosphatase and radiographic signs of osteodystrophy are present only in established renal disease. Bilaterally small kidneys are a characteristic of chronic disease. Hypertension may occur in either form. Production of dilute urine does not distinguish acute from chronic renal disease. *(Cecil, Chs. 110 and 117)*

18. **(A)–False; (B)–False; (C)–True; (D)–True; (E)–True.**
Discussion: The diagnosis of analgesic-associated nephropathy, which is often difficult to establish, has been made with increasing frequency in this country. It has been estimated to account for at least 20% of cases of chronic interstitial nephropathy. It is believed to arise from toxic effects of analgesics or their metabolites on the deep renal interstitium. Although phenacetin has been considered the most nephropathic analgesic compound, there is indication that use of combinations of analgesics is also significantly nephrotoxic. There is a female predominance. There is usually a history of consumption of more than 3 kg of analgesic, although this history is characteristically difficult to elicit. In the late stages, excretory urography usually shows small kidneys with cortical scarring and evidence of papillary necrosis. Anemia out of proportion to the degree of azotemia is common and is attributed to chronic gastrointestinal blood loss. *(Cecil, Ch. 120)*

19. **(A)–True; (B)–True; (C)–True; (D)–False; (E)–False.**
Discussion: Medullary sponge kidney is a disorder characterized by ectasia and calcification of medullary collecting tubules. It is usually diagnosed by the characteristic appearance on excretory urogram in an asymptomatic patient. It is probably a congenital rather than a hereditary disorder, although it occurs in several systemic diseases, including Ehlers-Danlos syndrome. Renal calculi, hypercalciuria, and urinary tract infection are common. A decreased urine concentrating ability is frequent, but other functional tubular abnormalities and renal insufficiency are not common in this disorder. *(Cecil, Ch. 127)*

20. **(A)–False; (B)–False; (C)–False; (D)–False; (E)–True.**
Discussion: Diabetic nephropathy presenting with azotemia and heavy proteinuria is generally observed to progress to end-stage renal disease at a predictable and inexorable rate. Virtually all patients with this diagnosis have hypertension and retinal vascular disease, and most have nephrotic-range proteinuria. The absence of these concomitant features should draw the diagnosis of diabetic nephropathy into question. Even with overt diabetic nephropathy, ACE inhibitors are efficacious by slowing loss of renal function. *(Cecil, Ch. 123)*

21. (A)–False; (B)–False; (C)–False; (D)–False; (E)–True.

22. (A)–False; (B)–False; (C)–False; (D)–True; (E)–False.
Discussion for questions 21 and 22: Rapidly progressive glomerulonephritis is a clinical syndrome that includes a heterogeneous group of disorders characterized by a rapid deterioration of renal function and proliferation of epithelial crescents affecting more than 50% (often more than 70%) of glomeruli. Etiologic disorders include Goodpasture's syndrome, Henoch-Schönlein purpura, post-streptococcal acute glomerulonephritis, a variety of immune-complex-mediated glomerular diseases, and primary crescentic glomerulonephritis. Post-streptococcal acute glomerulonephritis usually appears with a recent history of a streptococcal infection and is associated usually with an elevated antistreptolysin O titer. IgA nephropathy is characterized by prominent deposition of IgA in glomeruli. Wegener's granulomatosis is a systemic illness that consists of necrotizing granulomatous arteritis of the lung, along with other systemic features that include renal disease. The renal lesion can be identical to that described in this patient who had idiopathic crescentic glomerulonephritis. Because idiopathic crescentic glomerulonephritis is uncommon, there are no randomized, controlled studies on treatment. Most authors recommend combinations of glucocorticoids and cytotoxic agents, because this disease process progresses to end-stage kidney failure. Unlike Goodpasture's syndrome, which is generally responsive to removal of anti–glomerular basement antibodies with plasmapheresis, there is no clear role for plasma exchange in this group of patients who do not have demonstrable immunoglobulin deposition in the kidney. Patients with this form of crescentic glomerulonephritis may develop systemic manifestations of Wegener's granulomatosis, particularly if there is a high titer of antineutrophil cytoplasmic antibodies, suggesting this represents a "renal-limited" form of Wegener's granulomatosis. (*Cecil, Ch. 119*)

23. (A)–False; (B)–True; (C)–True; (D)–True; (E)–True.
Discussion: The acidosis of advanced uremia is a state in which renal compensatory mechanisms are inadequate to maintain external acid-base balance. Even before acidosis appears in uremia, careful balance studies indicate that there is net positive acid balance (i.e., body tissues, including bone, buffer acid). The normal renal compensatory mechanisms in acidosis include increased renal ammoniagenesis; ammonia is the major urinary buffer responsible for the increment in acid excretion. In addition, there is an increased fractional proximal reabsorption of bicarbonate. When uremic acidosis supervenes, the reduction in renal mass prevents an appropriate increment in urinary ammonia. When the GFR is below 20 to 25% of normal, there is an absolute retention of organic and inorganic acid anions, leading to an increased anion gap. At this point, although the urine is normally acid, a bicarbonate load cannot be adequately reabsorbed and bicarbonaturia on alkali loading will result. Hyperkalemia inhibits and hypokalemia stimulates renal ammoniagenesis. (*Cecil, Ch. 117*)

24. (A)–True; (B)–False; (C)–True; (D)–True; (E)–False.
Discussion: Aminoglycoside-induced nephrotoxicity is a common cause of acute renal failure, accounting for 10 to 15% of all cases in the United States. Functional tubule abnormalities may produce potassium and magnesium wasting and produce symptomatic hypokalemia and hypomagnesemia. Risk factors include an elderly age, preexisting renal failure, extracellular fluid volume depletion, administration of high doses of aminoglycosides, and prolonged duration of therapy. Generally, a nonoliguric type of acute renal failure occurs and the prognosis for recovery of renal function is excellent. Aminoglycosides are not equally nephrotoxic, although all can cause acute renal failure. (*Cecil, Ch. 116*)

25. (A)–True; (B)–True; (C)–False; (D)–False; (E)–True.
Discussion: Pregnancy-induced hypertension (preeclampsia) typi-

cally occurs in the third trimester, although it can rarely occur as early as the 24th week of gestation. The syndrome is characterized by hypertension, proteinuria (which can be nephrotic-range), edema, and reductions in GFR and renal blood flow. Uric acid levels increase because of decreased renal clearance. The clinical manifestations of preeclampsia generally resolve spontaneously within 4 to 6 weeks after delivery; persistence of renal abnormalities after 12 weeks suggests an underlying primary renal disease. (*Brenner and Rector's The Kidney*)

26. (A)–False; (B)–True; (C)–True; (D)–True; (E)–True.
Discussion: Most crystals seen on routine urinalysis are formed after voiding, when the urine cools and becomes alkaline. To demonstrate that crystals are formed in the kidney, examine a freshly voided urine sample. Hexagonal-shaped crystals are seen in cystinuria, a common aminoaciduria affecting about 1:7000 individuals. Cystine is the least soluble of the naturally occurring amino acids especially in acidic solutions, hence the tendency toward renal stone formation in these patients. Magnesium ammonium phosphate crystals (struvite) are associated with urinary tract infections with urea-splitting organisms. Treatment of all patients with renal calculi should include a high fluid intake (minimum 2 L) if tolerated. Successful therapy should produce at least one bout of nocturia, because the urine tends to become acidic when concentrated. Alkalinization of the urine with potassium citrate may be effective in preventing the formation of both uric acid and calcium stones; alkalinization will also help patients with cystinuria, but a urine pH of greater than 7.5 is necessary to produce the desired effect. (*Cecil, Ch. 126*)

27. (A)–True; (B)–True; (C)–True; (D)–False; (E)–True; (F)–True. *Discussion:* Autosomal-dominant polycystic kidney disease (ADPKD) is the most common hereditary disease in the United States, affecting 500,000 people. Although half of the offspring of one affected parent will inherit the gene that produces ADPKD, expression of the disease is variable. Renal failure, for example, can occur as early as the first decade of life in some patients; in others, renal function can remain well preserved throughout life. Patients can present with microscopic and macroscopic hematuria, renal calculi, hypertension, or subarachnoid bleeding from intracranial aneurysms, which may be found in 10 to 40% of patients with ADPKD. The presence of hepatic cysts on ultrasound supports the diagnosis of ADPKD. (*Cecil, Ch. 127*)

28. (**All True**). *Discussion:* Gross hematuria may occur from many sources along the urinary tract from the glomerulus to the urinary bladder. The most common glomerular source of gross hematuria is IgA nephropathy (Burger's disease). In this disorder, gross hematuria often follows upper respiratory infections and is generally transient. Schönlein-Henoch purpura has a renal lesion identical to IgA nephropathy but has additional clinical features of leukocytoclastic vasculitic purpura, arthralgias, and abdominal pain. Both chronic analgesic abuse and sickle cell disease can cause papillary necrosis, which can result in massive hematuria. Hemorrhagic cystitis is a known complication of cyclophosphamide therapy. (*Cecil, Chs. 119, 120, and 124*)

29. (A)–True; (B)–False; (C)–True; (D)–True; (E)–False.
Discussion: Acute glomerulonephritis is an important clinical syndrome that must be promptly recognized so an appropriate diagnosis can be established and therapy instituted. It is characterized by hematuria, edema (which occurs in the hands and face as well as the feet and ankles), azotemia, and decreasing urine output. The urinalysis demonstrates proteinuria and hematuria with red blood cell casts present on the microscopic examination. Hypercholesterolemia, hypoalbuminemia, and dependent edema are features of the nephrotic syndrome. (*Cecil, Ch. 119*)

30. (A)–True; (B)–True; (C)–False; (D)–True; (E)–False.
Discussion: Hypocomplementemia is present in those disorders,

which activate factors of the complement cascade at a rate greater than they are being produced. This is true of immune complex deposition disorders such as systemic lupus erythematosus, infective endocarditis, "shunt" nephritis, and cryoglobulinemia. Serum complement levels are also low in membranoproliferative glomerulonephritis (MPGN), although the mechanism is incompletely understood. MPGN is occasionally associated with an autoantibody (termed C_3 *nephritic factor*), which prolongs the half-life of C_3 convertase and in turn accelerates the consumption of C_3. (*Cecil, Ch. 119*)

31. (A)–True; (B)–False; (C)–False; (D)–True; (E)–True.
Discussion: Salt retention is present in disease states in which glomerular filtration is decreased in the presence of intact renal tubular function. Renal hypoperfusion of any cause, whether hypovolemia, relative renal vasoconstriction (hepatorenal syndrome), or poor cardiac performance (cardiogenic shock), leads to increased sodium and chloride reabsorption and a lower urinary sodium concentration. Disorders of renal tubular function such as ATN and acute interstitial nephritis are associated with renal salt wasting. In acute glomerulonephritis the glomerular pathology compromises the filtration rate, which results in increased tubular sodium reabsorption. (*Cecil, Chs. 116 and 120*)

32. (A)–False; (B)–True; (C)–False; (D)–True; (E)–False.
Discussion: Acute renal failure in the hospitalized patient is a common clinical problem. An accurate diagnosis is necessary so the appropriate therapy can be instituted and prognosis provided. ATN can result in profound renal dysfunction requiring dialytic support. Additionally, the overall prognosis for ATN approaches 60%. However if the patient recovers from his or her underlying illness, the chances of renal recovery exceed 90%. The diagnosis of ATN is established with a characteristic history, a fractional excretion of sodium that is greater than 1% in the setting of oliguria, and urinary findings of muddy brown granular casts and renal tubular epithelial cells. Radiocontrast agents, aminoglycoside antibiotics, renal ischemia, and sepsis are established causes of ATN. β-Lactam antibiotics are associated with allergic interstitial nephritis. Cholesterol embolic disease is associated with intravascular procedures as well as systemic anticoagulation and often follows an inexorable course to ESRD. Vancomycin was historically associated with ATN, but more purified products have virtually eliminated this side effect. (*Cecil, Ch. 116*)

33. (All True). *Discussion:* Radiocontrast poses virtually no risk of acute renal failure in patients with normal renal function. However in the presence of chronic renal insufficiency, several risk factors have been defined. Any clinical circumstance that results in decreased renal perfusion pressure increases the risk of acute renal failure. This includes volume depletion, nonsteroidal anti-inflammatory agents, cyclosporine, and hypercalcemia. Diabetes mellitus and multiple myeloma are two systemic diseases in which the incidence of radio-contrast nephropathy is increased. (*Cecil, Ch. 116*)

34. (A)–False; (B)–False; (C)–True; (D)–False; (E)–False.
Discussion: Many strategies have been employed in an attempt to decrease the risk of contrast nephropathy in high-risk patients. If the patient is not diabetic, all of these regimens (designed to increase urine flow rate) have proven modestly effective at decreasing risk. Diabetics represent a particularly high-risk group in whom most of these protocols actually increase the risk of developing acute renal failure after contrast procedures. The only protocol that does seem to decrease the risk of acute renal failure in diabetics is the infusion of 0.45% saline before and during the procedure. (*Cecil, Ch. 116*)

35. (A)–True; (B)–True; (C)–True; (D)–False; (E)–True.
Discussion: The cornerstones of treatment for nephrotic patients are blood pressure control and the use of an ACE-I. These two interventions appear to decrease the rate of loss of renal function. ACE inhibitors decrease protein excretion by changing glomerular hemodynamic features. Calcium-channel blockers (especially diltiazem) have similar effects, though the decrease in protein excretion is modest. Nonsteroidal anti-inflammatory agents decrease protein excretion by decreasing GFR. Low dietary protein intake decreases proteinuria but the overall effect on renal survival is modest and rarely outweighs the risk of malnutrition. α-Adrenergic receptor antagonists have no direct effect on renal protein excretion. (*Cecil, Ch. 119*)

36. (D); 37. (B); 38. (D). *Discussion:* This patient's acute renal failure is due to an intrinsic renal lesion. The differential diagnosis includes immune complex–mediated acute glomerulonephritis from a cutaneous bacterial infection, aminoglycoside-induced ATN, and allergic interstitial nephritis from β-lactam antibiotics. However, the clinical presentation, which consisted of hypertension, oliguria, and hematuria with red blood cell casts, is classic for the syndrome of acute glomerulonephritis. Acute glomerulonephritis may occur after pharyngeal or cutaneous streptococcal infections. The latent period between the onset of a streptococcal pharyngeal infection to clinically apparent acute nephritis is 6 to 20 days (average, 10 days), whereas for impetigo the latent period has been more difficult to determine but is probably longer. Postinfectious glomerulonephritis is generally associated with low serum complement levels. The prognosis for complete recovery from poststreptococcal glomerulonephritis is excellent in pediatric patients. The prognosis for renal recovery in adults is somewhat less predictable, although probably fewer than 5% of adult patients may have clinical evidence of persistent renal disease at follow up. (*Cecil, Ch. 119*)

39. (D) *Discussion:* IgA nephropathy is an intrinsic renal disease of undetermined cause. It represents the most common cause of primary glomerular disease in Europe, Australia, and the United States. The lesion is characterized by mesangial immune deposits composed of IgA, which are predominantly polymeric and of mucosal origin. (*Cecil, Ch. 119*)

40. (E); 41. (D). *Discussion:* The patient has sarcoidosis with systemic manifestations that include pulmonary and skin involvement. Renal lesions in sarcoidosis are variable but may involve glomeruli and the tubulointerstitium. Immune complex–mediated glomerulonephritis may be more common in those patients who have erythema nodosum. Granulomatous infiltration of the kidney may produce a variety of tubular abnormalities that include inability to concentrate the urine, nephrogenic diabetes insipidus, and renal tubular acidification defects. The hypercalcemia that occurs with sarcoidosis results from the presence in the macrophages of the enzyme that converts 25(OH) vitamin D to the metabolically highly active form, $1,25(OH)_2$ vitamin D (calcitriol), which facilitates gastrointestinal absorption of calcium. Prolonged hypercalcemia produces renal failure from nephrocalcinosis. Typically, hypercalcemia from sarcoidosis responds very well to prednisone. (*Cecil, Ch. 120*)

42. (B); 43. (A); 44. (D). *Discussion:* One of the challenges in the management of the patient with end-stage renal failure is acquired cystic kidney disease (ACKD). ACKD has a male predominance and occurs in patients who have received any form of renal replacement therapy, including hemodialysis and peritoneal dialysis. ACKD can also develop in any patient who has chronic renal failure (serum creatinine > 3 mg/dL) but is not yet on dialysis. Whereas successful renal transplantation retards or reverses ACKD, the associated renal cell carcinoma accounts for nearly 2% of deaths in renal transplant patients. Most patients with ACKD are asymptomatic, even when renal cell carcinoma develops. When symptomatic, a common manifestation is hematuria. Although ultrasound is convenient and relatively inexpensive, CT appears to be the best imaging tool to identify small tumors. Generally, tumors less than 3 cm do not metastasize but should be followed closely if elective nephrectomy is not performed. In almost 10% of patients, the tumors are bilateral and some have advocated elective bilateral nephrectomy even in those individuals with unilateral disease. Metastatic disease has a variable course, but some patients survive for several years despite metastases. Results of use of adjuvant chemotherapy have been disappointing. (Cecil, Ch. 127; Truong, 1995).

45. (F); 46. (E); 47. (D); 48. (D). *Discussion:* This patient has multiple myeloma and his renal failure most likely is related to overproduction of immunoglobulin light chains. He has anemia, a reduced anion gap, and reduction in creatinine clearance. In addition, he has significant proteinuria. Ordinarily, proteinuria in that range strongly suggests a glomerular lesion, but the patient has a normal serum albumin and therefore did not have nephrotic syndrome. Thus, the presence of low-molecular-weight protein that is readily filtered at the glomerulus, such as immunoglobulin light chain, could explain the proteinuria. Immunofixation electrophoresis of the serum and urine serves to sort out the proteinuria and establish the diagnosis. The diagnosis is then confirmed using bone marrow aspiration and biopsy and bone survey. There is no role for use of serum electrophoresis because this test is too insensitive to be used as a screening tool. The most common renal lesion of multiple myeloma is cast nephropathy, which results from precipitation of the immunoglobulin light chain in the tubule lumen. Other renal lesions include amyloidosis (type AL) monoclonal immunoglobulin light chain deposition disease, ATN, and tubulointerstitial nephritis. Although deposition of light chain also occurs in arterioles, a true vasculitis has not been described. (Cecil, Chs. 119 and 120)

49. (A); 50. (B); 51. (C). *Discussion:* This patient has a presentation typical of retroperitoneal fibrosis. These patients often present with diminished urine output, and despite careful evaluation, it is difficult to show significant obstruction, because the kidneys and ureters are often encased with fibrotic material in the retroperitoneal space. CT scanning generally confirms the diagnosis by showing medial deviation and extrinsic compression of the ureters (lateral deviation suggests retroperitoneal adenopathy). Retroperitoneal fibrosis is usually idiopathic, but radiation therapy, aortic aneurysm, and malignancy are other causes. Finally, a small percentage of patients develop retroperitoneal fibrosis from drugs, especially methysergide, an ergot alkaloid. (Cecil, Ch. 121)

52. (B); 53. (E); 54. (E). *Discussion:* Anti-GBM glomerulonephritis is a disease typically of young males. Patients often present after an upper respiratory tract infection with pulmonary hemorrhage and renal failure from glomerulonephritis. Because success of treatment is dependent on how early in the course it is initiated, the most appropriate initial study is percutaneous renal biopsy with indirect immunofluorescence staining that demonstrates the characteristic linear deposits of IgG in glomerular capillary loops. Although antibody to the glomerular basement membrane may be diagnostic of anti-GBM disease, this specialized test takes time to complete. Sampling lung tissue may not provide diagnostic results and therefore delay treatment, and this patient had evidence of significant renal involvement. Response to treatment is poor in patients who are oliguric on presentation or who have serum creatinine concentrations greater than 6 mg/dL. (Cecil, Ch. 119)

55. (D); 56. (E); 57. (E); 58. (D). *Discussion:* This patient had chronic renal failure with superimposed acute renal failure. Prerenal and postrenal factors as well as intrinsic renal diseases are possible causes of the acute renal failure, and further studies are needed to make the diagnosis. Because the patient was taking indomethacin, renal syndromes associated with nonsteroidal anti-inflammatory drugs (NSAIDs) are major considerations. One of these syndromes producing acute renal failure is renal ischemia from a hemodynamically mediated reduction in renal blood flow. This syndrome most often occurs in those conditions in which the renin-angiotensin system is activated, such as cirrhosis, severe congestive heart failure, and volume depletion. It also occurs in patients with preexisting intrinsic renal disease. NSAID-induced allergic interstitial nephritis can occur after 2 weeks to 18 months of therapy. Hematuria, pyuria, and proteinuria are frequently seen and serve to differentiate interstitial nephritis from hemodynamically mediated renal failure from NSAIDs. Occasionally, nephrotic-range proteinuria from a concomitant minimal change glomerulopathy is seen. Unlike antibiotic-associated allergic interstitial nephritis, eosinophilia, fever, and rash are generally not present. Although eosinophilia is also infrequent in this syndrome, when it is found it supports the diagnosis. A third syndrome is hyperkalemia, which usually occurs in patients with antecedent renal impairment. Prostacyclin inhibition decreases renin release by the kidney and aldosterone secretion by the adrenal gland through a decrease in angiotensin II formation and direct inhibition of potassium-mediated aldosterone secretion. This patient's hyperkalemia may have been due partially to decreased aldosterone activity, although urinary tract obstruction also produces a renal tubular acidosis with hyperkalemia. A fourth renal complication of NSAID use is chronic interstitial nephropathy often with papillary necrosis, probably the result of medullary ischemia from decreased medullary blood flow. This diagnosis is associated with a long-standing use of greater than 3 kg of combinations of analgesics. Along with a compatible history, this patient has small kidneys with hydronephrosis and demonstrated fragments of tissue in the urine. The findings support the diagnosis of chronic interstitial nephropathy from analgesic abuse and now superimposed urinary tract obstruction presumably from sloughing of the papillary tip into the ureters bilaterally. (Cecil, Ch. 120)

59. (C); 60. (E); 61. (D); 62. (D). *Discussion:* This description represents the classical presentation of ethylene glycol ingestion. The typical patient is usually an alcoholic who elects to substitute ethanol for antifreeze, which is another available alcohol-containing palatable solution. Symptoms of acute poisoning resemble those of alcoholic intoxication, but they progress to stupor, obtundation, coma, and seizures. In addition, a characteristic severe anion-gap metabolic acidosis develops as the ethylene glycol is metabolized to glycolic acid and oxalate. The metabolic acidosis is also aggravated by increased production of lactic acid due to alteration of the intracellular redox state. Acute renal failure develops early in the course of ethylene glycol overdose and is probably related to intratubular obstruction from oxalate, the end product of metabolism of ethylene glycol. Characteristic calcium oxalate crystals are present in the urine. If treatment is not instituted early in the course, renal failure can be permanent. Thus, it is important to recognize this clinical presentation. Treatment can consist of volume expansion and creation of an osmotic diuresis, intravenous infusion of ethanol or fomepizole to prevent the conversion of ethylene glycol to its toxic metabolites (glycolic acid), and hemodialysis to remove the toxic metabolites (glycolic acid, oxalate).

The patient presented with a mixed metabolic and respiratory acidosis. This conclusion is evident when the P_{CO_2} is examined, because in a simple metabolic acidosis the respiratory compensation is rapid and obeys the following relationship: for every 1 mEq/L decrease in $[HCO_3^-]$, the P_{CO_2} will fall 1.25 mm Hg. In this example, the P_{CO_2} should have been 25 mm Hg and instead was inappropriately elevated at 40 mm Hg. Most likely, the seizure produced this respiratory depression. The patient has a marked increase in his anion gap, suggesting the addition of unmeasured anions, in this case glycolic acid and lactic acid. Uremia is an unlikely cause of this degree of an elevated anion gap. (Cecil, Chs. 113 and 116)

63. **(E)** *Discussion:* Methanol and ethylene glycol are responsible for most alcohol poisonings. Both can cause severe morbidity and mortality, particularly if not detected early. Because these are osmotically active compounds, differences between the observed and expected serum osmolality (osmolal gap) can provide an early clue to their presence. In both cases, the arterial pH correlates with serum levels of products of alcohol dehydrogenase: formic acid (from methanol) and glycolic acid (from ethylene glycol). Fomepizole, an inhibitor of alcohol dehydrogenase, is a safe and effective treatment of methanol and ethylene glycol poisoning. *(Cecil, Ch. 113; Brent et al., 1999 and 2001)*

64. **(C)** *Discussion:* Type IV renal tubular acidosis (RTA) is probably better termed *tubular hyperkalemia*, because, unlike other types of RTA, type IV RTA is associated with hyperkalemia and the urine pH is often low. Renal ammoniagenesis is impaired in this syndrome and results in impairment of distal nephron hydrogen ion secretion; the urine pH is acid, but without the requisite buffer a hyperchloremic metabolic acidosis results. The etiology of type IV RTA includes diabetes, sickle cell disease, drugs (NSAIDs, cyclosporine), and tubulointerstitial diseases. *(Cecil, Ch. 113)*

65. **(D)**; 66. **(D)**; 67. **(A)**; 68. **(E)**. *Discussion:* The age at onset of hypertension and the patient's race make the diagnosis of essential hypertension very unlikely and suggest renal artery stenosis. Because ACE inhibition produced reversible acute renal failure, hemodynamically significant bilateral renal artery stenosis is probably present.

ACE inhibitors have revolutionized the management of hypertension and left ventricular failure, but the physician prescribing these agents should be aware of their potential side effects. The first widely recognized complication is acute severe hypotension that occurs when the blood pressure is dependent on the renin-angiotensin system, such as in those patients who have volume depletion or renal artery stenosis. When renal perfusion pressure is decreased, such as in bilateral renal artery stenosis, the intrinsic renin-angiotensin system of the kidney functions to maintain filtration fraction and thus GFR. Inhibition of this system can produce hemodynamically mediated depression of glomerular filtration and subsequent acute renal failure. This complication may occur more readily with the long-acting converting enzyme inhibitors. By preventing aldosterone release by the adrenal gland, hyperkalemia can develop independently of alteration in renal function. The new angiotensin II receptor antagonists are selective type II receptor blockers; with the exception of cough, they produce side effects that are identical to converting enzyme inhibitors.

Views on the emergent management of hyperkalemia have changed. Calcium and insulin are still recommended to antagonize the effects of hyperkalemia on the cardiac conduction system and to shift potassium into cells, respectively. Recently, selective β_2-agonists have been shown to shift effectively potassium into cells; β_2-agonists also potentiate the effect of insulin to lower the serum potassium concentration. The efficacy of bicarbonate administration to decrease the serum potassium has been questioned. Although many authorities still recommend the use of bicarbonate to treat hyperkalemia, it should not be the sole agent utilized and should not interfere with other more definitive therapies. *(Cecil, Chs. 112 and 124)*

69. **(D)**; 70. **(D)**; 71. **(D)**; 72. **(B)**. *Discussion:* This patient has reflux nephropathy, which is a preventable common cause of end-stage renal failure throughout the world. Estimates of the prevalence of reflux nephropathy among end-stage renal failure patients range from 9 to 21%. The pathophysiologic mechanisms of reflux nephropathy are thought to center on a defect in the vesicoureteral junction, which allows transmission of a high intravesical pressure to the ureter and kidney. With severe vesicoureteral reflux, urine may actually reflux into the kidney, so-called intrarenal reflux.

When the urine becomes infected, the intrarenal reflux of infected urine results in cortical scarring of the kidney. Thus, in the management of reflux nephropathy, early surgical correction of the abnormal vesicoureteral junction and prevention of recurrent urinary tract infections remains the mainstay of prevention of this lesion. Hypertension develops as nephrons become damaged. Reflux nephropathy is the most common cause of hypertension in children and adolescents. Finally, proteinuria develops and often can result in nephrotic syndrome. Renal biopsy at that time demonstrates focal segmental glomerulosclerosis with associated IgM and C3 deposition. Typically, renal failure then ensues. Renal failure is therefore due to the anatomic injury to the kidney, hypertension, and the glomerulopathy. As mentioned, reflux nephropathy is a preventable lesion, and for this reason it is suggested that all patients who have a urinary tract infection within the first 5 years of life be evaluated for vesicoureteral reflux. About 1.6% of children will have at least one urinary tract infection during the first 5 years of life, and between 30 and 50% of these will have vesicoureteral reflux. Of these patients who have vesicoureteral reflux, 19% have or will develop some renal scarring and half of these patients will also have hypertension before the age of 30. Approximately 1% of these children experience chronic renal failure and eventually require treatment for end-stage renal disease. *(Cecil, Ch. 128)*

73. **(A)**; 74. **(C)**; 75. **(E)**; 76. **(B)**. *Discussion:* This patient has a disorder of osmoregulation resulting in acute hypernatremia. The inappropriately low urine osmolality in the face of severe hypernatremia with an estimated serum osmolality of 352 mOsm/kg supports a diagnosis of diabetes insipidus, either central (absent ADH) or nephrogenic. The increase in urine osmolality with vasopressin confirms a central diabetes insipidus. Ordinarily, patients with diabetes insipidus do not manifest hypernatremia because of an intact thirst mechanism that allows repletion of excreted water losses. Thus, these patients usually present with symptoms of polydipsia and polyuria. With general anesthesia, this patient's thirst mechanism became impaired and she was unable to replete urinary losses of water; severe hypernatremia resulted. To calculate the deficit in free water, X, one assumes that total body water is 60% of body weight and there has been no loss of solute. That is,

$$\text{total body solute now} = \text{total body solute at baseline}$$
$$[\text{Na}]_{\text{now}} \times (\text{total body water})_{\text{now}}$$
$$= [\text{Na}]_{\text{baseline}} \times (\text{total body water})_{\text{baseline}}$$
$$170 \text{ mEq/L} \times (55 \times 0.6) = 140 \text{ mEq/L} \times [(55 \times 0.6) + X]$$

Rearranging this equation to solve for X:
$$X = (170 - 140)(33)/140 = 7 \text{ L}$$

Because the hypernatremia developed acutely, this severe water deficit, which was over 21% of her total body water, can be safely repaired rapidly. Appropriate management is free water because there was no apparent significant loss of solute that would manifest clinically as intravascular volume depletion. *(Cecil, Ch. 112)*

77. **(C)**; 78. **(B)**. *Discussion:* The likely diagnosis is acute tubulointerstitial nephritis. The presence of fever, rash, and eosinophilia is highly suggestive of, but not essential to, the diagnosis. Pyuria with eosinophiluria is very common in this disorder. Although most commonly associated with methicillin, it may occur as a consequence of other penicillin derivatives as well as many other drugs. Tubulointerstitial nephritis is often associated with mild proteinuria and renal tubular dysfunction out of proportion to the decrement in the GFR. These defects often include hyperchloremic acidosis with a normal anion gap, hyperkalemia, inappropriate renal salt loss, and inability to form a concentrated urine. *(Cecil, Ch. 120)*

79. **(C)**; 80. **(B)**. *Discussion:* The likely diagnosis is obstructive uropathy. The well-preserved hemoglobin concentration and only

slightly depressed calcium concentration suggest that the renal failure is of recent onset. The history of urinary hesitancy suggests that the patient has prostatism. The ultrasound examination that was normal initially, then showed signs of obstruction the next day, was caused by severe volume depletion resulting in inadequate urine flow and inadequate pressure to distend the renal pelvis. In the presence of anuria, bladder catheterization must be performed to eliminate lower urinary tract obstruction, a potentially reversible cause of acute renal failure. (*Cecil, Ch. 121*)

81. **(B)**; 82. **(E)**. *Discussion:* The patient's clinical and laboratory data are highly suggestive of the syndrome of inappropriate antidiuretic hormone (SIADH), a common consequence of small cell carcinoma of the lung. He has hyponatremia with a high urine osmolality. To make the diagnosis of SIADH, there must be no evidence of ECF concentration. Associated findings that support the notion of ECF *expansion* are a low BUN and serum creatinine and uric acid. The ADH elaborated by the tumor represents a nonphysiologic stimulus for continued urinary concentration in the face of hypo-osmolality. Thus, the patient has an impaired free water clearance and continues to retain free water despite hyponatremia. The presence of a high urine sodium concentration despite hyponatremia and hypo-osmolality underscores the fact that in SIADH there is *expansion* of the ECF. Therefore, the major physiologic stimulus to sodium retention—ECF volume depletion—is not present. In SIADH, sodium excretion reflects sodium intake and not plasma osmolality. (*Cecil, Ch. 112*)

83. **(B)**; 84. **(D)**. *Discussion:* The patient has renal atheroembolic disease. In this disorder, cholesterol microemboli from ragged atherosclerotic plaques in the major vessels are showered distally. They lodge in the kidney as well as other organs, where their effects may be silent or may produce cutaneous lesions, pancreatitis, or manifestations of central nervous system disease. In the kidney, cholesterol crystals may lodge in the small arterioles and produce an inflammatory perivascular reaction that ultimately leads to sclerosis of the blood vessel. This sclerosis, accompanied by varying degrees of inflammation, is often accompanied by the pathologic hallmark of the disease—the cholesterol cleft, a cleft-like area that was occupied by the cholesterol crystal. These clefts may be found in many organs. The precipitating events for cholesterol embolization may be found in many organs. The precipitating events of cholesterol embolization may be major trauma, major vessel angiography, or vascular surgery; it may occasionally occur spontaneously. The renal manifestations include hypertension, eosinophilia, and progressive renal impairment developing over weeks to months after the precipitating event. The azotemia is usually not reversible (although exceptions have been reported). Although not treatable, this disorder should be considered as an explanation for progressive azotemia and hypertension that develop weeks to months after an aortic angiogram or aortic surgery. (*Cecil, Ch. 124*)

85. **(D)**; 86. **(A)**. *Discussion:* In autosomal-dominant polycystic kidney disease the kidneys are massively enlarged with tubular cysts—dilatations of tubules that continue to enlarge over years. Among the complications of this disorder are bleeding and infection of the cysts. The typical presentation of cyst bleeding is flank or abdominal pain and hematuria, although blood loss is not usually severe and stops spontaneously. Because bacteriuria and urinary infection are also very common in polycystic kidney disease, the index of suspicion for urinary tract infection should be high. Renal ultrasound examination of polycystic kidneys usually shows masses of large overlapping cysts. The presence of cysts with complex echoes in this case is consistent with bleeding into a cyst. However, because bleeding or complex sonographic echoes may be a manifestation of renal cell carcinoma, a CT scan with contrast agent enhancement may be useful in ruling out a malignant process. (*Cecil, Ch. 127*)

87. **(D)**; 88. **(E)**. *Discussion:* This is an example of idiopathic focal segmental glomerulosclerosis that was initially misdiagnosed as minimal change disease, an occurrence that is not uncommon. The initial renal biopsy diagnosis was minimal change disease or nil lesion based on the absence of any specific light microscopic and immunofluorescence findings, along with the absence of any ultrastructural findings other than fusion of the glomerular epithelial foot processes. The treatment, prednisone, was appropriate for this diagnosis. However, the development of azotemia is not characteristic of minimal change disease. Focal segmental glomerulosclerosis is a common cause of nephrotic syndrome. It is usually idiopathic, although it can be associated with heroin abuse as well as long-term vesicoureteral reflux and human immunodeficiency virus infection. The process typically affects the juxtamedullary nephrons initially and causes focal and segmental sclerosis of the glomerular tuft without deposition of immune complexes. It is therefore not uncommon to miss this diagnosis on an initial renal biopsy and to diagnose minimal change disease, a diagnosis of exclusion. Focal segmental glomerulosclerosis can respond to steroid therapy but requires prolonged treatment with high doses of prednisone. Because of the absence of a significant response to treatment in this patient, the more appropriate treatment now might be ACE inhibitors or angiotensin II receptor antagonists. (*Cecil, Ch. 119*)

89. **(B)**; 90. **(B)**. *Discussion:* The patient's presentation is not unusual. Hypernatremia in adults, with rare exceptions of hypothalamic function, is a serious disorder with considerable mortality, precisely because to become hypernatremic considerable other pathology must be present. Although there may be an impairment of thirst sensation in the elderly, the urge to drink when plasma sodium is elevated is strong. Hypernatremia usually occurs in patients who have significant sensory impairment or inability to seek water. This patient's free water deficit is about 6 L. In addition, his physical examination shows that his total body sodium content is decreased. Depletion of sodium manifests clinically as extracellular fluid volume depletion. Intravascular volume depletion produces hypotension with hypoperfusion of vital organs. Therefore, isotonic saline should be started to repair the sodium content deficit. At the same time, correction of the water deficit will also be initiated because isotonic saline is dilute with respect to the serum sodium concentration of 162 mEq/L. In the treatment of hypernatremia it is important to consider that the brain is a major target of disorders of water metabolism. In hypernatremic conditions, to avoid cell shrinkage, the brain generates intracellular solute, often termed *idiogenic osmoles,* to offset plasma hyperosmolality. These osmotically active substances are generated after several hours of hypernatremia. Rapid reduction of plasma sodium will result in swelling of a brain in which intracellular solute has been generated. Therefore, correction of hypernatremia of more than a few hours' duration should be undertaken slowly. It has been suggested that the plasma sodium be decreased no more than about 2 mEq/hr. This generally translates to correction over about 48 hours. Seizures are the clinical manifestation of cerebral edema in overrapid correction of hypernatremia. (*Cecil, Ch. 112*)

91. **(A)**; 92. **(D)**. *Discussion:* This patient is losing gastric contents—sodium, chloride, and acid—and replacing them with fluids that are essentially free water. Although a normal individual will excrete free water to maintain plasma osmolality, volume depletion (as well as pain) is a potent nonosmotic stimulus to the release of ADH. ADH impairs free water clearance by preventing the formation of dilute urine. The final result in this patient will be loss of NaCl and HCl and retention of free water, producing hyponatremia and metabolic alkalosis. ECV depletion will cause renin and aldosterone production. This favors avid distal sodium reabsorption as well as potassium and proton secretion by the distal tubule. In addition, the incremental elevation of plasma bicarbonate after

each episode of vomiting may obligate further potassium loss. Hypokalemia and metabolic alkalosis will eventually result as well. (*Cecil, Ch. 112*)

93. (E); 94. (B). *Discussion:* The two major routes of magnesium loss are the urine and gastrointestinal tract. A normal individual placed on a magnesium-free diet will rapidly lower urinary magnesium losses to an almost negligible level. Hypomagnesemia will ensue because of persistent gastrointestinal losses. Renal magnesium wasting is seen in a variety of disorders, including diuretic use, Bartter's syndrome, hyperparathyroidism, hyperaldosteronism, and hyperthyroidism, and as a result of toxic injury by a variety of drugs, including aminoglycosides and cisplatin. Although the magnesium loss of cisplatin may be profound, it probably abates within 1 to 2 months. The patient in question has hypomagnesemia because of continued diarrheal gastrointestinal loss with poor oral intake. The contribution of cisplatin-induced renal magnesium wasting is highlighted by the elevated urinary magnesium concentration. When extrarenal magnesium loss is present, the normal renal response is avid magnesium conservation; 24-hour urinary magnesium excretion falls to a few milliequivalents per day within 1 week of extrarenal hypomagnesemia. Pure hypomagnesemia can cause hypocalcemia by impairment of parathyroid hormone release and action. (*Cecil, Ch. 115*)

95. (D); 96. (D); 97. (A); 98. (C). *Discussion:* This patient has a chronic systemic illness (manifested by months of constitutional symptoms) that now presents as a pulmonary-renal syndrome. This set of symptoms and signs in an elderly man is strongly suggestive of a systemic vasculitis such as Wegener's granulomatosis or microscopic polyarteritis nodosa (mPAN). In this context a renal biopsy is urgently performed to direct therapy. The biopsy findings presented are consistent with a systemic vasculitis, and early treatment with corticosteroids and cyclophosphamide is standard. Many forms of systemic vasculitis are associated with antineutrophil cytoplasmic antibodies (ANCA). ANCA can be divided into C-ANCA and P-ANCA. C-ANCA is more than 90% sensitive for Wegener's granulomatosis whereas P-ANCA may be positive in a large group of diseases (including Churg-Straus and mPAN) and is less sensitive or specific. Factors affecting prognosis include age at presentation, presenting serum creatinine, and the presence of oliguria. Patients can, however, recover sufficient renal function to discontinue dialysis, although it often takes months. Goodpasture's syndrome is associated with linear staining of the glomerular basement membrane with IgG on immunofluorescence microscopy. Post-streptococcal acute glomerulonephritis is usually sudden in onset and is not generally associated with alveolar hemorrhage. (*Cecil, Ch. 119*)

99. (D); 100. (A); 101. (B). *Discussion:* Obtaining a specific renal diagnosis is important because the intervention and prognosis may vary widely. In this oliguric patient, one must decide if he has prerenal azotemia, ATN, or HRS. Several characteristics help make this distinction. In ATN the urinary spot sodium concentration (U_{Na}) is usually greater than 10 and the fractional excretion of sodium (FeNa = $(U_{Na} \times S_{Cr})/(U_{Cr} \times S_{Na}) \times 100$) is greater than 1%. Both prerenal azotemia and HRS have low U_{Na} and FeNa less than 1%, but with prerenal azotemia the BUN:creatinine ratio is often greater than 20:1. This relationship may be altered in the presence of poor hepatic synthetic function, however. There is no structural renal abnormality in HRS. HRS represents a functional form of renal impairment that is fully reversible with liver transplantation. Oliguria, profound sodium retention, and a bland urinary sediment characterize HRS. Although HRS can be precipitated by events that reduce circulatory blood volume, it can also occur without an apparent precipitating factor. HRS usually occurs in the setting of severe hepatic dysfunction and is associated with a mortality rate in excess of 90%. Decreased effective circulatory volume

in cirrhotic patients leads to increased aldosterone production and increased salt and water retention. (*Cecil, Ch. 116*)

102. (C); 103. (E); 104. (E). *Discussion:* Urinary tract obstruction can occur at any level from the renal pelvis to the distal urethra and may be unilateral or bilateral. Animal experiments with acute obstruction demonstrate that renal recovery declines in inverse proportion to the degree and duration of the obstruction. Complete recovery is the rule if obstruction is relieved within 7 days but about 30% recovery in GFR can be expected if the obstruction persists for 28 days. Renal cortical thinning is ultrasonographic evidence for renal injury. Urinary obstruction leads to increased intratubular hydrostatic pressure, which favors the reabsorption of solutes and water and dissipates the medullary salt/urea gradient. When the obstruction is relieved, these factors as well as a functional resistance to ADH produce the well-described "post-obstructive diuresis." Urinary obstruction can result in chronic renal cortical injury. A common result is a type IV RTA as manifested by this patient. Injury to the renal parenchyma results in decreased renin production and therefore diminished serum aldosterone levels. This is distinguished from proximal (type II) and distal (type I) RTA by the presence of hyperkalemia. This defect can be partially overcome by presenting the distal convoluted tubule and cortical collecting duct with more sodium (e.g., through addition of a loop diuretic). This results in the exchange of urinary sodium for potassium and hydrogen ions. Because the acidosis is caused by the inability to secrete hydrogen ions instead of bicarbonate loss (as in proximal RTA), oral bicarbonate is not the initial therapy. Furthermore, avoiding agents that may worsen hyperkalemia (e.g., ACE inhibitors, NSAIDs, and trimethoprim) should be emphasized. (*Cecil, Ch. 121*)

105. (B); 106. (D); 107. (E). *Discussion:* Renal cell carcinoma (RCC) has been referred to as the "internist's tumor" because of its wide variety of clinical presentations, including anemia, polycythemia, hypertension, pyrexia, hypercalcemia, elevated erythrocyte sedimentation rate, abnormal liver function, myopathy/neuropathy, and weight loss. The classic triad of flank pain, hematuria, and a palpable mass is present in a minority of patients. The majority of RCCs are found incidentally during abdominal imaging for other reasons. CT offers an excellent method for assessing the anatomy and extent of the tumor. Currently the only effective treatment is surgical extirpation with improved survival after radical nephrectomy over any less extensive procedure. Percutaneous biopsy of RCC carries the risk of tumor seeding along the needle tract. Both acquired cystic renal disease and von Hippel-Lindau syndrome impose greater risk for the occurrence of RCC. Patients with autosomal-dominant polycystic kidney disease are at no greater risk than the general population. (*Cecil, Ch. 127*)

108. (C); 109. (A); 110. (B); 111. (E); 112. (E); 113. (C); 114. (E); 115. (E). *Discussion:* Impaired free water excretion is characteristic both of drugs causing inappropriate release of ADH, such as vincristine and chlorpropamide, and of drugs with intrarenal effects, such as the thiazide diuretics. Nephrogenic diabetes insipidus unresponsive to vasopressin and leading to polyuria and pure water loss may be a side effect of such drugs as lithium, demethylchlortetracycline, and vinblastine. Nephrotic syndrome can result from the administration of heavy metals, penicillamine, anticonvulsants, and NSAIDs. Hypokalemia from renal potassium loss can appear during therapy with both thiazides and loop diuretics. In susceptible individuals, hyperkalemia can occur during the course of treatment with trimethoprim, which can inhibit the epithelial sodium channel in the cortical collecting tubule and thereby impair potassium secretion. Cyclosporine can cause a renal tubular hyperkalemia syndrome. Spironolactone serves as a competitive antagonist for aldosterone and can cause hyperkalemia. In addition, depolarizing muscle relaxants such as succinylcholine can produce sudden hyperkalemia based on rapid shifts of potassium from muscle cells to the extracellular fluid space. (*Cecil, Ch. 112*)

116. (E); 117. (D); 118. (C); 119. (B); 120. (A). *Discussion:* Type IV RTA is characterized by hyperkalemia and hyperchloremic acidosis with a normal anion gap. Distal (type I) RTA is also characterized by hyperchloremic acidosis with a normal anion gap, and hypokalemia is often significant. Proximal (type II) RTA is again characterized by normal-anion-gap hyperchloremic acidosis. Hypokalemia from renal potassium wasting can become severe during attempts at correction, because inadequate reabsorption of bicarbonate in the proximal tubule results in presentation of this anion to the distal nephron, which cannot readily reabsorb it. In the steady state, however, there is no bicarbonaturia and hypokalemia can resolve. Uremic acidosis is caused both by a failure of ammoniagenesis and by renal net acid secretion (as in type IV RTA) but also by a net retention of nonmetabolizable acids, producing an elevated anion gap. Finally, in diabetic ketoacidosis, the clue is the elevated anion gap, as well as hyponatremia caused by hyperglycemia. (*Cecil, Ch. 112*)

121. (A); 122. (C); 123. (B); 124. (C); 125. (D). *Discussion:* Pharmacologic modulation of the immune response has dramatically improved morbidity and mortality of transplantation. OKT3 is a mouse monoclonal antibody directed against the CD3 antigen on T cells. Corticosteroids inhibit T cell activation primarily by inhibiting the synthesis of cytokines that include interleukin (IL)-1 and IL-6 production in antigen-presenting cells. Cyclosporine and tacrolimus inhibit calcineurin activation in T cells and thereby prevent IL-2 production, which activates T cells. Sirolimus binds to the same cytoplasmic protein (FKBP-12) as tacrolimus, but the complex does not inhibit calcineurin but instead inhibits the activation of mammalian target of rapamycin (mTOR), which suppresses cytokine-induced T cell proliferation. However, despite different mechanisms of action, tacrolimus and rapamycin are not synergistic because these molecules compete for binding to the same cytoplasmic protein in the T cell. (*Cecil, Ch. 118*)

BIBLIOGRAPHY

Brenner BM (ed): Brenner and Rector's The Kidney, 5th ed. Philadelphia, WB Saunders, 1996.

Brent J, McMartin K, Phillips S, et al. for The Methylpyrazole for Toxic Alcohols Study Group: Fomepizole for the treatment of methanol poisoning. N Engl J Med 2001;344:424-429.

Brent J, McMartin K, Phillips S, et al. for The Methylpyrazole for Toxic Alcohols Study Group: Fomepizole for the treatment of ethylene glycol poisoning. N Engl J Med 1999;340:832-838.

Goldman L, Ausiello D (eds): Cecil Textbook of Medicine, 22nd ed. Philadelphia, WB Saunders, 2004.

Haas M, Meehan SM, Karrison TG, Spargo BH: Changing etiologies of unexplained adult nephrotic syndrome: A comparison of renal biopsy findings from 1976-1979 and 1995-1997. Am J Kidney Dis 1997;30:621-631.

Truong LD, Krishnan B, Cao JT, et al: Renal neoplasm in acquired cystic kidney disease. Am J Kidney Dis 1995;26:1-12.

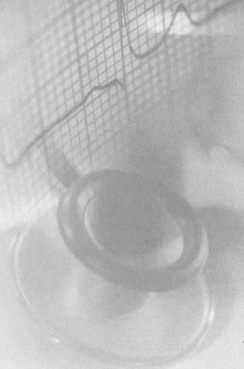

Part V
Oncology

Jeffrey R. George and Lisle M. Nabell

MULTIPLE CHOICE

DIRECTIONS: For questions 1–5, choose the best answer.

1. A 60-year-old woman with a history of recently diagnosed breast cancer currently on therapy with CMF (cyclophosphamide, methotrexate, 5-fluorouracil) presents with complaints of nausea and vomiting after chemotherapy and new-onset shortness of breath, mouth soreness, and fatigue. She is found on physical examination to have a new right pleural effusion and mucositis. Her laboratory studies are notable for:

Serum creatinine	2.4 mg/dL
BUN	25
WBC	1000/μL
Hgb	9.2 mg/μL
PCV	28%
Platelets	91,000/μL

   The most likely source of her discomfort is:
   A. Methotrexate toxicity
   B. Metastatic breast carcinoma
   C. 5-Fluorouracil toxicity
   D. Cardiomyopathy

2. A 55-year-old woman with a history of locally advanced, untreated carcinoma of the breast presents with complaints of progressive low back pain for 3 weeks. Her pain radiates into the left hip, and she has noted that she is weaker with walking but there is no history of bowel or bladder incontinence or loss of strength in either leg. A plain film of the thoracic/lumbar spine demonstrates multiple lytic abnormalities. You recommend which of the following studies?

   A. Electromyography of the left leg
   B. Bone scan
   C. Magnetic resonance imaging of the spine
   D. Lumbar puncture

3. The patient is later found to have spinal cord compression at L2. All of the following are true regarding the management of the patient *except*:

   A. The patient should begin emergent chemotherapy for treatment of her disease.
   B. The patient should be referred to a neurosurgeon for consideration of decompressive surgery.
   C. The patient should begin emergent therapy with high dose dexamethasone (Decadron).
   D. The patient should be seen in consultation by a radiation oncologist.

4. A 40-year-old woman presents with an enlarged, red, indurated right breast. Mammography reveals a large area of architectural distortion in the central portion of the breast. Biopsy of the breast and skin indicates infiltrating ductal carcinoma. The patient should be referred immediately for:

   A. Administration of preoperative chemotherapy
   B. Consideration of surgery with mastectomy and lymph node dissection
   C. High-dose chemotherapy with stem cell rescue
   D. External-beam radiation therapy

5. A healthy 67-year-old woman presents for an annual physical examination and is found to have palpable shotty cervical and axillary lymphadenopathy. She does not have a palpable spleen or liver on examination. Her laboratory studies are as follows:

Hemoglobin	12.0 g/dL
Hematocrit	36%
Leukocyte count	12,000/μL with 80% small lymphocytes
Platelet count	240,000/μL

To confirm suspected chronic lymphoid leukemia, blood is sent to the laboratory for flow cytometry, which returns positive for CD5+ B cells that express clonal λ light chains. Which of the following would be the optimal management for the patient at this time:

A. Chlorambucil and prednisone
B. Intravenous gamma globulin
C. Monoclonal antibody to CD52 (Campath)
D. Observation

MATCHING
QUESTIONS 6–10

DIRECTIONS: For questions 6–10, match the following agents to their best description:

A. Cyclophosphamide
B. Herceptin
C. Paclitaxel (Taxol)
D. Tamoxifen
E. Cisplatin
F. Amifostine (Ethyol)
G. 5-Fluorouracil (5-FU)
H. Methotrexate
I. Doxorubicin (Adriamycin)

6. Monoclonal antibody that targets the Her-2 protein

7. Use results in significant risk of nephrotoxicity

8. In high doses can result in risk of hemorrhagic cystitis

9. Derived from the yew tree and stabilizes microtubules during cell division; use may result in peripheral neuropathy

10. Significant cumulative usage may result in cardiomyopathy

MULTIPLE CHOICE
QUESTIONS 11–16

DIRECTIONS: For questions 11–16, choose the best answer.

11. A 50-year-old woman with metastatic, medullary thyroid cancer presents for a routine follow-up visit. She has never received therapy for her metastatic disease and is currently doing well. You note that she has never had any manifestations of pheochromocytoma or hyperparathyroidism. Nevertheless, you discuss genetic testing with her and recommend referral for testing for mutations in which gene?

A. *Her2/neu* oncogene
B. *RET* proto-oncogene
C. *BRCA1/2* gene mutation
D. *FAP* gene mutation
E. 9:22 gene translocation

12. A 69-year-old woman with a history of non–small cell lung cancer (NSCLC) status post resection 2 years ago is brought to medical attention by her family because of confusion. The family states that the patient has complained of fatigue, constipation, and loss of appetite. Physical examination is notable for a lethargic woman with no focal neurologic deficits.

Hemoglobin	12.8
Hematocrit	40%
Platelets	42,800/μL
Total bilirubin	1.0
Albumin	2.8
Calcium	12.6
BUN	36
Creatinine	1.3

What is the next best approach to this patient's management?

A. Intravenous furosemide (Lasix) every 6 hours to increase urinary excretion of calcium
B. Two-hour infusion of pamidronate to decrease osteoclastic activity, and serial monitoring of ionized calcium
C. Bone scan to look for recurrent NSCLC involving the axial skeleton
D. Vigorous hydration with normal saline at 200-400 mL/hour, with Lasix as needed to balance the intake and output after adequate rehydration

13. A 36-year-old woman presents with a complaint of a lump in her breast. Physical examination reveals an area of thickness in the upper outer quadrant of the left breast. The patient has a history of "lumpy breast" and no family history of breast cancer. Mammography is negative and ultrasound reveals a suspicious mass. Fine-needle aspiration of the mass is nondiagnostic. What is the most appropriate next step in management of this patient?

A. Reassure the patient that this is likely related to her fibrocystic disease and schedule a follow-up appointment.
B. Repeat ultrasound with biopsy in 3 to 6 months.
C. Immediately refer the patient to a surgeon for excisional biopsy.
D. Recommend a trial of birth control pills for fibrocystic disease and advise annual mammography.

QUESTIONS 14 AND 15

14. A 40-year-old premenopausal woman is found to have an early breast cancer (1.5 cm, node negative, ER/PR positive) on segmental mastectomy and sentinel lymph node biopsy. The patient is treated with four cycles of adjuvant Adriamycin and cyclophosphamide (Cytoxan) followed by local radiation therapy. She is then started on tamoxifen, 10 mg/day, for 5 years. What is the most appropriate follow-up for this patient?

A. Routine follow-up with no specific recommendations regarding her breast cancer
B. Routine follow-up including yearly mammography and yearly transvaginal ultrasound while on tamoxifen
C. Aggressive follow-up including tumor markers and liver function tests every 6 months, yearly mammography, bone scan, and CT scans of chest and abdomen
D. Routine follow-up including yearly mammograms and yearly pelvic examinations

15. The patient asks about the risks of taking tamoxifen for 5 years. Tamoxifen therapy carries all of the following risks *except*:

A. A 1/1000 chance of developing endometrial cancer
B. A 1/100 chance of developing a deep venous thrombosis
C. Increased chance of developing ovarian cancer
D. Fatty infiltration of the liver and abnormal results of liver function tests

16. A 60-year-old man presents with abdominal distention and early satiety. Physical examination reveals marked spleno-megaly. Laboratory results reveal: WBCs, 56,000/μL with 60% segmented granulocytes, 15% bands, 20% lymphocytes, and 5% basophils; the platelet count is elevated at 750,000/μL. The leukocyte alkaline phosphatase score was low. What is the most likely chromosomal abnormality?

    A. t(15,17), PML/RARa
    B. t(9,22), BCR-ABL
    C. t(14,18), bcl-2
    D. t(11,14), bcl-1

MATCHING
QUESTIONS 17–21

DIRECTIONS: For questions 17–21, match the infectious agent with the associated malignancy.

    A. Hepatitis B virus
    B. Human herpesvirus 8
    C. Human papillomavirus
    D. *Helicobacter pylori*
    E. Epstein-Barr virus
    F. Human T-lymphotrophic virus
    G. *Schistosoma haematobium*

17. Nasopharyngeal cancer

18. Hepatocellular carcinoma

19. Mucosa-associated gastric lymphoma

20. Kaposi's sarcoma

21. Cervical cancer

MULTIPLE CHOICE

DIRECTIONS: For questions 22–46, choose the best answer.

22. A 50-year-old man with a history of gastroesophageal reflux disease undergoes esophagogastroduodenoscopy for persist-ent symptoms despite medical management. Gastritis is found with a thickened mucosa. A biopsy of the thickened mucosa is taken, and pathology reveals mucosa-associated lymphoid tissue lymphoma. What is the most appropriate management for this patient?

    A. Multi-drug systemic chemotherapy such as CHOP
    B. Referral to surgeon for a partial or total gastrectomy
    C. Treatment to eradicate *H. pylori* infection
    D. Twice-daily proton pump inhibitor therapy

23. A 64-year-old man presents for an annual physical exami-nation. He is healthy except for a history of borderline hypertension and the examination is normal. Laboratory tests are remarkable only for a total protein level of 8.3 g/L. His serum albumin level is 5 g/dL, and his serum globulin level is 3.3 g/dL. His serum immunoglobulin levels are measured and the serum IgG is 2.4 g/dL. Which of the fol-lowing diagnostic tests would be the most likely to be help-ful in the assessment of possible multiple myeloma?

    A. Serum protein electrophoresis
    B. Immunoelectrophoresis of a concentrated 24-hour urine specimen

    C. Bone marrow aspirate and biopsy
    D. Bone scan
    E. Skeletal survey

QUESTIONS 24–26

A healthy 45-year-old man was seen at your office for evaluation of an upper respiratory tract infection. Laboratory studies were recently obtained at a comprehensive job physical examination; you review these studies and notice a screening prostate-specific antigen (PSA) level of 3.8 ng/mL (laboratory reference range, 0-4 ng/mL).

24. All of the following statements are true *except:*

    A. This PSA level may be abnormal because the reference range for PSA in this young age group is lower than the standard reference range.
    B. If the ratio of free to total PSA is low, the patient could be monitored with biannual PSA levels without further intervention at this time.
    C. If a PSA is repeated in 6 months, a PSA velocity could be calculated, which is helpful in determining whether the elevated PSA is representative of a malignant or benign process.
    D. The American Cancer Society (ACS) recommends PSA determinations starting at age 50.

25. If this patient has a repeat PSA value of 4.5 ng/mL in 6 months, which of the following is *true?*

    A. The patient should wait and have a repeat PSA test in 1 year regardless of further evaluation.
    B. A bone scan should be the next test ordered.
    C. A biopsy should be obtained regardless of further evalu-ation.
    D. If rectal examination and transrectal ultrasonogram are both normal, the patient should wait and repeat the PSA in 6 months.

26. One year later, with a PSA value of 6.0 ng/mL, a transrectal biopsy was obtained and revealed no evidence of malig-nancy. With these results, you should now suggest the fol-lowing:

    A. Repeat biopsy
    B. Magnetic resonance imaging (MRI)
    C. Radioimaging
    D. No further work-up at this time

QUESTIONS 27–29

A 45-year-old woman with a history of hemorrhoids noted rectal bleed-ing over the past 6 months. A flexible sigmoidoscopy revealed a polyp in the sigmoid colon without other polyps in the remainder of visible bowel. A biopsy was performed, and pathology revealed adenocarcinoma within a tubular adenoma. Limited bowel resection demonstrated the absence of cancer in the bowel wall or lymph nodes. The patient comes to discuss plans for follow-up.

27. All of the following statements about colorectal screening are true *except:*

    A. In the absence of any risk factors, the American Cancer Society recommends yearly fecal occult blood testing and sigmoidoscopy every 3 to 5 years beginning at age 50.
    B. Fewer than one third of patients with polyps have occult blood in stool.
    C. Studies demonstrated that screening for occult fecal blood increases the number of cancers detected at an earlier stage.

D. Flexible sigmoidoscopy can reach 45 cm above the anus and diagnose one third of all colorectal cancers and polyps.

28. The patient tells you that her mother had colorectal cancer at age 50 and her grandmother had colorectal cancer at the age of 45. All of the following statements are true about genetic risk factors for colorectal cancer *except:*

A. Although familial adenomatous polyposis (FAP) is an autosomal-dominant trait that increases the risk of colorectal cancer with greater than 90% penetrance, it is unlikely in this family because no other polyps were found.

B. Gardner's syndrome is an autosomal-recessive trait with polyps and is associated with an increased risk of colorectal cancer and osteomas.

C. The hereditary nonpolyposis colorectal cancer syndrome (HNPCC) is possible because this is an autosomal-dominant condition and those affected have cancer at a young age.

D. In patients with a family history of colorectal cancer or an autosomal-dominant cancer syndrome, screening should begin earlier than standard recommendations.

29. All of the following statements about colorectal polyps are true *except:*

A. Tubular adenomas are about four times more common than villous adenomas.

B. The likelihood of a polyp being cancerous is greater if it is villous, large, and multiple.

C. Patients with a history of resected colon cancer or polyps should have colonoscopy every 1 to 3 years after two colonoscopies are performed a year apart and are negative.

D. In this patient, no further follow-up is required because the only polyp to have cancer has been removed.

QUESTIONS 30 AND 31

A 65-year-old man with a history of asbestos exposure was noted to have a cough and pulmonary infiltrate with a small pleural effusion on the right side of the chest radiograph. Although he does not have a fever, the radiologist claims that the radiograph reveals a "pneumonia-like" process.

30. All of the following regarding lung cancer are true *except:*

A. Asbestos exposure increases the risk of both mesothelioma and primary lung cancer.

B. Screening chest radiography every year would have improved his chance of survival from a lung cancer, given his asbestos exposure.

C. The risk of lung cancer increases even more if he is a smoker.

D. Bronchoscopy is an appropriate procedure in this patient.

31. If this patient was diagnosed with a non–small cell lung cancer, all of the following are true *except:*

A. Mediastinoscopy is useful to stage more accurately.

B. If a CT scan of the chest and abdomen demonstrates enlarged mediastinal lymph nodes on the left side (N3), he should be considered for surgery.

C. Stage IIIB non–small cell lung cancer is best treated with combined radiation and chemotherapy.

D. If a thoracentesis is performed and the cytology of the pleural fluid is positive for malignancy, he does not require a mediastinoscopy.

32. Which of the following statements regarding ovarian carcinoma is true?

A. Use of oral contraceptive agents is a risk factor.

B. The CA-125 tumor-specific antigen test is a good screening test.

C. Those patients with complete primary surgical debulking have improved survival.

D. All patients should undergo a surgical re-exploration (second-look surgery) after chemotherapy.

QUESTIONS 33 AND 34

A 65-year-old woman was evaluated in your office after a recent surgery for adenocarcinoma of the rectum. The pathology revealed that the tumor was invading through the bowel wall and involved only one lymph node. You advise the patient about adjuvant therapy.

33. You should recommend all of the following for rectal carcinoma *except:*

A. Adjuvant treatment with only chemotherapy

B. Adjuvant treatment with combined radiation and chemotherapy

C. Rigorous follow-up with periodic colonoscopy after treatment

D. Continuation of yearly screening mammograms

34. If the tumor was located in the sigmoid colon, you would change your recommendations as follows:

A. You would not recommend follow-up with periodic colonoscopy.

B. Adjuvant therapy with only chemotherapy should be used, without radiation therapy.

C. Adjuvant therapy should include radiation therapy and chemotherapy.

D. Total colectomy should now be performed.

35. A 40-year-old woman was diagnosed with cancer of the breast. She asks you to test her 20-year-old daughter to determine whether she is at increased risk of breast cancer. All of the following are true *except:*

A. Because the mother is already known to have breast cancer, only the daughter should be tested for a *BRCA-1* mutation; the mother will need rigorous screening in the future regardless of testing.

B. The *BRCA* mutations present as an autosomal-dominant pattern of inheritance.

C. If the daughter has a *BRCA* mutation, her risk of breast cancer can be greater than 80% by age 65.

D. Carcinoma of the ovary and that of breast are often inherited in association.

QUESTIONS 36 AND 37

A 25-year-old woman was seen in the emergency department for fever and was noted to have an elevated WBC count of 160,000/μL with blasts. She is suspected of having leukemia. Other laboratory studies demonstrated a platelet count of 20,000/μL (normal > 120,000/μL), prothrombin time (PT) of 18 seconds (normal < 13), and fibrinogen of 40 (normal > 120).

36. All the following statements regarding the initial management are true *except:*

    A. One potential problem in this patient could be hyperviscosity syndrome related to the markedly elevated WBC count, which may require emergent plasmapheresis.
    B. This patient should immediately be started on antibiotics as a neutropenic patient because the abnormal WBCs may be ineffective at fighting infection.
    C. The elevated PT and low fibrinogen are common with all leukemias.
    D. A bone marrow aspirate with special stains would distinguish acute myelogenous leukemia (AML) from acute lymphocytic leukemia (ALL).

37. Which type of leukemia is most likely based on these laboratory studies?

    A. Promyelocytic leukemia (M3)
    B. Chronic lymphocytic leukemia
    C. Chronic myelocytic leukemia
    D. Hairy cell leukemia

38. Which of the following statements regarding bladder carcinoma is *true?*

    A. Risk factors include smoking and prior treatment with cyclophosphamide.
    B. Hematuria is an uncommon presenting symptom.
    C. Transurethral resection is the standard treatment used in patients with deep muscle invasion.
    D. Patients with metastatic disease are generally treated with combined radiation and chemotherapy.

39. A 50-year-old male smoker is noted to have a lung mass on a chest radiograph and a calcium level of 13 mg/dL (normal, 8.5-10.4). Which of the following statements is *true?*

    A. He likely has diarrhea and abdominal pain.
    B. Given the elevated calcium concentration, he most likely has a primary tumor of bowel origin with metastasis to the lung.
    C. If he has a lung primary tumor, this is more likely a non–small cell tumor than a small cell (oat cell) cancer.
    D. The most common cause of malignancy-associated hypercalcemia is the production of parathyroid hormone (PTH).

QUESTIONS 40 AND 41

40. All of the following statements regarding the biology and treatment of pancreatic carcinoma are true *except:*

    A. The only intervention that offers a chance for cure is surgical resection.
    B. A palpable gallbladder (Courvoisier's sign) is present in most patients.
    C. Cystadenocarcinoma histology indicates a favorable prognosis.
    D. Jaundice is a presenting symptom in most patients with a tumor at the head of the pancreas.

41. Which of the following statements regarding treatment of pancreatic carcinoma is *true?*

    A. Adjuvant chemotherapy plus radiation therapy does not improve survival compared with radiation or chemotherapy alone.
    B. Most patients with pancreatic carcinoma have resectable tumors.
    C. Most patients with metastatic pancreatic carcinoma have an initial response to 5-FU chemotherapy.

    D. Pancreaticoduodenectomy (Whipple procedure) is the surgical procedure of choice.

42. A 43-year-old woman was diagnosed with cancer of the ovary and underwent a surgical procedure to optimally debulk the disease. Which of the following is *true* regarding the surgical management of ovarian cancer?

    A. Patients with advanced disease (stage III or IV) should be treated with only chemotherapy, because there is no benefit from surgery.
    B. If the patient has a recurrence despite initial surgery and chemotherapy, there is no role for a second debulking surgery.
    C. Patients who have a successful initial surgery with optimal debulking have a better survival than those with less optimal debulking.
    D. Patients who have successful debulking surgery will not benefit from adjuvant chemotherapy.

43. The most correct statement regarding tumor markers is:

    A. The CA-125 value is normal in some patients with early-stage ovarian cancer.
    B. Patients with seminoma usually have elevated α-fetoprotein (AFP) levels.
    C. The AFP level is not useful as a screening test for any malignancy.
    D. Most tumor markers are useful as a screening test; few markers are of use to follow for a treatment response.

QUESTIONS 44–46

A 45-year-old woman had an excisional biopsy of a mammographic abnormality in the upper outer quadrant of the left breast. The initial pathology revealed ductal carcinoma in situ (DCIS) with positive surgical margins and a small amount of lobular carcinoma in situ (LCIS).

44. All of the following are *true* regarding in situ cancers of the breast *except:*

    A. DCIS, like LCIS, does not require further surgery because these abnormalities do not represent true malignancy.
    B. LCIS is a marker of high risk for breast carcinoma.
    C. This patient needs further surgery because DCIS, like invasive ductal cancer, needs to be completely excised.
    D. The prognosis for DCIS is better than for invasive ductal carcinoma.

45. The patient underwent a second excision because the surgical margins had tumor present. The pathology of the second excision revealed residual DCIS and an area of invasive ductal carcinoma measuring 1.2 cm. All of the following are *true* regarding the management of this patient *except:*

    A. The patient should undergo an axillary dissection to assess lymph node status.
    B. An axillary dissection would not be indicated if only noninvasive disease was found.
    C. A mastectomy is the option of choice at this point.
    D. Radiation therapy is standard after lumpectomy in patients with resected DCIS and those with invasive ductal cancer.

46. Which of the following is also *true?*

    A. A bone scan should be obtained in all patients such as those with stage I or II disease.
    B. If the patient had only LCIS, no further surgical treatment would be necessary, but the patient should be counseled for high risk.

C. The survival after mastectomy is better than of lumpectomy (complete excision of the tumor) and radiation to the breast.

D. There is no benefit of radiation in addition to mastectomy.

TRUE OR FALSE
QUESTIONS 47 AND 48

DIRECTIONS: For questions 47 and 48, decide whether *each* choice is true or false. Any combination of answers, from all true to all false, may occur.

47. Which of the following statements is/are *true* regarding brain metastasis?

A. The common sources include lung and breast cancer.

B. Melanoma is the tumor most likely to have brain metastasis.

C. Surgical resection should be considered in patients with solitary metastasis.

D. Chemotherapy is the primary treatment for most patients.

48. Which of the following statements is/are *true* regarding superior vena cava syndrome?

A. Infection is the most common cause.

B. The most common malignancy causing superior vena cava syndrome is gastric cancer.

C. Dyspnea is a common symptom.

D. Treatment should always include surgical resection.

MULTIPLE CHOICE
QUESTIONS 49–68

DIRECTIONS: For questions 49–68, choose the best answer.

QUESTIONS 49 AND 50

A 45-year-old man noted abdominal pain. A CT scan of the abdomen revealed a mass in the head of the pancreas. A fine-needle biopsy revealed adenocarcinoma.

49. Which of the following is *true* regarding the therapy of this patient?

A. The only chance of cure is surgical resection.

B. Adenocarcinoma is an uncommon histology with better prognosis.

C. Jaundice is a common sign of tumors in the pancreatic tail.

D. After resection, radiation therapy without chemotherapy should be considered.

50. All of the following regarding risk factors and prognosis for pancreatic cancer are true *except:*

A. Firmly established risk factors for pancreatic cancer include coffee and alcohol use.

B. Cigarette smoking is a risk factor implicated in 30% of pancreatic cancer cases.

C. Patients with cystadenocarcinoma pathology have a more favorable prognosis and are cured approximately 50% of the time by surgical resection, in contrast to adenocarcinoma in which cure is unlikely.

D. Only about 15% of patients with metastatic disease have temporary tumor shrinkage with chemotherapy.

51. You are recommending adjuvant therapy to a patient with early-stage breast cancer. Clearly, your recommendation depends on the risk of recurrence and the benefit of adjuvant therapy to your patient. Which of the following represents the most proven and important prognostic factor found in the initial surgery of breast cancer?

A. Percent S phase

B. DNA index

C. *HER-2* status

D. Lymph node status

52. Which of the following is *true* regarding the tumor markers AFP and β-hCG?

A. A falsely elevated β-hCG, secondary to increased luteinizing hormone (LH), can be discerned with testosterone injection.

B. Most patients with seminoma have an elevated AFP value.

C. The half-life of AFP is 1 day.

D. β-hCG is never elevated in seminoma.

QUESTIONS 53 AND 54

A 68-year-old smoker was diagnosed with a type of retroperitoneal sarcoma (malignant fibrous histiocytoma). Two years after complete surgical excision, he is seen in your office for evaluation of minimal hemoptysis.

53. All of the following are true regarding his subsequent management *except:*

A. A chest radiograph should be obtained.

B. If he is found to have a recurrent sarcoma with only a single pulmonary nodule, surgical resection is a reasonable treatment modality.

C. If a chest radiograph is normal, further evaluation with a CT scan is appropriate.

D. If a pulmonary nodule is noted on initial radiograph, chemotherapy should be initiated.

54. All of the following general statements about sarcomas are true *except:*

A. The main curative modality is surgical resection.

B. Small or round cell sarcomas such as osteosarcoma and Ewing's sarcoma are radiosensitive and chemosensitive, and combined-modality therapy (chemotherapy, irradiation, and surgery) is often used in an attempt to cure these tumors.

C. The lung is the most frequent metastatic site.

D. Adjuvant chemotherapy will improve survival of patients with retroperitoneal soft tissue sarcomas.

55. A 27-year-old man was diagnosed with testicular carcinoma by an orchiectomy. He was noted to have a markedly elevated AFP and normal β-hCG. You review the pathology, which states that he has seminoma, before making final plans for therapy. Which of the following is *true*?

A. The pathologic diagnosis of seminoma is incorrect.

B. If he has early-stage seminoma, chemotherapy is the only adjuvant option of therapy.

C. If he had early-stage nonseminoma, radiation therapy after orchiectomy would be a reasonable option of therapy.

D. He should undergo bilateral orchiectomy to exclude nonseminoma in the contralateral testis.

56. A 48-year-old man was noted to have hematuria, abdominal pain, and a palpable mass in the left upper quadrant of his abdomen. On review of systems, you find that he has a mild cough and a headache. He is also a smoker and does not have any family history of cancer. Which of the following is the most likely diagnosis in this patient?

    A. von Hippel-Lindau disease
    B. Lung carcinoma
    C. Renal cell cancer
    D. Bladder cancer

QUESTIONS 57 AND 58

A 79-year-old man underwent prostatectomy for an adenocarcinoma of the prostate. One year later his PSA was 1.0 ng/mL (normal, 0-4 ng/mL).

57. Which of the following is a factor that represents increased risk of prostate cancer?

    A. Smoking
    B. Alcohol consumption
    C. Black race, male gender
    D. Excessive tomato paste consumption

58. Which of the following could be considered in the management of this patient?

    A. Hormonal (androgen ablation) therapy
    B. Chemotherapy
    C. Repeat surgery
    D. Combined radiation and chemotherapy

59. A 45-year-old woman with a history of colon cancer was noted to have a carcinoembryonic antigen (CEA) level elevated to five times the upper limit of normal. All of the following are *true except:*

    A. CEA can be elevated from smoking.
    B. CEA can predict recurrence from colorectal cancer.
    C. Recurrence at the anastomotic site may be curable.
    D. A high preoperative level in patients with colon cancer does not correlate with prognosis.

60. All of the following are true regarding staging of prostate cancer *except:*

    A. Stage B represents disease defined only by PSA elevation.
    B. Stage D1 represents disease involving the lymph nodes.
    C. Stage D2 represents distant metastatic disease.
    D. Stage C represents seminal vesical involvement.

61. A 56-year-old male bartender chews tobacco and smokes cigarettes. He was noted to have a white patch in his mouth. All of the following are *true except:*

    A. In addition to lung cancer, he also has an increased risk of prostate cancer.
    B. Leukoplakia is a common manifestation in people who chew tobacco.
    C. If the plaque were red (erythroplakia), he would have a greater chance of malignancy than if the plaque is white.
    D. Secondary smoke at his occupation likely contributes to his cancer risk.

62. Which of the following is *true* about the management of metastatic prostate cancer?

    A. Data have proved that a second antiandrogen should be added to the primary hormonal therapy with orchiectomy or a luteinizing hormone-releasing hormone (LHRH) agonist.

    B. In patients who progress after initial androgen ablation therapy, chemotherapy has been proved to improve survival.
    C. Orchiectomy is superior to an LHRH agonist.
    D. After progression on double hormonal therapy, withdrawal of the antiandrogen (flutamide or bicalutamide [Casodex]) can result in a response in 25% of patients.

63. A 60-year-old man with a PSA of 10 ng/mL was just diagnosed with prostate cancer by transrectal biopsy. Before any further therapy, he experienced a decrease in PSA to 5 ng/mL over 1 month with the use of a herbal combination. On examination you notice left leg swelling. All of the following statements are *true except:*

    A. You should obtain a Doppler ultrasonogram to rule out a deep vein thrombosis.
    B. Measurement of the serum testosterone would be helpful in understanding the decrease in PSA.
    C. The decrease in PSA is secondary to the immune effects of the herbal medicine.
    D. Saw palmetto can decrease prostate size in patients with benign prostatic hypertrophy (BPH).

QUESTIONS 64–66

A 27-year-old man stated that a pigmented lesion on his ankle (Figure V-1) was present "all of his life" but increased in size over the course of 1 year. A biopsy revealed melanoma 1.5 mm thick.

64. All of the following statements regarding initial management are *true except:*

    A. Excision with wide margins should be performed.
    B. The melanoma may have started in a preexisting nevus.
    C. A lymph node dissection or sentinel node biopsy will give prognostic information.
    D. Adjuvant interferon therapy for 1 year has a substantial risk of inducing renal failure.

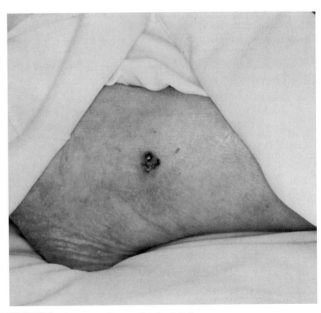

FIGURE V-1 • *(Courtesy of James Gaydos, MD.)*

65. All of the following are *true* regarding prognostic factors *except:*

    A. Ulceration is a poor prognostic sign.
    B. Superficial spreading melanoma has a worse survival compared with nodular melanoma.
    C. Tumor thickness is the most important prognostic sign.
    D. Elective lymph node dissection does not improve survival.

66. If this patient was found to have metastatic disease to the lung on further work-up, all of the following would be *true* *except:*

    A. Further work-up, including a bone scan and CT of the brain, is in order.
    B. The most common sites of metastasis include the skin, lung, liver, bone, and brain.
    C. Clinical trials are important to consider, because standard options such as interleukin (IL)-2 therapy are not curative.
    D. Bone marrow transplant should be considered.

67. All of the following are *true* regarding chemotherapy drug resistance *except:*

    A. A cell with increased multidrug resistance (P glycoprotein) fails to pump out chemotherapy agents such as mitomycin and doxorubicin.
    B. Paclitaxel and vincristine act to alter the microtubules of the cell.
    C. High levels of bcl-2 lead to chemotherapy resistance.
    D. P glycoprotein expression increases during chemotherapy administration.

68. A 27-year-old man was found to have a tumor arising from the mediastinum. Pathology revealed an undifferentiated tumor of unknown primary site. All of the following are *true* *except:*

    A. No treatment should be given without knowing the primary site.
    B. Unknown primary tumors comprise 5 to 10% of all tumors.
    C. For tumors above the diaphragm, lung cancer is the most common site of origin.
    D. Treatment with a platinum regimen may result in long-term survival in up to 15% of patients.

TRUE OR FALSE

DIRECTIONS: For questions 69–75, decide whether *each* choice is true or false. Any combination of answers, from all true to all false, may occur.

69. Which of the following statements is/are *true* regarding programmed tumor cell death (apoptosis)?

    A. Bcl-2 is a protein that blocks apoptosis.
    B. Bax helps bcl-2 to stop tumor cell death.
    C. Resistant tumors may have increased bcl-2 expression.
    D. Therapy that decreases the expression of bax may increase apoptosis.

70. Which of the following statements is/are *true* regarding seminoma compared with nonseminoma?

    A. Seminoma is a more radiosensitive tumor compared with nonseminoma.

    B. Chemotherapy is used in seminoma as the primary treatment if the initial tumor is extensively involving the retroperitoneal lymph nodes.
    C. Disease confined to the testis only (stage I) has a greater than 90% cure rate.
    D. The chemotherapy used to treat seminoma is similar to that used for nonseminoma.

71. Which of the following statements regarding cancer epidemiology is/are *true*?

    A. Prostate cancer incidence has increased recently compared with prior years secondary to the use of PSA testing.
    B. The leading cause of death from cancer in men and women is lung cancer.
    C. The incidence of cervical cancer has increased in the past 10 years.
    D. Breast cancer mortality would likely decrease in women if mammogram screening is performed on all women as recommended.

72. A 66-year-old patient with lung carcinoma was diagnosed with a malignant pericardial effusion. Which of the following statements is/are *true*?

    A. The ECG is likely to show increased voltage.
    B. Pericardiocentesis is likely to reveal a positive cytology.
    C. The most common tumors to cause pericardial effusion include lung, breast cancer, and lymphoma.
    D. A pericardiocentesis without a window may be ineffective.

73. A 70-year-old man with lung cancer notes proximal muscle weakness. Which of the following statements is/are *true*?

    A. Eaton-Lambert syndrome is a possible cause of the weakness.
    B. Eaton-Lambert syndrome usually involves the proximal muscles: ocular and bulbar muscles.
    C. Myasthenia gravis, in contrast to Eaton-Lambert syndrome, has abnormal deep tendon reflexes.
    D. This patient most likely has small cell lung cancer (oat cell).

74. Which of the following is/are *true* with regard to syndrome of inappropriate antidiuretic hormone (SIADH)?

    A. SIADH, like hypercalcemia, is most likely to occur in squamous cell carcinoma of the lung.
    B. Patients present with hyponatremia and low urine osmolality.
    C. A CT scan of the brain may be appropriate to determine whether brain metastases are present.
    D. SIADH can be caused by some chemotherapy agents.

75. Which of the following statements is/are *true* regarding Hodgkin's disease?

    A. The finding of a Reed-Sternberg cell is pathognomonic for Hodgkin's disease.
    B. The histologic subtypes can predict prognosis.
    C. "B" symptoms include fever, weight loss, and night sweats.
    D. Patients with early-stage disease (local disease) can be treated with radiation therapy only.

MATCHING

DIRECTIONS: The following are matching questions. For each numbered item, choose the most likely associated lettered item from those provided. Each numbered item has *only one* answer. Within each set of questions, each lettered item may be used once, more than once, or not at all.

QUESTIONS 76–80

Match the following tumor markers with the appropriate description.

    A. CA-125
    B. CEA
    C. β-hCG
    D. AFP
    E. PSA

76. May be elevated in seminoma testicular cancers.

77. Ratio of the free to total protein may distinguish benign versus malignant disease.

78. Used in follow-up after colectomy for colorectal adenocarcinoma.

79. Elevated in some lung carcinomas and choriocarcinoma.

80. Often elevated with any peritoneal malignancy.

QUESTIONS 81–87

Match the following paraneoplastic syndromes with the appropriate description.

    A. SIADH
    B. Erythrocytosis
    C. Necrolytic migratory erythema
    D. Acanthosis nigricans
    E. Sign of Leser-Trélat
    F. Eaton-Lambert syndrome
    G. Flushing of the face

81. Carcinoid

82. Hyponatremia seen in a patient with small cell lung cancer

83. Gastric cancer

84. Renal cell carcinoma

85. Islet cell tumor of the pancreas (glucagonoma)

86. Proximal muscle weakness in a patient with lung cancer

87. Seborrheic keratosis and diagnosis of adenocarcinoma

QUESTIONS 88–95

Match the following oncologic emergencies to the most appropriately numbered choice.

    A. Spinal cord compression
    B. Elevated PTH-related protein
    C. Superior vena cava syndrome
    D. Solitary brain metastasis
    E. Lytic bone lesion of the humerus
    F. Neutropenia
    G. Hypercalcemia of malignancy
    H. Multiple brain metastasis

88. This is best evaluated by plain radiography.

89. CT and plain radiography are inadequate for diagnosis.

90. This is a major cause of hypercalcemia of malignancy.

91. Surgery may be the best option of therapy.

92. If a diagnosis of the tumor primary is not yet made, a biopsy should be performed before treatment.

93. This is most commonly seen in squamous cell malignancies.

94. This is associated with an absolute neutrophil count less than 1000.

95. This is best treated initially with radiation therapy.

QUESTIONS 96–100

Match the following site of metastasis of gastrointestinal malignancy with the correct name.

    A. Left axillary lymph node
    B. Peritoneal implant palpable on rectal examination
    C. Large ovarian metastasis
    D. Left supraclavicular lymph node
    E. Periumbilical lymph node

96. Blumer shelf

97. Virchow's node

98. Irish's node

99. Sister Mary Joseph node

100. Krukenberg's tumor

Part V
Oncology
Answers

1. **(A)** *Discussion:* Methotrexate inhibits the enzyme dihydrofolate reductase. This inhibition blocks the production of the reduced *N*-methylenetetrahydrofolate, the coenzyme in the synthesis of thymidylic acid. Although used frequently as a neoplastic agent in the treatment of cancers of the breast and head and neck, methotrexate is also employed in the treatment of autoimmune diseases such as rheumatoid arthritis. Methotrexate affects renal function, and most episodes of severe methotrexate toxicity occur after an event that results in lowered excretion of the drug. The most common of these toxicities is dehydration, which can be caused by nausea and vomiting, decreased oral intake, or mucositis from prior drug administration. Third-space reservoirs created by pleural effusions or ascites are another potential method by which toxicity may be increased due to delayed clearance and prolonged serum drug levels. This toxicity is most typically manifested by myelosuppression and mucositis. Patients who are on methotrexate need to be followed closely for any change in renal function or development of fluid accumulations that may alter the drug's half-life. In addition, numerous drug interactions have been reported that may alter renal clearance of methotrexate including nonsteroidal anti-inflammatory agents, sulfonamides, and antibiotics. (*DeVita et al, 2001*)

2. **(C); 3. (A).** *Discussion:* Almost any tumor can result in the symptoms of spinal cord compression, although statistically the most common tumors to do so include breast, lung, prostate, and kidney cancers as well as lymphomas and plasma cell dyscrasias. The symptoms of spinal cord compression are typically manifest first by pain most commonly in the thoracic spine where the cord is narrowest. Pain may precede other symptoms of cord compression by several weeks, but once motor impairment develops the symptoms typically progress rapidly. Plain radiographs and radionucleotide bone scans can be useful but fail to pick up evidence of cord compression in 15-20% of cases. Magnetic resonance imaging (MRI), however, is extremely sensitive and specific for evidence of cord impingement and has largely replaced CT and myelography in the diagnosis of epidural metastasis. Improvement in symptoms is best if there are minimal signs of cord dysfunction, and it is important to begin a diagnostic evaluation promptly. If cord compression is suspected, then high-dose glucocorticoids should begin immediately while arranging for the imaging study. Doses over 10 mg of dexamethasone every 6 hours have not been conclusively shown to be superior to lower doses. If a patient has a known cancer, then radiation therapy (a total dose of 3000 cGy) has been the mainstay of treatment. In the absence of a preexisting cancer diagnosis then a biopsy of the epidural mass is required. Surgery, either a laminectomy or decompression, is also considered in the setting of progression of symptoms despite radiation or if the area under treatment has already undergone radiation therapy. A study comparing radiation therapy alone to decompression surgery followed by radiation therapy found a strong benefit in favor of the combined approach, with a significant improvement in the number of patients who could ambulate at the end of treatment. In

the future, for selected patients, this combined approach may provide more functional benefit then the sole use of radiation therapy. While chemotherapy may be used to treat the systemic disease there is no benefit in its use for treatment of a cord compression. (*DeVita et al, 2001; Patchell et al, 2003*)

4. **(A)** *Discussion:* Inflammatory breast cancer is generally suspected based on the clinical findings of brawny edema of the skin of the breast with reddened, roughened skin described as peau d'orange changes. The clinical picture of inflammatory breast cancer is due to the presence of tumor cells within the dermal lymphatics of the breast. Historically, individuals who presented with inflammatory breast cancer had an extremely high recurrence rate with traditional surgery followed by systemic therapy, owing in large part to problems with clearing the skin margins and local recurrence. Current treatment programs with primary chemotherapy followed by surgery and radiation therapy have yielded significantly better survival rates. Individuals whose tumors respond completely appear to have a better overall survival. High-dose chemotherapy has been employed in several randomized trials with no evidence of a superior disease-free or overall survival as compared with traditional systemic therapy. At this time in the absence of any apparent benefit, high-dose chemotherapy should be employed only in the setting of a controlled clinical trial. (*DeVita et al, 2001*)

5. **(D)** *Discussion:* Despite steady improvements in therapeutic modalities for lymphoma, there remains no evidence that early treatment of low-grade lymphoma or chronic lymphocytic leukemia (CLL) improves overall survival. This patient has evidence of a clonal CD5+ B cell population consistent with the diagnosis of CLL. Over half of patients with CLL are diagnosed in the absence of any disease-related symptoms and are picked up during a routine physical examination with lymphadenopathy or an abnormal CBC. CLL can be distinguished from other related lymphoproliferative disorders on the basis of immunophenotyping with flow cell cytometry. CLL cells most commonly express the B-cell antigens CD19, CD20, and CD23 and coexpress CD5 in the absence of T cell markers. The cells are monoclonal with respect to their expression of either κ or λ light chains. As no therapy has been shown to impact survival, the decision about when to initiate therapy is a critical one. Molecular analysis of CLL cells has demonstrated that markers can be used to divide patients into two very different groups. In the more favorable group, CLL cells express the cell marker CD38 (ectopepidase) and immunoglobulin genes are mutated, appearing similar to germline sequence. This group can be typified by a relatively indolent disease course, good response to therapy, and survival of over 20 years on average. In contrast, the second group has a weaker expression of CD38 and cells with unmutated immunoglobulin genes (naive B cells). This group is characterized by having more males vs. females, advanced clinical stage, progressive course with poorer response to therapy, and worse median survival around 8 years.

When therapy is indicated for CLL due to disease progression, single-agent chlorambucil or fludarabine are the most effective choices. The use of combination therapy has been associated with higher response rates but no change in survival and may actually increase the infectious complications that are frequently encountered in this disease. (*DeVita et al, 2001; Hamblin et al, 1999*)

6. **(B)**; 7. **(E)**; 8. **(A)**; 9. **(C)**; 10. **(I)**. *Discussion:* Herceptin is a monoclonal antibody targeting the HER-2 gene product. Use of this agent in combination with chemotherapy has produced significant improvements in response to treatment in the setting of metastatic breast cancer. This agent has been associated with an increased risk of cardiomyopathy. Cisplatin is extremely active in the treatment of many tumors but has undesirable effects, including ototoxicity and risk of renal toxicity, which may result in a chronic potassium and magnesium wasting process. Taxol (and a similar agent, Taxotere) bind to the microtubules during cell division, acting to stabilize them and prevent division. Peripheral neuropathy is dose limiting. Cyclophosphamide binds to and cross links DNA, resulting in cell death. Its use has been associated with hemorrhagic cystitis and the syndrome of inappropriate antidiuretic hormone. The drug amifostine is a thiol compound that scavenges free radicals and is used as a protective agent from the effects of cisplatin and also as a radioprotectant. The anthracyclines including doxorubicin, idarubicin, and daunorubicin are antitumor antibiotics, which all have the capacity for producing a delayed, dose-dependent, generally irreversible cardiomyopathy. (*DeVita et al, 2001*)

11. **(B)** *Discussion:* The multiple endocrine neoplasia (MEN) syndromes consist of MEN 2A, MEN 2B, and familial medullary thyroid cancer (FMTC). The major disease characterizing these syndromes is medullary thyroid cancer (MTC), which occurs in all affected individuals. The syndromes are caused by a germ-line mutation in the *RET* proto-oncogene and are inherited in an autosomal dominant fashion. The MEN syndromes differ with regard to the site of the mutation along the *RET* gene, age at onset of MTC, and manifestation of other features outside of MTC. MEN2A is characterized by onset of bilateral MTC at a young age, generally before age 30. Pheochromocytomas develop in around 40% of patients, and one third of patients also develop parathyroid hyperplasia resulting in hyperparathyroidism. Individuals with MEN2B tend to develop MTC also at a young age, with 50% also developing pheochromocytomas. These patients tend to have a fairly characteristic physical appearance with a marfanoid habitus, including elongated skeletal features, an enlarged tongue, and hyperflexible joints. Hyperparathyroidism is not a feature of MEN2B. FMTC is characterized by the development of MTC in the absence of any other endocrinopathies or other clinical features. In FMTC onset of MTC tends to occur at a later age and is generally indolent. Genetic testing for *RET* mutations should be undertaken in any individual who develops MTC. If positive, these individuals should be counseled about risks to other related family members.

BRCA-1/2 mutations have been associated with early onset breast and ovarian carcinoma in women. Mutations in these genes are thought to account for around 5-8% of all cases of breast cancer. Individuals at greater risk for BRCA-1/2 mutations include having a first-degree relative develop breast cancer before age 40, the appearance of ovarian cancer in the family, and being of Ashkenazi Jewish descent. The *HER*-2 oncogene is amplified in approximately 30% of all cases of invasive breast cancer and has been associated with a worse prognostic outcome. Herceptin, a monoclonal antibody that targets the *HER*-2 protein, is now used clinically for patients with metastatic breast cancer whose tumors overexpress the *HER*-2 gene. Mutations in the familial adenomatous polyposis (FAP) gene have been associated with the clinical appearance of hundreds of polyps though the colon and early-onset colorectal carcinoma. The 9:22 translocation juxtaposes the *abl* oncogene on chromosome 9 with *bcr* on chromosome 22, creating a constitutively active tyrosine kinase. (*DeVita et al, 2001*)

12. **(D)** *Discussion:* Hypercalcemia is a common oncologic emergency in patients with malignancy. It is common in patients with myeloma, breast, and lung cancer. Symptoms from hypercalcemia include fatigue, constipation, diminished appetite, nausea, urinary frequency, and increased thirst. Cancers that produce hypercalcemia often produce a parathyroid protein-related hormone (PTH-rP) and growth factors such as tumor necrosis factor and interleukin-6. Patients with hypercalcemia should be aggressively rehydrated with normal saline. Lasix can be used to balance intake and output after adequate hydration. Bisphosphonates inhibit osteoclast activity and decrease bone resorption of calcium. Bisphosphonates reduce hypercalcemia over 24 to 48 hours. (*DeVita et al, 2001*)

13. **(C)** *Discussion:* Approximately 183,000 women are diagnosed with breast cancer each year, and nearly 41,000 will die of the disease. Early detection of breast cancer improves the chance for successful treatment. A suspicious breast mass requires immediate and systematic evaluation. A negative mammogram or needle aspirate does not ensure that a mass is not malignant. Fine-needle aspiration has demonstrated false-negative rates of 4 to 9.6%. In patients proven to have malignancy, 20 to 30% of mammograms are nondiagnostic. Therefore, a suspicious mass requires referral to a qualified surgeon for an excisional biopsy. (*Cecil, Ch. 208.5; DeVita et al, 2001*)

14. **(D)**; 15. **(C)**. *Discussion:* Women with a history of breast cancer are at increased risk for developing recurrence, metastasis, and contralateral cancers. Routine checkups, with special attention to the emotional concerns related to cancer diagnosis and treatment, management of the problems related to menopause, yearly mammography, and yearly pelvic examinations are important. Extensive testing to identify early metastatic disease, however, is not warranted. Early diagnosis of metastatic disease by doing frequent, invasive, and expensive tests does not improve survival. Several randomized trials have been performed to compare routine physical examinations and mammography to more intensive follow-up. The intensive follow-up resulted in earlier detection of metastatic disease but did not change survival.

Tamoxifen therapy has been shown to be of substantial benefit in the adjuvant setting in patients with receptor positive disease. Tamoxifen has three major side effects, which fortunately are rare: thromboembolic events, endometrial cancer, and cataracts. The risk of developing endometrial cancer on tamoxifen is about 1/1000, whereas the risk of developing a clot is about 1/100. Tamoxifen is not associated with ovarian cancer and helps to prevent accelerated bone loss. Less serious but more common side effects of tamoxifen include fatty liver, abnormal liver function tests, hot flashes, vaginal discharge, and sexual dysfunction. Most women on tamoxifen therapy will develop endometrial thickening. The risk of developing endometrial cancer is about 1/1000. Women need routine yearly pelvic examinations, but in the absence of symptoms (i.e., abnormal uterine bleeding), routine pelvic or transvaginal ultrasounds are not warranted. (*DeVita et al, 2001*)

16. **(B)** *Discussion:* Chronic myeloid leukemia accounts for about 20% of leukemias. The leukocyte alkaline phosphatase level is low in CML and is helpful in determining benign from malignant cause for leukocytosis. The Philadelphia chromosome (BCR-ABL) is present in more than 90% of patients with CML. This translocation brings the *abl* oncogene on chromosome 9 into proximity with the *bcr* region on chromosome 22. The gene formed by this translocation produces an abnormal tyrosine kinase protein capable of inducing CML. Chromosome 14 contains a site responsible for encoding the immunoglobulin heavy chain. Translocations from chromosome 11 and 14 juxtapose the *bcl-1* and *bcl-2* genes with

the immunoglobulin heavy chain, resulting in overexpression of *bcl-1* and *bcl-2*. Both *bcl-1* and *bcl-2* inhibit apoptosis and are associated with low-grade lymphomas and CLL. The t(15,17) results in the fusion of the retinoic acid receptor (RAR) and the promyelocytic leukemia gene, which is found in the M3 subtype of acute myelogenous leukemia. *(DeVita et al, 2001)*

17. **(E)**; 18. **(A)**; 19. **(D)**; 20. **(A)**; 21. **(C)**. *Discussion:* Many infectious agents have been implicated as causal or associated factors in many malignancies. Epstein-Barr virus has been implicated in multiple malignancies, including post-transplant lymphomas, Burkitt's lymphoma, and nasopharyngeal carcinoma, which is common in many Asian populations. Hepatitis B and Hepatitis C are common causes of cirrhosis and are associated with hepatocellular carcinoma. *Helicobacter pylori* is associated with peptic ulcer disease and an increased risk of gastric carcinoma and gastric lymphoma. Eradication of *H. pylori* infection with antibiotic therapy results in regression of gastric lymphoma in a majority of patients. Kaposi's sarcoma and certain non-Hodgkin's lymphomas have been associated with human herpesvirus 8 infection in patients with HIV. Human papillomavirus is a major cause of carcinoma of the uterine cervix as well as squamous cell cancer of the anus in men with HIV infection. *(DeVita et al, 2001)*

22. **(C)** *Discussion:* Gastric MALT lymphomas are frequently associated with chronic gastritis and *H. pylori* infection. Eradication of *H. pylori* infection has led to tumor regression in the majority of patients. In one study from Germany, patients treated with antibiotics, more than 70% remained in complete remission at 1 year. The standard of care for patients with *H. pylori* infection and gastric MALT lymphoma should be antibiotics with a follow-up esophagogastroduodenoscopy in 3 and 6 months. Patients who are in complete remission do not need further treatment. Patients who have a partial response should receive a second course of antibiotic therapy. Patients who fail to achieve a response, relapse, or progress need definitive therapy in the form of irradiation, surgery, or chemotherapy. *(DeVita et al, 2001)*

23. **(E)** *Discussion:* A serum protein electrophoresis demonstrates a monoclonal spike in patients with either myeloma or monoclonal gammopathy of uncertain significance (MGUS). In general, the level of the monoclonal protein is less than 3 g/dL in patients with MGUS, but follow-up is necessary to ensure that the monoclonal immune globulin does not change significantly over the next 12 months. Approximately 3% of normal individuals older than the age of 70 have a monoclonal protein in the serum; and although the majority will never develop myeloma, around 15% will develop the disease eventually, and follow-up is mandatory. In a long-term study by Kyle and colleagues, the initial concentration of the serum monoclonal protein was the most important risk factor for progression to overt myeloma. A bone marrow aspirate and biopsy can be useful if the percentage of plasma cells exceeds 10%. However, in patients with low levels of protein this test is not likely to be informative. The finding of light chains in the urine can discriminate between myeloma and MGUS, but this test is likely to be uninformative given the small amount of protein seen. The finding of lytic bone lesions on a skeletal survey is a reliable indicator of the presence of myeloma. A bone scan is not helpful in the evaluation of MGUS/myeloma. *(Cecil, Ch. 50; Kyle et al, 2002)*

24. **(B)**; 25. **(C)**; 26. **(A)**. *Discussion:* Screening for prostate cancer has become popular with the advent of PSA blood testing. As more patients have PSA blood testing, all physicians need to be comfortable with the management of abnormalities in PSA. Although screening recommendations are controversial, the American Cancer Society recommends annual PSA determinations for patients 50 years of age and older. Once a PSA is obtained, the value must be interpreted with regard to the age-specific reference

ranges. Because PSA normally increases with age and most laboratory references ranges were derived from a relatively older population than this patient, the normal laboratory range is likely to be misleading. In fact, one study defined a normal reference range of 0 to 2.5 ng/mL for the 40- to 49-year age group. Therefore, the value of 3.8 is abnormal in this 45-year-old patient. Because other causes of PSA elevation could be involved, such as BPH or prostatitis, other studies are often ordered to distinguish a benign from a malignant process. For example, the ratio of free to total PSA is one method used to distinguish benign versus malignant disease. Because more PSA is complexed in patients with cancer compared with BPH and this ratio is independent of age, this ratio has been studied to distinguish these conditions. When a cutoff of 18% or more free PSA is used, this test has a sensitivity of 71% and a specificity of 95% in predicting malignant versus BPH. However, final recommendations for the use of the ratio of free to total PSA have not yet been made. The velocity of rise of PSA is also predictive of malignant vs. benign disease. An increase of 0.75 ng/mL/year or more has a sensitivity of 72% and a specificity of 90% in distinguishing malignant disease versus BPH. Therefore, in question 26, the likelihood of a missed cancer despite a negative initial biopsy is high. Repeated biopsy with special attention to the transition zone (a common site where tumor is often found when a biopsy has been negative despite a high clinical suspicion) could be performed. *(Cecil, Ch. 180)*

27. **(D)**; 28. **(B)**; 29. **(D)**. *Discussion:* Screening with stool testing and sigmoidoscopy every 3 to 5 years for colorectal cancer is reasonable and recommended by the American Cancer Society for those 50 years of age and older. The stool testing for occult blood has been shown to increase the number of early cancers diagnosed, but effects on mortality are currently unproved. The predictive value of a positive test is only 20%, but all patients with positive testing need further evaluation, even with a history of hemorrhoids. It is also true that fewer than one third of patients with polyps are positive for blood. Flexible sigmoidoscopy is useful because it reaches approximately 45 cm above the anus and diagnoses two thirds of all colorectal cancers. The familial risk factors for colorectal cancer have been well studied. The polyposis syndromes include FAP, which is the most common autosomal-dominant polyposis syndrome. Polyps are noted by late adolescence throughout the colon, and the risk of colorectal cancer is greater than 90%. Gardner's syndrome is a similar autosomal-dominant syndrome associated with desmoid tumors, lipomas, sebaceous cysts, and osteomas. Turcot's syndrome is an autosomal-recessive syndrome associated with central nervous system malignancy and bowel polyposis. Unlike patients with these syndromes, however, the patient in question does not have multiple adenomatous polyps. A hereditary process with a high frequency of colon cancer without adenomatous polyposis is HNPCC and occurs in 1 to 6% of all colorectal cancers. The syndromes are divided into Lynch I and II; Lynch I is characterized by an autosomal-dominant pattern. Multiple genes have been described that are mutated in germline cells of families with HNPCC. Screening and management of patients with familial syndromes must be rigorous. Patients with FAP often undergo a total colectomy. Patients with Lynch syndromes require frequent screening with colonoscopy every 3 to 5 years starting at age 30. In contrast to these syndromes with an increased risk of cancer, Peutz-Jeghers syndrome and juvenile polyposis, which are characterized by hamartomatous polyps, have only a small risk of cancer. Adenomatous polyps may be villous or tubular. Although tubular polyps are more common, villous polyps are 8 to 10 times more likely to be cancerous. *(Cecil, Ch. 37; Toribara and Sleisenger, 1995)*

30. **(B)**; 31. **(B)**. *Discussion:* The risk of lung cancer increases with exposure to smoking, radon, and asbestos. Asbestos also increases the risk of mesothelioma. The histologies of primary lung

cancers include non–small cell lung cancer (75%) and small cell lung cancer (25%). The most common histologies of non–small cell carcinoma include squamous cell cancer, adenocarcinoma, and large cell carcinoma. Bronchoalveolar histology is a category of adenocarcinoma, which can present as a more diffuse infiltrate mimicking pneumonia. Staging evaluation should include a CT scan of the chest and abdomen and a bone scan. Staging for patients with small cell cancer needs to distinguish only between extensive (involving more than one lung) and limited (involving one lung) disease. Small cell lung cancer is very sensitive to chemotherapy and radiation; if small cell lung cancer is limited in extent, both chemotherapy and radiation are administered; if the disease is extensive, only chemotherapy is administered. In contrast to staging small cell lung cancer, non–small cell lung cancer (squamous, adenocarcinoma, large cell) is more involved. An important point to understand in the staging of non–small cell lung cancer is that stage IIIA is a gray zone in which treatment could consist of surgery, neoadjuvant chemotherapy followed by surgery, or radiation combined with chemotherapy. Stage IIIA includes either a T3 tumor (tumor extending to the pleura, chest wall, or pericardium) or N2 nodes (nodes in the ipsilateral mediastinum). Stage IIIB is defined by a T4 tumor (tumor involving the mediastinal organs or the pleural fluid) or N3 nodes (nodes on the contralateral side, as choice B in question 31 describes). Treatment approaches in non–small cell cancer depend on the stage of the tumor. In stage I and stage II disease (which represent tumor within the lung without extension, 2 cm or more from the carina, and at most involving the hilar or bronchopulmonary lymph nodes [N1]), complete excision gives a chance of cure. Therefore, in a patient without mediastinal lymphadenopathy (N2) and with a tumor less than 3 cm (T1), the proper management should be surgery, with a 5-year survival rate of greater than 50%. Stage IIIA can be treated with any of three approaches, as mentioned. If the mediastinal lymph node involvement is minimal (N2), surgical resection could still be possible. Some have been evaluating the role of chemotherapy before surgical resection (neoadjuvant) in stage IIIA. Patients with more extensive mediastinal involvement or tumors extending to the pleura, chest wall, or pericardium (T3) may be treated with chemotherapy and radiation therapy because surgical resection may not be possible. Stage IIIB is considered unresectable and is treated with radiation and chemotherapy. An example of a planning radiograph of the chest for a stage IIIB tumor is shown in Figure V-2. Figure V-2

demonstrates the area (port) in which radiation will be administered (outlined in black) to the tumor and mediastinal lymph nodes. This patient will also receive chemotherapy because studies demonstrated a survival benefit of adding chemotherapy to radiation in stage IIIB. (*Cecil, Ch. 183; DeVita et al, 2001; Dillman et al, 1990*)

32. (C) *Discussion:* Risk factors for ovarian carcinoma have included a lower mean number of pregnancies and a history of infertility. Oral contraceptives may actually reduce the risk of ovarian cancer. The risk of ovarian cancer is also increased in women who have had breast cancer. The CA-125 test is useful to follow patients undergoing or completing treatment for ovarian carcinoma. In fact, most studies show that failure of the CA-125 levels to return to normal by the fourth treatment course is a bad prognostic sign. The usefulness of CA-125 as a screening test, however, has not been proven. In fact, only 50% of patients with clinically detectable ovarian cancer have elevated CA-125 levels. Patients with residual disease after initial surgery have decreased survival. However, some have argued that patients who can be optimally cytoreduced represent a different population of patients with improved survival related to the tumor biology and not the technique of cytoreduction. Although initial (primary) cytoreduction appears to be important, the importance of a second-look surgical reassessment and cytoreduction in patients who have completed a planned course of treatment is not clear. It is true, however, that the second-look operation can yield more accurate information about the disease status. Approximately 50% of patients who are clinically without evidence of disease still have residual disease on surgical re-exploration. A second exploration and cytoreduction may be important as new second-line therapies are tested. Therefore, it is reasonable to perform a second-look surgery in various clinical trials testing new agents. (*Cecil, Ch. 208; DeVita et al, 2001*)

33. (A); 34. (B). *Discussion:* Adjuvant therapy is given in addition to local therapy in an attempt to eradicate any unseen tumor cells (micrometastasis) that may have escaped local control. If unaffected, these tumor cells will eventually grow as a tumor recurrence, which is incurable. Adjuvant therapy has been proved to decrease recurrence in some tumor types, including breast, colon, and rectal cancer. Adjuvant therapy in colon cancer (tumor greater than 12 cm above the anus) differs from that of rectal cancer because rectal tumors recur more locally and benefit from radiation therapy in addition to chemotherapy. Studies in colon carcinoma have demonstrated that patients with Duke's stage C colon carcinoma (tumor involving the lymph nodes) have improved survival with adjuvant 5-FU based treatment. These treatments included 5-FU combined with levamisole or combined with leucovorin, although levamisole is not believed to have significant antitumor activity and is now rarely prescribed. A landmark study evaluated treatment of patients with stage B colon cancer (with tumor invading the muscularis propria but not the lymph nodes) and stage C colon cancer (with tumor involving the lymph nodes). Patients with stage C disease had a significantly reduced rate of death (by 33%) with treatment using 5-FU and leucovorin compared with no adjuvant treatment. More recent data support the use of chemotherapy in patients with Duke's stage B disease, but further studies are ongoing. Many patients have stage B disease with poor prognostic factors and have a risk of recurrence similar to that of stage C patients; these stage B patients are often treated as stage C with adjuvant chemotherapy. Factors indicating poor prognosis include presentation with obstruction, perforation, and tumor that has invaded through the serosa. Rectal cancer is defined as tumor occurring below 12 cm from the anal verge or below the peritoneal reflection; therefore, the rectal wall does not have a serosal surface because the peritoneal reflection occurs above the rectum. Because of these differences anatomically, patients with rectal cancer have a greater risk of local recurrence compared with those with colon

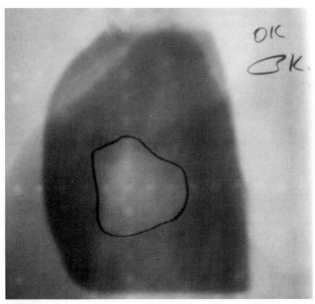

FIGURE V-2 • *(Courtesy of Parvish Kumar, MD.)*

carcinoma and benefit from combined adjuvant chemotherapy and radiation therapy. Studies demonstrated a survival benefit of combined chemotherapy and radiation therapy for stage B and stage C rectal cancer. (*DeVita et al, 2001; Moertel et al, 1990*)

35. (A) *Discussion:* A gene responsible for inherited breast cancer called *BRCA* appears to code for a tumor suppressor protein (a protein that acts as a negative regulator of tumor growth). The predisposition to cancer is inherited in an autosomal-dominant fashion in about 5% of all breast cancers. The testing of this abnormality is difficult because many mutations exist, and the test may not detect all mutations found in a family. Therefore, testing begins with the affected relative to determine whether the current testing can detect the abnormality found in a family. Once the test is validated in the affected relative, it can be used to screen family members. If the test is negative in the affected member, then either the member does not have the gene abnormality or the test is unable to detect that specific mutation; when the test is negative, it is not useful to screen unaffected members of that family. Mutations in the gene have been linked to cancer of both the breast and ovary. Other inherited predispositions to breast cancer also exist. One example is the Li-Fraumeni syndrome, which is caused by an abnormality in the *TP53* gene, a common tumor suppressor gene. Families with this syndrome have a high rate of female breast cancer along with other tumors. Currently, all patients with potential genetic risk factors should be referred to a high-risk breast center for evaluation and counseling. (*Cecil, Ch. 179; Miki et al, 1994*)

36. (C); 37. (A). *Discussion:* The French-American-British Cooperative Group established a classification system for acute leukemia. AML is categorized as M0-M7. M3, or acute promyelocytic leukemia (APL), is characterized by numerous promyelocytes (with heavily granulated cells) and accounts for 20 to 30% of adult AMLs. APL has distinctive clinical and molecular features. This subtype often manifests with disseminated intravascular coagulation (DIC), especially after the initiation of treatment. DIC usually presents with elevated fibrin split products and reduced fibrinogen, as in this patient. This can be treated with blood product support (transfusion platelets, cryoprecipitate, and fresh-frozen plasma to correct the thrombocytopenia, hypofibrinogenemia, and coagulation factors, respectively). APL is characterized at a molecular level by the reciprocal fusion of the promyelocytic leukemia (PML) gene on chromosome 15 and the retinoic receptor α (RARA) gene on chromosome 17. Differentiation therapy has revolutionized the treatment of APL. All-*trans*-retinoic acid (ATRA) can induce a morphologic remission in APL by targeting the PML/RARA fusion protein for degradation and inducing terminal differentiation of the APL cells.

Potential complications of induction chemotherapy include tumor lysis syndrome. This is characterized by the elevation of uric acid and phosphate and ultimately can result in renal failure. In an effort to reduce tumor lysis, allopurinol and hydration are started before treatment. Additionally, alkalinization of the urine with IV bicarbonate will decrease the precipitation of uric acid stones. Other complications of leukemia include hyperviscosity syndrome when the WBC count is markedly elevated. This complication can be very serious and requires attention with possible plasmapheresis and/or immediate treatment with chemotherapy to control the disease. (*Cecil, Ch. 47: DeVita et al, 2001*)

38. (A) *Discussion:* Etiologic agents implicated in bladder carcinoma include smoking, occupational exposures (chemicals, dyes, leather, paints, rubber, and plastics), pelvic irradiation, and cyclophosphamide chemotherapy. Smoking is responsible for about 45% of male and 37% of female bladder carcinoma deaths. The most common presenting symptom is hematuria, which occurs in approximately 80% of patients. The standard treatment for superficial bladder carcinoma is transurethral resection; in

patients at high risk of recurrence, adjuvant intravesicular treatment (with agents such as BCG) is often added. Most patients with deep muscle invasion should be treated with cystectomy. Increasingly, however, trimodality therapy with transurethral resection and chemotherapy/radiotherapy is being used for bladder-sparing therapy. Patients with metastatic disease are treated with combination chemotherapy agents such as MVAC (methotrexate, vincristine, doxorubicin [Adriamycin], and cisplatin). (*DeVita et al, 2001*)

39. (C) *Discussion:* Hypercalcemia of malignancy is a life-threatening metabolic disorder. It is most common in myeloma, breast cancer, and non–small cell lung cancer (most likely squamous cell). It is uncommon in colon and small cell lung cancer. Symptoms usually include pruritus, dehydration, constipation, lethargy, and coma. Mechanisms of hypercalcemia include the production of a PTH-related protein (not PTH itself), prostaglandins, and cytokines. Treatment of hypercalcemia includes fluid hydration, diuretics, corticosteroids (which inhibit gastrointestinal calcium resorption and osteoclast-mediated resorption), plicamycin (Mithracin), and bisphosphonates such as etidronate and pamidronate. (*Cecil, Ch. 184; DeVita et al, 1996*)

40. (B); 41. (D). *Discussion:* Risk factors for pancreatic cancer include smoking and chronic pancreatitis. Most are ductal adenocarcinomas (80%). Although 5-year survival in these patients is about 17% with surgical resection, those with cystadenocarcinoma have a better prognosis and are cured with surgery about 50% of the time. At presentation, fewer than 33% have a palpable gallbladder, and jaundice is common for tumors at the head of the pancreas, where most occur. Surgical excision is the only chance for cure, and the Whipple procedure is the procedure of choice. Most patients are not resectable. In fact, only 25% of those explored are resected. In patients who undergo surgical resection, survival is improved with combined chemotherapy and radiation after surgery. Only about 15% of patients with metastatic disease respond to standard chemotherapy. (*Cecil, Ch. 108; Kalser and Ellenberg. 1985; DeVita et al, 2001*)

42. (C) *Discussion:* Stage III (disease with peritoneal implants outside the pelvis or involved nodes, superficial liver metastases) and stage IV ovarian cancer (disease with distant metastasis) represent advanced disease. The primary treatment for advanced ovarian cancer is optimally to debulk the disease surgically followed by adjuvant chemotherapy. Patients whose tumors can be optimally debulked (leaving less than 1 cm of residual tumor) have better survival. Patients with residual disease after initial surgery have decreased survival. Some researchers argue that patients who can be optimally cytoreduced represent a different population of patients with improved survival related to the tumor biology and not the technique of cytoreduction. Although initial (primary) cytoreduction appears to be important, the importance of a second-look surgical reassessment and cytoreduction in patients who have completed a planned course of treatment is not clear. However, one randomized trial was completed in which 425 patients who had more than 1 cm of residual tumor left after primary surgery received three cycles of chemotherapy and were randomized to undergo secondary cytoreduction surgery or no surgery. The overall survival was improved significantly in the group that underwent secondary cytoreductive surgery. (*Cecil, Ch. 183; DeVita et al, 1996*)

43. (A) *Discussion:* Tumor markers are measured in the blood and often represent products secreted by malignant cells. Most have not been useful as a screening test but can be useful to follow treatment. CA-125 recognizes an antigen secreted by ovarian cancer. This test is not specific and, therefore, is of little use as a screening test. For example, the CA-125 value is normal in up to 50% of patients with stage I ovarian cancers. The CA-125 value can be used to follow response to chemotherapy. In patients with testicular cancer, high levels of hCG or any elevation of AFP indicates a nonseminomatous tumor, because patients with seminoma do not have elevated AFP and have only modest elevations of hCG. Either marker is elevated in most patients with nonseminomatous tumors and can be used to follow response of treatment. AFP is useful as a screening test for hepatoma in patients at high risk in Asian countries. (*Cecil, Ch. 208; DeVita et al, 2001*)

44. (A); 45. (C); 46. (B). *Discussion:* Pathologic findings in breast disease include in situ carcinoma (DCIS and LCIS) and invasive cancer (invasive ductal cancer and invasive lobular cancer). Ductal carcinoma in situ is defined by demonstrating carcinoma within breast ducts, not penetrating the basement membrane. DCIS represents a good prognosis pathology but if unresected completely has a high chance of developing into an invasive tumor. After an initial biopsy finding of DCIS, most patients have the option of a conservative approach (lumpectomy) or mastectomy. The conservative approach includes complete removal of the tumor (lumpectomy) with clear surgical margins. In patients with pure DCIS, the likelihood of axillary lymph node involvement is low and an axillary lymph node dissection is not recommended. Adjuvant chemotherapy is also not standard treatment for DCIS. Standard therapy for DCIS also includes radiation to the breast when lumpectomy is elected. LCIS, in contrast to DCIS, is a marker for high risk. Patients are at just as high a risk for invasive cancer in the breast with LCIS as in the contralateral breast. LCIS does not need to be surgically resected, but the patient needs to be counseled about her increased risk of breast cancer. Included in that counseling is the possibility of preventive agents such as tamoxifen; a recent trial demonstrated the benefit of tamoxifen in reducing the risk of breast cancer in such patients at an early time interval. In contrast to DCIS and LCIS, invasive tumor (defined as tumor penetrating through the basement membrane of the mammary ducts) should undergo complete excision and an axillary dissection. Patients who elect to undergo a lumpectomy should also receive a course of radiation therapy as is standard in DCIS because it has been demonstrated to decrease the risk of in-breast recurrence in both in situ and invasive cancer. Most patients with invasive carcinoma also have the option of lumpectomy or mastectomy, with equal survival rates. Therefore, in appropriately selected patients, the option of lumpectomy with radiation is a reasonable alternative to mastectomy. Additional radiation therapy in patients who undergo lumpectomy is important because studies comparing lumpectomy alone with lumpectomy with radiation reveal a significant decrease in local recurrence for those who receive radiation. In fact, 90% of the women treated with breast irradiation after lumpectomy remained free of ipsilateral breast tumor compared with 61% of those not treated with radiation after lumpectomy. One study also demonstrated a survival benefit to giving radiation after mastectomy for some patients with node-positive disease. Because this patient likely has stage I or II disease, a bone scan is not necessary. Bone scans are often used as a preoperative screening test to identify patients with metastatic disease. However, a positive bone scan is found in less than 5% of patients with stage I or II breast cancer. Given the low likelihood of positive scans in this early-stage group of patients, it is reasonable not to obtain them as part of a routine metastatic evaluation. Additionally, the false-positive rate is high, particularly for older patients. Patients with stage III disease (tumor > 5 cm), in contrast, have positive bone scans 20 to 25% of the time. If this patient had an abnormal bone scan, however, it should not be ignored. Plain radiographs of the bone or MRI may be helpful studies to evaluate these lesions further. If a lesion appears to be suspicious for metastatic disease, a biopsy should be considered to document metastatic disease. (*Cecil, Ch. 178; DeVita et al, 2001; Fisher et al, 1989, 1993; Silverstein et al, 1992*)

47. (A) True; (B) True; (C) True; (D) False. *Discussion:* Brain metastasis occurs in about one fourth of all patients with cancer. The most common primary tumors include lung, breast, gastrointestinal, urinary, and melanoma in order from most to least common. However, the tumor type most likely to have cerebral spread is melanoma, with 65% of patients developing this during the course of the disease. Treatment consists of steroids, radiation, and, in patients with solitary metastases, surgery. (*Cecil, Ch. 163*)

48. (A) False; (B) False; (C) True; (D) False. *Discussion:* Superior vena cava syndrome is the obstruction of blood flow through the superior vena cava. The first case ever described was a case of syphilitic aortic aneurysm in 1757. Now malignancy is the most common cause. Lung cancer represents 65% of malignant causes. Small cell lung cancer is the most common histologic subtype, found in 38% of patients who have lung cancer with the superior vena cava syndrome. The second most common subtype is squamous cell cancer. Lymphoma is the third most common. The most common symptom is dyspnea, occurring in 63% of patients. A biopsy should be attempted. Treatment depends on the tumor type. With small cell lung cancer, both chemotherapy and radiation are often given. For lymphoma, chemotherapy alone is usually sufficient. Surgery is rarely indicated when malignancy causes superior vena cava syndrome. (*Cecil, Ch. 163*)

49. (A); 50. (A). *Discussion:* Risk factors for pancreatic cancer include smoking (as the most firmly established risk factor), dietary factors (high-fat diets are generally associated, whereas coffee and alcohol have not been clearly implicated), and chronic pancreatitis. Cigarette smoking has been implicated as a cause of 30% of pancreatic cancer cases. Most are ductal adenocarcinomas (80%). Although 5-year survival in these patients is about 17% with surgical resection, those with cystadenocarcinoma have a better prognosis and are cured with surgery about 50% of the time. At presentation, fewer than 33% have a palpable gallbladder, and jaundice is common for tumors at the head of the pancreas, not the tail. Surgical excision is the only chance for cure, and the Whipple procedure is the procedure of choice, although unfortunately most cases are not resectable. In fact, only 25% of those explored are resected. In patients who undergo surgical resection, survival is improved with combined chemotherapy and radiation after surgery. Only about 15% of patients with metastatic disease respond to standard chemotherapy. (*DeVita et al, 2001; Kalser and Ellenberg, 1985*)

51. (D) *Discussion:* Prognostic factors in breast cancer are important because they often guide adjuvant therapy. Patients with a higher risk of recurrence derive greater potential benefit and should be considered for adjuvant therapy. For example, because adjuvant chemotherapy reduces the risk of recurrence by about 30%, a patient with a 60% chance of recurrence after initial local therapy will reduce that chance to 40%. In contrast, a patient with only a 12% chance of recurrence after local therapy will reduce the risk of recurrence to 8% with adjuvant therapy (30% less recurrence). Therefore, adjuvant chemotherapy saves 20 people of 100 at a 60% risk and 4 people of 100 at a 12% risk. In general, most patients are offered adjuvant therapy if the risk of recurrence is greater than 10%. Prognostic factors at the time of surgery help in deciding the ultimate risk of recurrence. Despite continued research in new prognostic factors, the number of involved lymph nodes remains the most important prognostic factor. (*Cecil, Ch. 183*)

52. (A) *Discussion:* Seminoma is the most common single germinal cell tumor, accounting for 40% of such tumors. Nonseminoma subtypes include embryonal cell carcinoma, teratocarcinoma, and choriocarcinoma, or combined histologies. In about 85% of patients with nonseminomatous testicular cancer, the β-hCG or AFP level is elevated. In contrast, in patients with seminoma, the

AFP level is always normal and the β-hCG level may be elevated in about half. In fact, patients with the diagnosis of seminoma with an elevated AFP level should be suspected of having nonseminomatous tumor, as was discussed in detail in question 43. The half-life of AFP is 5 to 7 days and that of β-hCG is 24 to 36 hours. β-hCG may be elevated in other malignancies, in pregnancy, and with marijuana use. One cause of a false-positive hCG assay is an increased LH level. This can be distinguished by repeating the hCG assay after an injection of testosterone. (*Cecil, Ch. 180; DeVita et al, 2001*)

53. (D); 54. (D). *Discussion:* Of primary importance, this patient with a smoking history may have a separate lung primary, and biopsy is critical before further management can be started. Although his primary tumor was a pleomorphic sarcoma, histologically there are three categories of sarcoma: spindle cell (which tend to be radiation and chemotherapy resistant), small or round cell (which are radiation sensitive and chemotherapy sensitive), and pleomorphic (which is a variant histologically between the other two). Both the small cell and pleomorphic variants are always high grade, whereas the spindle cell variant can be of low or high grade (such as fibrosarcoma or malignant fibrous histiocytoma, as in this case). High-grade soft tissue pleomorphic sarcomas such as malignant fibrous histiocytoma in this patient are treated by complete surgical excision. Although almost half of the patients will acquire metastatic disease, the use of adjuvant chemotherapy has not been shown to improve survival in patients with soft tissue sarcoma of the retroperitoneum. The treatment of low-grade malignant spindle cell sarcomas also involves wide surgical excision. In contrast to spindle cell and pleomorphic sarcomas, the treatment of small and round cell sarcomas is more intense. Small or round cell sarcomas, such as osteosarcoma or Ewing's sarcoma, are treated with combined chemotherapy, radiation, and surgical excision, with improved survival compared with surgery alone. The lung is the most frequent site of distant metastases, followed by the bone and liver. Resection of isolated pulmonary recurrences is important. In some series, about one third of patients with isolated metastasis were disease free at 3 years after surgical resection. (*DeVita et al, 2001*)

55. (A) *Discussion:* The two main categories of testicular primary tumors are seminoma and nonseminoma, and cure is obtained in more than 90% in either group. The differentiation between seminoma and nonseminoma on pathology can be difficult. A pearl often touted is that seminoma does not present as an elevated AFP (although liver dysfunction can mildly elevate AFP as a separate cause of such an abnormality). The pathologic diagnosis in this case is in question then because the AFP is elevated, and it is likely that this patient has nonseminoma. Patients with early-stage non-seminoma are treated adjuvantly with chemotherapy. Patients with early-stage seminoma (stage IIB or less, which can include disease in the retroperitoneal lymph nodes of < 5 cm) are often treated with radiation therapy, given the sensitivity of seminoma to radiation. (*DeVita et al, 2001*)

56. (C) *Discussion:* The usual presenting symptoms of renal cell carcinoma include hematuria, abdominal mass, and pain (the classic triad). The classic triad with all three presenting symptoms occurs in only 9% of patients. Renal cell carcinoma occurs in sporadic and familial forms. Although uncommon, patients can have familial renal cell carcinoma inherited in an autosomal-dominant fashion or associated with von Hippel-Lindau disease, which results from mutations at a tumor-suppressor locus on chromosome 3p25-p26. In the latter, renal cell carcinoma develops in as many as 35% of patients, and some have associated pheochromocytoma, cerebellar hemangioblastoma, and retinal angiomas. In inherited renal cell carcinoma, the tumor is often bilateral. This patient does not have any family history to suggest such a familial

cancer. Possible etiologic factors include cigarette smoking and use of phenacetin-containing analgesics. The 5-year survival for stage I is 66%; stage II, 64%; stage III, 42%; and stage IV, 11%. After surgical excision in early-stage patients, adjuvant chemotherapy or radiation therapy has not been conclusively shown to be of benefit. Although some advocate resection of the involved kidney in those patients with metastatic disease who have not undergone nephrectomy, this has not been shown to improve survival. Nephrectomy in this setting is performed to decrease symptoms such as pain and hemorrhage. Patients with a solitary metastasis can have a good 5-year survival rate after surgical resection. Success of systemic treatment for metastatic disease has been limited. Renal cell carcinoma is chemotherapy resistant. Vinblastine has been used but is associated with only a 7% response rate. Other therapies have been used, including biologic agents. Interferon has had response rates of 15 to 20%. IL-2 in combination with lymphokine-activated killer cell therapy has had a response rate similar to that of its use as a single agent (15-20%). (*Cecil, Ch. 183; DeVita et al, 2001*)

57. (C); 58. (A). *Discussion:* Prostate carcinoma is the most common cancer in men. It is second only to lung carcinoma as a cause of cancer death in men. Studies failed to demonstrate socioeconomic status, alcohol, cigarette smoking, or occupational exposure as risk factors, although patients with a family history and black men are at increased risk. One study demonstrated that tomato paste might be preventive, not a risk factor, although this is still controversial. Currently, for initial screening, PSA and rectal examination have been used in patients older than 50 years, although trials are ongoing to determine whether survival is improved with the addition of PSA to the screening. PSA is a serine protease secreted into the seminal fluid. It has a half-life of 2 to 4 days. PSA has greater sensitivity, although less specificity, compared with prostatic acid phosphatase. A PSA value greater than 10 ng/mL has a positive predictive value of 65% (the normal range for patients without cancer is 0-4 ng/mL). A certain level of PSA density (PSA per prostate weight measured by ultrasonography) may be more predictive of cancer. PSA increases with age and should be adjusted to age. In patients with cancer who undergo prostatectomy, detectable levels present 6 to 8 weeks after surgery represent persistent disease (because undetectable levels are expected in a patient after prostatectomy). A PSA value that does not fall after radiation therapy also predicts persistent disease. When PSA increases in patients after prostatectomy, options include radiation therapy (although only a small subgroup with low levels of PSA increase appear to benefit), androgen ablation (although no data are clear on when to initiate such therapy because eventually resistance develops), and watchful waiting. (*Cecil, Chs. 180 and 181; DeVita et al, 2001*)

59. (D) *Discussion:* CEA levels are elevated in many types of carcinoma and can be elevated in smokers, although not to such an extreme as in this case. Because both limited recurrence of colorectal cancer in the liver and local recurrence can be curable, and elevated CEA levels might precede other evidence of recurrence, patients like this should undergo further evaluation. However, there is no evidence that monitoring CEA levels postoperatively identifies a salvageable group. High preoperative levels in patients with colorectal cancers correlate with a worse prognosis. (*Cecil, Ch. 180; DeVita et al, 2001*)

60. (A) *Discussion:* Stage B prostate cancer represents tumor clinically limited to the prostate (the tumor is palpable on examination). Stage A represents tumor that is found during a non–cancer-related procedure such as a transurethral prostate resection or by transrectal biopsy, when the tumor is not palpable in the prostate as in stage B. Within category A, a stage T1C is defined as elevated PSA, no palpable nodule, but biopsy-positive tumor. T1C now represents the most commonly diagnosed stage, given the frequency with which PSA is tested. Stage C represents invasion of the seminal vesicles, prostatic apex, or bladder neck. Stage D1 represents lymph node involvement, and stage D2 indicates metastatic disease. Patients with early disease (stage B) are usually considered for treatment with radiation or radical prostatectomy. Both approaches appear equally successful, and a decision is made on the basis of the various risks involved in each approach and the patient's ability to undergo surgery. New nerve-sparing techniques cause impotence in less than 50% of patients, incontinence in 5%, and a 0.3% mortality rate. If the tumor is more extensive (stage C), radiotherapy is often given. Chemotherapy is considered for those patients whose tumor is unresponsive to hormonal manipulation. (*Cecil, Ch. 177; DeVita et al, 2001*)

61. **(A)** *Discussion:* Premalignant lesions found in the aerodigestive tract include leukoplakia and erythroplakia. Each has a propensity for malignant transformation . Leukoplakia is often found on the mucous membranes of the oral cavity, tongue, oropharynx, and larynx. It presents as small white patches. If biopsy is performed, the pathology specimen can reveal hyperkeratosis, hyperplasia, carcinoma in situ, or invasive carcinoma. Erythroplakia is characterized by red, superficial patches. It is more commonly associated with dysplasia and carcinoma in situ or malignancy than is leukoplakia. Leukoplakia is found in up to 50% of people who chew tobacco. Smoking cigarettes is the primary cause of cancer of the lung, larynx, oral cavity, and esophagus. However, it is not a known risk factor for prostate carcinoma. Environmental smoke also increased the risk of lung carcinoma in nonsmokers. (*Cecil, Ch. 20; DeVita et al, 2001*)

62. **(D)** *Discussion:* Patients with metastatic prostate cancer can be treated with antiandrogen therapy. The goal of any antiandrogen therapy is to remove the effect of testosterone on tumor cells because their growth is initially dependent on this male hormone. The primary antiandrogen therapy uses an agent that reduces testosterone levels (castration or an LHRH agonist). A second agent is often added to block the effect of testosterone at the androgen receptor (flutamide or bicalutamide [Casodex]). The use of one of these second antiandrogen agents for a combined therapy is controversial, however. In one trial, 603 men with stage D2 disease were randomized to leuprolide (an LHRH agonist), which will decrease testosterone levels, or leuprolide and flutamide. The progression-free response was increased by 3 months and survival by 7 months. The benefit was not seen in patients with poor performance status and severe osseous disease. A more recent study showed no benefit to adding flutamide to orchiectomy. In patients who progress after attempts at antiandrogen therapy, agents such as ketoconazole, steroids, and aminoglutethimide have been tried with minimal response. After progression on double hormonal therapy (LHRH agonist or orchiectomy with an antiandrogen such as flutamide or Casodex), withdrawal of the antiandrogen (flutamide or Casodex) can result in a response in 25% of patients. Currently, chemotherapy has little role in the treatment of metastatic prostate cancer outside of clinical trials. Cytotoxic agents such as estramustine and vinblastine or estramustine and docetaxel (Taxotere) have been used with some response, but it is unclear whether survival is improved. Alternative therapies include strontium 89, which can reduce the need for analgesics and prolong the period before pain progression. (*Crawford et al, 1989; DeVita et al, 2001; Porter et al, 1993*)

63. **(C)** *Discussion:* This patient clearly has shown a lower PSA. Although you cannot be sure of the cause of this effect, you should know that the most effective means to lower PSA in such a patient is with androgen ablation. Therefore, it is appropriate to determine whether something the patient is consuming is lowering the serum testosterone level. One possibility is an estrogen because these are

often found in herbs and can affect the level of testosterone in men, as was demonstrated in a study of an herbal combination used by men with cancer of the prostate. Estrogens lower testosterone levels in men by inhibiting LH. Prior studies comparing pharmaceutical doses of estrogen as a form of androgen ablation to standard forms such as leuprolide demonstrated equal efficacy but more toxicity with the use of estrogen, including blood clots. Regardless of the clinical scenario, a patient with unilateral leg swelling should be evaluated for a deep vein thrombosis before starting anticoagulants. Importantly, estrogen treatment in men is associated with a substantial risk of deep vein thrombosis. Studies of herbs continue to demonstrate potent effects, as do drugs. For example, saw palmetto has been studied for its ability to reduce prostate size in BPH. As studies demonstrate potent effects of many alternative medicines, it is important to evaluate patients carefully with the same consideration as patients consuming medicines. (*DeVita et al, 1996; DiPaola et al, 1998*)

64. **(D)**; 65. **(B)**; 66. **(D)**. *Discussion:* Most melanomas arise from a preexisting nevus (see Figure V-1). Poor prognostic features include increased vertical height and deeper level of invasion. A tumor that is 4 mm or less in thickness is associated with a 5-year survival rate of 37%. Ulceration is also a poor prognostic sign. The four major growth patterns are superficial spreading melanoma (70%), nodular melanoma, lentigo maligna melanoma, and acral lentiginous melanoma. Nodular melanoma has the worst survival. For initial lesions, surgical excision is important, and at least a 1-cm margin is removed. Elective lymph node dissection is controversial. However, one randomized trial demonstrated improved survival with adjuvant therapy with interferon in patients with disease involving lymph nodes, leading some physicians to treat patients with disease that involved the nodes (one trial that attempted to repeat these results did not fully confirm these findings). Therefore, a lymph node dissection may help in deciding on adjuvant interferon if that was the accepted plan by the physician and patient. Some centers are performing a sentinel node biopsy. This procedure consists of the injection of a tracking substance (dye or radioactive material) into the primary tumor site. After a short time, the surgeon dissects the draining lymph node bed and removes the first "marked" lymph node. The status of this node predicts the status of the whole lymph node bed with more than 90% accuracy and may avoid full lymph node dissections in most patients. The risks of adjuvant interferon include flulike symptoms and, rarely, liver failure, not renal failure. All patients on such therapy require careful follow-up of liver function studies. Metastasis occurs, from most common to least, in the skin and subcutaneous tissues, lungs, liver, brain, and bone. Serum lactate dehydrogenase is a useful marker for metastatic disease. Treatment includes surgical excision in superficial lesions and solitary brain metastasis. No initial therapy may be an option in patients with favorable sites such as the lung or bone but not the liver. Therapy for metastatic disease may consist of combination chemotherapy with agents such as dacarbazine, cisplatin, carmustine, and tamoxifen. No role for high-dose therapy and bone marrow transplant has been found. Biologic agents such as IL-2 and interferon have activity. Of note, the incidence of melanoma has increased. The cause of this increase is unclear but may be secondary to increased sun exposure. Risk factors include red hair with a threefold risk, fair skin, and family history. Antigenic markers are important in the pathologic evaluation. The S-100 and HMB-45 markers can be used to confirm the diagnosis; HMB-45 is more specific than S-100. (*Cecil, Chs. 177 and 183; DeVita et al, 2001; DiPaola et al, 1997*)

67. **(A)** *Discussion:* Multidrug resistance represents the ability of tumor cells to resist the lethal effects of multiple chemotherapeutic agents of different structure and mechanism. One mechanism of multidrug resistance is the expression of the P glycoprotein pump. P glycoprotein is a pump coded by the *mdr-I* gene. It acts as a trans-

porter protein and actively pumps out various chemotherapeutic agents, clearing the cell from lethal exposure to the drug. P glyco-protein is found in leukemia, lymphoma, breast cancer, and renal cell carcinoma. The expression appears to increase after the insti-tution of chemotherapy. Agents that appear to be substrates include anthracyclines (e.g., doxorubicin), epipodophyllotoxins (e.g., etoposide), *Vinca* alkaloids (e.g., vincristine), paclitaxel (Taxol), and mitomycin C. Studies are ongoing in a effort to alter this form of resistance. Another mechanism of resistance is the alteration of topoisomerase II and overexpression or alteration of genes that control programmed cell death (apoptosis) such as *bcl-2*. (*Cecil, Ch. 179*)

68. **(A)** *Discussion:* Patients with metastatic carcinoma from an unknown primary tumor comprise 5 to 10% of all cancer patients. Pathologic evaluation should be performed and should include immunostains, electron microscopy, and genetic analysis. The his-tologic categories include poorly differentiated neoplasms (in about 40%), well and moderately differentiated adenocarcinoma (accounting for 40% of all carcinomas of unknown primary site), and squamous cell carcinoma (10-15%). Above the diaphragm, lung cancer is the most common primary tumor found; below the diaphragm, a metastasis is most likely pancreatic in origin. Radiographic evaluation could include mammography and CT of the chest, abdomen, and pelvis. However, CT scans usually detect untreatable malignancies. For patients with poorly differentiated cancers, multiple causes are possible. All patients should have β-hCG, AFP, and PSA markers checked. Certainly, the possible presence of treatable tumors such as germ cell, breast, prostate, and lymphoma should be evaluated. Treatment of well- and moderately differentiated tumors usually consists of 5-FU combinations. Treatment for certain subtypes of tumors is more specific. For example, peritoneal carcinomatosis in women is treated as ovarian cancer, with surgery and a cisplatin chemotherapy regimen. In patients with poorly differentiated carcinoma, treatment with a cis-platin regimen can result in a good response and long-term sur-vival in a subset. (*Cecil, Chs. 177 and 180; Greco et al, 1986*)

69. **(A) True; (B) False; (C) True; (D) False.** *Discussion:* Apoptosis is an energy-dependent process of programmed cell death. The bcl-2 protein is a mitochondrial membrane protein that appears to block apoptosis; bcl-2 may, therefore, act to prolong tumor cell life. Bcl-2 dimerizes with a protein bax, which counter-acts the effect of bcl-2 in that it promotes the process of apoptosis. The current thinking is that bcl-2 blocks the leakage of cytochrome c from the mitochondria. The release of cytochrome c appears to start a series of reactions that lead to apoptosis. The expression of bcl-2 also confers resistance to chemotherapy in a tumor. For example, patients with prostate cancer before the use of androgen ablation therapy have very little bcl-2. In contrast, tumors that are resistant to androgen ablation therapy have increased expression. Clinical trials are ongoing to target therapies against bcl-2. (*Cecil, Ch. 179*)

70. **(A) True; (B) True; (C) True; (D) True.** *Discussion:* About 80% of seminomas are stage I (disease confined to the testis) on presentation. Patients with stage I disease have a long-term survival rate of greater than 90%. Seminoma is very radiosensitive, unlike nonseminoma. It is standard to treat patients with stage I disease with prophylactic irradiation to the regional lymphatics. Patients with stage II seminoma with extensive disease (defined as greater than 5 cm) are at risk for failure with radiotherapy alone. It is, therefore, reasonable to treat these patients with chemotherapy ini-tially, with a cure rate of approximately 90%. Alternatively, patients may be monitored after irradiation of the infradiaphragmatic lym-phatics, with follow-up and plans to treat with chemotherapy in the event of relapse. The chemotherapy used in seminoma is simi-lar to that used in nonseminoma. Bleomycin, etoposide, and cis-

platin (BEP) chemotherapy is standard. Some groups will not use bleomycin, given the concern for pulmonary toxicity based on some studies. Nonseminomatous testicular carcinoma stage A (Walter Reed stage I) has spread to the retroperitoneum, and stage C (Walter Reed stage III) indicates metastatic disease. The treat-ment of stage I nonseminomatous germ cell tumors is controver-sial. Because of the inaccuracy of clinical staging, retroperitoneal lymphadenectomy remains the standard surgical therapy. The 2- to 5-year survival rate in patients after orchiectomy and retroperi-toneal lymph node dissection is greater than 90%. Approximately 25% of clinical stage I tumors are understaged. Because 75% of clinical stage I patients who undergo retroperitoneal lymph node dissection are found to have pathologic stage I disease, most undergo this procedure without therapeutic benefit. In some patients, a surveillance program is initiated instead of retroperi-toneal lymph node dissection. However, this requires rigorous fol-low-up, including tumor marker evaluations each month for the first year and CT scans every 2 to 3 months for the first 2 years. Among patients with pathologically negative retroperitoneal lymph nodes, only 10% will experience recurrence. In patients with pathologically staged stage II disease, 50% will have no recurrence without any postoperative treatment. The group that has recur-rence can be treated with chemotherapy at that time, and so some advocate either treatment with chemotherapy postoperatively or close surveillance. Treatment for disseminated (stage III) disease has included systemic chemotherapy with bleomycin, etoposide, and cisplatin (BEP), as noted previously. This regimen will cause a response in about 70% of patients, with long-term survival in about 60%. (*DeVita et al, 2001*)

71. **(A) True; (B) True; (C) False; (D) True.** *Discussion:* In the United States, about 1 million people develop cancer each year. The incidence of prostate cancer and melanoma increased over the past 10 years, although the increase in prostate cancer incidence appears to be due to PSA testing with early detection. The leading causes of cancer among men (in order from most to least common) are prostate, lung, and colorectal carcinoma. The leading cancers seen in women are breast, lung, and colorectal carcinoma. For men and women, lung cancer is the leading cause of death. For women, the second most common cause of death is breast cancer and for men colorectal cancer. Mammogram screening can decrease the mortality rates of breast cancer by 20 to 30% in women older than 50. Rates of gastric and cervical cancer have declined, although proximal gastric cancers are increasing (gastric cardia). (*Cecil, Ch. 181; DeVita et al, 2001*)

72. **(A) False; (B) True; (C) True; (D) True.** *Discussion:* Malignant pericardial effusion occurs most commonly in lung can-cer, breast cancer, melanoma, lymphoma, and leukemia. The usual presentation is neck vein distention and pulsus paradoxus. The ECG usually has low voltage and may demonstrate electrical alter-nans (a periodic change of amplitude secondary to heart motion within the fluid). Symptoms include dyspnea. An echocardiogram is the initial diagnostic study of choice. Local treatment includes pericardiocentesis, or the formation of a pericardial window. Cytologic examination will demonstrate malignant cells in 80 to 90% of patients. After pericardiocentesis, the fluid often reaccu-mulates and may require a more definitive procedure such as a pericardial window. (*DeVita et al, 2001*)

73. **(A) True; (B) False; (C) False; (D) True.** *Discussion:* Proximal muscle weakness with reduced deep tendon reflexes, along with autonomic dysfunction, such as incontinence, and spar-ing of the ocular and bulbar muscles, is characteristic of Eaton-Lambert syndrome. Myasthenia gravis, in contrast, is characterized by preserved sensation and deep tendon reflexes and commonly results in ocular or bulbar manifestations. The diagnosis is aided by an electromyogram that reveals an increased muscle response to

each stimulation secondary to the accumulation of acetylcholine in the synaptic cleft. The Tensilon test has a poor response in Eaton-Lambert syndrome, unlike in myasthenia gravis. Eaton-Lambert syndrome is most commonly seen in small cell carcinoma of the lung. Therapy mainly consists of initiation of treatment of the primary cancer. Paraneoplastic syndromes do not affect the staging of a cancer. (*Cecil, Ch. 180*)

74. **(A) False; (B) False; (C) True; (D) True.** *Discussion:* SIADH can occur in patients with small cell lung cancer or brain metastases, in patients with pulmonary infection, or during treatment with cyclophosphamide and vincristine. Squamous cell lung cancer is more likely to cause hypercalcemia, not SIADH. The usual presentation of SIADH is hyponatremia, high urinary osmolality (higher than the plasma osmolality), and high urinary sodium concentration. Tumor-associated SIADH should be treated by treating the underlying cancer. (*Cecil, Ch. 182; DeVita et al, 2001*)

75. **(A) False; (B) True; (C) True; (D) True.** *Discussion:* The unique pathologic finding in Hodgkin's disease is the Reed-Sternberg cell or a variant among normal lymphocytes, plasma cells, and fibrous stroma. These cells are important for the diagnosis, but cells simulating these cells have also been found in reactive lymphoid hyperplasia so they should not be considered pathognomonic. The histologic types of Hodgkin's disease include nodular sclerosing (70%), lymphocyte predominant (15%), mixed cellularity, and lymphocyte-depleted disease, which are more commonly seen in advanced stages. Stage I represents involvement of two or more lymph node regions on the same side of the diaphragm. Stage II disease represents involvement on both sides of the diaphragm, and Stage III disease refers to the presence of lymph node involvement on both sides of the diaphragm. Stage IV is diffuse or disseminated disease involving extranodal organs. The classification A represents no symptoms and B represents fever, drenching sweats, or weight loss. Pruritus is associated with Hodgkin's disease but does not influence the staging. Staging laparotomy is important for patients being considered for radiation therapy because some will be upstaged by the procedure and require chemotherapy. Patients with stage IA or IIA disease can be treated with radiation therapy only. Patients with classification B symptoms consisting of fever or weight loss should be treated with chemotherapy because there is a higher rate of recurrence with radiation alone. Patients with stage III or IV disease are generally treated with chemotherapy. Patients with large mediastinal masses, defined as greater than one third of the thoracic width, are treated with chemotherapy followed by mediastinal radiation. (*DeVita et al, 2001*)

76. **(C); 77. (E); 78. (B); 79. (C); 80. (A).** *Discussion:* Tumor markers are measured in the blood and often represent products secreted by malignant cells. Most have not been useful as a screening test but can be useful to follow treatment. CA-125 recognizes an antigen secreted by ovarian cancer. This test is not specific and, therefore, is of little use as a screening test. CA-125 is usually elevated in any peritoneal malignancy. The CA-125 value can be used, however, to monitor response to chemotherapy. In patients with testicular cancer, high levels of hCG or any elevation of AFP indicates a nonseminomatous tumor because patients with seminoma do not have elevated AFP and have only modest elevations of hCG. Either marker is elevated in most patients with nonseminomatous tumors and can be used to monitor response to treatment. AFP is also useful as a screening test for hepatoma in patients at high risk in Asian countries. CEA, although not an effective screening marker for colorectal carcinoma, can be used in follow-up. The ratio of free to total PSA is used to distinguish benign versus malignant prostate disease. More PSA is complexed in patients with cancer compared with BPH (see also discussion to questions 1 to 3). (*Cecil, Ch. 180; DeVita et al, 2001*)

81. **(G); 82. (A); 83. (D); 84. (B); 85. (C); 86. (F); 87. (E).** *Discussion:* Paraneoplastic syndromes are often seen with many malignancies and may be the first manifestation of a cancer. SIADH was first reported in 1957 in two patients with lung cancer and hyponatremia. This syndrome is secondary to the ectopic production of ADH. Like the syndrome of ectopic production of corticotropin, small cell lung cancer is the most likely malignancy to be associated. Seventy-five percent of all cases of SIADH secondary to malignancy are caused by small cell lung cancer. Other malignancies include head and neck cancer and primary brain tumors. SIADH, however, is often caused by nonmalignant causes such as central nervous system abnormalities, pneumonia, and drugs. Erythrocytosis is often seen with renal cell carcinoma and is associated with elevated erythropoietin levels. Cutaneous paraneoplastic syndromes are also common. Acanthosis nigricans presents as gray-brown velvety plaques on the neck, axilla, flexor areas, and anogenital region. This syndrome is associated with adenocarcinoma mostly from gastric origin. The sign of Leser-Trélat is characterized by the development of large numbers of seborrheic keratoses and is associated with adenocarcinoma of the stomach, lymphoma, and breast cancer. Eaton-Lambert syndrome is a disorder of the myoneural junction that results in proximal muscle weakness. Sixty percent have an underlying cancer; two thirds are caused by small cell lung cancer. This syndrome is caused by an antibody to the presynaptic nerve terminal. Unlike classic myasthenia gravis, the weakness usually does not involve the bulbar muscles, and nerve conduction velocities show a characteristic pattern. Necrolytic migratory erythema is classic for glucagonoma or islet cell tumor of the pancreas. This presents as circinate and gyrate areas of blistering and erythema on the face, abdomen, and limbs. Flushing or episodic reddening of the face and neck is classic for carcinoid or medullary carcinoma of the thyroid and is thought to be secondary to the secretion of serotonin or other vasoactive peptides. (*Cecil, Ch. 182*)

88. **(E); 89. (A); 90. (B); 91. (D); 92. (C); 93. (G); 94. (F); 95. (H).** *Discussion:* Fever in neutropenic patients is a medical emergency. Risk of infection increases with a neutrophil count of less than 1000 (the absolute neutrophil count is calculated as the percentage of neutrophils and bands times the total WBC count). A culture should be performed immediately and patients started on broad-spectrum antibiotics. The coverage must include *Pseudomonas* and other gram-negative organisms. Additionally, if infection of a catheter is suspected or fever persists after initiation of antibiotics, coverage for gram-positive cocci should be added with drugs such as vancomycin. If fever persists after 5 to 7 days and the patient is still neutropenic, coverage for fungi should be added. The use of granulocyte colony-stimulating factor is best after the next cycle of treatment in patients who have had fever and neutropenia. In this setting, it has been shown to decrease duration of hospitalization and number of infections. It should not be given during the administration of chemotherapy because it could increase myelotoxicity. Its use at the time of neutropenia is not generally recommended. Back pain in patients with metastatic disease can be a symptom of spinal cord compression. Patients are treated in an emergent fashion because generally ambulation is maintained best in patients treated before paralysis. Evaluation usually consists of obtaining MRI to define the relationship of the tumor with the spinal cord. Both standard radiographs and CT are inadequate to demonstrate cord compression. Before MRI, a myelogram was the imaging method of choice. Treatment consists of radiation therapy. If compression occurs in an area of prior irradiation or worsens through radiation, surgery is the next option. Brain metastasis occurs in about one fourth of all patients with cancer. The most common primary tumors include lung, breast, gastrointestinal, urinary, and melanoma, in order from most to least common. However, the tumor type most likely to have cerebral spread is melanoma; 65% of patients experience this during the course of the disease. CT with contrast medium enhancement or an MRI needs to be performed. Nonenhanced CT may miss small

lesions. Treatment consists of corticosteroids, radiation, and, in patients with solitary metastases, surgery. In fact, one study demonstrated that resection of patients with a solitary metastasis improved survival when disease was not rapidly progressing elsewhere. A lytic bone lesion in a critical area, although not a true emergency, requires urgent management because a pathologic fracture can be debilitating. Although an MRI is the diagnostic procedure of choice for cord compression and CT (enhanced) or MRI for brain metastasis, standard bone radiographs are sufficient to rule out bone metastasis that may be unstable requiring orthopedic repair or radiation. If a lesion is believed to be unstable, orthopedic repair may be necessary before radiation because radiation can weaken the lesion a few days after initiation before its therapeutic effect. Superior vena cava syndrome is the obstruction of blood flow through the superior vena cava. The first case described involved syphilitic aortic aneurysm in 1757. Now malignancy is the most common cause; lung cancer represents 65% of malignant causes. Small cell lung cancer is the most common histologic subtype followed by squamous cell cancer of the lung and lymphoma. The most common symptom is dyspnea, occurring in 63% of patients. A biopsy should always be attempted. Treatment depends on the tumor type. With small cell lung cancer, both chemotherapy and radiation are used. For lymphoma, chemotherapy alone is usually sufficient. Surgery is rarely indicated when malignancy causes superior vena cava syndrome. Hypercalcemia can be secondary to malignancy or other causes (endocrine, infection, sar-

coid, vitamin D or A intoxication, lithium). Hypercalcemia of malignancy is caused most commonly by a PTH-related peptide (not elevation of PTH itself), and most commonly occurs in patients with squamous carcinomas. This is also elevated in about half of the patients with breast cancer. Patients often present with constipation and lethargy. Treatment consists of hydration, diuretics, and bisphosphonates. The bisphosphonates such as pamidronate are commonly used, and data support the use of pamidronate in patients with lytic bone metastasis from breast cancer to decrease progression. (*Cecil, Ch. 182; DeVita et al, 2001; Silber et al, 1998*)

96. **(B)**; 97. **(D)**; 98. **(A)**; 99. **(E)**; 100. **(C)**. *Discussion:* The names of common sites of metastasis serve to emphasize the importance of a complete physical examination in patients suspected of having a gastrointestinal malignancy. Most patients with gastric cancer, for example, have a combination of signs and symptoms such as weight loss, anorexia, and abdominal pain. On examination, a large peritoneal implant in the pelvis (Blumer shelf), a large ovarian mass (Krukenberg's tumor), a left supraclavicular lymph node (Virchow's node), a left anterior axillary lymph node (Irish's node), or a lymph node at the umbilicus (Sister Mary Joseph node) may be palpable. Distant sites of recurrence of gastric cancer include the liver, lungs, omentum, peritoneum, spleen, and adrenals. (*Cecil, Chs. 180, 185; DeVita et al, 2001*)

BIBLIOGRAPHY

Crawford ED, Eisenberger MA, McLeod DG, et al: A controlled trial of leuprolide with and without flutamide in prostatic carcinoma. N Engl J Med 1989;321:419.

DeVita VT Jr, Hellma S, Rosenberg SA (eds): Cancer: Principles and Practice of Oncology, 6th ed. Philadelphia, JB Lippincott, 2001.

Dillman R, Seagren S, Proprert D, et al: A randomized trial of induction chemotherapy plus high-dose radiation versus radiation alone in stage II non-small cell lung cancer. N Engl J Med 1990;323:940.

DiPaola RS, Goodin S, Ratzell M, et al: Chemotherapy for metastatic melanoma during pregnancy. Gynecol Oncol 1997;66:526.

DiPaola RS, Zhang H, Lambert G, et al: Clinical and biological activity of an estrogenic herbal combination (PC-SPES) in prostate cancer. N Engl J Med 1998;339:785.

Early Breast Cancer Trialists Collaborative Group: Systemic treatment of early breast cancer by hormonal, cytotoxic, or immune therapy. Lancet 1993;339:71.

Fisher B, Costantino J, Redmond C, et al: Lumpectomy compared with lumpectomy and radiation therapy for the treatment of intraductal breast cancer. N Engl J Med 1993;328:1581.

Fisher B, Redmond C, Poisson R, et al: Eight-year results of a randomized clinical trial comparing total mastectomy and lumpectomy with or without irradiation in the treatment of breast cancer. N Engl J Med 1989;320:822.

Goldman L, Ausiello D (eds): Cecil Textbook of Medicine, 22nd ed. Philadelphia, WB Saunders, 2004.

Greco FA, Vaughn WK, Hainsworth JD: Advanced poorly differentiated carcinoma of unknown primary site: Recognition of a treatable syndrome. Ann Intern Med 1986;104:547.

Hamblin TJ, Davis Z, Gardiner A, et al: Unmutated Ig VH genes are associated with a more aggressive form of chronic lymphocytic leukemia. Blood 1999;94:1848-1854.

Herskovic A, Matz K, Al-Sarraf M, et al: Combined chemotherapy and radiotherapy compared with radiotherapy alone in patients with cancer of the esophagus. N Engl J Med 1992;326:1563.

Kalser MH, Ellenberg SS: Pancreatic cancer: Adjuvant combined radiation and chemotherapy following curative resection. Arch Surg 1985;120:899.

Kyle RA, Therneau TM, Rajkumar SV, et al: A long-term study of prognosis in monoclonal gammopathy of undetermined significance. N Engl J Med 2002;346:564-569.

Miki Y, Swensen J, Sattuck-Eidens D, et al: A strong candidate for the breast and ovarian cancer susceptibility gene BRCA1. Science 1994;266:66.

Moertel CG: Chemotherapy for colorectal cancer. N Engl J Med 1994;330:1136.

Moertel CG, Fleming TR, MacDonald JS, et al: Levamisole and fluorouracil for adjuvant therapy of resected colon carcinoma. N Engl J Med 1990;322:352.

Patchell R., Tibbs PA, Regine WF, et al: A randomized trial of direct decompressive surgical resection in the treatment of spinal cord compression caused by metastasis. Proc Am Soc Clin Oncol (22, abstract #2), 2003.

Porter AT, McEwan AJB, Powe JE, et al: Results of a randomized phase-III trial to evaluate the efficacy of strontium-89 adjuvant to local field external beam irradiation in the management of endocrine resistant metastatic prostate cancer. Int J Radiat Oncol Biol Phys 1993;25:805.

Silber JH, Fidman M, DiPaola RS, et al: First cycle blood counts and subsequent neutropenia, dose reduction or delay in early stage breast cancer therapy. J Clin Oncol 1998;16:2392.

Silverstein MJ, Cohlan BF, Gierson ED, et al: Duct carcinoma in situ: 227 cases without microinvasion. Eur J Cancer 1992;28:630.

Toribara NW, Sleisenger MH: Screening for colorectal cancer. N Engl J Med 1995;332:861.

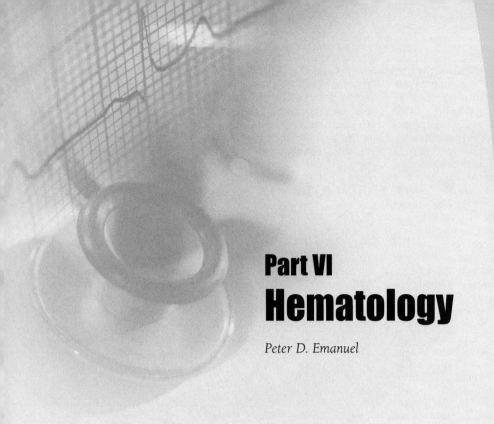

Part VI
Hematology

Peter D. Emanuel

MULTIPLE CHOICE

DIRECTIONS: For questions 1 to 90, choose the *best* answer to each question.

1. All of the following are characteristics of hematopoietic stem cells *except*:

   A. They are capable of self-renewal.
   B. They are relatively resistant to radiation.
   C. They adhere to marrow stroma.
   D. They have inherent homing mechanisms to the marrow.
   E. They are capable of giving rise to cardiac myocytes, hepatocytes, and neural cells.

2. Choose the correct combination for the lifespans of various blood cells and components:

   A. Red cells (10 days), platelets (9 hours), granulocytes (years), B lymphocytes (120 days), T lymphocytes (hours)
   B. Red cells (9 hours), platelets (10 days), granulocytes (years), B lymphocytes (hours), T lymphocytes (120 days)
   C. Red cells (10 days), platelets (9 hours), granulocytes (years), B lymphocytes (120 days), T lymphocytes (hours)
   D. Red cells (120 days), platelets (10 days), granulocytes (hours), B lymphocytes (hours), T lymphocytes (years)

3. All of the following mature cells are considered to be part of the myeloid cell compartment *except*:

   A. Neutrophils, monocytes, and dendritic cells
   B. Red cells
   C. B cells
   D. Platelets
   E. Eosinophils

4. Food and Drug Administration (FDA)–approved indications for therapy with erythropoietin include all of the following *except*:

   A. Anemia of inflammation (rheumatoid arthritis and inflammatory bowel disease)
   B. Chemotherapy-induced anemia
   C. Anemia with HIV induced by zidovudine with erythropoietin levels less than 500 U/mL
   D. Anemia of renal failure
   E. Perioperative setting

5. The initial diagnosis of anemia should be based on all of the following *except*:

   A. Complete history and physical examination (with emphasis on past medical history, family history, and evaluation of absence/presence of splenomegaly)
   B. Complete blood cell count
   C. Microscopic evaluation of the peripheral blood smear
   D. Hemoglobin electrophoresis
   E. Reticulocyte count

6. Inherited or congenital forms of hemolytic anemia include all of the following *except*:

   A. Red cell membrane abnormalities (membranopathies)
   B. Red cell enzyme abnormalities (enzymopathies)
   C. Paroxysmal nocturnal hemoglobinuria
   D. Hemoglobinopathies

7. Target forms of red blood cells can be found in all of the following conditions *except*:

   A. Liver disease
   B. Abetalipoproteinemia
   C. Chronic blood loss
   D. Hemoglobinopathies

8. Schistocytes and other forms of fragmented red blood cells are specifically found in which of the following categories of diseases?

   A. Hypersplenism
   B. Traumatic hemolysis
   C. Red cell membranopathies
   D. Lead poisoning
   E. Myelofibrosis

9. An infectious agent that can cause significant pure red blood cell aplasia in persons with underlying hemolysis is:

   A. *Mycoplasma*
   B. HIV
   C. *Escherichia coli*
   D. Fifth disease virus
   E. *Pneumococcus*

10. Bone marrow transplantation offers the best therapy for young aplastic anemia patients, with a 65 to 90% survival rate in patients younger than 20 years of age. Graft rejection is a major determinant of successful clinical outcome in aplastic anemia. Which of the following is a highly significant factor contributing to graft rejection?

    A. Sex
    B. Concomitant medical problems
    C. Number of infections associated with transplant
    D. Number of blood cell transfusions before transplant

11. Which of the following is considered the standard therapy for patients with severe aplastic anemia who lack a histocompatible sibling or who are older than 40 years of age?

    A. Antithymocyte globulin (ATG) therapy alone
    B. Androgen therapy alone
    C. Cyclophosphamide therapy alone
    D. ATG + androgens
    E. ATG + cyclosporine

12. All of the following are *true* statements regarding the term *megaloblastic except:*

    A. Megaloblastic anemias are caused by various defects in DNA synthesis.
    B. Megaloblastic and macrocytic refer to a similar state.
    C. Megaloblastic refers to a morphologic abnormality of cell nuclei.
    D. Etiology of megaloblastic anemia includes cobalamin deficiency, folate deficiency, and chemotherapeutic drugs.

13. All of the following are manifestations of folate deficiency *except:*

    A. Reticulocytopenia
    B. Neuropsychiatric abnormalities
    C. Bone marrow hypercellularity
    D. Elevated serum lactate dehydrogenase (LDH)
    E. Neutropenia

14. A 42-year-old African American nurse comes to your office complaining of a several-month history of fatigue, weight gain, constipation, and pedal edema. She has tried a high-carbohydrate diet program with no success. She was found to have a macrocytic anemia 2 years ago and says she faithfully gives herself monthly vitamin B_{12} shots for this. Her initial laboratory results from this visit are normal except for a hemoglobin of 11 g/dL, mean corpuscular volume (MCV) of 99 fL, and serum total protein level of 5.0. The best action to take at this point is:

    A. Perform endoscopy to rule out a gastric cancer.

    B. Obtain a serum vitamin B_{12} level and give the patient a 1000-μg vitamin B_{12} injection.
    C. Prescribe oral folic acid, 1 mg daily.
    D. Obtain thyroid function tests.
    E. Suspect Munchausen's syndrome and get a psychiatric evaluation.

15. A married, 25-year-old white schoolteacher is undergoing a work-up for infertility. During a laparoscopic procedure to evaluate her ovaries and fallopian tubes, splenomegaly is noted. Her laboratory test results include a hematocrit of 35% and normal MCV and ferritin values. Physical examination reveals no peripheral adenopathy, and a subsequent abdominal CT scan shows mild to moderate homogeneous splenomegaly and normal liver, gallbladder, pancreas, stomach, and intestines with no significant adenopathy. The next most appropriate action to take is:

    A. Obtain an osmotic fragility test.
    B. Perform a bone marrow aspirate and biopsy.
    C. Refer her to a surgeon for a splenic biopsy.
    D. Refer her to a surgeon for a splenectomy.
    E. Perform hepatic ultrasonography, looking for evidence of cirrhosis and portal venous hypertension.

16. A 35-year-old African American woman says she saw another doctor recently for a several-day history of malaise, myalgias, and fevers. His physical examination was apparently normal. Her complete blood cell count was normal, and her urinalysis showed a few white blood cells (WBCs). The patient says she told the doctor that she suffered from chronic urinary tract infections. He prescribed trimethoprim-sulfamethoxazole (Septra) for a 21-day course. Four days later she returned to him complaining of increased fatigue and now the complete blood cell count showed an anemia with a hemoglobin of 10 g/dL. He told her that the anemia was due to the urinary tract infection or possibly that this whole episode was a viral infection and that the anemia was due to the virus. She now comes to see you 14 days into the Septra course. Her hemoglobin now has increased to 13 g/dL. The best action to take at this point is:

    A. Tell her to continue the Septra because it looks like the other doctor was correct about the anemia being due to infection.
    B. Switch her from Septra to a cephalosporin.
    C. Order a methemoglobin reduction test.
    D. Tell her to stop the Septra and return to see you in 3 months.

17. Autoimmune hemolytic anemias are, in general, due to two major classes of antierythrocyte antibodies in humans, IgG and IgM. Determining which class is the cause for a specific case of autoimmune hemolytic anemia is important because of all the following *except:*

    A. The response to therapy
    B. The overall prognosis
    C. The pattern of red cell clearance
    D. The site of organ sequestration
    E. The presence of complement in the process

18. Glucocorticoids decrease hemolysis in IgG-induced hemolytic anemia by all of the following mechanisms *except:*

    A. They decrease production of the abnormal IgG antibody.
    B. They increase renal clearance of the abnormal IgG antibody.
    C. They induce a decrease in antibody affinity.
    D. They interfere with the macrophage Fc receptors.

19. Evans' syndrome refers to the combination of:

    A. Autoimmune hemolytic anemia and thrombotic thrombocytopenic purpura (TTP)
    B. Autoimmune hemolytic anemia and idiopathic thrombocytopenic purpura (ITP)
    C. Autoimmune hemolytic anemia and autoimmune neutropenia
    D. TTP and ITP

20. Presenting features of paroxysmal nocturnal hemoglobinuria include all of the following *except*:

    A. Chronic intravascular hemolysis
    B. Musculoskeletal pain
    C. Leukocytosis
    D. Budd-Chiari syndrome
    E. Iron deficiency

21. Which one of the following statements regarding paroxysmal nocturnal hemoglobinuria is *not true*?

    A. It is caused by mutations in the gene for a phosphatidylinositol glycan anchor, responsible for the attachment of at least 19 proteins to blood cells.
    B. It is most often diagnosed in young adults, but it can occur at any age and in individuals of either sex.
    C. Prednisone is the usual initial therapy, but many patients do not respond.
    D. It is an inherited disorder, following an autosomal dominant pattern of inheritance.
    E. Flow cytometry analysis of glycosylphosphatidylinositol (GPI)-anchored cell surface proteins (e.g., CD55, CD59) are the most sensitive and specific tests presently available for diagnosis.

22. You are asked to see a 25-year-old white man who developed marked weakness and dyspnea 4 days after being admitted for a compound arm fracture after falling from a tree. Estimated blood loss from the initial fracture episode was 600 mL and the patient was transfused with 1 unit of packed erythrocytes. The initial crossmatch was reported as compatible by the transfusion service. The patient has never been transfused before this incident and has no other serious medical illnesses. The patient's arm fracture was treated with surgical pinning and prophylactic antibiotics consisting of cefotetan, 2 g intravenously every 12 hours. When you examine the patient he is febrile, mildly tachycardic, with no evidence of wound infection or compartment syndrome. Laboratory data show a hematocrit of 15%, absolute reticulocyte count of 600,000/μL, and total bilirubin of 4.1 mg/dL with direct bilirubin of 0.5 mg/dL. The peripheral smear shows many spherocytes. There is no hemoglobinemia or hemoglobinuria seen on visual inspection of the plasma and urine. The transfusion service reports that the direct Coombs test is now strongly positive using anti-IgG and only weakly positive with anti-C3d antisera. They further report that routine compatibility tests show no new erythrocyte antibodies in the patient's serum and that when they attempted to elute antibody from the patient's red cells and test against normal red cells the results were negative. What is the most likely diagnosis?

    A. Hemolytic transfusion reaction caused by an ABO incompatibility
    B. Delayed hemolytic transfusion reaction
    C. Autoimmune hemolytic anemia of warm antibody type
    D. Autoimmune hemolytic anemia of cold antibody type
    E. Drug-induced immune hemolytic anemia

23. All of the following cause microangiopathic hemolytic anemia *except*:

    A. Thrombotic thrombocytopenic purpura
    B. Hemolytic-uremic syndrome
    C. Vasculitis
    D. Venoms
    E. Disseminated intravascular coagulation

24. Which of the following statements is *true*?

    A. Thalassemias are quantitative disorders of hemoglobin whereas hemoglobinopathies are qualitative disorders of hemoglobin.
    B. Thalassemias are qualitative disorders of hemoglobin whereas hemoglobinopathies are quantitative disorders of hemoglobin.
    C. Thalassemias are always inherited disorders.

25. A 52-year-old African-American woman comes to you for another opinion regarding a history of anemia that has been unresponsive to oral iron supplementation. She sought out your opinion because her other physician was recommending intravenous iron supplementation. She has been on nearly continuous iron supplementation therapy ever since her second child was born 23 years ago. Over the years she says her doctors have prescribed her to take anywhere from one to three pills daily, sometimes with vitamin C concomitantly. Although she has never needed a transfusion, she says she has been told that her red blood cell count has never completely normalized. She is otherwise healthy and has no unusual dietary habits. Her menstrual history reveals relatively normal menstrual periods until about 3 years ago, when she attained menopause. The patient believes that her mother was also iron deficient. Results of the physical examination are normal. Laboratory values show a hemoglobin of 11.6 g/dL, hematocrit of 33%, MCV of 70 fL, a normal WBC with differential, normal platelet count, serum iron of 70 μg/L, iron binding capacity of 255 μg/dL, and ferritin of 158 μg/L. At this point your next recommendation should be:

    A. Agree with the other physician and recommend intravenous iron supplementation because she does not appear to be absorbing enough oral iron to totally correct her anemia
    B. Perform a hemoglobin electrophoresis
    C. Obtain a serum erythropoietin level
    D. Discontinue iron supplementation
    E. Perform a bone marrow aspirate and biopsy

26. A 25-year-old white woman presents to the emergency department with complaints of extreme shortness of breath of acute onset. She was actually seen in the same emergency department 24 hours previously where she was diagnosed with a urinary tract infection and given prescriptions for Pyridium and sulfamethoxazole. She is overweight, sedentary, and smokes 2 packs of cigarettes a day. On physical examination she is markedly dyspneic and extremely cyanotic. An arterial blood gas analysis fails to reveal any hypoxia but a ventilation/perfusion scan is obtained anyway that is read as low probability. What should be the next course of action?

    A. Repeat the arterial blood gas analysis to look for progression and development of hypoxia.
    B. Proceed to pulmonary arteriography.
    C. Begin anticoagulation.
    D. Administer methylene blue.
    E. Transfuse 2 units of packed red blood cells.

27. A 50-year-old white man comes to see you because he was told he had "high blood." Physical examination is normal except for a ruddy complexion, which he says he has had most of his adult life. He has smoked two packs of cigarettes per day since he was 16 years old. A complete blood cell count shows a normal WBC count and differential, normal platelet count, a hemoglobin of 18.4 g/dL, and a hematocrit of 57%. To work up this elevated hematocrit what is the next most appropriate test to order?

   A. Serum erythropoietin level
   B. Arterial blood gas analysis
   C. Red cell mass study
   D. Bone marrow aspirate and biopsy
   E. Pulmonary function tests

28. For the patient described in question 27, the next set of tests to order following the preliminary assessment would include all of the following *except*:

   A. Serum erythropoietin level
   B. A venous P_{50} determination
   C. Arterial oxygen saturation determination
   D. Carbon monoxide determination
   E. Bone marrow aspirate and biopsy

29. The wide variation in the clinical severity of patients with hemoglobin SS disease is attributed to:

   A. Different point mutations in the hemoglobin gene
   B. Different lengths of gene deletions in the hemoglobin gene
   C. Lack of early intervention in the cases with the most severe clinical consequences
   D. The rate at which a patient "auto-splenectomizes" themselves
   E. Unknown causes

30. Causes of the "acute chest syndrome" in sickle cell disease include all of the following *except*:

   A. Vaso-occlusion
   B. Prolonged pain crisis
   C. Infection
   D. Fat embolus

31. Which of the following statements regarding sickle cell trait is *true*?

   A. It is a benign carrier condition with no known clinical complications.
   B. Despite being considered a benign carrier condition, rare complications do occur, such as hematuria
   C. It is associated with an increased incidence of anesthetic complications.
   D. Sickle cell forms are occasionally seen on the peripheral smear from sickle cell trait patients.

32. Which of the following statements regarding Hb SC disease is *false*?

   A. Hb SC red cells have a longer circulatory survival than Hb SS red cells (27 days vs. 17 days).
   B. Target cells are generally more prominent on the peripheral smear than sickle cells.
   C. Hb SC patients have a higher rate of splenic sequestration crisis than Hb SS patients.
   D. Sickle cell painful crises are always much milder as compared to Hb SS patients.
   E. The life expectancy of Hb SC patients is longer than Hb SS patients.

33. In the United States, the prevalence of sickle cell trait is 8 to 10% among black newborns. Given that the incidence of one- or two-gene α-thalassemia is greater than 20%, a significant number of individuals have sickle cell anemia coexistent with α-thalassemia. This combination results in which of the following?

   A. Less rapid hemolysis and milder anemia than in Hb SS disease
   B. Decreased incidence of leg ulcers
   C. Increased incidence of osteonecrosis
   D. Increased incidence of acute painful episodes
   E. All of the above

34. The most significant advancement in recent years in the management of sickle cell acute painful episodes has been the development of which of the following?

   A. The potent nonsteroidal anti-inflammatory drug ketorolac (Toradol)
   B. The orally administered, centrally acting analgesic tramadol, which binds to the μ-opioid receptor, causing minimal respiratory depression and low abuse potential
   C. Butyric acid
   D. Hydroxyurea
   E. The efficacy of bone marrow transplant

35. A 39-year-old black woman presents with a 3-month history of increasing fatigue and dyspnea on exertion. Over the last few weeks she thinks that she has noticed her complexion becoming more pale. She takes no medications and does not abuse alcohol. Her past medical history is unremarkable. She lives alone so she admits that her diet is not always as good as it should be. On physical examination she has no orthostatic changes. Her respiratory rate is 18 breaths/minute and pulse rate is 90 beats/minute. Laboratory values show a hemoglobin of 4.7 g/dL, MCV of 124 fL, WBC of 3800/μL, platelet count of 118,000/μL, and LDH of 3180 U/L. The electrocardiogram (ECG) is normal. Stool guaiac test for occult blood is negative. Blood is drawn for vitamin B_{12} and folate determinations. The most appropriate immediate management is:

   A. Transfuse 1 unit of packed red blood cells.
   B. Transfuse as many units of red blood cells necessary to bring the hemoglobin up to 8 g/dL.
   C. Transfuse as many units of red blood cells necessary to bring the hemoglobin up to 10 g/dL.
   D. Do not transfuse but immediately start subcutaneous erythropoietin.
   E. Do not transfuse but begin vitamin treatment and monitor the patient closely.

36. The most frequent, and usually one of the first, signs of an adverse reaction to blood transfusion is:

   A. Nausea and vomiting
   B. Wheezing/dyspnea
   C. Discomfort at the infusion site
   D. Fever
   E. Back/lumbar pain

37. Which of the following is a disease with a 90% mortality rate that can occur in bone marrow transplant recipients, patients with congenital immunodeficiency syndromes, Hodgkin's disease patients, and even under certain circumstances in normal individuals?

   A. *Pneumocystis carinii* infection
   B. *Mycobacterium kansasii* infection
   C. Transfusion-related graft vs. host disease
   D. Veno-occlusive disease
   E. Epstein-Barr virus–related non-Hodgkin's lymphoma

38. Eosinophilia can be associated with all of the following *except*:

    A. Parasitic infections
    B. Aspergillosis
    C. Churg-Strauss vasculitis
    D. Exogenous administration of Leukine (granulocyte-macrophage colony-stimulating factor [GM-CSF])
    E. Exogenous administration of Neupogen (granulocyte colony-stimulating factor [G-CSF])

39. A 53-year-old woman comes to see you regarding a possible diagnosis of essential thrombocytosis. She says her gynecologist has noted a platelet count of more than 550,000/μL on three separate occasions over the past 2 years. Apart from two uneventful childbirths the woman says she really has no significant past medical history. She says she has never been told she was anemic. Laboratory values reveal a normal hemoglobin, hematocrit, and MCV. The platelet count is 580,000/μL. Your review of the peripheral smear reveals no microcytosis or hypochromia but does show red cell Howell-Jolly bodies. The platelet count on the smear appears elevated, but there are no giant platelets or platelet clumps. What is the next most appropriate step in your diagnostic work-up?

    A. Perform bone marrow aspirate and biopsy.
    B. Obtain a C-reactive protein and a sedimentation rate looking for a state of chronic inflammation.
    C. Obtain a ferritin level to confirm that there is no iron deficiency.
    D. Go back and obtain a more thorough history and repeat the physical examination.
    E. Perform chest, abdominal, and pelvic CT scans searching for an occult malignancy.

40. A 62-year-old woman with a platelet count of 1.35 million/μL has been diagnosed with essential thrombocytosis after an exhaustive search has failed to reveal any reactive causes for the elevated platelet count. Her platelet count has been over 1 million for over 6 months. The most appropriate therapy now that a diagnosis of essential thrombocytosis has been established is:

    A. Plateletpheresis
    B. Aspirin
    C. Anagrelide
    D. Hydroxyurea
    E. Interferon-α

41. A 54-year-old white man is admitted to the hospital because of abdominal pain and "black stools." He has not seen a doctor in years. He smokes two packs of cigarettes daily. Physical examination reveals poor dentition, a normal cardiovascular examination, moderate splenomegaly with mild epigastric and left upper quadrant tenderness, and a guaiac-positive stool test for occult blood. Laboratory values reveal a hemoglobin of 9.5 g/dL, hematocrit of 29%, WBC count of 14,500/μL with a fairly normal differential, a platelet count of 540,000/μL, and a ferritin level of 4 μg/L. Serum vitamin B_{12} levels are elevated. A bone marrow examination shows hypercellularity without other specific findings, and chromosomes are reported as normal. Endoscopy reveals a gastric ulcer, and biopsies are negative for malignancy but positive for *Helicobacter pylori* infection. Appropriate management at this stage should be:

    A. Splenectomy
    B. Transfusion of 2 units of packed red blood cells

    C. Observation
    D. Antibiotic treatment for the *H. pylori* infection and iron supplementation for the iron deficiency anemia
    E. Antibiotic treatment for the *H. pylori* infection

42. Which of the following is the best clue that one is dealing with a myelophthisic disorder?

    A. Nucleated red blood cells on the peripheral smear
    B. Teardrop-shaped red blood cells on the peripheral smear
    C. The magnitude of splenic enlargement
    D. Anemia with constitutional symptoms (weight loss, fevers, sweats)
    E. Leukocytosis with anemia and thrombocytopenia

43. A 60-year-old man comes to you with symptoms that you correctly diagnose as erythromelalgia and aquagenic pruritus. He has been hospitalized three times in the past 2 years, twice for a deep venous thrombosis in the left leg and once for an arterial thrombosis in the right hand, both of which were successfully treated. His physical examination is relatively normal except for a palpable spleen tip. His laboratory values show a hematocrit of 55%, WBC count 14,000/μL, and platelet count of 525,000/μL. His prothrombin time (PT) and activated partial thromboplastin time (aPTT) are normal. The most likely diagnosis is:

    A. A myeloproliferative disorder
    B. Systemic lupus erythematosus
    C. Antiphospholipid antibody syndrome
    D. Hereditary resistance to activated protein C
    E. Antithrombin III deficiency

44. A 64-year-old woman comes to see you for fatigue symptoms over the past 4 months. She has a long-standing history of breast cancer initially diagnosed 10 years ago. She initially underwent mastectomy and then adjuvant chemotherapy with cyclophosphamide and doxorubicin (Adriamycin). Three years later she suffered a relapse with pulmonary metastases and a lesion in the opposite breast. She underwent a mastectomy on the other side, more chemotherapy, and then subsequently received an autologous bone marrow transplant, attaining a complete remission. She has been free of disease and feeling quite well the past several years. On physical examination there is no adenopathy and no signs of local recurrence in the chest area. Abdominal examination shows no hepatosplenomegaly. Chest radiography shows no signs of pulmonary recurrence of her metastases. Chemistry profile is normal. The WBC count is 2200/μL with 35 segmented neutrophils, 45 lymphocytes, 14 monocytes, 2 basophils, 2 eosinophils, and 2 atypical lymphocytes; the platelet count is 38,000/μL; hematocrit is 24% and the MCV is 106 fL. Review of the peripheral smear reveals anisocytosis, rare macro-ovalocytes, and hypogranulated neutrophils. What is the most likely diagnosis?

    A. Relapsed breast cancer with marrow invasion
    B. Aplastic anemia
    C. Systemic lupus erythematosus
    D. Delayed graft failure from the marrow transplant
    E. Myelodysplasia

45. The International Prognostic Scoring System for Myelodysplasia incorporates all of the following variables *except*:

    A. Percentage of bone marrow blasts
    B. Age and sex
    C. Karyotype
    D. Number of cytopenias

46. The current "standard of care therapy" for myelodysplasia is:

    A. Low dose chemotherapy with subcutaneous cytarabine
    B. High-dose chemotherapy similar to induction type regimens for acute myelogenous leukemia (AML)
    C. Hematopoietic growth factor support
    D. A trial of pyridoxine, followed by corticosteroids if pyridoxine fails
    E. Supportive care only

47. A 38-year-old woman presents with leukocytosis with numerous immature forms and basophils, thrombocytosis, and splenomegaly. A bone marrow examination shows a hypercellular marrow and is indicative of chronic myelogenous leukemia, but the chromosome analysis comes back and does not show the Philadelphia chromosome. The next most appropriate step to take is:

    A. Repeat the marrow biopsy and do another chromosome analysis.
    B. Initiate chemotherapy.
    C. Initiate interferon-α therapy.
    D. Refer for consideration of bone marrow transplantation.
    E. Perform polymerase chain reaction analysis for presence of the fusion *BCR/ABL* gene.

48. The following scenario is most typical for which of the diagnoses listed below: a 50-year-old white man with fever, weight loss, unusual infections, no adenopathy, pancytopenia, and splenomegaly.

    A. Chronic myelogenous leukemia
    B. Chronic lymphocytic leukemia
    C. Low grade non-Hodgkin's lymphoma
    D. Hairy cell leukemia
    E. Acute T-cell lymphocytic leukemia

49. A previously healthy 66-year-old white man comes in for his annual physical examination. He has no complaints and has been healthy the entire past year. Physical examination is unremarkable. Laboratory values are normal except for a WBC count of 18,500/µL with 10% segmented neutrophils and 90% lymphocytes. Which of the following tests will best help to definitively diagnose chronic lymphocytic leukemia (CLL)?

    A. Bone marrow aspirate and biopsy
    B. Lymph node biopsy
    C. Chromosomal analysis
    D. Peripheral blood cell surface marker analysis

50. Which of the following has been associated with an increased risk of acute leukemia?

    1. Benzene and benzene-containing compounds
    2. Ionizing radiation
    3. Tobacco
    4. Genetics
    5. Prior exposure to alkylating agents
    6. Certain viruses

    A. 1, 2, 4, and 5
    B. 1, 2, 3, and 5
    C. 1, 2, 4, 5, and 6
    D. 1, 2, and 5
    E. 1, 2, 3, 4, 5, and 6

51. Of all of the forms of AML, which one is clearly the most curable?

    A. M0, acute undifferentiated leukemia
    B. M3, acute promyelocytic leukemia
    C. M4, acute myelomonocytic leukemia
    D. M4E, acute myelomonocytic leukemia, eosinophilic variant

52. What percentage of patients with acute leukemia present with total WBC counts that are in the normal range?

    A. 0%
    B. 5%
    C. 20%
    D. 50%

53. So-called sanctuary sites that can be the site of an isolated relapse of acute lymphocytic leukemia include all of the following *except*:

    A. Pericardium
    B. Gonads
    C. Central nervous system
    D. Joints

54. Which of the following is the worst prognostic sign in adult acute lymphocytic leukemia (ALL)?

    A. High initial WBC count
    B. Central nervous system involvement at diagnosis
    C. Presence of Philadelphia chromosome
    D. Age older than 30 years
    E. Male sex

55. Infectious agents known to be linked with the development of non-Hodgkin's lymphomas (NHL) include all of the following *except*:

    A. Epstein-Barr virus
    B. Cytomegalovirus
    C. *Helicobacter pylori*
    D. HIV
    E. Kaposi's sarcoma–associated herpesvirus

56. Which of the following non-Hodgkin's lymphomas has emerged in recent years as a particularly aggressive indolent (low grade) lymphoma that can be quite resistant to therapy?

    A. Follicular lymphoma
    B. Extranodal marginal zone B-cell (MALT) lymphoma
    C. Mantle cell lymphoma
    D. Small lymphocytic lymphoma

57. The International Prognostic Index (IPI) has been developed for aggressive non-Hodgkin's lymphoma and incorporates all of the following variables *except*:

    A. Age
    B. Sex
    C. Serum LDH
    D. Stage
    E. Number of extranodal disease sites

58. The monoclonal antibody (rituximab) has received FDA approval for use in patients with chemotherapy-refractory or resistant indolent B-cell non-Hodgkin's lymphoma. The antibody is directed at which specific cell surface marker?

    A. CD19
    B. CD20
    C. CD5
    D. CD23
    E. CD43

59. All of the following can be late complications of Hodgkin's disease, depending on the therapy administered *except:*

    A. Breast cancer
    B. Myelodysplasia and acute myeloid leukemia
    C. Herpes zoster
    D. Infertility
    E. Central nervous system relapses

60. Therapy for multiple myeloma has for many years traditionally involved the use of melphalan and prednisone. Two significant developments in the therapy for multiple myeloma have occurred in just the past few years. Those developments are:

    1. The demonstration that VAD (vincristine, Adriamycine, Decadron) chemotherapy produces longer remissions than melphalan and prednisone chemotherapy
    2. The demonstration that autologous marrow transplantation cures a majority of patients
    3. The use of erythropoietin to relieve anemia symptoms
    4. The demonstration that autologous marrow transplantation results in a longer survival benefit than conventional therapy for multiple myeloma
    5. The demonstration that pamidronate results in fewer skeletal complications and improved quality of life in patients with myelomatous skeletal involvement

    A. 1 and 3
    B. 4 and 5
    C. 2 and 3
    D. 2 and 5

61. Peripheral blood stem cell harvesting has become the preferred method versus marrow harvesting for most autologous transplants and is rapidly increasing in popularity for allogeneic transplants. Some of the reasons for this include all of the following *except:*

    A. No need for general anesthesia or a hospital stay
    B. Much faster time to engraftment
    C. A potential of less contamination with infiltrating tumor cells in patients with solid tumor malignancies
    D. Decreased numbers of T lymphocytes

62. The first four tests that should be ordered in the initial evaluation of patients with a suspected coagulopathy are all of the following *except:*

    A. Platelet count
    B. Bleeding time
    C. Platelet aggregation studies
    D. Prothrombin time (PT)
    E. Activated partial thromboplastin time (aPTT)

63. In screening a patient with an acute thrombosis for the possibility of a hypercoagulable state, all of the following tests can be performed while the patient is on heparin *except:*

    A. Protein C level
    B. Protein S level
    C. Antithrombin III level
    D. Factor V mutations

64. Standard of care therapy for idiopathic thrombocytopenic purpura is the following sequence:

    A. Administer IVIG initially; if a relapse occurs then try prednisone followed by splenectomy within 3 weeks.
    B. Administer prednisone until remission occurs; if a relapse occurs re-treat with prednisone.
    C. Administer prednisone until remission occurs; if a relapse occurs initiate long-term anti-Rh antibody therapy.
    D. Use combined therapy with cyclophosphamide and prednisone initially until remission occurs.
    E. Administer prednisone until remission occurs; if a relapse occurs then use IVIG or anti-Rh antibody therapy temporarily to increase the platelet count sufficiently such that splenectomy can be performed.

65. A previously healthy 43-year-old black woman presents with a several-day history of malaise, fevers, and poor appetite. On initial examination it is thought that she may have a pneumonia or a viral syndrome. Chest radiography showed questionable atypical infiltrates. Laboratory values showed a WBC count of 11,000/μL with a normal differential, platelet count of 78,000/μL, and hematocrit of 32%. Serum LDH was elevated at 1500 U/L, but other liver function studies were normal. The serum creatinine concentration was 1.2 mg/dL. Antibiotic therapy and intravenous fluids are initiated, but 2 days later she is not improved. She has continued to have daily fevers to 104° F and as a result is starting to become delirious and have altered mental status. Her pulmonary status has not significantly worsened. All cultures are negative thus far. However, because of the severity of her illness, her hematocrit has dropped to 27%, platelet count has dropped to 42,000 /mL, and her renal function is now also deteriorating; her creatinine is now 2.3 mg/dL. The blood bank is reporting abnormal red blood cell forms on her peripheral smear. The next most appropriate intervention is to:

    A. Switch the antibiotic regimen to make sure there is broad coverage but try to avoid aminoglycosides if at all possible because of the deteriorating renal status.
    B. Perform a bronchoscopy to obtain adequate material for proper cultures to be performed.
    C. Discuss code status and end of life issues because the situation could obviously get worse much faster.
    D. Review the abnormal peripheral smear and initiate plasmapheresis.
    E. Obtain a urinalysis and increase the rate of intravenous fluids to make sure the patient is not intravascularly depleted.

66. A patient is described in his medical record as having lifelong moderate hemophilia A (factor VIII deficiency). Presuming that he has not been treated with any factor VIII recently, what is his factor VIII level likely to be?

    A. 50-70%
    B. 30-50%
    C. 10-25%
    D. 5-10%
    E. 1-5%

67. The patient described in question 66 has a brother who is 5 years younger who also has hemophilia. Which of the following statements is *true*?

    A. All four brothers in this family are likely to have hemophilia
    B. This patient's severity of hemophilia cannot be predicted from his brother's course. He could have mild, moderate, or severe hemophilia.

C. The two sisters in this family are likely to have moderate hemophilia.

D. This patient's endogenous factor VIII levels will be exactly the same as his brother's factor VIII activity level.

68. A 54-year-old white man is diagnosed with a colon cancer in his sigmoid colon and scheduled to undergo resection. Preoperative laboratory results show a normal platelet count, normal PT and aPTT, but a slightly prolonged bleeding time. The patient is on no prescription medications and denies use of any over-the-counter medications apart from rare use of acetaminophen. He does say that he seems to have bruised easily for as long as he can remember. Further laboratory tests obtained show a decreased von Willebrand factor antigen and decreased cofactor. Platelet aggregation studies show decreased response to ristocetin. Multimeric analysis shows a uniform decrease in all multimers. A safe and effective therapy for this patient for protection against hemorrhage associated with his upcoming surgery is:

A. Factor VIII concentrates
B. Cryoprecipitate
C. Desmopressin (DDAVP)
D. Activated factor IX complex concentrates

69. A 28-year-old white woman is trying to conceive a child. She has had no fertility problems but has already suffered from three spontaneous abortions. Vaginal ultrasonography and other evaluations from her gynecologist have revealed no anatomic reasons for the repeated spontaneous abortions. She is basically healthy otherwise but does admit to easy bruising since she was a teenager. Results of platelet count, bleeding time, PT, and aPTT are all normal. Which of the following factor deficiencies is she most likely to have?

A. Factor XIII
B. Factor VIII
C. Factor XII
D. Factor IX
E. Factor II

70. Which of the following known abnormalities has the highest prevalence in patients with venous thromboembolism?

A. Protein C deficiency
B. Protein S deficiency
C. Antithrombin III deficiency
D. Inherited activated protein C resistance
E. Prothrombin gene mutation

71. A 70-year-old previously healthy black man is admitted to the hospital with an apparent pneumococcal pneumonia. His only medication on admission is hydrochlorothiazide for mild hypertension. This is continued and he is treated with intravenous ceftriaxone (Rocephin) and ticarcillin/clavulanate (Timentin) antibiotics. He is also given nasal cannula oxygen at 2 L/minute and twice-daily subcutaneous heparin prophylaxis. His admission complete blood cell (CBC) count showed a WBC count of 15,000 with 80 segmented neutrophils and 13 bands. Five days later he is clearly improving but slowly. A repeat CBC count is ordered to monitor his WBC count. The WBC count now is 12,400/μL with 74 segmented granulocytes and 2 bands, but his platelet count is noted to be 65,000/μL. Review of the platelet count from the CBC on admission showed that it was not counted but estimated to be "adequate." The most likely diagnosis of the thrombocytopenia is:

A. Disseminated intravascular coagulation
B. Antibiotic suppression
C. Heparin-associated thrombocytopenia
D. Myelodysplasia (admit platelet estimate was inaccurate)
E. Developing ITP

72. Which of the following risk factors can predispose to either AML or chronic myelogenous leukemia (CML)?

A. Ionizing radiation
B. Benzene
C. Tobacco exposure
D. Previous chemotherapy
E. Family history of leukemia

73. Which therapy is currently considered "standard of care" for newly diagnosed CML patients who are not transplant candidates?

A. Interferon + cytarabine
B. Interferon alone
C. Imatinib (STI571) alone
D. Imatinib + interferon
E. Imatinib + cytarabine

74. Of the bone marrow failure syndromes, which form has the highest incidence rate?

A. Fanconi's anemia
B. Schwachman-Diamond syndrome
C. Paroxysmal nocturnal hemoglobinuria
D. Idiopathic
E. Epstein-Barr virus

75. When an individual becomes iron deficient, the first manifestation of iron deficiency noted in regard to erythropoiesis is which of the following?

A. Normochromic, normocytic anemia
B. Microcytosis without anemia
C. Microcytic anemia
D. Formation of target cells
E. Formation of pencil cells

76. A woman develops ITP during her pregnancy. She is wondering what decisions she should make regarding her pregnancy. In general, what can you tell her regarding her delivery risk and the outcome of the infant?

A. She is at low risk for complications and the infant stands a very good chance of a normal outcome, but she needs to be monitored closely through pregnancy.

B. She is at moderate to high risk for complications and she needs to begin therapy to raise her platelet count immediately.

C. She is at severely high risk for complications to herself and her fetus, and she should consider immediate termination of the pregnancy.

77. The current mean survival for both men and women with sickle cell anemia is which of the following age groups?

A. 20s
B. 40s
C. 30s
D. 50s

78. Partial exchange transfusions are not indicated in which of the following sickle cell disease patient scenarios?

   A. In the early management of a cerebrovascular accident
   B. In the management of a severe osteonecrosis episode
   C. In the management of sickle chest syndrome when arterial oxygen tension cannot be maintained above 70 mm Hg
   D. In the management of priapism when local measures fail

79. Which of the following features identifiable on the peripheral smear are *not* characteristic for myelodysplasia?

   A. Pseudo Pelger-Huët neutrophils
   B. Neutrophils with agranular cytoplasm
   C. Basophilia
   D. Thrombocytopenia with small platelet volumes

80. In reviewing a peripheral smear you note Howell-Jolly bodies in the red cells. You can immediately assume that the patient has had what performed in the past?

   A. Chemotherapy administration for acute leukemia
   B. Cholecystectomy
   C. Plasmapheresis for multiple myeloma
   D. Splenectomy

81. The presentation of a middle to elderly aged patient with splenomegaly and minimal lymphadenopathy can be typical for all of the following disorders *except*:

   A. Hairy cell leukemia
   B. Marginal zone leukemia/lymphoma
   C. CLL/SLL
   D. Waldenström's macroglobulinemia

82. Which of the following are associated with indolent disease and a favorable prognosis in CLL?

   1. Mutated Vh genes and low CD38 expression
   2. Unmutated Vh genes and high CD38 expression
   3. Mutated Vh genes and high CD38 expression
   4. Unmutated Vh genes and low CD38 expression
   5. Chromosome 17p deletions
   6. Chromosome 13q deletions

   A. 1, 5, and 6
   B. 2 and 6
   C. 3 and 6
   D. 4 and 6
   E. 1 and 6

83. CLL patients are at risk for all of the following *except*:

   A. Second malignant tumors including skin cancers, colorectal and lung cancers, and sarcomas
   B. Transformation to ALL
   C. Autoimmune disorders, especially ITP and immune hemolytic anemia
   D. Hypogammaglobulinemia

84. Alemtuzumab (Campath 1-H) is a monoclonal antibody that is FDA-approved for use in fludarabine-refractory CLL. It is directed against which cell surface antigen?

   A. CD20
   B. CD22
   C. CD52
   D. CD4
   E. Her 2-neu

MATCHING

DIRECTIONS: In questions 85–90, match the following patient descriptions with their likely clinical outcome scenarios.

   A. An ALL patient with a *BCR/ABL* fusion gene product
   B. A CML patient with a *BCR/ABL* fusion gene product
   C. An AML patient with a *PML/RAR* fusion gene product
   D. A patient treated for Hodgkin's lymphoma 5 years ago, now with pancytopenia and chromosome 5 and 7 abnormalities
   E. An AML patient with an *AML/ETO* fusion gene product
   F. A patient with a chloroma treated with radiation therapy only

85. High likelihood for complete remission and long-term survival with a combination of all-trans retinoic acid (ATRA) and chemotherapy

86. Very good likelihood for complete remission and long-term survival when treated with high dose chemotherapy alone

87. Likely will attain a complete remission with conventional chemotherapy but will relapse during chemotherapy and needs a stem cell transplant to have any hopes of long-term survival

88. Has a high likelihood of attaining a complete normalization of blood cell counts when treated with an oral, nonchemotherapeutic agent

89. Likely will respond poorly even to initial chemotherapeutic attempts at intervention

90. Likely will suffer a relapse in the bone marrow within 1 to 2 years

QUESTIONS 91–100

Each group of items in this section consists of lettered options followed by a set of numbered items. For each item, select the one lettered option that is most clearly associated with it. Each lettered option may be selected once, more than once, or not at all.

	Hemoglobin (g/dL)	MCV (fL)	Total WBC (/μL)	Platelet Count (/μL)	Reticulocyte Count (cells/μL)	Total Bilirubin	Direct Bilirubin	Serum LDH
A.	5.0	108	3,500	45,000	50,000	2.5	0.2	620
B.	5.0	108	1,500	20,000	20,000	0.5	0.2	220
C.	5.0	108	7,000	400,000	240,000	2.5	0.2	620
D.	5.0	108	7,000	45,000	240,000	2.5	0.2	620
E.	14.0	108	7,000	90,000	50,000	1.0	0.2	220

91. Acute alcohol abuse

92. Paroxysmal nocturnal hemoglobinuria

93. Autoimmune hemolytic anemia

94. Myelodysplasia

95. Thrombotic thrombocytopenic purpura

	Platelet Count (/μL)	Bleeding Time	aPTT	PT	Thrombin Time	D-Dimer
A.	50,000	Normal	Normal	Normal	Normal	Negative
B.	50,000	Prolonged	Prolonged	Prolonged	Prolonged	Increased
C.	250,000	Prolonged	Normal	Normal	Normal	Negative
D.	250,000	Normal	Prolonged	Slightly prolonged	Prolonged	Negative
E.	85,000	Normal	Prolonged	Prolonged	Normal to prolonged	Negative

96. Continuous intravenous infusion therapy for lower extremity deep venous thrombosis

97. Chronic renal failure

98. Thrombotic thrombocytopenic purpura

99. Disseminated intravascular coagulation

100. Chronic liver disease

Part VI
Hematology
Answers

1. **(C)** *Discussion:* Multipotent hematopoietic stem cells generally exist in a resting state and thus are relatively resistant to the effects of chemotherapy and radiation. They can self-renew and thus perpetuate the marrow environment over a lifetime. Recent studies indicate that bone marrow–derived hematopoietic stem cells are capable of giving rise to cardiac myocytes, keratinocytes, pneumocytes, hepatocytes, neural cells, skeletal muscle, and a variety of mesenchymal cells, including cartilage, fat, and bone. They are not adherent to marrow stroma, and thus we are able to mobilize them in clinical situations and harvest them from the peripheral circulation for transplantation purposes. *(Cecil, Ch. 159; Hoffman et al, 2000; Lee et al, 1999)*

2. **(D)** *Discussion:* The production of active blood cell types occurs predominantly in the bone marrow. Hematopoiesis is a tightly regulated system with different cell types responding to various but specific stimuli. Under the appropriate stress situations, the marrow can increase the production of cells by many fold. Mature cells are released into the bloodstream through largely unknown regulatory mechanisms. In normal, nonstressed situations, the average lifespan of red blood cells is 120 days; platelets, 10 days; granulocytes, 9 hours; and B and T lymphocytes are highly variable, but, in general, B cells have half-lives ranging in hours whereas the T cell half-life is measured in years. *(Cecil, Ch. 159; Hoffman et al, 2000; Lee et al, 1999)*

3. **(C)** *Discussion:* Multipotent lymphohematopoietic stem cells can commit to the lymphoid stem cell compartment, which leads to the production of mature B cells, plasma cells, CD4 and CD8 T cells, and NK cells. Alternatively, multipotent stem cells can commit to the myeloid stem cell compartment, which leads to the production of mature basophils, eosinophils, red cells, platelets, neutrophils, and monocyte/macrophage/dendritic cells. *(Cecil, Ch. 159; Hoffman et al, 2000; Lee et al, 1999)*

4. **(A)** *Discussion:* Erythropoietin (EPO) was the first cytokine (synonyms: colony-stimulating factor, hematopoietic growth factor) to gain FDA approval for patient use in the therapy for a cytokine deficiency state. Its initial success fueled the original tremendous growth of the biotech company, Amgen. The original approval indication was for the treatment of anemia of renal failure. Ninety percent of EPO production occurs in the kidney (the remainder primarily in the liver) in response to hypoxemia. Thus, patients with end-stage renal disease and on chronic dialysis therapy are not capable of producing even baseline levels of EPO. Since this initial approval, clinical benefit has been demonstrated to one degree or another in all of the other answers except for anemia of inflammation wherein EPO increases the hematocrit but without clinical benefit. *(Cecil, Ch. 159; Hoffman et al, 2000; Lee et al, 1999)*

5. **(D)** *Discussion:* A hemoglobin electrophoresis should not be considered part of the initial work-up for the patient with newly diagnosed anemia. The first distinction to be made in an anemia work-up is whether the primary cause of the anemia is due to a bone marrow failure state wherein insufficient numbers of erythrocytes are produced or due to a state of accelerated loss or destruction of erythrocytes. In this regard, the reticulocyte count is often very informative. An elevated reticulocyte count indicates an intact bone marrow capable of increasing red cell production at times of stress, whereas a normal to low reticulocyte count is indicative of a probable intrinsic marrow problem as the primary cause for anemia. *(Cecil, Ch. 160; Hoffman et al, 2000; Lee et al, 1999)*

6. **(C)** *Discussion:* Paroxysmal nocturnal hemoglobinuria is a form of membrane abnormality, but it is an acquired hemolytic anemia not inherited or congenital. Other acquired membrane abnormalities of hemolytic anemia include acanthocytes (spur cells), echinocytes (burr cells), and thermal injury (burns). Other acquired forms of hemolytic anemias include various types of immune hemolysis, traumatic hemolysis, hypersplenism, infection, and osmotic damage. Inherited red cell membranopathies include spherocytosis, elliptocytosis, pyropoikilocytosis, and stomatocytosis. Inherited red cell enzymopathies include G6PD deficiency, pyruvate kinase deficiency, and other rarer forms. Inherited hemoglobinopathies include thalassemias; hemoglobins S, C, D, and E; unstable hemoglobins; and other rarer hemoglobinopathies. *(Cecil, Ch. 169; Hoffman et al, 2000; Lee et al, 1999)*

7. **(C)** *Discussion:* Target cells are not seen in any form of blood loss anemia. They are specific to hemoglobinopathies such as thalassemias and hemoglobins S, C, D, and E and to liver disease and lipoprotein disorders. *(Cecil, Chs. 160 and 161; Hoffman et al, 2000; Lee et al, 1999)*

8. **(B)** *Discussion:* Schistocytes (red cell fragments) can be seen on the peripheral smear in various types of traumatic hemolysis, including thrombocytopenic purpura (TTP)/hemolytic-uremic syndrome (HUS), disseminated intravascular coagulation (DIC), the HELLP syndrome, vasculitis, eclampsia, malignant hypertension, prosthetic heart valves, and arterial grafts. They can occasionally be seen, albeit at much lower frequency, after thermal injuries and in postsplenectomy states. Membranopathies are more likely to produce specific red cell shapes dependent on the specific membrane defect: spherocytes in spherocytosis, elliptocytes in elliptocytosis,

and flame-shaped cells in pyropoikilocytosis. Lead poisoning typically gives rise to basophilic stippling, Myelofibrosis and myelophthisic states (marrow infiltration by neoplastic cells) are generally the only disorders that produce significant numbers of teardrop cells. (*Cecil, Chs. 160 and 161; Hoffman et al, 2000; Lee et al, 1999*)

9. (D) *Discussion:* Parvovirus B19 causes fifth disease, a benign exanthem of childhood and a polyarthralgia syndrome in adults. In persons with any number of underlying hemolytic disorders, such as sickle cell disease, immune hemolytic anemia, or spherocytosis to name a few, parvovirus infection causes temporary but abrupt worsening of anemia. This is due to the extreme tropism of the parvovirus specifically for erythroid progenitors because the parvovirus uses the P antigen on the red cell surface as its cellular receptor. Normal individuals can tolerate the temporary cessation of erythropoiesis until new erythroid progenitors are generated. However, individuals with underlying hemolytic processes depend on increased production of red cells to keep up with their increased destruction rate. Therefore, even a temporary lack of erythropoiesis in these patients can be devastating. Normally the parvoviral infection is a short-lived one, but it can persist in immunosuppressed individuals and may require immunoglobulin infusions. (*Cecil, Ch. 174; Hoffman et al, 2000; Lee et al, 1999*)

10. (D) *Discussion:* The number of units transfused between the time of initial diagnosis and the time of marrow transplantation directly and significantly correlates with the incidence of graft rejection. Therefore, children and young adults up to about age 30 should be considered for very early transplantation if they have a suitable donor. The incidence of graft-versus-host disease increases dramatically in older adults, and thus marrow transplantation for aplastic anemia for patients older than 45 to 50 years of age is generally discouraged. (*Cecil, Ch. 174; Hoffman et al, 2000; Lee et al, 1999*)

11. (E) *Discussion:* The combination of antithymocyte globulin (ATG) plus cyclosporine, which is superior to ATG alone in severe aplastic anemia, produces hematologic responses in about 70% of cases, with long-term survival rates approaching 80 to 90%. Importantly, the response can take up to 2 months, so patients and clinicians should not be overly anxious to attempt subsequent therapies and abandon the ATG combination. Occasional patients can show responses to androgen therapy, but it should not be considered a front-line option. Cyclophosphamide also offers effective immunosuppressive therapy and may have the advantage of avoiding late clonal evolution to other hematologic disease, which ATG and cyclosporine cannot do. Nevertheless, it is not considered first-line therapy by today's standards. (*Cecil, Ch. 174; Hoffman et al, 2000; Lee et al, 1999*)

12. (B) *Discussion: Megaloblastic* and *macrocytic* are distinctly different terms and refer to different states even though they, at times, can be found in the same disease situation. The term *megaloblastic* refers to a morphologic abnormality of cell nuclei that is caused by various defects in DNA synthesis. The most common causes are cobalamin deficiency, folate deficiency, metabolic inhibitor-type chemotherapeutic agents, and, less commonly, inborn errors and other unexplained disorders. *Macrocytic* is a specific term that refers only to the size of red cells. Young, normal red cells can be macrocytic, as can be red cells that are abnormal due to disorders of DNA synthesis. (*Cecil, Chs. 160 and 175; Hoffman et al, 2000; Lee et al, 1999*)

13. (B) *Discussion:* The neuropsychiatric abnormalities caused by cobalamin deficiency are not seen in folate deficiency, even though methionine synthesis appears to be equally impaired in both vitamin deficiencies. The cytopenias and bone marrow hypercellularity that results from either cobalamin or folate deficiency can be so severe that patients are rarely misdiagnosed with myelodysplasia or even leukemia. Because cobalamin and folate deficiencies are so easy to correct with replacement therapy, it is imperative that these disorders be ruled out. Serum LDH levels can be excessively elevated in cobalamin- and folate-deficient states. (*Cecil, Ch. 175; Hoffman et al, 2000; Lee et al, 1999*)

14. (D) *Discussion:* Recognize that pernicious anemia is more common than originally thought in black women in their 40s. This woman has developed autoimmune hypothyroidism. Development of other autoimmune disorders is a common feature of pernicious anemia. She concomitantly developed a low serum protein from the strict diet she had placed herself on trying to overcome the hypothyroid effects. Although a gastric cancer could have been the underlying cause for her pernicious anemia, at this stage one would expect a microcytic, iron deficiency anemia and weight loss rather than the opposite. Mild macrocytic anemia can be seen in hypothyroid and other endocrine disorder states. A folic acid deficiency would not explain all of her symptoms. (*Cecil, Ch. 175; Hoffman et al, 2000; Lee et al, 1999*)

15. (A) *Discussion:* Recognize the patient with undiagnosed mild hereditary spherocytosis. An osmotic fragility test will be abnormal, and a review of the peripheral smear would reveal spherocytes. Because of the mild nature of her hereditary spherocytosis, this woman has reached maturity without the development of sequelae of her spherocytosis, including gallstones and severe hemolytic anemia. If a diagnosis of spherocytosis had been ruled out, then tests such as a bone marrow examination or splenectomy looking for types of lymphoma would be potentially appropriate. Given her other lack of signs and symptoms, hepatic cirrhosis is much less likely. (*Cecil, Ch. 170; Hoffman et al, 2000; Lee et al, 1999*)

16. (C) *Discussion:* Recognize the prevalence of, and the clinical course of, G6PD deficiency in black African populations. These patients are typically hematologically normal in the absence of an exogenous oxidant stress. Unlike the Mediterranean forms of G6PD deficiency, these individuals, when exposed to oxidant drugs, develop an acute hemolysis episode which then abates despite continuation of the drug because the bone marrow is able to compensate by producing new young red cells that compensate for the ongoing hemolysis. The red blood cells of Mediterranean individuals are more susceptible to oxidant-induced hemolysis, and even the new young red cells cannot compensate for the brisk hemolysis. (*Cecil, Ch. 172; Hoffman et al, 2000; Lee et al, 1999*)

17. (E) *Discussion:* Complement is involved with both types of antibody hemolysis: IgG and IgM. Two molecules of IgG antibody need to be in close proximity to one another on the red cell surface to bind the first component of complement, C1. On the other hand, a single molecule of IgM can bind C1 and activate the classic complement pathway. Splenic macrophages, owing to their abundant receptors for the Fc domain of the IgG antibody, are the primary site of clearance of IgG-coated red cells. But they do not have receptors for the Fc domain of the IgM antibody. Consequently, the pattern of clearance of IgM-coated erythrocytes is entirely different from that of IgG-coated cells. IgM-coated cells are cleared rapidly by hepatic macrophage C3 receptors. The clearance is entirely complement dependent. This difference in the mechanism of clearance explains the difference in response to splenectomy between IgG- and IgM-mediated autoimmune hemolysis, as well as the overall prognosis of the diseases. (*Cecil, Ch. 169; Hoffman et al, 2000; Lee et al, 1999*)

18. (B) *Discussion:* Glucocorticoids are believed to decrease hemolysis in IgG-induced hemolytic anemia by three major mechanisms. Increased renal clearance is not a mechanism. However, the other three listed mechanisms all contribute to improved erythrocyte survival despite the continued presence of IgG on the red cell surface. Therefore the Coombs test, which is one of the easiest tests to obtain if autoimmune hemolytic anemia is suspected, may remain positive despite improvements in the level of anemia. This combined effect of these three mechanisms may take effect within a matter of a few days after initiation of glucocorticoid therapy. (*Cecil, Ch. 169; Hoffman et al, 2000; Lee et al, 1999*)

19. (**B**) *Discussion:* Autoimmune hemolytic anemia occurring concurrently with immune thrombocytopenia is termed *Evans' syndrome*. It occurs in a small percentage of both adults and children with autoimmune hemolytic anemia. Many patients have associated disorders such as chronic lymphadenopathy or dysgammaglobulinemia. Glucocorticoid therapy is usually effective at controlling acute episodes. Because of the patient usually having an underlying disorder, splenectomy is associated with more infections and more relapses. (*Cecil, Ch. 169; Hoffman et al, 2000; Lee et al, 1999*)

20. (**C**) *Discussion:* Patients with paroxysmal nocturnal hemoglobinuria (PNH) typically present with chronic intravascular hemolysis. It is a primary bone marrow disorder affecting the hematopoietic stem cell and all cell lineages. Thus, patients often present with pancytopenia but not with leukocytosis. Frequent clinical complaints include abdominal, back, and musculoskeletal pain. Thrombosis of various venous systems, such as the hepatic veins (Budd-Chiari syndrome) is a common cause of death. (*Cecil, Ch. 169; Hoffman et al, 2000; Lee et al, 1999*)

21. (**D**) *Discussion:* Paroxysmal nocturnal hemoglobinuria (PNH) is an acquired (not inherited) disorder that affects hematopoietic stem cells and cells of all blood lineages due to mutations in the gene encoding a phosphatidylinositol glycan anchor responsible for the attachment of at least 19 proteins to blood cells. This abnormal anchoring mechanism results in an unusual susceptibility to lysis of red cells, white cells, and platelets. The Ham test (acid hemolysis) or the sugar water test (sucrose hemolysis) traditionally was used to rule out paroxysmal nocturnal hemoglobinuria; however, flow cytometry analysis of glucosylphosphatidylinositol (GPI)-anchored cell surface proteins (e.g., CD55, CD59) is rapidly replacing these tests as much more sensitive and specific for a diagnosis of PNH. Therapy with prednisone may decrease the rate of hemolysis in some, but certainly not all, patients. Because this is an acquired genetic disorder, corticosteroids will not fix the disorder and the aberrant stem cells can eventually evolve into other hematopoietic disorders, including aplastic anemia, myelodysplasia, myelofibrosis, and acute leukemia. For this reason, young patients who are diagnosed with PNH should be considered for allogeneic bone marrow transplantation to replace the defective stem cells. (*Cecil, Ch. 169; Hoffman et al, 2000; Lee et al, 1999*)

22. (**E**) *Discussion:* Recognize drug-induced immune hemolytic anemia of the hapten type, classically developing in patients exposed to high doses of penicillin. The other types of drug-induced immune hemolytic anemia are the α-methyldopa type (the most common) and the quinidine type (occurring with quinidine, quinine, stibophen, chlorpromazine, and sulfonamides). In this patient the strongly positive direct Coombs test shows that this is an immune hemolytic anemia. Three findings suggest the diagnosis of a drug-induced mechanism rather than an autoimmune mechanism: (1) the patient received a cephalosporin, known to induce a hapten-type reaction, (2) routine tests for red cell antibodies in the patient's serum were negative even though the patient's red cells were strongly coated for antibody, and (3) eluate from the patient's red cells was not reactive with normal red cells. In most cases of drug-induced immune hemolytic anemia, the red cell antibodies are detectable only if the offending drug is added to the in vitro system. (*Cecil, Ch. 169; Hoffman et al, 2000; Lee et al, 1999*)

23. (**D**) *Discussion:* Venoms cause intravascular hemolysis but not by a mechanism of microangiopathic fibrin deposition. Other causes of intravascular hemolysis but not by a mechanism of microangiopathic hemolytic anemia include valve hemolysis, exertional hemolysis, chemical agents, osmotic lysis, thermal injury, infections, paroxysmal nocturnal hemoglobinuria, and cold agglutinin disease. (*Cecil, Ch. 177; Hoffman et al, 2000; Lee et al, 1999*)

24. (**A**) *Discussion:* In the general classification schema, thalassemias can be classified as disorders of quantitative abnormalities of hemoglobin, wherein the morbidity of the disease is usually a result of the excess globin chains of the unaffected gene (e.g., α-thalassemia results in decreased α chains and excess β chains with the precipitated excess β chains causing the problems). Hemoglobinopathies (e.g. SS, SC hemoglobin) are qualitative abnormalities of the hemoglobin chains usually as a result of point gene mutations. Thalassemias are generally inherited, but acquired cases have been reported. (*Cecil, Chs. 168 and 171; Hoffman et al, 2000; Lee et al, 1999*)

25. (**D**) *Discussion:* Recognize a clinical history suspicious for two-gene α-thalassemia. Deletion of two α genes ($-\alpha/-\alpha$ or $--/\alpha\alpha$) results in mild to moderate microcytosis and mild anemia, rarely with any progression or development of other signs or symptoms. It is probably the most common hemoglobinopathy in the world and the combination of one-gene or two-gene α-thalassemia has an incidence of 20% or more of African-American populations. It is often mistaken for iron deficiency anemia, and menstruating women with 2-gene alpha thalassemia are often treated for prolonged periods with iron supplementation because it is presumed that the mild microcytic anemia is due to iron deficiency. A hemoglobin electrophoresis is a useful test for β-thalassemia wherein one looks for increased levels of Hb A_2 and Hb F. However, hemoglobin electrophoresis is generally not helpful for the diagnosis of an α-thalassemia disorder. A globin chain synthesis study is generally required for a conclusive diagnosis. Because these studies are not routinely available, α-thalassemias are often diagnosed presumptively by ruling out other possibilities. (*Cecil, Ch. 168; Hoffman et al, 2000; Lee et al, 1999*)

26. (**D**) *Discussion:* Recognize an individual with methemoglobinemia who has been exposed to an offending agent. Rapid development of extreme dyspnea and cyanosis, in the setting of no hypoxia, should be the clue to consider methemoglobinemia. In this case the patient was exposed to two different known medications (Pyridium and sulfamethoxazole) associated with increased levels of methemoglobin in susceptible individuals. Methemoglobin is the derivative of hemoglobin in which the iron of the heme group is oxidized from the ferrous to the ferric state. It is the oxidation status that determines the oxygen-carrying capacity of hemoglobin. When iron is in the ferrous form (deoxyhemoglobin), oxygen can easily bind, in contrast to the inability to bind, to the ferric hemes of methemoglobin. Steady-state methemoglobin levels in the blood are usually less than 1% but can increase markedly when susceptible individuals (heterozygotes for methemoglobin reductase deficiency) are exposed to certain medications or chemicals. Correct therapy is prompt institution of methylene blue, which individuals will respond rapidly to, with resolution of cyanosis. (*Cecil, Ch. 172; Hoffman et al, 2000; Lee et al, 1999*)

27. (**C**) *Discussion:* A red cell mass study is the next most appropriate test to order to determine whether the elevated hematocrit is a true polycythemia (erythrocytosis) or a spurious elevation (due to reduced plasma volume). Because of the significant smoking history, this patient may have evidence of chronic obstructive pulmonary disease with resultant abnormal arterial blood gases and pulmonary function tests, but these tests will not distinguish a true polycythemia from a spurious one. An erythropoietin level may be

indicated later in the work-up once a true polycythemia has been documented. (*Cecil, Ch. 176; Hoffman et al, 2000; Lee et al, 1999*)

28. **(E)** *Discussion:* Once a true red cell mass elevation has been documented, a search for a cause must ensue. The patient's history of nearly life-long ruddy complexion could be due to tobacco abuse but may also suggest a congenital polycythemia. Most congenital polycythemias are due to hemoglobin mutants with high oxygen affinity. These abnormal hemoglobin affinities as well as abnormal levels of 2,3-diphosphoglycerate (2,3-DPG) can be detected by measuring a P_{50} level on the oxygen saturation/desaturation curve. Tumors and other disorders can lead to elevated levels of endogenous erythropoietin. Arterial oxygen saturation and carbon monoxide determinations can rule out pulmonary and environmental conditions. A bone marrow examination is rarely useful in the work-up of erythrocytosis, even for a potential diagnosis of polycythemia rubra vera, in which culture of erythroid progenitor cells for the detection of erythropoietin-independent colony growth is at present the closest thing to a diagnostic test for this disease. (*Cecil, Chs. 172 and 176; Hoffman et al, 2000; Lee et al, 1999*)

29. **(E)** *Discussion:* Hb S is the cause of only one known mutation with a subsequent cascade: an A to T nucleotide substitution in the sixth codon of the β-globin gene; a resultant β-globin gene Val to Glu substitution on the surface of the Hb S tetramer; the abnormal solubility and polymerization of Hb S when deoxygenated; the impaired deformability and sickling of polymer-containing erythrocytes; and the occlusion of the microvasculature by poorly deformable red cells. There are compound heterozygosities with other mutant β-globin genes including sickle cell-$β^0$ thalassemia (HbS-$β^0$ thal), sickle cell-Hb C disease (Hb SC disease), and sickle cell-$β^+$ thalassemia (HbS-**B**$^+$ thal). These compound heterozygosities can affect disease severity. However, little is known regarding the reasons for the wide clinical heterogeneity observed in Hb SS disease with all cases caused by the single point mutation and subsequent cascade as just described. (*Cecil, Ch. 171; Hoffman et al, 2000; Lee et al, 1999*)

30. **(B)** *Discussion:* The "acute chest syndrome" of sickle cell disease is characterized by dyspnea, chest pain, fever, tachypnea, leukocytosis, and pulmonary infiltrates. Approximately one third of all sickle cell disease patients will experience at least one episode of acute chest syndrome. Causative factors include pulmonary vaso-occlusion, infection (especially *S. pneumoniae, H. influenzae, Mycoplasma pneumoniae, Chlamydia pneumoniae,* and *Legionella*), and pulmonary fat embolus from infarcted marrow (a result of vaso-occlusion in the marrow and parvovirus infection). The length and/or severity of a pain crisis is not a direct causative factor for acute chest syndrome unless it precipitates pulmonary vaso-occlusion or results in an infection. (*Cecil, Ch. 171; Hoffman et al, 2000; Lee et al, 1999*)

31. **(B)** *Discussion:* Despite its label as a benign carrier condition, rare complications of sickle cell trait are known to occur including hematuria. There is also a 30-fold greater frequency of unexplained death in military recruits during basic training as a result of exercise-induced vaso-occlusion and rhabdomyolysis. Nevertheless, the few rare complications do not justify a reclassification from a benign carrier condition. There is no increased incidence of anesthetic complications. Sickle cell trait has no hematologic manifestations. Sickle cell forms are not seen on the peripheral smear. (*Cecil, Ch. 171; Hoffman et al, 2000; Lee et al, 1999*)

32. **(D)** *Discussion:* Hb C does not participate directly in polymerization but does sustain potassium-chloride leading to cellular desiccation, thereby raising intraerythrocytic Hb S concentrations. Hb SC red cells live longer than Hb SS red cells and make more target cell shapes. Hb SC patients live longer (on average 20 years

longer) and because splenic function persists longer into adult life they are at higher risk for splenic sequestration crises. Although the overall disease course is milder, isolated painful crises can be just as severe as in patients with Hb SS disease. (*Cecil, Ch. 171; Hoffman et al, 2000; Lee et al, 1999*)

33. **(E)** *Discussion:* Sickle cell anemia coexistent with α-thalassemia produces a variety of conflicting clinical correlates that are hard to explain from a pathophysiologic basis. These patients have less rapid hemolysis, milder anemia, fewer reticulocytes, less sickle cells, and a decreased incidence of leg ulcers. Paradoxically, there is an increased incidence of osteonecrosis, frequency of acute painful episodes, incidence of cerebrovascular accidents, and higher mortality rate after 20 years of age. (*Cecil, Chs. 168 and 171; Hoffman et al, 2000; Lee et al, 1999*)

34. **(D)** *Discussion:* The search for an agent capable of increasing Hb F (fetal hemoglobin) production, thereby reducing the sickling rate of red cells in Hb SS patients, led to the discovery of the significant efficacy of hydroxyurea in reducing the frequency of acute painful episodes, decreasing the episodes of acute chest syndrome, and diminishing transfusion requirements in some sickle cell patients. Although developed as an agent to increase Hb F production, the exact mechanism of action through which hydroxyurea exerts these tremendous beneficial effects in sickle cell patients is still unknown. Toradol, tramadol, butyric acid, and bone marrow transplantation all may have application in some sickle cell patients, but none has exerted a significant impact on the management of sickle cell disease to anywhere near the degree that hydroxyurea has in the past several years. (*Cecil, Ch. 171; Hoffman et al, 2000; Lee et al, 1999*)

35. **(E)** *Discussion:* This patient almost certainly has a megaloblastic anemia due to either vitamin B_{12} deficiency or folate deficiency. Although not distinguishable by the given data, vitamin B_{12} deficiency is more likely. In either event, the anemia has likely developed slowly and at present the patient shows no significant signs of cardiovascular distress. Immediate transfusion is therefore not necessary. In patients who are suffering from cardiovascular symptoms of anemia, it is better to transfuse until symptoms abate rather than to pick an arbitrary hemoglobin level to shoot for. Administration of erythropoietin is not indicated because the endogenous erythropoietin levels are likely already quite elevated. Instead the ingredient lacking for appropriate red cell production is either vitamin B_{12} or folate. Once replaced, reticulocytosis should ensue within a matter of days. (*Cecil, Ch. 175; Hoffman et al, 2000; Lee et al, 1999*)

36. **(D)** *Discussion:* Fever is the most frequent sign of an adverse reaction to blood transfusion. Because it is also one of the earliest signs of a problem during transfusion, prompt recognition of fever and discontinuation of transfusion if there are more ominous signs can prevent further morbidity. It is because of this that routine use of acetaminophen and diphenhydramine (Benadryl) as premedications for a transfusion are discouraged. All of the other answers are adverse reactions that occur with an acute hemolytic transfusion reaction, whereas only some of these problems occur in febrile, nonhemolytic reactions. (*Cecil, Ch. 165; Hoffman et al, 2000; Lee et al, 1999*)

37. **(C)** *Discussion:* Transfusion-related graft versus host disease occurs in immunocompromised individuals receiving blood product transfusions and occasionally in normal individuals who receive transfusions from blood relatives. The pathogenesis involves the transfusion of T lymphocytes that are able to survive the transfusion and engraft in the recipient. Four to 30 days after the infusion, pancytopenia, infections, and hemorrhage ensues. By the time it is recognized it is generally too late to save the individual from the relentless process. This problem can be completely

eliminated if the unit of blood is irradiated with 2500-3000 cGy γ-irradiation before transfusion. A common misconception is that irradiation is superior to filtration for removing lymphocytes to prevent alloimmunization. Although irradiation can kill the lymphocytes, it does not remove the antigens that give rise to alloimmunization. Therefore, immunocompromised patients and patients receiving family-directed donations should receive blood products that have been filtered and irradiated. (*Cecil, Ch. 165; Hoffman et al, 2000; Lee et al, 1999*)

38. **(E)** *Discussion:* Eosinophilia can occur in association with a wide variety of conditions, notably parasitic and specific fungal infections. It can be associated with many other conditions, including various rheumatologic diseases such as Churg-Strauss vasculitis. GM-CSF affects many cell lineages, including neutrophils, monocytes, and eosinophils. Transient eosinophilia can be a consequence of GM-CSF administration but will quickly abate after discontinuation of the drug. To the contrary, Neupogen (G-CSF) affects only the neutrophil series and eosinophilia is not seen after its administration. (*Cecil, Ch. 184; Hoffman et al, 2000; Lee et al, 1999*)

39. **(D)** *Discussion:* The red cell Howell-Jolly bodies should be the tipoff that the patient has had a prior splenectomy. Further questioning would reveal that the patient failed to mention a splenectomy at the age of 14 after splenic injury in a motor vehicle accident. You missed the surgical scar on physical examination. Postsplenectomy patients can sometimes have life-long mild elevations of either their WBC count or their platelet count. The gynecologist was correct to obtain several platelet counts over time to make sure the platelet elevation was persistently increased. Reasons for reactive thrombocytosis include iron deficiency, splenectomy, postsurgical state, infection or inflammation, and occult malignancy. There is at present no diagnostic test for essential thrombocytosis. It remains a diagnosis of exclusion and can be entertained only after all forms of reactive thrombocytosis have been ruled out. (*Cecil, Ch. 183; Hoffman et al, 2000*)

40. **(C)** *Discussion:* Anagrelide is an oral imidazoquinazolin derivative that has been approved by the FDA as a platelet-lowering agent in essential thrombocythemia. It appears to lower the platelet count by interfering with the maturation of megakaryocytes. There are some side effects, but they are relatively mild in most cases. It should not be administered in cases of reactive thrombocytosis because the risk of complications from thrombocytosis is much less than in patients with thrombocytosis owing to an inherent marrow disorder. Because patients with essential thrombocytosis are at risk for hemorrhage as well as thrombosis, aspirin is not indicated in all cases. Hydroxyurea has a potential leukemogenic risk because it is a chemotherapeutic agent, although this risk has not been substantiated. Anagrelide lacks this potential risk because it is not a chemotherapeutic agent. Interferon has many more associated side effects with less efficacy. Thus, anagrelide appears to offer the best therapeutic window with the fewest risks and is the treatment of choice for essential thrombocythemia as long as it is tolerated by the patient. (*Cecil, Ch. 183; Hoffman et al, 2000*)

41. **(E)** *Discussion:* Recognize that this patient has all of the manifestations of polycythemia rubra vera except that his bleeding gastric ulcer has masked the development of polycythemia. Because of his bleeding gastric ulcer he has already made himself iron deficient, which is the goal of the cornerstone phlebotomy therapy for polycythemia vera. Instituting iron supplementation at this point may very well give the patient more morbidity because it could cause a rebound erythrocytosis. Rather, the *H. pylori* infection should be treated to cure the gastric ulcer and a further work-up for a probable diagnosis of polycythemia vera should ensue, including culture of the patient's erythroid progenitor cells looking

for erythropoietin-independent colony growth, a hallmark for the diagnosis of polycythemia vera. (*Cecil, Ch. 176; Hoffman et al, 2000*)

42. **(B)** *Discussion:* Teardrop-shaped red blood cells are rarely seen in any other disorders other than those that cause marrow fibrosis. Schistocytes and other red cell fragments can be seen in several other types of disorders, but true teardrop-shaped cells without other types of fragments are a good tip-off to a marrow fibrosis (myelophthistic) problem. A number of hematologic as well as nonhematologic disorders can cause marrow fibrosis. The rest of the potential answers are all other signs and symptoms of agnogenic myeloid metaplasia (myelofibrosis) but are nonspecific. (*Cecil, Ch. 183; Hoffman et al, 2000*)

43. **(A)** *Discussion:* Erythromelalgia is painful erythematous swelling of the fingers and toes often relieved by aspirin. Aquagenic pruritus is itching of the skin after bathing. Both symptoms frequently accompany patients who have myeloproliferative disorders or occasionally those with other forms of erythrocytosis. Lupus does not have these manifestations. The normal aPTT makes antiphospholipid antibody syndrome less likely, and this syndrome would not cause the erythromelalgia or aquagenic pruritus. Patients with hereditary resistance to activated protein C have predisposition to venous, but not arterial, thrombosis. Antithrombin III deficiency does not fit the constellation of signs and symptoms. (*Cecil, Ch. 183; Hoffman et al, 2000*)

44. **(E)** *Discussion:* Recognize treatment-related myelodysplasia. This distinct entity, whose incidence is rising rapidly as chemotherapy is being dose-escalated for many cancer therapies, is particularly difficult to treat when it occurs. The clues in this patient include the lag time until the development of pancytopenia, the lack of any signs for breast cancer relapse, and the macro-ovalocytes and hypogranulated neutrophils on the peripheral smear, which are both strong indicators for myelodysplasia. Aplastic anemia would be a possibility, but there is no good reason to suspect the patient to develop aplastic anemia at this stage. Treatment-related myelodysplasia is a real possibility given the significant exposure she has had to chemotherapy. Late graft failure would be distinctly unusual especially since this was an autologous transplant. Autologous graft failures are rarely reported to occur but only in the early post-transplant setting. (*Cecil, Ch. 182; Hoffman et al, 2000*)

45. **(B)** *Discussion:* The International Scoring System for evaluating prognosis in myelodysplastic syndromes was developed during the 1990s and gives the most reliable estimates to date regarding survival and likelihood of progression to AML. It is based on a scoring system that assigns values according to the percentage of bone marrow blasts, the complexity of karyotype abnormalities, and the number of cytopenias present in the peripheral circulation. Age and sex were not found to be predictive prognosticators. (*Cecil, Ch. 182; Hoffman et al, 2000*)

46. **(E)** *Discussion:* Numerous agents have been tested for efficacy in myelodysplasia, including pyridoxine, vitamins, androgens, corticosteroids, differentiating agents, hematopoietic growth factors, and various doses of chemotherapy. Although some responses have been noted with all of the above, none is considered standard of care. A trial of pyridoxine is warranted in refractory anemia with ringed sideroblasts but should be discontinued if no response is noted. Likewise, trials of androgens or corticosteroids, if attempted, should have set criteria for discontinuation. Bone marrow transplantation remains the only known cure for myelodysplasia and should be considered in young patients with suitable donors. However, the relapse rate is significantly high. Supportive care with transfusions and antibiotics when necessary remains the standard of care at present. (*Cecil, Ch. 182; Hoffman et al, 2000*)

47. (E) *Discussion:* This patient has a classic presentation for CML including all immature forms of WBCs on the peripheral smear, presence of basophils, splenomegaly, and so on. The lack of the Philadelphia chromosome on karyotype analysis does not completely rule out a diagnosis of CML. Polymerase chain reaction analysis should be performed to investigate the possibility of *bcr* +, Philadelphia − CML. Accurate diagnosis is essential because *bcr*− CML has a far worse prognosis than *bcr* + CML. No therapy should be initiated until the diagnostic work-up is complete unless the patient's condition is rapidly deteriorating. (*Cecil, Ch. 192; Hoffman et al, 2000*)

48. (D) *Discussion:* This scenario is typical for a presentation of hairy cell leukemia, a B-lymphocyte disorder with a 4:1 male predominance. Clinical lymphadenopathy is distinctly uncommon and if present is likely caused by the opportunistic infections these patients are prone to rather than by the leukemia itself. CML rarely presents as pancytopenia. CLL would have more predilection to produce lymphadenopathy than splenomegaly. Low-grade lymphomas do not generally produce pancytopenias and would likely have clinical lymphadenopathy. T-cell acute lymphocytic leukemia does not present as splenomegaly and pancytopenia. (*Cecil, Ch. 192; Hoffman et al, 2000*)

49. (D) *Discussion:* Typical CLL cells express the pan–B-cell antigens CD19 and CD20 and in addition, aberrantly express CD-5, a pan–T-cell antigen. There are several other antigens that can be expressed, including CD23, CD24, and CD21. However, the co-expression of CD19, CD20, and CD5 is seen in 95% of cases of CLL. Unless there are other unusual features, demonstration of this cell surface marker pattern is generally diagnostic for CLL and marrow examinations, node biopsies, and other procedures can be avoided initially. (*Cecil, Ch. 192; Hoffman et al, 2000*)

50. (E) *Discussion:* All of the listed factors have been associated with the development of acute leukemias in humans. Atomic bomb survivors and patients exposed to high doses of ionizing radiation are at increased risk for AML, ALL, and CML. Low-frequency non-ionizing electromagnetic fields such as those emitted by high-voltage electrical lines were reported to have an increased incidence and raised much public concern. However, the investigator who published that report has been found to have falsified the data. HTLV-I and HTLV-II are oncogenic viruses found in parts of Japan but also reported in the United States. A link between tobacco and leukemia has been reported. Prior exposure to certain chemotherapeutic agents, especially alkylating agents such as melphalan and nitrosoureas, are associated with an increased risk of AML. (*Cecil, Ch. 193; Hoffman et al, 2000*)

51. (B) *Discussion:* With conventional chemotherapy, M3 AML or APL had an increased cure rate somewhat above that of the other forms of AML. However, in the past decade all-*trans* retinoic acid (a vitamin A derivative) has proven its ability to induce complete remissions in APL patients. This response to all-*trans* retinoic acid is specific for APL and is related to the known cytogenetic translocation (t15;17) that is present in the majority of APL and involves one of the nuclear retinoic acid receptors. By using a combination of all-*trans* retinoic acid and chemotherapy, the cure rate of APL has increased significantly and now appears to be more than 80%. The optimal sequencing and length of therapy with all-*trans* retinoic acid and chemotherapy is still being defined. (*Cecil, Ch. 193; Hoffman et al, 2000*)

52. (D) *Discussion:* Contrary to popular belief, many (50%) of patients with acute leukemia actually present with a total WBC count that is in the normal range. The differential will be abnormal, which points out the importance of doing and checking the entire complete blood cell count in anyone suspected of having hematologic problems. About 25% of patients with acute leukemia will present with a low total WBC count, and only 25% will present with the more commonly described elevated WBC count. Acute leukemia should definitely be part of the differential diagnosis in a patient presenting with pancytopenia. (*Cecil, Ch. 193; Hoffman et al, 2000*)

53. (A) *Discussion:* The so-called sanctuary sites of ALL are areas in which leukemic lymphoblasts can apparently evade the effects of chemotherapy and have a high predilection for relapse. The pericardium is not one of these known sites. The predilection for a CNS relapse is so high that most ALL regimens include specific measures for CNS prophylaxis, including intrathecal chemotherapy and craniospinal radiation. Any ALL patient in remission who presents with testicular swelling or joint effusions should be suspected of having an isolated relapse until proven otherwise. (*Cecil, Ch. 193; Hoffman et al, 2000*)

54. (C) *Discussion:* Adult patients with ALL and whose karyotype is positive for the Philadelphia chromosome (usually the p190 variant) are at extremely high risk for relapse of ALL, even during chemotherapy. Every attempt should be made to treat these patients with bone marrow transplantation as soon as possible. Other significant poor prognostic factors do include advanced age and high white cell count at diagnosis, but neither is as ominous as the presence of the Philadelphia chromosome. (*Cecil, Ch. 193; Hoffman et al, 2000*)

55. (B) *Discussion:* Epstein-Barr virus is implicated in the pathogenesis of African Burkitt's lymphoma as well as NHL in immunocompromised patients. *H. pylori* infection has been linked to the development of MALT and gastric lymphomas. HIV and the Kaposi's sarcoma–associated herpesvirus are known to be involved in HIV-related lymphomas. Cytomegalovirus, while often complicating the course of organ transplant patients, is not associated with the development of NHL. (*Cecil, Ch. 195; Hoffman et al, 2000*)

56. (C) *Discussion:* Over 75 to 80% of indolent B-cell lymphomas are follicular lymphomas. They are typically quite indolent and most often occur primarily in older adults. Marginal zone (MALT) lymphomas can often arise in lymphoepithelial tissue and be associate with either *H. pylori* infections or autoimmune diseases. Small lymphocytic lymphomas are the equivalent of chronic lymphocytic leukemia and are also quite indolent. Mantle cell lymphomas can be distinguished on cell surface pattern analysis from the other low grade lymphomas by bright surface immunoglobulin expression and lack of CD23 expression. In addition, mantle cell lymphoma is usually CD10− and CD43+, in contrast to follicular lymphoma. Mantle cell lymphomas are typically more aggressive than other indolent lymphomas, prompting some people to reclassify them as intermediate-grade lymphomas. In addition, mantle cell lymphoma in general is also one of the worst NHLs in terms of responsiveness to therapy, although a small percentage of mantle cell patients appear responsive to some therapies. Complete remissions are rare. Bone marrow transplantation is being attempted for mantle cell lymphoma, but results are still under evaluation. (*Cecil, Ch. 195; Hoffman et al, 2000*)

57. (B) *Discussion:* The patterns of disease spread in Hodgkin's and non-Hodgkin's lymphomas are distinctly different. Hodgkin's lymphomas tend to spread more locally first, with wider dissemination usually occurring as a later manifestation. Non-Hodgkin's lymphomas, on the other hand, are rarely found to be locally isolated because they spread more diffusely by means of the blood and lymphatic systems. Because of this characteristic of NHL the Ann Arbor staging system is less accurate in NHL than in Hodgkin's lymphoma. As a result, the International Prognostic Index was developed for aggressive NHL but also has predictive outcome for more indolent NHLs as well. The scoring system is set up on: age = 60 vs. > 60; serum LDH normal vs. 1× > normal;

performance status 0 or 1 vs. 2-4; stage I or II vs. III or IV; and extranodal involvement = 1 site vs. > 1 site. Sex is not a prognostic determining factor. *(Cecil, Chs. 194 and 195; Hoffman et al, 2000)*

58. **(B)** *Discussion:* Rituximab is directed against the CD20 antigen present on the surface of normal B cells and most indolent B-cell non-Hodgkin's lymphomas. In clinical trials it demonstrated significant effectiveness in inducing responses in patients who had become refractory or resistant to conventional chemotherapy. The exact mechanism by which it exerts this effect is unknown, just as the exact function of the CD20 antigen in B cells is also unknown. Rituximab should only be used in lymphomas that are proven to be CD20+. It should also not be used in patients with significant levels of circulating lymphoma cells or in CLL patients because of unproven effectiveness and increased toxicity in this patient population. Other monoclonal antibodies directed against the CD20 antigen are nearing FDA approval. After years of investigation and development, it appears that monoclonal antibodies have finally carved a niche in oncology therapy. *(Cecil, Chs. 194 and 195; Hoffman et al, 2000)*

59. **(E)** *Discussion:* Involvement of the central nervous system is distinctly unusual for Hodgkin's disease. Hodgkin's patients can be at risk for complications of suppressed cell-mediated immunity for a significant length of time even after complete remission has been attained, often developing shingles after all therapy has ended months or years earlier. Patients treated with MOPP chemotherapy are prone to develop myelodysplasias, leukemias, and non-Hodgkin's lymphoma from exposure to the nitrogen mustard. MOPP also causes a high rate of infertility, although other treatments or even the Hodgkin's disease itself can play a role in infertility. Young males who desire sperm banking should be checked for motility and then deposit specimens in a sperm bank before therapy. High-dose radiation therapy is associated with an increased risk for second tumors, primarily solid tumors in the field of the radiation, including thyroid, breast, lung, and mediastinal tumors. *(Cecil, Chs. 194 and 195; Hoffman et al, 2000)*

60. **(B)** *Discussion:* Autologous marrow transplantation has been demonstrated to have a definite survival benefit over conventional chemotherapy in multiple myeloma. It is unclear yet if it results in any significant proportion of patients achieving a cure of disease. VAD chemotherapy is an effective alternative to melphalan and prednisone chemotherapy for multiple myeloma but does not clearly produce longer remissions. If one is contemplating a potential autologous marrow transplant, then VAD should be used and melphalan therapy avoided because the latter damages hematopoietic stem cells. Erythropoietin can alleviate some anemia symptoms but has not had a major impact on the disease. Pamidronate on the other hand has shown an unexpected benefit of fewer skeletal complications and significantly improved quality of life in myeloma patients with skeletal involvement. *(Cecil, Ch. 196; Hoffman et al, 2000)*

61. **(D)** *Discussion:* Because of the larger cell yield, which can be obtained from peripheral blood stem cell harvesting, engraftment times are usually much shorter than with typical marrow harvests. This reduces costs significantly because of shorter hospital stays, lack of need of general anesthesia, and so on. There are some reports that show less tumor contamination in peripheral blood stem cell harvests as compared with marrow harvests. Whether this will lead to a decreased relapse rate is as yet unknown. There are increased numbers (not decreased) of T lymphocytes in a peripheral blood stem cell harvest as compared with a marrow harvest. While this may be desirable for a significant graft vs. tumor effect, until we can effectively control graft vs. host disease it makes increased numbers of T lymphocytes a more dangerous situation. *(Cecil, Ch. 196; Hoffman et al, 2000)*

62. **(C)** *Discussion:* Platelet aggregation studies would only be employed after a prolonged bleeding time had been demonstrated and the patient had discontinued any drugs that might interfere with platelet function. The bleeding time is prolonged in (1) thrombocytopenia, (2) qualitative platelet abnormalities, (3) defects in platelet-vessel wall interactions (e.g. von Willebrand's disease), and (4) primary vascular disorders. The bleeding time is usually not prolonged in patients with coagulation factor deficiencies. However, the test is highly operator-dependent and should be performed only by well-trained personnel. The PT and aPTT detect only severe deficiencies of coagulation factors, generally those with levels 30% or less than normal. If an elevated PT or aPTT test is detected, the next step is generally to do a mixing study with normal plasma to evaluate for the presence of an inhibitor. *(Cecil, Chs. 162 and 177; Hoffman et al, 2000)*

63. **(C)** *Discussion:* Heparin therapy significantly decreases plasma antithrombin activity while warfarin therapy lowers the functional levels of protein C and protein S. However, the timing of all of these tests is critical to avoid erroneous diagnoses. An acute thrombosis, in and of itself, can cause transient decreases in the levels of all three—antithrombin III, protein C, and protein S. Because activated protein C resistance is caused by mutations in the factor V gene this test can be performed at any point because a genetic mutation is being searched for and not a functional level. Factor V mutations, therefore, are not affected by the presence of an acute thrombosis or anticoagulants. *(Cecil, Ch. 180; Hoffman et al, 2000)*

64. **(E)** *Discussion:* The American Society of Hematology has developed practice guidelines for the proper management of ITP. Prednisone as the initial therapy results in increases in platelet counts in 80 to 90% of patients. Unfortunately, after the prednisone is tapered off most patients (90%) suffer a relapse of thrombocytopenia. IVIG and anti-Rh antibody therapy are the most active agents to rapidly induce a rise in the platelet count. However, the response is quite transient in both, and these agents cannot be considered definitive therapy unless all other maneuvers have failed. Rather, one of these agents should be used to transiently increase the platelet count such that the patient can safely go to surgery for splenectomy. Splenectomy improves the platelet count in 70% of patients, with 60% having a sustained remission. Therefore, splenectomy should be considered the therapy of choice after a relapse from prednisone. Re-treatment with prednisone is not effective for inducing lasting remissions. *(Cecil, Ch. 177; George et al, 1996; Hoffman et al, 2000)*

65. **(D)** *Discussion:* Recognize the progressive development of thrombotic thrombocytopenic purpura (TTP). TTP is characterized by a pentad of features—micoangiopathic hemolytic anemia, thrombocytopenia, fever, renal involvement, and neurologic impairment. The neurologic features can fall under a very wide spectrum. Not all patients exhibit the pentad at initial presentation. In fact, patients do not have to have all five features at all to have a diagnosis of TTP established. Quite often patients are admitted with a possible unrelated diagnosis and when they do not improve or develop more multisystem failure, the features of TTP are often overlooked and the diagnosis is not entertained in the differential diagnosis. Disseminated intravascular coagulation must be ruled out. If it is and if there are schistocytes on the peripheral smear, then a diagnosis of TTP seems likely. Prompt institution of plasmapheresis is the treatment of choice and has significantly improved the mortality rate from this obscure disease. *(Cecil, Ch. 177; Hoffman et al, 2000)*

66. **(E)** *Discussion:* Patients with either factor VIII or IX hemophilia who are described as having moderate clinical courses typically have endogenous factor levels in the 1 to 5% range. Severe hemophiliacs typically have less than 1% activity. Spontaneous

hemorrhages are uncommon, with mild deficiencies having more than 5% normal activity, but mild hemophiliacs can bleed excessively with trauma or surgery. (*Cecil, Ch. 178; Hoffman et al, 2000*)

67. (**D**) *Discussion:* The genes for factor VIII and IX are located on the X chromosome and therefore these are sex-linked recessive diseases. Affected males will transmit the disorder to half of their sons, and their daughters will be carriers but will not ever be affected by hemophilia themselves. Because hemophilias are specific genetic mutations, affected family members within the same family will inherit the same mutation and thus have exactly the same reduced level of factor activity. (*Cecil, Ch. 178; Hoffman et al, 2000*)

68. (**C**) *Discussion:* This patient almost certainly has type 1 von Willebrand's disease. Type 1 accounts for up to 75 to 80% of all cases of von Willebrand's disease, which has emerged as the most common bleeding disorder with a prevalence of 1 to 3%. Some patients with mild von Willebrand's disease can go nearly a lifetime without being diagnosed. They can suffer from easy bruising and bleeding but until they are challenged with a significant event such as major surgery the diagnosis may not be made. Desmopressin (DDAVP) is the initial treatment of choice except for patients with type 2B von Willebrand's disease. These patients can have thrombocytopenia, which can be made much worse by administration of desmopressin. Factor VIII concentrates and cryoprecipitate therapy can also be used but is not as safe as desmopressin owing to potential infectious concerns. Activated factor IX complex concentrates are generally reserved for hemophiliac patients with inhibitors. (*Cecil, Ch. 178; Hoffman et al, 2000*)

69. (**A**) *Discussion:* Easy bruising and repeated spontaneous abortions are hallmarks for factor XIII deficiency. The diagnosis must be suspected on clinical grounds because screening coagulation assays are most often normal. The euglobulin clot lysis assay can be used for detection in suspected cases. (*Cecil, Chs. 178-180; Hoffman et al, 2000*)

70. (**D**) *Discussion:* Totaled together, deficiencies of protein C and S and antithrombin III combine for about a 10% incidence in patients with venous thromboembolism. Prothrombin gene mutation, a newly identified cause for hypercoagulable state, is found in 6 to 18% of patients with venous thromboembolism. Inherited activated protein C resistance, due to factor V mutations, are found in a wide range (10-64%) of patients with venous thromboembolism. All of these as well as hyperhomocysteinemia should be checked in patients with suspected hypercoagulable states. (*Cecil, Ch. 180; Hoffman et al, 2000*)

71. (**C**) *Discussion:* Heparin-associated thrombocytopenia occurs in 1 to 3% of patients treated with heparin. It can occur at any dose, including low-dose subcutaneous prophylaxis doses. It generally manifests after several days of therapy. If a platelet count is not checked 4 to 5 days after heparin initiation, the thrombocytopenia can become quite severe. Low-molecular-weight heparins have about one tenth the frequency of inducing thrombocytopenia but cannot be used as a replacement after the development of heparin-associated thrombocytopenia because of some inherent cross-reactivity. Alternatives to heparin for acute anticoagulation of patients who absolutely need anticoagulation due to active thrombosis include new thrombin inhibitors or heparinoids. (*Cecil, Ch. 177; Hoffman et al, 2000*)

72. (**A**) *Discussion:* Atomic bomb survivors had a clear-cut increased risk of subsequent CML, with a peak occurring 5 to 12 years after exposure and seeming to be dose related. No familial association of CML has been noted. Benzene exposure increases the risk of AML but not CML. CML is not a frequent secondary leukemia after the treatment of other cancers with radiation and/or alkylating agents. (*Cecil, Chs. 192 and 193; Hoffman et al, 2000*)

73. (**A**) *Discussion:* After the publication of the IRIS trial, the results were so compelling that most hematologists now regard that sole therapy with imatinib should be the new standard of care for newly diagnosed CML patients who are not transplant candidates. Having said this, as the data continue to emerge, it is clear that imatinib as a single agent likely will not be curative for most CML patients, even though more than 95% of patients achieve a hematologic remission. Therefore, imatinib combinations are now being tested but none has yet emerged as better than sole imatinib therapy. (*O'Brien et al, 2003*)

74. (**D**) *Discussion:* Idiopathic aplastic anemia is far more common than the other marrow failure syndromes listed as answers. Aplastic anemia is a disease of the young, with a median age at onset of 25 years. There are mild, moderate, and severe forms that are classified primarily on the severity of the peripheral cytopenias. Diepoxybutane (DEB) and mitomycin-C (MMC) testing for chromosomal stability will help rule out Fanconi's anemia. The Ham's test (acid hemolysis) or the sugar water test (sucrose hemolysis) traditionally were used to rule out paroxysmal nocturnal hemoglobinuria; however, flow cytometry analysis of GPI-anchored cell surface proteins (e.g., CD55, CD59) is rapidly replacing these tests as much more sensitive and specific for a diagnosis of paroxysmal nocturnal hemoglobinuria. (*Cecil, Ch. 174; Hoffman et al, 2000*)

75. (**A**) *Discussion:* A normochromic, normocytic anemia is the earliest form of anemia with iron deficiency. Only when the hematocrit falls below 31 to 32% do the red cells start to become microcytic. Other manifestations of iron deficiency can include sore tongue (glossitis), atrophy of the lingual papillae, erosions at the corners of the mouth (angular stomatitis), atrophy of the gastric mucosa with achlorhydria, atrophic rhinitis with a foul nasal discharge (ozena), greenish hue to the complexion (chlorosis), and nail spooning (koilonychia). (*Cecil, Ch. 160; Hoffman et al, 2000*)

76. (**A**) *Discussion:* Somewhat surprisingly, recent studies show that ITP in pregnancy carries a relatively low risk with good chances that for many women the pregnancy will be uneventful. However, approximately 20% of women will experience moderate to severe bleeding and approximately 30% will require treatment to increase platelet counts. On the other hand, the initial diagnosis of ITP in pregnancy is no reason to panic and start immediate therapy or, worse yet, consider pregnancy termination. Close, careful monitoring is warranted. (*Cecil, Chs. 162 and 177; Webert et al, 2003*)

77. (**B**) *Discussion:* The improvement in life expectancy for patients with sickle cell disease compared with earlier eras is primarily due to improvements in the general medical care of these patients, such as prophylactic penicillin therapy in children. (*Cecil, Ch. 171; Hoffman et al, 2000*)

78. (**B**) *Discussion:* Partial exchange transfusions have proven benefit in cerebrovascular accidents and in acute chest syndrome when hypoxia cannot be corrected by other measures. Although sometimes used in difficult cases of priapism, partial exchange transfusion has limited or questionable benefit and local measures usually better relieve the urologic problem. Partial exchange transfusion is not indicated for treatment of osteonecrosis in sickle cell disease. (*Cecil, Ch. 171; Hoffman et al, 2000*)

79. (**C**) *Discussion:* Basophilia on the peripheral smear is a typical finding in the myeloproliferative disorders not the myelodysplastic syndromes. Basophilia is particularly prominent in chronic myelogenous leukemia, but it may also be seen in the other myeloproliferative disorders. Pseudo–Pelger-Huët cells are indicative of myelodysplasia. Other prominent dysplastic features include agranular cytoplasm. (*Cecil, Chs. 182 and 183; Hoffman et al, 2000*)

80. **(D)** *Discussion:* Howell-Jolly bodies are fragments in red blood cells that are normally removed by a functioning spleen. If Howell-Jolly bodies are observed on the peripheral smear, you can be fairly sure that the patient does not have a functioning spleen and either has hyposplenism or more likely had a splenectomy at some point in the past, either due to disease or trauma. *(Cecil, Ch. 161; Hoffman et al, 2000)*

81. **(D)** *Discussion:* Waldenström's macroglobulinemia, just as with multiple myeloma, is typically not associated with splenomegaly. A patient with hairy cell leukemia will have prominent splenomegaly but should not have much lymphadenopathy. If there is prominent lymphadenopathy in a suspected hairy cell leukemia, reconsider some type of lymphoma or search for an infectious cause for the lymphadenopathy in hairy cell leukemia. Patients with CLL/SLL can occasionally present with more prominent splenomegaly than lymphadenopathy, but they will usually also have a concomitant peripheral lymphocytosis. *(Cecil, Chs. 164 and 192)*

82. **(E)** *Discussion:* Hypermutation of the Ig heavy chain sequences is indicative of a postgerminal center mutational event in CLL. Because Vh gene mutational analysis is cumbersome to perform, CD38 expression appears to be a useful surrogate marker for Vh mutational status. Low CD38 expression correlates to a mutated Vh gene status and both are indicative of indolent disease and a favorable prognosis. Deletions of chromosome material from 11q and 17p are associated with a poor prognosis, whereas it is likely that chromosome 13q deletion results in the deletion of a tumor suppressor gene. *(Cecil, Ch. 192)*

83. **(B)** *Discussion:* Five to 10% of CLL patients are at risk of developing a large cell lymphomatous transformation (Richter's syndrome), but this is not equivalent to a transformation to ALL. CLL patients are often hypogammaglobulinemic. Ten to 20% of CLL patients develop secondary solid tumors, presumably owing to their defective immune systems, which also put them at risk for many autoimmune disorders but especially ITP and autoimmune hemolytic anemia. *(Cecil, Ch. 192)*

84. **(C)** *Discussion:* Rituximab is directed against CD20, as are some newly FDA-approved radioimmunoconjugates. Antibodies are in development that target CD22. Herceptin targets the Her 2-neu receptor. Alemtuzumab is directed against CD52, which is present on virtually all CLL cells as well as on normal B and T lymphocytes. Alemtuzumab is extremely active in fludarabine-refractory CLL but also very immunosuppressive owing to its effects on normal B and T lymphocytes. *(Cecil, Ch. 192)*

85. **(C)**; 86. **(E)**; 87. **(A)**; 88. **(B)**; 89. **(D)**; 90. **(F)**. *Discussion:* Recognize different scenarios of leukemias and their relative prognoses. Answer C describes a patient with acute promyelocytic leukemia who stands an excellent chance of remission and cure if treated with all-*trans*-retinoic acid and chemotherapy. Answer E describes an AML patient, likely of FAB M2 category, who has a reasonable chance for long-term survival treated with conventional chemotherapy alone, rather than a stem cell transplant for AML. Answer A describes a patient with a very poor prognosis with Philadelphia chromosome–positive ALL who is highly likely to undergo relapse even while on chemotherapy. This patient's only hope for survival is an early allogeneic stem cell transplant. Answer B describes a Philadelphia chromosome–positive CML patient who is likely to respond very well, at least initially, to oral therapy with imatinib. Answer D describes a patient who likely has therapy-related MDS/AML. These patients are often resistant to therapy even at the outset. Their overall prognosis is very poor. Answer F describes a patient with AML cells growing in the skin (chloroma or granulocytic sarcoma). These cells are virtually always of marrow origin, so if only local therapy is administered to the chloroma, the patient is highly likely to suffer a relapse in the skin or marrow within a short period of time. These patients should almost always receive systemic therapy. *(Cecil, Ch. 193; Hoffman et al, 2000)*

91. **(E)**; 92. **(A)**; 93. **(C)**; 94. **(B)**; 95. **(D)**. *Discussion:* Acute alcohol abuse often leads to transient macrocytic red cell changes and transient thrombocytopenia. More chronic alcohol abuse can lead to more prolonged and more profound marrow suppression affecting other cell lines. Paroxysmal nocturnal hemoglobinuria (PNH) and autoimmune hemolytic anemia both cause macrocytic anemia with evidence of hemolysis, but only in PNH will other cell lines be decreased and there be a blunted reticulocyte response due to the marrow failure state. Myelodysplasia also shows signs of marrow failure with a more profound lack of reticulocytosis and no signs of hemolysis generally. TTP does not generally affect the WBC count but does have significant hemolysis and thrombocytopenia. *(Cecil, Chs. 160, 163, 165, 166, 174, and 175)*

96. **(D)**; 97. **(C)**; 98. **(A)**; 99. **(B)**; 100. **(E)**. *Discussion:* TTP gives thrombocytopenia with microangiopathic hemolytic anemia but coagulation screening assays and D-dimer assays must be negative for a diagnosis of TTP. On the other hand, DIC will also give thrombocytopenia and microangiopathic hemolytic anemia but with abnormalities in coagulation assays and increased D-dimers. Chronic renal failure will inhibit platelet function, but other parameters will be normal. Chronic liver disease will not affect platelet function but will decrease platelet numbers and will affect coagulation assays due to several reasons, including lack of production of vitamin K–dependent factors. Heparin therapy, in the absence of heparin-associated thrombocytopenia, will mostly affect the aPTT but also has some influence on the PT and other coagulation screening assays. *(Cecil, Chs. 164, 166, 183, 184, 185, and 186)*

BIBLIOGRAPHY

George JN, Woolf SH, Raskob GE, et al: Idiopathic thrombocytopenic purpura: A practice guideline developed by explicit methods for the American Society of Hematology. Blood 1996;88:3.

Goldman L, Ausiello D (eds): Cecil Textbook of Medicine, 22nd ed. Philadelphia, WB Saunders, 2004.

Hoffman R, Benz EJ Jr, Shattil SJ, et al: (eds): Hematology Basic Principles and Practice, 3rd ed. New York, Churchill Livingstone, 2000.

Lee GR, Foerster J, Lukens J, et al (eds): Wintrobe's Clinical Hematology, 10th ed. Baltimore, Williams & Wilkins, 1999.

O'Brien SG, Guilhot F, Larson RA, et al: Imatinib compared with interferon and low-dose cytarabine for newly diagnosed chronic-phase chronic myeloid leukemia. N Engl J Med 2003;348:994-1004.

Webert KE, Mittal R, Sigouin C, et al: A retrospective 11-year analysis of obstetric patients with idiopathic thrombocytopenic purpura. Blood 2003; 102:4306-4311.

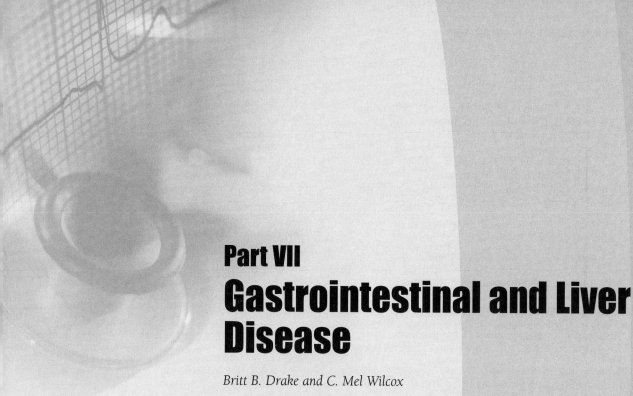

Part VII
Gastrointestinal and Liver Disease

Britt B. Drake and C. Mel Wilcox

MULTIPLE CHOICE

DIRECTIONS: For questions 1–52, choose the best answer to each question.

1. The best radiologic modality to diagnose gallbladder stones is:

   A. Computed tomography (CT)
   B. Ultrasonography
   C. HIDA scan (technetium 99–labeled iminodiacetic acid)
   D. Percutaneous transhepatic cholangiography (PTC)
   E. Kidney-ureter-bladder (KUB) radiograph

2. All of the following are indications for the use of endoscopic retrograde cholangiopancreatography (ERCP) *except*:

   A. Evaluation of jaundiced patient suspected of having biliary obstruction
   B. Evaluation of recurrent pancreatitis of unknown cause
   C. Relief of biliary ductal obstruction caused by gallstones
   D. Evaluation of known metastatic pancreatic carcinoma
   E. Placement of plastic stents across biliary strictures

3. Acute or chronic liver disease may cause an abnormal prothrombin time (PT). All of the following statements are correct *except*:

   A. The PT depends on plasma concentration of prothrombin; factors V, VII, IX, and X; and fibrinogen.
   B. The synthesis of prothrombin and factors V, VII, IX, and X depends on vitamin K.
   C. Malabsorption of vitamin K can lead to prolonged PT.
   D. Prolonged PT seen in fulminant hepatic failure can be corrected by parenteral administration of vitamin K.

4. A 68-year-old white man presents with chills and right upper quadrant abdominal pain for 6 hours. On examination the patient is icteric. His serum transaminase levels are mildly elevated, the direct bilirubin level is 6 mg/dL, and the leukocyte count is 18,000/µL. Of the following options, which one is the most appropriate first therapeutic approach?

   A. Obtain a magnetic resonance imaging (MRI) study of the liver.
   B. Order viral hepatitis serologic studies.
   C. Perform an ERCP.
   D. Obtain a CT scan of the liver.
   E. Administer broad-spectrum IV antibiotics.

5. Which of the following statements about acute pancreatitis is *false*?

   A. The most common causes of acute pancreatitis are gallstones and alcohol.
   B. Pancreatic necrosis is best diagnosed by contrast medium–enhanced dynamic CT.
   C. Most systemic complications occur during the third week of the illness.
   D. Transient, mild hyperglycemia is common and does not require insulin therapy.

6. Which statement about *Helicobacter pylori* infection is *true*?

   A. Antibiotic therapy should be based on results from culture and sensitivity.
   B. After successful *H. pylori* eradication ulcer recurrence is decreased to less than 5%.
   C. Long-term maintenance with antisecretory therapy is mandated.
   D. In peptic ulcer–related *H. pylori* infection it is recommended to perform endoscopy with antral biopsy before and after eradication therapy.
   E. There is no difference in eradication rates between dual- and triple-drug regimens.

121

7. Hepatitis C virus (HCV) is currently the most common cause of chronic liver disease in the United States. All of the following statements about HCV are correct *except*:

   A. IV drug use is the most common mode of transmission.
   B. In 40% of sporadic cases of acute hepatitis C the mode of transmission is unknown.
   C. Vertical transmission from mother to child is universal.
   D. With anti-HCV screening the incidence of post-transfusion hepatitis has significantly declined.
   E. Among healthy blood donors, 0.5% in the United States have HCV antibodies.

8. Which of the following statements regarding gastrointestinal hemorrhage is *false*?

   A. The most accurate noninvasive indicator of the severity of blood loss is the presence of orthostatic hypotension.
   B. The presence of hematemesis indicates upper gastrointestinal bleeding.
   C. Peptic ulcer disease is the most common cause of upper gastrointestinal bleeding.
   D. Endoscopy is useful for diagnosis and therapy.
   E. Diverticular bleeding is associated with abdominal pain.

9. Patients with ileitis or ileal resection may develop chronic diarrhea. Which statement regarding this type of diarrhea is *true*?

   A. The degree of steatorrhea is independent of the amount of resected or diseased ileum.
   B. Choleretic diarrhea occurs when more than 100 cm of ileum have been resected.
   C. When bile acid absorption in the ileum is reduced as a result of regional ileitis, the elevated levels of bile acids in the colon will trigger steatorrhea.
   D. Cholestyramine is useful for the management of steatorrhea secondary to extensive (i.e., >100 cm) ileal resection.
   E. Choleretic diarrhea is due to increased colonic secretion of water by colonic mucosal cells.

10. A 27-year-old man with a history of IV drug use was found to have abnormal results of liver function tests. Further work-up including serologic tests for viral hepatitis show:

    Hepatitis B surface antibody (HBsAb) negative
    Hepatitis B surface antigen (HBsAg) positive
    Hepatitis core antibody (HBcAb) positive
    Hepatitis B e antibody (HBeAb) positive
    Hepatitis B e antigen (HBeAg) negative

    Which of the following statements is *true* regarding this patient?

    A. He is a chronic hepatitis B virus (HBV) carrier with high infectivity.
    B. He is in the incubation period of HBV infection.
    C. He is a chronic HBV carrier with low infectivity.
    D. He has recovered from HBV infection and is immune to HBV.

11. A 23-year-old woman experienced watery diarrhea, nausea, vomiting, and abdominal cramps 6 hours after eating a salad and a hamburger in a local restaurant. The most likely organism causing her disease is:

    A. *Vibrio vulnificus*
    B. *Listeria monocytogenes*
    C. *Yersinia enterocolitica*
    D. *Escherichia coli* 0157:H7
    E. *Staphylococcus aureus*

12. A 35-year-old man presents with diarrhea for 10 days, characterized by frequent, low-volume stools with the presence of mucus. He also complained of subjective fever and lower abdominal pain. The presence of leukocytes in stool is consistent with which organism?

    A. *Clostridium perfringens*
    B. *S. aureus*
    C. *Giardia lamblia*
    D. *Enterobius vermicularis*
    E. *Entamoeba histolytica*

13. Acetaminophen is an important cause of acute hepatic failure. All of the following statements about acetaminophen toxicity are correct *except*:

    A. Significant liver injury usually occurs with doses of more than 10 to 15 g.
    B. Alcoholics are more susceptible to liver injury even with a low dose.
    C. N-Acetylcysteine is most effective when administered within 10 hours of ingestion.
    D. Hemodialysis is effective in the management of hepatotoxicity.
    E. Survivors of acetaminophen-induced hepatotoxicity typically do not experience any progressive or residual liver damage.

14. Which statement about esophageal cancer is *true*?

    A. Dysphagia is an early manifestation.
    B. Squamous cell carcinoma is associated with intestinal metaplasia of the esophagus.
    C. Incidence of squamous cell carcinoma has increased significantly over the past 30 years.
    D. Most esophageal cancers are not resectable for cure at presentation.
    E. Adenocarcinoma is related to alcohol and tobacco use.

15. A 42-year-old man presents with intermittent dysphagia to solids and liquids and regurgitation of food. He has lost 4 pounds in 2 months. His physical examination is normal. A barium swallow reveals a dilated esophageal body, with the distal esophagus terminating in a narrow end. All of the following are treatment options *except*:

    A. Nifedipine
    B. Metoclopramide
    C. Heller myotomy
    D. Pneumatic dilation
    E. Botulinum toxin

16. A 45-year-old male executive comes to your office complaining of epigastric pain for 2 months. His primary physician prescribed him H_2-blockers 3 weeks ago, which have produced only partial relief of his symptoms. His weight is stable. His physical examination is normal. An upper endoscopy reveals a 1-cm duodenal ulcer. Which of the following risk factors is *not* associated with the development of ulcer disease?

    A. Daily use of nonsteroidal anti-inflammatory drugs (NSAIDs)
    B. Gastric infection with *H. pylori*
    C. Alendronate
    D. Cigarette smoking
    E. Gastrin-secreting tumors

17. A 20-year-old white woman presents with jaundice and malaise of 2 weeks' duration. Her boyfriend had some form of hepatitis several months before. Initial laboratory studies reveal alanine transaminase (ALT) of 211 U/L, aspartate

transaminase (AST) of 194 U/L, and bilirubin of 5.4 mg/dL. HBsAg and anti-HBc IgM are positive. Which of the following statements regarding acute hepatitis B is *false?*

A. About 90% of patients with acute hepatitis B will recover completely.
B. About 1% of patients with acute hepatitis B can experience fulminant hepatic failure.
C. Chronic hepatitis B carrier state will develop in 10% of patients.
D. Interferon administration in the acute phase of infection prevents the development of the chronic hepatitis B carrier state.
E. Patients with positive HBV DNA levels 6 weeks after symptom onset frequently develop chronic disease.

18. Which of the following features best distinguishes Crohn's disease from ulcerative colitis?

A. Oral ulcers
B. Rectal bleeding
C. Continuous colonic involvement on endoscopy
D. Noncaseating granulomas
E. Crypt abscesses

19. A 49-year-old man presents to the emergency department because of melena of 3 days' duration. He denies abdominal pain. Vital signs reveal a resting pulse of 104 beats/minute and a 25-mm Hg orthostatic drop in blood pressure. Physical findings include bilateral temporal wasting, pale conjunctivae, spider angiomas on his upper torso, muscle wasting, hepatosplenomegaly, and hyperactive bowel sounds without abdominal tenderness to palpation. His stool is melenic. Nasogastric tube aspiration reveals coffee grounds material. Hematocrit is 31%. The appropriate next step in the management of this man's illness would be to:

A. Pass a Sengstaken-Blakemore tube.
B. Obtain an upper gastrointestinal series.
C. Insert a transjugular intrahepatic portosystemic shunt (TIPS).
D. Obtain immediate visceral angiography.
E. Perform upper endoscopy.

20. Colonoscopy is indicated in all of the following situations *except:*

A. A 63-year-old woman with ulcerative colitis of 21 years' duration and now presenting with toxic megacolon
B. A 65-year-old woman with acute colonic pseudo-obstruction (Ogilvie's syndrome)
C. A 26-year-old HIV-positive man (CD4 count of 89) with diarrhea for 4 weeks, abdominal pain, and fever
D. A 62-year-old man with microcytic anemia and Hemoccult-positive stools
E. A 42-year-old man whose brother and father had colon cancer at ages 51 and 60, respectively

21. A 48-year-old woman has had profuse, watery diarrhea for 3 months. Laboratory studies of fecal water show the following:

Sodium   39 mmol/L
Potassium   96 mmol/L
Chloride   15 mmol/L
Bicarbonate 40 mmol/L
Osmolality 270 mmol/kg H_2O (serum osmolality, 280 mOsm/kg H_2O)

The most likely diagnosis is

A. Villous adenoma
B. Lactose intolerance

C. Follicular carcinoma of the thyroid
D. Pancreatic insufficiency
E. Celiac disease (nontropical sprue)

22. A 32-year-old man presents with self-limited recurrent episodes of right upper quadrant pain accompanied with chills and fever for the past 6 months. He was diagnosed with ulcerative colitis about 6 years ago. Currently he is in remission and taking sulfasalazine (Azulfidine), 2 g/day. On physical examination his sclera are icteric, and he has hepatosplenomegaly. Laboratory studies show total bilirubin of 3.2 mg/dL, AST of 110 U/L, ALT of 98 U/L, and alkaline phosphatase of 476 U/L. What is the most likely diagnosis?

A. Primary sclerosing cholangitis
B. Primary biliary cirrhosis
C. Choledocholithiasis
D. Autoimmune hepatitis
E. Drug-related injury

23. A 41-year-old woman presents with a chronic watery diarrhea over the past 4 years. The diarrhea occurs mainly in the mornings; she never has nocturnal diarrhea. On abdominal examination she has tenderness in the left lower quadrant (LLQ); the rectal vault is empty. On sigmoidoscopy the mucosa appears normal but there is an excess of mucus. Barium enema evaluation is normal, and examination of a stool specimen reveals soft feces that are negative for occult blood, pathogenic bacteria, and parasites. Results of thyroid studies are normal. A trial of milk restriction results in no change in symptoms. At this point you should:

A. Consider a trial of diphenoxylate or paregoric to control symptomatic diarrhea.
B. Tell the patient that her symptoms are largely emotional in origin.
C. Consider a trial of psyllium to increase stool bulk.
D. Obtain stool electrolytes and osmolality.
E. Perform a jejunal aspirate and analyze the fluid for parasites.

24. Which one of the following statements about achalasia is *false?*

A. A tumor at the gastroesophageal junction (GEJ) can cause secondary achalasia.
B. Dysphagia, chest pain, and regurgitation are the predominant symptoms.
C. Chest x-ray films often reveal a large gastric air bubble.
D. Nifedipine is effective for the control of symptoms in some patients.
E. Manometry reveals a normal or elevated pressure of the lower esophageal sphincter.

25. A 17-year-old boy is brought to the emergency department in the morning because of right lower quadrant abdominal pain of 4 to 6 hours. The day before he had periumbilical pain and nausea. He vomited three times during the night. Physical examination discloses tenderness in the right lower quadrant; bowel sounds are normal. His leukocyte count is 10,000/μL. Urinalysis shows 5 to 10 WBC per high-power field. The most appropriate statement regarding surgical consultation is that:

A. Surgical consult is not necessary.
B. Surgical consultation should be requested if fever develops.
C. Surgical consultation should be requested if rebound tenderness develops.
D. Surgical consultation should be requested if the leukocyte count rises above 15,000/μL.
E. Surgical consultation should be arranged promptly.

26. A 26-year-old man who has had type I diabetes mellitus for 15 years complains of postprandial epigastric discomfort, nausea, and bloating. An upper gastrointestinal series fails to reveal an ulcer, but the fluoroscopist notes delayed gastric emptying. These results are confirmed by a gastric emptying study. Which of the following therapies would be best at this stage of the man's illness?

    A. Percutaneous endoscopic gastrostomy
    B. Proton pump inhibitors
    C. Metoclopramide
    D. Propantheline
    E. Liquid antacids

27. A 50-year-old man has had watery diarrhea and weight loss (20 pounds) for the last 6 months. He also complains of night sweats and arthralgias of the knees, wrists, and elbows. Stool fat content is 35 g/24 hours. A peroral small bowel biopsy reveals subtotal villous atrophy and infiltration of the lamina propria with macrophages that stain positively with periodic acid–Schiff (PAS) stain. The most appropriate management is:

    A. Start him on a gluten-free diet.
    B. Prescribe a lactose-free diet.
    C. Prescribe 5-aminosalicylic acid.
    D. Prescribe trimethoprim-sulfamethoxazole.
    E. Perform exploratory laparotomy with biopsy of retroperitoneal nodes.

28. A 63-year-old man presents to your office complaining of malaise, anorexia, and weight loss of 15 pounds for the last 4 months. On examination he appears chronically ill. He has various verrucous, hyperpigmented skin lesions on the flexor surfaces of his body. An upper gastrointestinal series reveals a large gastric ulcer along the greater curvature. An upper endoscopy with biopsies confirms the diagnosis of gastric cancer. What is the diagnosis of the skin lesions?

    A. Dermatitis herpetiformis
    B. Pyoderma gangrenosum
    C. Linitis plastica
    D. Acanthosis nigricans
    E. Erythema nodosum

29. A 45-year-old man presents with a 1-year history of increasing fatigue for the past year. Physical examination is unremarkable. Laboratory studies show the following: total bilirubin, 0.8 mg/dL; AST, 84 U/L; ALT, 104 U/L; and alkaline phosphatase, 124 U/L. The viral hepatitis serologic profile is as follows: HBsAg positive, HBc IgM negative, HBc IgG positive, HCV antibody negative, and HAV IgG negative. The most likely diagnosis is:

    A. Acute hepatitis A
    B. Acute hepatitis B
    C. Chronic hepatitis B
    D. Chronic hepatitis C
    E. Acute hepatitis C

30. A 72-year-old man presents with massive rectal bleeding of 4 hours' duration. On admission he is hypotensive and tachycardic. His physical examination is otherwise unremarkable. His hemoglobin is 7 g/dL. After adequate fluid resuscitation and blood transfusion, the patient is stabilized and undergoes a colonoscopy, which discloses several small "spider-like" erythematous lesions in the cecum consistent with colonic vascular ectasia. Which statement is *true* regarding these lesions?

    A. Colonic vascular ectasias can be diagnosed by angiography.
    B. Colonic vascular ectasias can be diagnosed with a technetium-99m bleeding scan.
    C. Colonic vascular ectasias are associated with cutaneous vascular malformations.
    D. Colonic vascular ectasias occur most often in the left colon.
    E. Subtotal colectomy is the preferred therapy for bleeding colonic vascular ectasias.

31. All of the following are treatment options for actively bleeding colonic vascular ectasias *except:*

    A. Argon plasma coagulation
    B. Embolization
    C. Hormonal therapy
    D. Colonic resection
    E. Endoscopic application of heater probe

32. A 65-year-old white man with a history of congestive heart failure and peripheral vascular disease presents with a sudden onset of severe and persistent abdominal pain associated with bloody stools. He is afebrile, and abdominal examination reveals only very mild tenderness to deep palpation in the mid abdomen. Laboratory studies reveal leukocytosis with left shift. The lactate level is normal. Which of the following is the next appropriate step?

    A. Colonoscopy
    B. Exploratory laparotomy
    C. Angiography
    D. Upper gastrointestinal small bowel series
    E. Indium scan

33. A 38-year-old white woman with an 18-year history of heavy alcohol use presents with nausea and epigastric pain radiating to the back worsened by eating for 2 weeks. Plain x-ray films of the abdomen reveal diffuse calcifications in the region of the pancreas. Upper endoscopy shows nonspecific "gastritis." Which of the following is indicated to confirm a diagnosis of chronic pancreatitis?

    A. Abdominal CT scan
    B. ERCP
    C. Secretin tests with duodenal aspiration
    D. Stool trypsin concentration
    E. No further testing is necessary.

34. Which of the following is *not* a local complication of acute pancreatitis?

    A. Acute renal failure
    B. Gastrointestinal hemorrhage
    C. Pseudocyst
    D. Splenic vein thrombosis
    E. Ascites

35. A 32-year-old phlebotomist sustained a percutaneous needle stick while caring for a patient who is HBsAg positive. She has not previously undergone hepatitis B vaccination. Which of the following should be done now?

    A. Immediate administration of hepatitis B immunoglobulin (HBIG) and hepatitis B vaccination
    B. Immediate administration of HBIG only
    C. Start lamivudine, 100 mg/day for 2 weeks.
    D. Administer hepatitis B vaccination.

36. Which of the following is *not* considered a risk factor for gastric adenocarcinoma?

A. Long-term use of proton pump inhibitors (e.g., omeprazole)
B. Gastric adenomatous polyp(s)
C. *H. pylori* infection
D. Common variable immunodeficiency
E. Previous gastric surgery for peptic ulcer disease

37. A 65-year-old woman had four bloody bowel movements accompanied by left-sided crampy abdominal pain. She arrived at the emergency department and feels somewhat better. On physical examination her vital signs are stable, her abdomen is tender in the LLQ, bowel sounds are normal, and there is no rebound tenderness. What is the most likely diagnosis?

A. Ischemic colitis
B. Diverticulosis
C. Diverticulitis
D. Peptic ulcer with bleeding

38. All of the following influence the risk of cancer in colonic polyps *except*:

A. Villous histology
B. Size greater than 1 cm
C. Dysplasia
D. Polyp location
E. Tubular adenoma

39. A 52-year-old woman underwent a colonoscopy for Hemoccult-positive stools. A 2-cm pedunculated polyp was found in the transverse colon; it was resected with a snare and electrocautery. The pathologist reports that the polyp is adenomatous with dysplastic changes. Which statement is *true*?

A. The patient should undergo partial colectomy.
B. Repeat colonoscopy should be performed to review the polyp site for remnant tissue.
C. Flexible sigmoidoscopy should be done every 6 months for 2 years.
D. Colonoscopy should be repeated in 3 years.
E. No further surveillance endoscopies are indicated.

40. A 55-year-old man is referred for evaluation of weight loss and weakness. He noticed the onset of fatigue 6 months ago. During this time he has lost 25 pounds. In addition, he has been complaining of small volume diarrhea. He was diagnosed with insulin-requiring diabetes mellitus 1 year ago. On physical examination he appears wasted. A raised, scaly erythematous rash is observed over the buttocks, inner thighs, and groins. Laboratory examination is significant for anemia (hemoglobin, 9 g/dL). A CT scan of the abdomen revealed a large pancreatic mass with hepatic metastasis. The most likely diagnosis is:

A. Somatostatinoma
B. VIPoma
C. Glucagonoma
D. Insulinoma
E. Zollinger-Ellison syndrome

41. A 25-year-old man presents with rectal bleeding described as the presence of streaks of blood mixed with stool and proctalgia. In addition, the patient complains of intermittent crampy abdominal pain and a 20-pound weight loss over 6 months. On physical examination, you discover a 0.5-cm anteriorly located anal fissure. Which statement regarding anal fissures is *false*?

A. Anal fissures present with painful defecation.
B. Anal fissures are associated with increased anal sphincter tone.
C. Sphincterotomy is the treatment of choice.
D. Anal fissures may be a manifestation of Crohn's disease.
E. Anal fissures may be associated with a sentinel skin tag at the anal verge.

42. The diarrhea associated with nontropical sprue (celiac disease) is secondary to:

A. Disordered motility
B. Mucosal damage
C. Carbohydrate malabsorption
D. PAS-positive microorganism
E. Increased concentration of cholecystokinin (released from enterocytes)

43. A small bowel biopsy was performed in a 6-year-old child with chronic diarrhea, weight loss, malabsorption, lower extremity edema, and ataxia. The mucosal biopsy disclosed normal intestinal villi; the enterocytes had multiple fat particles. What is the diagnosis?

A. *G. lamblia*
B. Radiation enteritis
C. Whipple's disease
D. Intestinal lymphangiectasia
E. Abetalipoproteinemia

44. All of the following factors are used to establish a prognosis during an attack of acute pancreatitis *except*:

A. Hypoxia
B. Hyperbilirubinemia
C. Hypoalbuminemia
D. Hypocalcemia
E. Hyperglycemia

45. A 34-year-old bricklayer comes to the emergency department with a history of passing black, tarry stools for 2 days. He has no other medical problems. He takes over-the-counter aspirin for headaches. His blood pressure is 95/40 mm Hg, with a resting pulse of 106 beats/minute. Blood is drawn and sent for study. The next step should be:

A. Place two large-bore peripheral catheters and bolus with IV crystalloids.
B. Transfuse with two units of packed RBCs.
C. Determine his BP and pulse in the sitting and standing positions.
D. Await the results of his hemoglobin and hematocrit tests before further action.
E. Order an emergency bleeding scan.

46. A 60-year-old white man presents with LLQ pain, loose stools, and fever. He has no significant medical history. Physical examination reveals normal vital signs except for a temperature of 38.7° C. On abdominal examination there is guarding and tenderness to palpation in the LLQ but no definite mass can be palpated. Laboratory evaluation is normal except for a WBC count of 15,000 cells/µL. Plain and upright abdominal radiographs are normal. All of the following would be reasonable parts of an initial plan *except*:

A. Empirical therapy with broad-spectrum antibiotics
B. Surgical consultation
C. Flexible sigmoidoscopy
D. Barium enema
E. CT scan of abdomen and pelvis

47. A 50-year-old white man is admitted because of jaundice and pruritus. A CT scan reveals a large pancreatic mass causing biliary obstruction and multiple filling defects in the liver consistent with metastasis. A metal stent is placed during ERCP. One week after stent placement, he returns for follow-up. The patient feels well but he continues to be jaundiced. Laboratory tests show the following:

	Before Stent Placement	7 Days Later
Bilirubin	14.0 mg/dL	7.0 mg/dL
AST	89 IU/L	41 IU/L
Serum alkaline phosphate	725 IU/L	496 U/L
Urine bilirubinogen	Positive	Negative

Which one of the following options is the most appropriate action?

A. Obtain a sonogram to assess duct size.
B. Replace the stent because it is probably occluded.
C. Establish drainage by a percutaneous transhepatic route.
D. Consider surgery to create a choledochoenterostomy.
E. Continue observation without therapeutic intervention at this time.

48. A 45-year-old man presents to your office with intermittent epigastric pain for 8 months. The pain is partially relieved with the ingestion of food and antacids. He frequently awakens at night with "nagging" epigastric pain and heartburn. He has had no nausea, vomiting, hematemesis, melena, diarrhea, or weight loss. He has been treated intermittently with H$_2$-blockers and proton pump inhibitors with some relief of his symptoms. His medical history is significant for peptic ulcer disease. He does not smoke or drink alcohol. He does not take aspirin or other NSAIDs. Physical examination is negative. The stool is Hemoccult positive. An upper endoscopy shows erosive esophagitis. A 1.0-cm clean-based ulcer is identified in the duodenal bulb, prominent gastric folds were noted, but no other abnormalities were identified. The second duodenum was normal. Histologic assessment of antral biopsy specimens demonstrates no gastritis or *H. pylori* infection. Which of the following would you do next?

A. Upper gastrointestinal series
B. *H. pylori* serology
C. Serum gastrin level
D. Empirical treatment for *H. pylori*
E. Radiolabeled (technetium) gastric-emptying study

49. A 34-year-old man with AIDS complains of odynophagia for solids and liquids. On physical examination the patient has oropharyngeal thrush. You prescribe fluconazole for presumed candidiasis, but after 3 days on therapy the symptoms have become worse. Upper endoscopy reveals a deep 2 × 3-cm ulcer in the mid esophagus. The most likely diagnosis is:

A. Herpes simplex virus (HSV) esophagitis
B. Resistant *Candida* esophagitis
C. Reflux esophagitis
D. Cytomegalovirus esophagitis
E. Histoplasmosis of the esophagus

50. Which statement about acute colonic pseudo-obstruction (Ogilvie's syndrome) is *true?*

A. If cecal distention is more than 7 cm, urgent laparotomy should be considered.

B. Ogilvie's syndrome is precipitated by serious illnesses, medications, or metabolic conditions.
C. Ogilvie's syndrome has a high mortality rate as a result of colonic perforation.
D. Ogilvie's syndrome is caused by malignant strictures of the colon.
E. Colonoscopy is contraindicated in Ogilvie's syndrome.

51. A 25-year-old man presents with lower abdominal pain, chronic diarrhea, and weight loss. Physical examination reveals oral aphthous ulcers and a genital ulcer. You order baseline laboratory data and schedule him to have a lower endoscopy. What is the most likely diagnosis?

A. Crohn's disease
B. Pemphigoid
C. Behçet's syndrome
D. Henoch-Schönlein purpura
E. Whipple's disease

52. Each of the following is associated with an increased risk of gastric and/or small bowel adenocarcinoma *except*:

A. AIDS
B. Common variable immunodeficiency
C. Crohn's disease
D. Peutz-Jeghers syndrome
E. Familial adenomatous polyposis

TRUE OR FALSE
QUESTIONS 53–67

DIRECTIONS: For questions 53–67, determine whether *each* choice is true or false. Any combination of answers, from all true to all false, may occur.

53. A 40-year-old man presented to the emergency department after an episode of massive hematemesis. On examination he had a heart rate of 112 beats/minute and a blood pressure of 90/40 mm Hg. After initial hemodynamic stabilization, an urgent endoscopy was done, which revealed large esophageal varices. Which of the following statements regarding the management of acute variceal bleeding are *true?*

A. Balloon tamponade with a Sengstaken-Blakemore tube should be performed immediately.
B. Endoscopic variceal ligation and endoscopic sclerotherapy are equally effective in the control of variceal hemorrhage.
C. Octreotide (somatostatin analogue) is highly effective in controlling acute hemorrhage.
D. β-Blockers given after the control of hemorrhage reduce the risk of rebleeding.
E. TIPS should be used as a first option in the patient who is bleeding severely.

54. A 25-year-old male college student was found to have mild jaundice on routine physical examination. He is asymptomatic and has a normal physical examination. His liver chemistry profile is normal except for total bilirubin of 2.8 mg/dL and a direct bilirubin level of 0.3 mg/dL. Which of the following statements are *true?*

A. The most common cause of these abnormalities is Gilbert's syndrome.
B. Chronic hemolysis can give a similar picture.
C. Liver biopsy is likely to show normal histology.
D. His urine will be positive for bilirubin.

55. Which of the following statements is/are *true* concerning the eradication of *H. pylori*?

    A. Most individuals with non-ulcer dyspepsia and *H. pylori* infection have symptomatic cures when the organism is eradicated.
    B. Elimination of *H. pylori* is associated with a very low rate of ulcer recurrence.
    C. Treatment of *H. pylori* decreases the risk of gastric cancer.
    D. Successful treatment can be documented by repeating serologic testing in 4 to 6 weeks.
    E. Appropriate triple-antibiotic therapy leads to *H. pylori* eradication in greater than 80% of cases.

56. Which of the following are considered to be extraintestinal manifestations of inflammatory bowel disease (IBD)?

    A. Ankylosing spondylitis
    B. Sclerosing cholangitis
    C. Uveitis
    D. Erythema nodosum
    E. Large joint arthritis

57. Which of the following statements concerning ulcerative colitis is/are *true*?

    A. Toxic megacolon may complicate severe ulcerative colitis.
    B. Corticosteroids are useful as maintenance therapy.
    C. Proctocolectomy represents a cure.
    D. The duration of disease and extent of colonic involvement influences long-term colon cancer risk.
    E. Ulcerative colitis typically extends from the rectum in a continuous manner.

58. A 35-year-old woman has a 12-year history of ulcerative colitis. She underwent a screening colonoscopy and was found to have severe dysplasia on random biopsies of the colon. One month later she had proctocolectomy with ileoanal anastomosis. On the 5th postoperative day, she started having bleeding per rectum. Laboratory studies revealed the following:

Hemoglobin	6.8 g/dL
Prothrombin time	35 seconds (control, 12 seconds)
Partial thromboplastin time	95 seconds (control, 35 seconds)
Total bilirubin	4.5 mg/dL
Direct bilirubin	2.8 mg/dL
AST	256 U/L
ALT	345 U/L
Alkaline phosphatase	456 U/L

    Which of the following statements are *true*?

    A. Immediate exploration of the abdomen is required to determine the source of bleeding.
    B. Coagulopathy should be corrected by infusion of fresh-frozen plasma and vitamin K.
    C. Prolonged prothrombin time is more likely due to malabsorption of vitamin K resulting from associated cholestasis.
    D. Vitamin K given parenterally will correct the prolonged prothrombin time.
    E. The cholestatic biochemical profile may be due to associated primary sclerosing cholangitis (PSC).

59. Which of the following statements regarding medical therapy of IBD is/are *true*?

    A. Topical mesalamine (enema) therapy is effective in treating distal proctocolitis.
    B. Metronidazole is useful in inducing remission of active ulcerative colitis.
    C. Elemental diets have therapeutic benefit in active Crohn's disease.
    D. Corticosteroids should be discontinued in pregnant women with IBD.
    E. Therapy with sulfasalazine may be limited by allergy to the sulfa moiety.

60. Which of the following statements concerning Zenker's diverticulum is/are *true*?

    A. It is most commonly seen in the mid esophagus.
    B. It is classically seen in patients with scleroderma.
    C. It may present with recurrent aspiration.
    D. The patient with Zenker's diverticulum is at increased risk of perforation during upper endoscopy.
    E. Zenker's diverticulum should not be treated surgically.

61. Which of the following statements about laboratory tests used to assess liver disease is/are *true*?

    A. Elevation of ALT is generally more sensitive and specific for liver injury than is elevation of AST.
    B. Increases in serum alkaline phosphatase activity can be attributed to a hepatobiliary origin if there is also an elevation in serum levels of 5′-nucleotidase or γ-glutamyltransferase (GGT).
    C. GGT is a sensitive and specific test for hepatobiliary disease.
    D. Acute biliary obstruction, as may occur during passage of a gallstone, can cause transient elevation of serum transaminases (AST and/or ALT) levels of 1000 U/L or more.
    E. In about one third of patients with isolated elevation of alkaline phosphatase, no demonstrable cause of liver or biliary disease can be detected.

62. Which of the following is/are indications for colonoscopy?

    A. A 28-year-old woman with a 5-year history of left-sided ulcerative colitis confirmed on flexible sigmoidoscopy 1 year ago and asymptomatic on conservative medical therapy
    B. A 45-year-old woman with guaiac-positive stools
    C. A 60-year-old man with a single 1-cm sessile polyp in the descending colon found on screening sigmoidoscopy
    D. A 70-year-old asymptomatic man 1 year after right hemicolectomy for colon cancer

63. Which of the following is/are *true* statements concerning radiation enterocolitis?

    A. Injury usually develops when total radiation dose exceeds 5000 rads.
    B. Stricture formation is a late complication.
    C. Surgical resection should routinely be recommended.
    D. Arteritis and mucosal ischemia may result from significant exposure levels.

64. With regard to HCV, which of the following are *true*?

    A. Acute infection progresses to chronic hepatitis in more than two thirds of patients.
    B. HCV is associated with hepatocellular carcinoma.
    C. A sustained response to interferon treatment is seen in about two thirds of patients.
    D. Chronic infection is characterized by fluctuations in serum transaminase levels.
    E. Chronic HCV is associated with mixed cryoglobulinemia.

65. Which of the following statements is/are *true* about the epidemiology of pancreatic cancer?
    A. Carcinoma of the pancreas is more common in men than women.
    B. Coffee consumption is a strong risk factor in the development of pancreatic cancer.
    C. The incidence of pancreatic cancer has increased recently.
    D. The vast majority of pancreatic cancers are derived from the cells of the pancreatic duct.
    E. With new surgical techniques, the 5-year survival rate of pancreatic cancer now approaches 50%.

66. A 28-year-old female student from Ecuador comes to the student health service complaining of abdominal pain for the past 2 to 3 months. She describes the pain as being crampy and associated with increased flatus. She does not have nausea, vomiting, weight loss, or intolerance to any specific food. She has frequent loose bowel movements (4-6 per day) and none at night. She admits she has stress and insomnia related to completing her graduate studies. On physical examination she has mild LLQ tenderness without rebound. A stool test for occult blood is negative. Which of the following should be done?
    A. Obtain colonoscopy.
    B. Obtain stool studies for ova and parasites.
    C. Refer patient to gastroenterologist.
    D. Refer patient for psychological testing.
    E. Begin a therapeutic trial with psyllium.

67. A 59-year-old man who underwent a right hemicolectomy 5 years ago for adenocarcinoma of the colon comes to the office to review the results of a routine barium enema performed 3 days ago. The x-ray film shows a 1.5-cm pedunculated polyp in the splenic flexure and multiple diverticula. The most appropriate management is to advise him that:
    A. This single polyp is not likely to be a problem; thus, nothing should be done.
    B. A laparotomy will be required both to excise the polyp and ensure that no metastases are present.
    C. Colonoscopy with polypectomy is likely to be adequate therapy.
    D. Colonoscopy with biopsy is the next step, with segmental resection if villous elements are found.
    E. A repeat barium study will be necessary in 3 months, and excision of the polyp will be necessary if it has changed in size.

MATCHING
QUESTIONS 68–115

DIRECTIONS: Questions 68–115 are matching questions. For each numbered item, choose the most likely associated lettered item from those provided. Each item has *only one* correct answer.

For each of the following risk factors for gallstone formation, select the mechanism for this increased risk.

   A. Increased biliary secretion of cholesterol
   B. Bile salt deficiency
   C. Poor gallbladder emptying
   D. Chronic biliary infection and stasis
   E. Increased biliary secretion of unconjugated bilirubin

68. Obesity

69. Chronic hemolysis

70. Parenteral alimentation

71. Bile duct strictures

72. Female sex or estrogen use

73. Ileal inflammation or ileal resection

Match each of the following statements with the type of hepatitis described.

   A. Hepatitis A
   B. Hepatitis B
   C. Hepatitis C
   D. Hepatitis D
   E. Hepatitis E

74. This virus is most readily transmitted by sexual contact.

75. This epidemic form of acute hepatitis carries a very high mortality in pregnant women.

76. This is an incomplete virus that requires another hepatitis virus to infect and replicate.

77. This virus is the most common cause of chronic liver disease in the United States.

78. This virus is transmitted by fecal-oral route and is the most common cause of point source epidemics in the United States.

Match the following mechanisms of diarrhea with the stool fluid electrolyte results: Na^+ (mEq/L), K^+ (mEq/L), and stool osmolarity (mOsm/kg H_2O).

	Na+ (mEq/L)	K+ (mEq/L)	Stool Osmolarity (mOsm/kg H₂O)
A.	5	5	22
B.	90	35	280
C.	40	20	280
D.	40	20	500

79. Osmotic diarrhea caused by a nonmetabolizable substance (e.g., magnesium citrate)

80. Osmotic diarrhea caused by a metabolizable substance (e.g., lactose malabsorption)

81. Secretory diarrhea (e.g., cholera)

82. Dilution of stool by added water

For each type of liver disease shown, select the most likely causative drug.

   A. Didanosine
   B. Amoxicillin-clavulanate
   C. Acetaminophen
   D. Isoniazid

83. Acute hepatitis

84. Fulminant hepatic failure

85. Cholestasis

86. Microvesicular steatosis

Match the following causes of esophagitis with the best option.

   A. Ganciclovir
   B. Penicillin
   C. Cowdry-type A inclusion bodies
   D. Refractory *Candida* esophagitis
   E. Involves mid-esophagus

87. HSV

88. Actinomycosis

89. Cytomegalovirus

90. Aspergillosis

91. Pill induced

Match the following manometric pattern with the esophageal disorders.

    A. Aperistalsis, poor lower esophageal sphincter (LES) relaxation
    B. High LES pressures, poor LES relaxation
    C. High esophageal body pressures, normal motility
    D. Low LES pressures, poor peristalsis
    E. Simultaneous contraction, preserved peristalsis

92. Achalasia

93. Nutcracker esophagus

94. Diffuse esophageal spasm

95. Scleroderma

96. Hypertensive lower esophageal sphincter

Match the following liver chemistry tests to the corresponding disease.

    A. AST, 295 U/L; ALT, 120 U/L; total bilirubin, 3.2 mg/dL; alkaline phosphatase,150 U/L; GGT, 100 g/dL
    B. AST, 85 U/L; ALT, 104 U/L; total bilirubin, 1.4 mg/dL; alkaline phosphatase, 570 U/L; GGT, 425 g/dL
    C. AST, 4200 U/L; ALT, 3875 U/L; total bilirubin, 1.2 mg/dL; alkaline phosphatase, 57 U/L; GGT, 76 g/dL
    D. AST, 54 U/L; ALT, 75 U/L; total bilirubin, 1.2 mg/dL; alkaline phosphatase, 65 U/L; GGT, 45 g/dL

97. Tylenol overdose

98. Primary biliary cirrhosis (PBC)

99. Chronic hepatitis C

100. Alcoholic hepatitis

Match the following hepatitis serology panels to the corresponding disease.

    A. HBsAg+, HbeAg+, anti-HBs−, anti-HBc IgM+
    B. HBsAg+, HbeAg+, anti-HBs−, anti-HBc IgM−, anti-HBc IgG+
    C. HBsAg−, HBeAg−, anti-HBc IgM+, anti-HBs+
    D. HbsAg−, anti-HBs+, anti-HBc IgM−, anti-HBc IgG−
    E. Anti-HCV IgM+, anti-HCV IgG+

101. Hepatitis B vaccination

102. Chronic hepatitis C

103. Chronic hepatitis B

104. Acute hepatitis B

105. Resolved hepatitis B infection

Indicate if the following characteristics are associated with primary sclerosing cholangitis, primary biliary cirrhosis, or both.

    A. Primary sclerosing cholangitis
    B. Primary biliary cirrhosis
    C. Both primary sclerosing cholangitis and primary biliary cirrhosis

106. Associated with positive anti-mitochondrial antibody (AMA)

107. Increased risk of cholangiocarcinoma

108. Ursodeoxycholic acid is the only medication with proven benefit

109. Women affected more frequently than men

110. Associated with inflammatory bowel disease

111. Cholangiogram reveals multifocal structuring and irregularity of the bile ducts

112. Treatment of end-stage disease is liver transplant

113. Characterized by inflammatory destruction of the interlobular and septal bile ducts

114. Associated with positive P-ANCA

115. Symptoms include pruritus and jaundice

For each of the following patients, select the next most appropriate diagnostic test.

    A. Serum ferritin and total iron-binding capacity
    B. Serum ceruloplasmin
    C. Antimitochondrial antibody
    D. Anti–smooth muscle antibody
    E. α-Fetoprotein

116. A 52-year-old man presents with increasing fatigue. Physical examination demonstrates hyperpigmentation of the skin, tenderness, and deformity of the metacarpophalangeal and interphalangeal joints of both hands. Abdominal examination reveals hepatosplenomegaly. Liver chemistry profile shows the following: AST, 66 U/L; ALT, 76 U/L; alkaline phosphatase, 132 U/L; all hepatitis viral serologic studies are negative.

117. A 19-year-old previously healthy college student is found to have hepatosplenomegaly on routine physical examination. Chemistry profile shows the following: AST, 96 U/L; ALT, 86 U/L; alkaline phosphatase, 152 U/L. All hepatitis serologic studies are negative.

118. A 45-year-old white woman presents with pruritus and increasing fatigue for 6 months. On examination her sclera are icteric, and she has multiple small xanthomas on her eyelids. Abdominal examination reveals hepatosplenomegaly. Liver chemistry profile shows the following: AST, 96 U/L; ALT, 106 U/L; alkaline phosphatase, 162 U/L.

119. A 46-year-old man with a history of IV drug use presents with recent onset of jaundice associated with marked fatigue, anorexia, and weight loss. On physical examination his sclera are deeply icteric. He has an enlarged, nodular liver, a palpable spleen, and ascites. Liver chemistry profile shows the following: AST, 146 U/L; ALT, 176 U/L; and alkaline phosphatase, 232 U/L. Hepatitis B surface antigen is positive.

120. A 28-year-old white woman presents with fatigue and complains of pain and swelling of the wrist, elbow, and ankle joints. On examination she has a rash over the face and has hepatosplenomegaly. Liver chemistry profile shows the following: AST, 66 U/L; ALT, 106 U/L; alkaline phosphatase, 162 U/L; albumin, 4.2 g/dL; and gamma globulin, 4.6 g/dL; all viral hepatitis serologic studies are negative, and the antinuclear antibody (ANA) test is positive.

For each condition, select the most closely associated diagnosis.

    A. Transient cystic duct obstruction
    B. Cystic duct obstruction
    C. Common bile duct obstruction
    D. Common bile duct obstruction with infection
    E. Cholecystolithiasis

121. Acute cholecystitis

122. Obstructive jaundice

123. Cholangitis

124. No symptoms

125. Biliary pain or colic

For each condition, select the most closely associated characteristic.

    A. Desmoid tumors and mandibular osteomas
    B. Melanotic spots on the lips, buccal mucosa, and skin
    C. Medulloblastoma
    D. Fingernail dystrophy, alopecia, hypoalbuminemia, and cutaneous hyperpigmentation

126. Gardner's syndrome

127. Cronkhite-Canada syndrome

128. Peutz-Jeghers syndrome

129. Turcot's syndrome

Match the following effects with the associated compounds.

    A. Sulfasalazine (Azulfidine)
    B. Azathioprine
    C. Glucocorticosteroids
    D. Metronidazole
    E. Olsalazine (Dipentum)

130. Competitively inhibits intestinal folate absorption

131. Reversible sperm abnormalities

132. Peripheral neuropathy

133. Pancreatitis

134. Secretory diarrhea

MULTIPLE CHOICE

DIRECTIONS: For questions 135–149, choose the best answer to each question.

135. A 28-year-old white man presents because his father was diagnosed as having hereditary hemochromatosis. His father is a 54-year-old whose liver biopsy showed increased hepatic iron with a hepatic iron index of 5.5. His son feels well and has a normal physical examination. He takes no medications and has no significant medical history. His serum transaminase levels and liver biochemistries are normal. What is the most appropriate approach to decide whether the son has hemochromatosis?

    A. Do human leukocyte antigen (HLA) typing on father and son and look for identical alleles.
    B. Measure iron, transferrin saturation, and ferritin level.
    C. Obtain a CT scan of the liver.
    D. Obtain an MRI of the liver.
    E. Screening of any type is inappropriate because only homozygotes are affected and siblings are more commonly affected than the proband children.

136. All of the following are indications for cholecystectomy in a patient with gallstones *except*:

    A. Vague abdominal discomfort, bloating, and flatulence
    B. Biliary colic
    C. Acute cholecystitis
    D. Calcification of the gallbladder (porcelain gallbladder)
    E. Acute pancreatitis without other obvious causes

137. All of the following are true statements regarding Crohn's disease *except*:

    A. An increased prevalence is seen among Ashkenazi Jews.
    B. Incidence has been rising steadily over the past 20 years.
    C. Cigarette smoking is a risk factor for disease.
    D. An autosomal recessive pattern of inheritance is seen.

138. Upper endoscopy is indicated in all of the following situations *except*:

    A. A 62-year-old man with a nonhealing gastric ulcer on upper gastrointestinal series after 6 weeks of acid suppressive therapy
    B. A 26-year-old HIV-positive woman with odynophagia
    C. A 32-year-old man with newly diagnosed familial adenomatous polyposis
    D. A 65-year-old woman with absent bowel sounds, rigid abdomen, rebound tenderness, and a history of peptic ulcer disease

139. All of the following statements about α_1-antitrypsin deficiency are correct *except*:

    A. Liver involvement occurs almost entirely in PiZZ homozygotes.
    B. Males are at higher risk for cirrhosis than females.
    C. Those with liver involvement have an unusually low incidence of liver cancer.
    D. A1AT deficiency should be considered in adults with cirrhosis of unknown cause.
    E. The only treatment for cirrhosis due to A1AT deficiency is liver transplant.

140. All patients with new-onset ascites should undergo diagnostic paracentesis. A serum-ascites albumin gradient (SAAG) greater than 1 is associated with:

    A. Malignancy
    B. Pancreatitis
    C. Spontaneous bacterial peritonitis
    D. Cirrhosis
    E. Tuberculosis

141. All of the following statements about *E. coli* 0157:H7 are true *except*:

    A. It is the most common cause of bloody diarrhea in the United States.
    B. Average incubation time is 3 to 4 days.
    C. Hemolytic-uremic syndrome is a known complication.
    D. Treatment includes supportive care and antibiotics.
    E. A KUB radiograph often reveals thumbprinting of the ascending and transverse colon.

142. Which of the following is *not true* regarding celiac disease?

    A. If there is a high clinical suspicion of sprue, serologic markers (anti-gliadin, anti-endomysial, and anti-tissue transglutaminase) can confirm the diagnosis.
    B. Treatment involves a gluten-free diet.
    C. It is characterized by blunted villi and increased intraepithelial lymphocytes on biopsy.
    D. Extraintestinal manifestations include anemia, osteopenia, and dermatitis herpetiformis.
    E. Most symptoms result from intestinal malabsorption.

143. A 27-year-old man with HIV disease and recent CD4 count of 28 cells/mm^3 presents with a 1-week history of worsening odynophagia and rare dysphagia. Physical examination shows oropharyngeal candidiasis and a suggestion of Kaposi's sarcoma on the lower extremities. Which of the following is the best approach for his esophageal complaints?

A. Upper endoscopy
B. Barium swallow
C. Mediastinal chest CT scan
D. Fluconazole therapy
E. Proton pump inhibitor therapy

144. Which of the following is the most appropriate surveillance strategy for hepatocellular carcinoma in patients with cirrhosis?

    A. Liver function tests (LFTs) alone
    B. α-Fetoprotein (AFP) alone
    C. Three-phase CT scan of abdomen and LFTs
    D. Angiography and LFTs
    E. Ultrasound and AFP

145. A 42-year-old woman presents with two episodes of rectal bleeding. On questioning, the blood is described as filling the toilet bowl but the stool itself is brown. She also noted a large amount of blood on the tissue paper. Her stool the next day was normal color. Physical examination including digital rectal examination is normal. Which of the following is the best approach?

    A. Flexible sigmoidoscopy
    B. Anoscopy
    C. Colonoscopy
    D. Air contrast barium enema
    E. Stool guaiac cards on the appropriate diet

146. A 72-year-old man presents with a 1-week history of low-grade fevers and vague upper abdominal pain. Work-up including abdominal CT scan shows three hyperdense lesions in the right lobe of the liver and one in the left lobe, the largest of which is 2 cm. The pattern is most suggestive of liver abscess. Laboratory studies include WBC of 15,000/μL and normal results of liver function tests. Which of the following is not an appropriate management strategy?

    A. Percutaneous drainage
    B. Blood cultures

C. Broad spectrum antibiotics
D. ERCP
E. Aspiration of the abscess with cultures

147. A 58-year-old man complains of progressive weight loss and jaundice. He denies a past history of liver disease, increasing abdominal girth, fever, or right upper quadrant pain. Laboratory studies include total bilirubin, 24 mg/dL; alkaline phosphatase, 475 U/L; GGT, 560; AFP, 2; AST, 25 U/L; and ALT, 30 U/L. CT scan reveals multiple liver nodules, no evidence of underlying cirrhosis, dilated intrahepatic bile ducts, a large perihilar mass encircling the bile duct and increased intra-abdominal lymphadenopathy. The next step in the management of this patient would be:

    A. Radiation
    B. Chemotherapy
    C. Liver transplant
    D. IV antibiotics
    E. ERCP

148. A 24-year-old man presents complaining of fatigue, anorexia, and depressed mood. Examination reveals hepatomegaly and elevated transaminase levels. His history is of concern for Wilson's disease. All of the following test results can be seen with Wilson's disease except:

    A. Elevated ceruloplasmin
    B. Kayser-Fleisher rings on slit lamp examination
    C. Elevated 24-hour urinary copper
    D. Negative C282Y mutation
    E. Normal iron indices

149. Which of the following is/are risk factors for squamous cell cancer of the esophagus?

    A. Tobacco
    B. Lye ingestion
    C. Achalasia
    D. Alcohol
    E. Squamous papilloma

Part VII
Gastrointestinal and Liver Disease
Answers

1. **(B)** *Discussion:* Because of the superb ability to demonstrate gallstones, ultrasonography has replaced oral cholecystography for the diagnosis of cholelithiasis. PTC is used to visualize the intrahepatic and extrahepatic biliary tree. CT is useful in the evaluation of the acute abdomen, providing excellent visualization of the pancreas, mesentery, liver, retroperitoneum, and gallbladder. Although CT will allow excellent visualization of the gallbladder wall, its sensitivity for the detection of gallstones is poor. *(Cecil, Chs. 131 and 158; Johnston and Kaplan, 1993)*

2. **(D)** *Discussion:* ERCP has emerged as a major diagnostic and therapeutic tool for pancreatobiliary disorders. In evaluating suspected biliary obstruction, a cholangiogram is indicated before deciding on therapy. Placement of plastic stents will decompress the biliary tree in the case of benign or malignant biliary obstruction or ascending cholangitis. Endoscopic sphincterotomy is useful for the removal of common bile duct stones. In the presence of *known* metastatic pancreatic carcinoma, ERCP will not add major diagnostic information. ERCP is useful in the diagnosis of suspected pancreatic head carcinoma. *(Cecil, Ch. 131)*

3. **(D)** *Discussion:* Prothrombin time depends on the plasma concentration of prothrombin and the other clotting factors V, VII, IX, and fibrinogen. The synthesis of prothrombin and factors V, VII, IX, and X depend on an adequate supply of vitamin K. Prothrombin time is abnormal in the setting of reduced synthesis (liver failure, vitamin K deficiency) and increased consumption (disseminated intravascular coagulation) of clotting factors. Vitamin K is a fat-soluble vitamin, and deficiency is seen most commonly in malabsorption syndromes. In fulminant hepatic failure, administration of vitamin K does not correct a prolonged prothrombin time. *(Cecil, Chs. 148 and 149)*

4. **(C)** *Discussion:* This patient has the classic clinical findings of ascending cholangitis: fever, abdominal pain, and icterus (Charcot's triad). These clinical findings alone strongly suggest biliary tract infection resulting from benign (stones) or malignant (cancer) obstruction. In this clinical scenario, the most important diagnostic and therapeutic intervention is aimed at the relief of biliary obstruction. This can be accomplished with ERCP, PTC, or surgery with sphincteroplasty. Although the administration of antibiotics may be helpful to treat biliary sepsis resulting from the biliary obstruction, failure to relieve the obstruction will lead to progressive sepsis and possibly death. Common viral hepatitides rarely present with mildly abnormal transaminases. CT and MRI are useful in the evaluation of parenchymal liver disease and are not helpful in the initial management of a patient with ascending cholangitis. *(Cecil, Ch. 158)*

5. **(C)** *Discussion:* Most systemic complications of acute pancreatitis occur during the *first* week of illness and include circulatory shock, acute renal failure, adult respiratory distress syndrome, and sepsis. They are treated by standard medical measures. Close patient monitoring is the key in their timely recognition. Transient hyperglycemia is common during an attack of pancreatitis and usually does not require therapy with insulin. The most common causes of acute pancreatitis are gallstones and alcohol. The best modality to diagnose pancreatic necrosis is contrast medium–enhanced CT. Ultrasound is insensitive for the diagnosis of pancreatic necrosis. *(Cecil, Ch. 145; Baron and Morgan, 1999)*

6. **(B)** *Discussion:* With eradication of *H. pylori* infection, *H. pylori* ulcers are cured and ulcer recurrence is decreased to less than 5% in developing countries. The best eradication results for *H. pylori* are achieved with triple-antibiotic regimens; dual therapies rarely achieve cure rates of more than 80%. Despite increasing evidence of *H. pylori* resistance to metronidazole and clarithromycin, currently it is not necessary to base antibiotic therapy on culture and sensitivity results. In patients with uncomplicated *H. pylori*–related peptic ulcer disease, it is not necessary to maintain the patient on long-term antisecretory therapy after uncomplicated *H. pylori* eradication therapy. *(Cecil, Ch. 137; National Institutes of Health Consensus Statement, 1994; Walsh and Peterson, 1995)*

7. **(C)** *Discussion:* HCV RNA is readily detected in the serum of infected individuals but at a much lower concentration than generally found with other hepatitis viruses such as hepatitis B. The concentration of HCV RNA in other body fluids is much lower or undetectable. HCV is readily transmitted by a large-volume inoculum (e.g., transfusion) but is less likely to be spread by perinatal or sexual contact. IV drug use with sharing of contaminated needles is the most common mode of transmission in the United States. Approximately 0.5% of healthy blood donors in the United States are HCV antibody positive. About 40% of acute sporadic cases of HCV are not associated with any recognizable risk factors. *(Cecil, Chs. 151 and 152; Sjögren, 1996)*

8. **(E)** *Discussion:* Bleeding associated with diverticular diseases is painless. Colonic diverticula are responsible for nearly one fourth of all episodes of hemodynamically significant bleeding from the lower gastrointestinal tract. The most accurate noninvasive indicator of the severity of blood loss is the presence of shock and the presence of postural vital signs changes. Hematemesis is always associated with an upper gastrointestinal bleeding source. Peptic ulcer disease is the most common cause of upper gastrointestinal bleeding, followed by esophageal varices and Mallory-Weiss tears. Endoscopy is performed as soon as the patient has undergone resuscitation and correction of any underlying coagulopathy. *(Cecil, Ch. 133; Laine and Peterson, 1994)*

9. **(E)** *Discussion:* Disease of the distal ileum leads to an interruption of the enterohepatic circulation of conjugated bile acids, resulting in a diminished bile acid pool and steatorrhea. The degree

of steatorrhea is proportional to the amount of diseased or resected intestine. When less than 100 cm of intestine is damaged or resected, proximal to the ileocecal valve, the steatorrhea is mild (the liver can compensate by increasing the production of bile salts and prevent fat malabsorption), and choleretic diarrhea tends to be the most frequent problem. The malabsorbed bile acids dump into the colon, exerting a secretory effect on the colonic mucosa and impairing water and electrolyte absorption. Choleretic diarrhea usually can be managed with cholestyramine. When more than 100 cm of small intestine is resected, the steatorrhea is large. The liver is not able to compensate by increased bile salt synthesis, and malabsorption occurs. In addition, other factors such as a loss of absorptive function of the ileum and bacterial overgrowth make this diarrhea worse. (*Cecil, Ch. 141*)

10. (C) *Discussion:* In the interpretation of results of hepatitis B serologic tests, the following facts should be considered: during the incubation period (i.e., before the onset of clinical manifestations) HbsAg, HbeAg, and HBV DNA become detectable in the serum. At the onset of clinical symptoms (e.g., jaundice), an increase in the serum transaminases occurs and antibodies to HBc become detectable (HBc antibodies). Initially, the HBc antibodies are IgM and thereafter IgG; these latter antibodies persist for years. HBs antibodies become detectable late in convalescence. A rise in HBs antibodies in combination with a loss of HbsAg, HbeAg, and HBV DNA indicate the presence of immunity to HBV. HbeAg and HBV DNA are markers of active viral replication and thus indicate high infectivity. The loss of HbeAg and appearance of anti-HbeAb indicates a less infective stage. (*Cecil, Chs. 151 and 152; Sjögren, 1996*)

11. (E) *Discussion:* Staphylococcal food poisoning is manifested 2 to 6 hours after eating food (salad, potato salads) contaminated by a preformed enterotoxin. *Yersinia* is most commonly associated with the ingestion of improperly cooked meat, but symptoms generally begin more than 1 day after ingestion of the contaminated food. Symptoms resulting from *L. monocytogenes* also occur more than 24 hours after the ingestion of contaminated foods (milk, ice cream, and poultry). *V. vulnificus*–associated food poisoning presents usually 24 to 48 hours after the ingestion of contaminated seafood (usually oysters). *E. coli* 0157:H7 typically causes symptoms 3 to 4 days after ingestion and often progresses to bloody diarrhea. (*Cecil, Ch. 141*)

12. (E) *Discussion:* The presence of large numbers of leukocytes in stool is diagnostic of colonic mucosal inflammation and should suggest infection with enteroinvasive organisms such as *Shigella, E. histolytica, Salmonella, Campylobacter,* invasive *Escherichia coli,* or *Y. enterocolitica.* Those organisms that cause diarrhea by a noninvasive mechanism (*Giardia lamblia,* enterotoxigenic *E. coli, Vibrio cholerae*) are not associated with leukocytes in the stool. (*Cecil, Ch. 141*)

13. (D) *Discussion:* Acetaminophen overdose causes acute liver failure. Significant liver injury usually occurs with doses of more than 10 to 15 g, most frequently taken in a suicide attempt. The liver injury is caused by toxic metabolites of acetaminophen formed by the microsomal cytochrome P-450–dependent drug-metabolizing system. Because ethanol induces this cytochrome P-450 system, severe hepatotoxicity can be seen in alcoholics, even with lower dosages of acetaminophen. *N*-Acetylcysteine administered early after ingestion (i.e., <24 hours) reduces the severity of liver necrosis. Acetaminophen and its metabolites are not cleared by hemodialysis. Survivors of acute acetaminophen toxicity usually recover completely without progressive or residual liver damage. (*Cecil, Ch. 150*)

14. (D) *Discussion:* Most esophageal cancers are asymptomatic, and at the time of diagnosis most are unresectable. Barrett's syndrome is squamous metaplasia of the distal esophagus that can develop into *adenocarcinoma.* The number of adenocarcinoma

cases has been increasing and now equals squamous cell carcinoma in prevalence. Squamous cell typically involves the proximal two thirds of the esophagus while adenocarcinoma involves the distal third. Risk factors for squamous cell carcinoma of the esophagus include tobacco and alcohol use. (*Cecil, Ch. 136*)

15. (B) *Discussion:* Goal of treatment for achalasia is symptomatic relief. Four treatments are available: pharmacotherapy, botulinum toxin injection, dilation, and myotomy. Dilation and myotomy offer the longest-lasting benefits. Promotility agents like metoclopramide increase the lower esophageal sphincter pressure and thus are contraindicated in achalasia. (*Cecil, Ch. 136; Sleisenger and Fordtran, 2002*)

16. (C) *Discussion:* Alendronate has been shown to cause esophageal ulcers, not large solitary duodenal ulcers. Daily NSAID use significantly increases the risk of ulcer disease (risk ratio, 10- to 20-fold). Gastric infection with *H. pylori* increases risk about five- to sevenfold. Cigarette smoking doubles the risk of duodenal ulcer. At least 90% of those patients with Zollinger-Ellison syndrome have duodenal ulcer. (*Cecil, Ch. 138; Walsh and Peterson, 1995*)

17. (D) *Discussion:* Ninety to 95% of otherwise healthy adult patients with acute hepatitis B recover completely and become HBsAg negative. About 1% experience massive necrosis, and 5 to 10% of patients who remain HBV DNA and/or HBeAg positive beyond 6 weeks are at increased risk of chronic hepatitis. Interferon given during acute hepatitis B infection has not shown any benefit. (*Cecil, Ch. 151*)

18. (D) *Discussion:* Oral ulcerations can occur both in Crohn's disease and ulcerative colitis. Rectal bleeding and continuous involvement of the colon may also be seen in both Crohn's disease and ulcerative colitis. The presence of crypt abscesses does not distinguish ulcerative colitis from Crohn's disease; however, noncaseating granulomas, when present, are pathognomonic of Crohn's disease. (*Cecil, Ch. 142*)

19. (E) *Discussion:* After this patient has been hemodynamically stabilized, the next most important step is to perform a diagnostic/therapeutic upper endoscopy. If the source of his bleeding is from esophageal varices, then these can be obliterated with sclerosis or, preferably, endoscopic band ligation. The use of a Sengstaken-Blakemore tube should be reserved for patients in whom upper endoscopy was unsuccessful in controlling the hemorrhage. A TIPS should be considered in patients in whom medical and endoscopic therapy have failed. Barium studies have no role in the evaluation of patients with suspected variceal hemorrhage. (*Cecil, Chs. 133 and 156; Sleisenger and Fordtran, 2002*)

20. (A) *Discussion:* Although colonoscopy is also the preferred method to perform surveillance in patients with long-standing ulcerative colitis, it is *contraindicated* in the presence of toxic megacolon because of the high risk of colonic perforation. Colonoscopy is the method of choice to evaluate patients with guaiac-positive stools and to screen patients at high risk for colon cancer. In patients with acute colonic pseudo-obstruction (Ogilvie's syndrome), a colonoscopy may be helpful to decompress the colon. Up to 65% of AIDS patients with chronic diarrhea and negative stool studies may have a diagnosis made by colonoscopy and/or EGD with biopsies (*Cecil, Ch. 132; Kornbluth and Sacchar, 1997; Levin et al, 1991; Wilcox, 1997*)

21. (A) *Discussion:* The laboratory values of the stool analysis are consistent with secretory diarrhea. The osmolality of fecal water is approximately equal to serum osmolality. Furthermore, there is no osmotic "gap" in the fecal water: the osmolality of the fecal water can be accounted for by the stool electrolyte composition: $[2 \times ([Na^+] + [K^+])] = [2 \times (39 + 96)] = 270$. A villous adenoma of the colon can induce a *secretory* diarrhea. Inhibition of absorption or a net luminal gain of water and electrolytes will also result in secretory diarrhea. In pancreatic cholera, high levels of vasoactive intestinal peptide cause intestinal and electrolyte secretion that results in large-volume diarrhea. Enterotoxigenic *E. coli* can induce secretory diarrhea through various enterotoxins. Endocrine causes of secretory diarrhea include Zollinger-Ellison syndrome, carcinoid tumors, and *medullary* carcinoma (not follicular) of the thyroid. Lactose intolerance, nontropical sprue, and excessive use of milk of magnesia produce *osmotic* diarrhea with osmotic "gaps" caused by lactose, carbohydrates, and magnesium, respectively. Pancreatic insufficiency causes steatorrhea, not watery diarrhea. *(Cecil, Ch. 141; Donowitz et al, 1995; Eherer and Fordtran, 1992)*

22. **(A)** *Discussion:* This patient has increased bilirubin, elevated transaminases, and very high alkaline phosphatase concentration suggestive of cholestasis. Cholestasis may result from conditions affecting large bile ducts (choledocholithiasis), disorders of small bile ducts and canaliculi (PSC, primary biliary cirrhosis [PBC]), or hepatocytes (drugs). This patient has IBD, and PSC is often associated with it. About 15% of patients with PSC have clinical manifestations suggestive of recurrent bacterial cholangitis. PBC is more common in females, and the diagnosis is made by a positive antimitochondrial antibody. *(Cecil Ch. 158; Kaplan, 1996)*

23. **(C)** *Discussion:* This presentation is classic for one of the three clinical variants of the irritable bowel syndrome, each associated with abnormal colonic motility. Other groups have chronic abdominal pain and constipation or alternating constipation and diarrhea. The chronic nature of the condition and the presence of formed stool make a work-up for secretory or osmotic diarrhea rather low yield. Giardiasis, although typically occult and requiring jejunal sampling for diagnosis, usually presents with belching and pain, not diarrhea of 4 years' duration. The absence of discernible significant organic pathology should not prompt a discussion with the patient that centers on a psychogenic cause of her problem; such an approach will frequently lead to alienation of the patient. Instead, an effort to effect safe symptomatic improvement of the diarrhea with antispasmodics is worthwhile. To increase stool bulk, psyllium is a good choice for patients with irritable bowel syndrome who complain of both diarrhea and constipation. *(Cecil, Ch. 135; Camilleri and Prather, 1992; Lynn and Friedman, 1993)*

24. **(C)**. *Discussion:* Achalasia is a motor disorder of esophageal smooth muscle in which the LES does not relax properly in response to swallowing, and normal esophageal peristalsis is replaced by abnormal contractions. Tumors of the GEJ can mimic achalasia. In achalasia or pseudoachalasia secondary to GEJ tumor, manometry reveals a normal or elevated LES pressure and a reduced or absent swallow-induced relaxation. Dysphagia, chest pain, and regurgitation are the predominant symptoms. The chest x-ray film often reveals absence of the gastric air bubble, and the barium swallow reveals a dilated esophagus. Calcium-channel antagonists such as nifedipine relax smooth muscle and have been effective in controlling symptoms in some patients. Alternative treatment options include Botox injection, myotomy, and dilation *(Cecil, Ch. 136; Sleisenger and Fordtran, 2002)*

25. **(E)** *Discussion:* This patient likely has a classic presentation of appendicitis, and an early surgical consultation is mandatory. Delay in surgical intervention may have deleterious consequences. Some nonsurgical conditions such as Crohn's disease of the terminal ileum, *Y. enterocolitica* gastroenteritis, mesenteric lymphadenitis, or, in female patients, ovarian torsion or infection may present as right lower quadrant pain. In any event, early surgical consultation is mandatory because a delay in recognition of surgical conditions can lead to an intra-abdominal catastrophe. *(Cecil, Ch. 143)*

26. **(C)** *Discussion:* Persons who have long-standing diabetes mellitus may experience autonomic and visceral neuropathy (gas-

troparesis). These patients not commonly display clinical symptoms and radiologic findings suggestive of gastric retention. A gastric emptying study is the preferred way to confirm the diagnosis and to quantify the response to therapy. Metoclopramide, a stimulant of gastric motility, often can help relieve symptoms of retention. Poor gastric emptying that is not due to ulceration would be unlikely to respond to antacids or proton-pump inhibitors. The use of propantheline might aggravate the condition, considering that anticholinergic medications tend to retard gastric emptying. Placement of a percutaneous endoscopic gastrostomy tube is rarely necessary and should not be considered unless an adequate trial of nonsurgical therapy is unsuccessful. *(Cecil, Ch. 134; Sleisenger and Fordtran, 2002)*

27. **(D)** *Discussion:* This patient has Whipple's disease, a bowel disorder associated with dilated gut lymphatics and characterized by weight loss, abdominal pain, diarrhea, malabsorption, and arthralgias. Histologic examination of the small bowel reveals that the macrophages contain PAS-positive granules and are filled with rod-shaped organisms (*Tropheryma whippleii*). Given the infectious nature of this disorder, the treatment of choice is at least 1 year of therapy with antibiotics, with trimethoprim-sulfamethoxazole as first-line therapy. Clinical recovery is accompanied by the disappearance of the bacilliform bodies. Other differential diagnoses in a patient like this include tuberculosis, lymphoma, and celiac disease, but in none of these disorders do the macrophages have the characteristic PAS-positive staining. *(Cecil, Ch. 143; Sleisenger and Fordtran, 2002)*

28. **(D)** *Discussion:* Acanthosis nigricans is one of several extragastric signs that may precede or occur after the diagnosis of gastric cancer. Acanthosis nigricans is a verrucous, dark, hyperpigmented elevated skin lesion involving primarily the axilla or the flexor surfaces of the body. It has been associated with other malignancies such as pancreatic and colon cancer. Pyoderma gangrenosum is a round to oval lesion with ulcerated center and covered with yellow exudate or crust that typically occurs in association with IBD. Erythema nodosum can occur in association with a wide variety of infectious and inflammatory conditions (e.g., leprosy, tuberculosis, histoplasmosis, IBD). Dermatitis herpetiformis is an erythematous papular eruption occurring in the extensor surfaces of elbows and knees in patients with celiac disease (nontropical sprue). Linitis plastica refers to a thickening and hardening of the stomach wall as a result of diffuse infiltration of the tumor, most commonly gastric adenocarcinoma. *(Sleisenger and Fordtran, 2002)*

29. **(C)** *Discussion:* This patient has chronic hepatitis B infection. HBc IgM antibody is positive during the acute phase of hepatitis B, and HBc IgG antibody appears later and persists for years. This patient has negative antibodies for hepatitis A and hepatitis C. *(Cecil, Chs. 151 and 152; Sjögren, 1996)*

30. **(A)** *Discussion:* Colonic vascular ectasias are the most common vascular abnormality of the GI tract; they can be diagnosed by angiography and/or colonoscopy. These are vascular lesions associated with aging and are not associated with other cutaneous or visceral lesions. They are almost always confined to the cecum or ascending colon, are usually multiple, and rarely can be identified surgically or on routine histologic sections. *(Cecil, Ch. 133)*

31. **(C)** *Discussion:* Bleeding can be controlled nonsurgically in most patients. Argon plasma coagulation and the heater probe are both endoscopic techniques used to control active bleeding. If the bleeding vessel can be identified by angiogram, embolization of the vessel can halt bleeding. Colonic resection should be used as a last resort. Although hormonal therapy, usually with conjugated estrogens, has been used to empirically treat chronic bleeding, its role in the management of *acute* lower gastrointestinal bleeding is limited. *(Cecil, Ch. 144; Sleisenger and Fordtran 2002)*

32. (C) *Discussion:* Acute onset of severe abdominal pain disproportional to physical findings associated with gastrointestinal bleeding in an elderly patient with atherosclerosis should suggest the diagnosis of acute mesenteric ischemia. Early use of mesenteric angiography is critical for diagnosis and therapy. Failure to diagnose this disorder before intestinal infarction occurs is associated with a mortality rate of 70 to 90%. The intra-arterial use of papaverine during mesenteric angiography may be helpful in both occlusive and nonocclusive mesenteric ischemia. *(Cecil, Ch. 144)*

33. (E) *Discussion:* Diagnosis of chronic pancreatitis requires positive documentation of two of the following: symptoms, abnormal test(s) of pancreatic function (bentiromide test, secretin test, 13 C-breath test), and radiologic studies. The presence of pancreatic calcifications on plain abdominal x-ray films in a patient with epigastric pain radiating to the back worsened by eating is highly suggestive for the diagnosis of chronic pancreatitis (in the absence of peptic ulcer disease). *(Cecil, Ch. 145; Steer et al, 1995)*

34. (A) *Discussion:* Direct (local) complications of pancreatitis may include pseudocyst formation, pancreatic abscess, pancreatic ascites, splenic vein thrombosis, and gastrointestinal hemorrhage. Gastrointestinal hemorrhage can occur from gastric varices (as a result of splenic vein thrombosis) or from direct invasion and erosion of the gastrointestinal wall by the inflammatory pancreatic tissue. Acute renal failure is an indirect result (systemic complication) of pancreatitis and may be caused by circulatory shock and an elevation in renal vascular resistance. *(Cecil, Ch. 145; Baron and Morgan, 1999)*

35. (A) *Discussion:* For the prophylaxis of acute hepatitis B infection, it is recommended to institute passive immunization with HBIG (0.6 mL/kg), combined with active immunization using HBV vaccine, administered at a separate site, as early as possible. *(Cecil, Ch. 151)*

36. (A) *Discussion:* The use of proton pump inhibitors is not associated with gastric carcinoma. Laboratory experiments with rats demonstrated an increased incidence of gastric carcinoid tumors, but long-term clinical and endoscopic follow-up in patients taking proton pump inhibitors has not demonstrated an increased incidence of carcinoid tumors in humans. Peptic ulcer disease is not a risk factor for gastric cancer, although gastric adenocarcinoma may present as a gastric ulcer. Dietary nitrosamines are powerful carcinogens in animal studies and are thought to be important as a cause of gastric cancer. Gastric adenomatous polyps are rare; however, they occasionally give rise to carcinoma. Subtotal gastric resection for benign peptic ulcer disease may result in a chronic atrophic gastritis, which is a long-term risk factor for gastric cancer. Immunologic deficiencies such as common variable immunodeficiency may predispose to gastric cancer and lymphoma. *(Cecil, Ch. 138)*

37. (A) *Discussion:* This patient has the classic clinical presentation of left-sided ischemic colitis. The segment of colon typically involved is the "watershed area," which corresponds to the splenic flexure. In most cases the symptoms subside gradually in a few days. In contrast to acute mesenteric artery ischemia (which requires emergent angiography with papaverine infusion), the management of left-sided colonic ischemia is expectant. Laparotomy is only indicated when there is significant ischemic damage, as manifested by a deteriorating clinical course (persistent abdominal pain and distention, leukocytosis, fever, and lactic acidosis). *(Cecil, Ch. 144)*

38. (D) *Discussion:* Size, histologic type, and epithelial dysplasia are important factors in the transformation of adenomatous polyps to carcinomas. The frequency of cancer in adenomas less than 1 cm is 1 to 3%, those between 1 to 2 cm have a rate of 10%, whereas those larger than 2 cm have a rate of malignancy greater than 40%.

The location of polyps in the colon does not appear to influence the risk of cancer. *(Cecil, Ch. 132)*

39. (D) *Discussion:* After endoscopic removal of a large neoplastic polyp, continued surveillance is indicated because the patient is now identified as being at increased risk of colon cancer; a repeat surveillance colonoscopy is warranted in 3 to 5 years. Most pedunculated polyps are completely removed during endoscopy; thus, a partial colectomy is not indicated unless the polyp had invasive carcinoma extending beyond the margins of the resected specimen. A flexible sigmoidoscopy is warranted 3 to 6 months after the surgical resection of a rectosigmoid carcinoma. *(Cecil, Ch. 200, Sleisenger & Fordtran, 2002)*

40. (C) *Discussion:* The rash described in this patient is characteristic of that associated with glucagonoma. It typically develops in the intertriginous areas of the body (e.g., groins, axillae) as a raised scaly rash that eventually forms bullae that burst and crust over. Hyperpigmentation results after healing of the lesions. Glucose intolerance, weight loss, and anemia are also common in these patients. Patients with insulinoma present with syncope, sweating, and hypoglycemia. VIPomas are associated with severe watery diarrhea. Patients with Zollinger-Ellison syndrome typically present with peptic ulcer disease and severe reflux disease; diarrhea is not uncommon. *(Cecil, Ch. 140)*

41. (C) *Discussion:* Anal fissures are located in the posterior midline in more than 90% of cases as a result of straining during defecation or passing hard stools. A sentinel tag at the anal verge is frequently a herald to the presence of an anal fissure. The presence of an anal fissure posteriorly or laterally should alert the clinician to the possibility of Crohn's disease, sexually transmitted disease, or anal cancer. Treatment should begin with medical management such as sitz baths, topical anesthetics, and stool softeners. Approximately 70% will heal with conservative measures. Those who fail can be treated with botulinum injections or with surgical sphincterotomy. *(Cecil, Ch. 147)*

42. (B) *Discussion:* The most accepted theory is that metabolites of gluten initiate an immunologic reaction leading to strikingly damaged enterocytes. Malabsorption is secondary to the impaired transport of nutrients through the damaged enterocyte. In addition, a net secretory state for water and electrolytes has been noted in the jejunum, and pancreatic exocrine function may be secondarily diminished owing to a decreased release of secretin and cholecystokinin from the damaged small bowel mucosa. *(Cecil, Ch. 141)*

43. (E) *Discussion:* In abetalipoproteinemia, the intestinal cells are lacking apoprotein B; therefore, fat absorption cannot occur normally (lack of chylomicron formation). Biopsy of the small intestine shows the epithelial cells to be engorged with fat even after an overnight fast. Primary or congenital lymphangiectasia is characterized by diarrhea, mild steatorrhea, edema, and protein-losing enteropathy. Biopsy of small bowel shows abnormally dilated lymphatic channels. The hypoplastic lymphatics lead to an obstruction in lymph flow, increased pressure within lymphatics, dilated lymphatic channels in the intestine, and finally rupture of the lymphatic channels, discharging lymph into the bowel lumen. Radiation enteritis is characterized by extensive mucosal damage, vasculitis, and extensive lymphangiectasia. In Whipple's disease, the small bowel biopsies demonstrate heavy infiltration of the mucosa and lymph nodes by macrophages that stain positive with PAS and are filled with rod-shaped bacilli (*T. whippleii*). The enterocytes have blunted villi and dilated lymphatics. *(Cecil, Ch. 141)*

44. (B) *Discussion:* Several scoring systems exist that predict the morbidity and mortality of acute pancreatitis. These are based on clinical and laboratory observations obtained during the first 48 hours after admission to the hospital. The most commonly used prognostic scores are Ranson's, Glasgow's and Imrie's criteria. The bilirubin is not valuable in assessing prognosis of an attack of pancreatitis. (*Baron and Morgan, 1999; Cecil, Ch. 145*)

45. **(A)** *Discussion:* In upper gastrointestinal tract bleeding, immediate resuscitation is the first goal, with specific diagnosis postponed until the patient is hemodynamically stable. Before diagnostic procedures such as endoscopy or upper gastrointestinal series are undertaken, the placement of a large-bore intravenous catheter and commencement of volume replacement therapy are mandatory. The decision whether to transfuse immediately is made after assessing the degree of volume loss, presence of anemia or underlying coronary artery disease, and whether bleeding continues or has stopped. Our patient had resting tachycardia and a low blood pressure; therefore, measurement of orthostatic blood pressure change to assess the severity of blood loss (tilt test) is completely unnecessary in this patient. The presence of shock indicates an acute blood volume loss of at least 15 to 20%. Postural decreases in blood pressure indicate an acute loss of 10 to 15%. In acute bleeding, the hemoglobin may not reflect the degree of volume loss. Bleeding scans with technetium-99m may be helpful if the bleeding source has not been determined with the use of endoscopy. (*Cecil, Ch. 133; Laine and Peterson, 1994*)

46. **(C)** *Discussion:* Endoscopy is contraindicated in the presence of diverticulitis because of the possibility of perforation. Diverticulitis typically presents as fever and constant LLQ pain in older patients. IV antibiotic therapy is appropriate for moderate to severe disease, whereas mild disease may be managed with oral antibiotics on an outpatient basis. Abdominal CT is the diagnostic test of choice and may reveal thickened colonic wall or abscess formation. Barium enema can be complementary because CT is not 100% sensitive or specific. If x-ray films raise the possibility of colon cancer or IBD, endoscopy may be appropriate later once the inflammatory process has subsided. (*Cecil, Chs. 131 and 143*)

47. **(E)** *Discussion:* Chronic biliary obstruction (or hepatitis) can lead to a substantial amount of bilirubin becoming bound to albumin. This tightly bound bilirubin is cleared slowly, with a half-life similar to that of albumin: 17 days. Because it is tightly bound to albumin, bilirubin is not filtered at the glomerulus and does not appear in the urine. Because such protein-bound bilirubin can account for varying amounts of the total bilirubin (8-90%), a slow resolution of hyperbilirubinemia alone does not imply stent failure. In this patient, because the bilirubinuria has cleared and all other parameters of cholestasis are improving, no further intervention is necessary. (*Cecil, Ch. 158; Zakim and Boyer, 1990*)

48. **(C)** *Discussion:* Zollinger-Ellison syndrome accounts for less than 1% of peptic ulcers, but it should be considered in patients with recurrent peptic ulcer disease in whom there is no evidence of *H. pylori* infection or history of NSAID use. Furthermore, suspicion is warranted in any patient with associated erosive esophagitis, an ulcer complication, ulcers distal to the duodenal bulb, ulcers refractory to routine therapy, rapid ulcer recurrences, or kidney stones. Zollinger-Ellison syndrome should also be considered in patients with unexplained chronic diarrhea or family histories suggesting peptic ulcer disease, parathyroid disease, or pituitary disease (multiple endocrine neoplasia type I). Patients with sporadic Zollinger-Ellison syndrome should undergo imaging with CT, MRI, endoscopy, and selective angiography to localize the gastrinoma and to look for evidence of metastasis. (*Cecil, Ch. 138*)

49. **(D)** *Discussion:* The most common causes of solitary esophageal ulceration in HIV-infected patients are cytomegalovirus and idiopathic esophageal ulceration. Various HIV-related medications have been associated with pill-induced esophagitis. HSV is usually associated with multiple small shallow esophageal ulcerations. Gastroesophageal reflux disease can present with distal ulcerations (not mid esophagus). Fungi like *Candida* and *Histoplasma* are rarely associated with esophageal ulcers. (*Cecil, Ch. 136; Monkemuller and Wilcox, 1999; Wilcox and Monkemuller, 1997*)

50. **(B)** *Discussion:* Ogilvie's syndrome is a form of primary colonic pseudo-obstruction, most commonly precipitated by serious illnesses, medications, and metabolic disturbances. Because this is a pseudo-obstruction, the presence of a colonic stricture is not part of the syndrome. Therapy for Ogilvie's syndrome is directed at correcting the precipitating factors. Patients with Ogilvie's syndrome can benefit from colonoscopic decompression when conservative measures have failed. In contrast to other causes of colonic obstruction, urgent laparotomy is seldom necessary, even when the diameter of the cecum has reached more than 7 cm. (*Cecil, Ch. 134*)

51. **(C)** *Discussion:* Patients with Behçet's disease characteristically have oral and genital ulcerations. The gastrointestinal findings and therapy are similar to those of IBD. Other diseases that can affect the gastrointestinal tract and can present with oral aphthous ulcerations include pemphigus, celiac disease, vitamin deficiencies, malabsorptive states associated with macrocytic anemias, herpes simplex virus, and HIV. Patients with Henoch-Schönlein purpura (HSP) can present with abdominal pain and/or intussusception; however, the skin lesions associated with HSP are petechiae in the lower extremities secondary to a leukocytoclastic vasculitis. (*Sleisenger and Fordtran, 2002*)

52. **(A)** *Discussion:* Patients with regional enteritis, especially those who have had segments of intestine surgically bypassed, have an increased incidence of small bowel carcinoma. Individuals with Gardner's syndrome (familial adenomatous polyposis) have an increased risk of periampullary adenocarcinoma. In patients with Peutz-Jeghers syndrome, the relative risk of small bowel cancer is 16 times that expected, with a lifetime prevalence of 2%. Patients with common variable immunodeficiency have an increased incidence of gastric carcinoma. Although patients with AIDS are at increased risk for gastrointestinal lymphoma, the incidence of gastric or small bowel adenocarcinoma is not increased in these patients. (*Rustgi, 1994; Sleisenger and Fordtran, 2002*)

53. **(A) True; (B) True; (C) True; (D) True; (E) False.** *Discussion:* Squamous papillomas of the esophagus are papillary structures lined by normal squamous epithelium and do not have malignant potential. (*Cecil, Ch.136; Sleisenger and Fordtran, 2002*)

54. **(A) True; (B) True; (C) True; (D) False.** *Discussion:* Gilbert's syndrome is the most common cause of an isolated elevation of unconjugated bilirubin. It occurs in up to 7% of the general population. Type I Crigler-Najjar syndrome is almost uniformly lethal and presents in neonates with very high levels of bilirubin. Chronic hemolysis can also present with hyperbilirubinemia resulting from increased production of bilirubin. Because unconjugated bilirubin is very poorly soluble in water, it circulates bound to albumin and is not filtered by glomeruli. Histologic examination does not show any abnormality in Gilbert's syndrome. (*Cecil, Ch. 154; Zakim and Boyer, 1990*)

55. **(A) False; (B) True; (C) True; (D) False; (E) True.** *Discussion:* Most studies on eradication of *H. pylori* in patients with nonulcer dyspepsia have not shown significant symptomatic improvement. In those with duodenal ulcer in whom *H. pylori* is eradicated, the recurrence rate is less than 5% at 12 months as opposed to 85% in those in whom *H. pylori* has persisted. Epidemiologic evidence associates *H. pylori* infection with gastric adenocarcinoma of the body and antrum. However, gastric cancer occurs in individuals with no evidence of *H. pylori* infection. In the United States, fewer than 1% of *H. pylori*–infected individuals acquire gastric cancer. However, current guidelines suggest the

elimination of the organism in anyone with documented infection. Antibody levels to *H. pylori* decrease slowly after successful eradication. A dramatic fall 6 to 12 months after treatment indicates successful eradication. Urea breath testing is currently the best noninvasive test documenting successful eradication; however, it is not routinely indicated. The issue of which antimicrobial regimen is best is still unclear. The best results have occurred with triple therapy: bismuth subsalicylate, tetracycline, and metronidazole for 2 weeks. Antimicrobial therapy is usually combined with antisecretory. *(Cecil, Chs. 137 and 138; National Institutes of Health Consensus Statement, 1994; Laine and Peterson, 1994; Walsh and Peterson, 1995)*

56. (All True) *Discussion:* All these disorders are associated with IBD. Large joint arthritis and erythema nodosum generally coincide with active bowel disease and will respond to treatment of intestinal inflammation. Uveitis and ankylosing spondylitis are associated with the HLA-B27 haplotype and may run a course independent of the activity of bowel disease. Sclerosing cholangitis is more frequently associated with ulcerative colitis than Crohn's disease, and its progression is not affected by treatment of intestinal inflammation, including colectomy. *(Cecil, Ch. 142; Kornbluth and Sacchar, 1997)*

57. (A) True; (B) False; (C) True; (D) True; (E) True. *Discussion:* Severe colitis or toxic megacolon are medical emergencies that may complicate ulcerative colitis. Patients who have not been treated with steroids may be treated with corticotropin or IV corticosteroids. Patients with evidence of transmural disease, such as abdominal tenderness, fever, and leukocytosis, should receive broad-spectrum antibiotics. Corticosteroids are effective in controlling active disease and inducing remission; however, they have not been shown to prevent relapse in ulcerative colitis or Crohn's disease and have significant long-term side effects. Ulcerative colitis, but not Crohn's disease, is cured by proctocolectomy. Indications for surgery include toxic megacolon, perforation, intractable hemorrhage, and evidence of confirmed dysplasia or cancer. Pancolitis represents a greater risk for colon cancer than left-sided disease. Cancer risk increases with increasing duration of disease as well. *(Cecil, Ch. 142; Elson, 1996; Kornbluth and Sacchar, 1997; Podolsky, 1991)*

58. (A) False; (B) True; (C) True; (D) True; (E) True. *Discussion:* This patient experienced bleeding in the immediate postoperative period. Laboratory data reveal the presence of a significant coagulopathy. First, attempts should be made to correct the coagulopathy by giving fresh-frozen plasma and vitamin K. The cholestatic biochemical pattern is likely due to associated primary sclerosing cholangitis, which is seen in about 3% of all patients with ulcerative colitis. Cholestasis causes significant malabsorption of all fat-soluble vitamins, including vitamin K. Parenteral administration of vitamin K will only correct the prolonged prothrombin time. *(Cecil, Ch. 158)*

59. (A) True; (B) False; (C) True; (D) False; (E) True. *Discussion:* Mesalamine and corticosteroid enemas are effective in treating active proctocolitis. Metronidazole may successfully induce remission of active Crohn's disease, especially with parenteral involvement, but is not helpful in ulcerative colitis. Active Crohn's disease responds favorably to elemental diets as well as to parenteral nutrition. Pregnant women with active IBD may be safely treated with corticosteroids and/or sulfasalazine. Sulfasalazine is cleaved by colonic bacteria to its active moiety, 5-aminosalicylic acid, and a sulfa moiety, which may cause allergic reactions in patients with sulfa sensitivity. *(Cecil, Ch. 142; Das, 1989; Elson, 1996)*

60. (A) False; (B) False; (C) True; (D) True; (E) False. *Discussion:* Zenker's diverticula occur above the upper esophageal sphincter at the level of the pharynx and may present as recurrent aspiration of undigested food particles hours after eating. Scleroderma is generally associated with multiple wide-mouth diverticula throughout the length of the esophagus. When large enough to be clinically problematic, Zenker's diverticula are effectively treated with a diverticulectomy and cricopharyngeal transection. *(Cecil, Chs. 134 and 136)*

61. (A) True; (B) True; (C) False; (D) True; (E) True. *Discussion:* AST is commonly elevated in diseases of skeletal or cardiac muscle, whereas ALT elevation is more often seen with hepatocellular necrosis. Alkaline phosphatase activity mainly reflects hepatic and bone isoenzymes. When the source is less apparent, measurement of 5'-nucleotidase, leucine aminopeptidase or γ-glutamyltranspeptidase (GGTP) will help to differentiate a hepatobiliary from bone source of alkaline phosphatase. GGTP is a very sensitive test for hepatobiliary disease, but it is present in other tissues and can be induced by ingestion of alcohol or other microsomal inducers such as in the absence of liver disease. Acute biliary obstruction caused by common bile duct stones can cause transient elevation in transaminases to more than 1000 U/L. As many as one third of patients with isolated elevation of alkaline phosphatase activity have no demonstrable liver or hepatobiliary cause. *(Cecil, Chs. 149 and 158)*

62. (A) False; (B) True; (C) True; (D) True. *Discussion:* Endoscopic screening for dysplasia should begin after 7 years of extensive colitis. Left-sided disease may have a lower risk for carcinoma, and later initiation of surveillance colonoscopy (after 12-15 years of disease) may be reasonable. Guaiac-positive stools, screening for synchronous polyps in patients in whom a polyp has been found on sigmoidoscopy, and 1-year follow-up after colorectal cancer resection are accepted indications for colonoscopy. *(Cecil, Ch. 132; Kornbluth and Sacchar, 1997; Levin et al, 1991)*

63. (A) True; (B) True; (C) False; (D) True. *Discussion:* At higher doses of radiation (>5000 rads), submucosal damage and arteritis may result in late complications, including stricture formation and bleeding from diffuse vascular ectasias. Such patients are at an increased risk of operative resection because of damage to adjacent bowel segments leading to problems with reanastomosis of the bowel. As a result, patients should be referred to surgery only when more conservative measures have failed. *(Cecil, Ch. 144; Sleisenger and Fordtran, 2002)*

64. (A) True; (B) True; (C) False; (D) True; (E) True. *Discussion:* HCV infection progresses to chronic liver disease in more than two thirds of patients. About 20% of patients progress to cirrhosis and are at increased risk for hepatocellular carcinoma. Chronic infection with HCV is known to be associated with mixed cryoglobulinemia. The recent introduction of pegylated interferon, when used in combination with ribavirin, has increased the sustained response rate from 45 to 47% to 54 to 56%. Factors associated with better outcome include low serum HCV RNA levels, viral genotype other than 1, absence of cirrhosis, female gender, and age younger than 40. Chronic infection is characterized by fluctuating serum transaminase levels. *(Cecil, Ch. 151 and 152; Sleisenger and Fordtran, 2002; Zakim and Boyer, 1990)*

65. (A) True; (B) False; (C) True; (D) True; (E) False. *Discussion:* The male-female sex ratio is 2:1 in most studies of pancreatic cancer. Whereas early epidemiologic studies showed an association, multiple studies showed no association between pancreatic cancer and coffee consumption. The incidence of pancreatic cancer has increased, and the reason for this increase is not clear. Ninety percent of adenocarcinomas are of ductal origin and 5% are of islet cell origin. The 5-year survival is less than 2%. There have not yet been proven therapeutic breakthroughs in the management of pancreatic cancer. *(Cecil, Ch 201; Warshaw and Fernandez-Del Castillo, 1992)*

66. **(A) False; (B) True; (C) False; (D) False; (E) True.** *Discussion:* This patient has irritable bowel syndrome (IBS). Her symptoms are mild and have not interfered with her daily routine. A flexible sigmoidoscopy is usually indicated, whereas a colonoscopy is not. Testing her stools for ova and parasites is important; giardiasis is an endemic disorder in the United States, and it can be easily treated with metronidazole. Pharmacologic therapy for IBS should be reserved for a limited trial for patients with intractable symptoms. It is best tailored to the specific symptom: constipation or diarrhea. Bulk-forming agents such as psyllium may be helpful to regulate her bowel habits; thus, a therapeutic trial is warranted in this patient. Mild IBS is best treated by a primary care physician who will develop a therapeutic relationship with the patient. Psychological testing is not indicated at this stage of her disease. Consultants should be reserved for confirmation in difficult cases or for intractable cases. (*Cecil, Ch. 135; Camilleri and Prather, 1992; Drossman and Thompson, 1992; Lynn and Friedman, 1993*)

67. **(A) False; (B) False; (C) True; (D) False; (E) False.** *Discussion:* Whenever a polyp is found during colonoscopy it should be resected; biopsy is only recommended if a single polyp less than 1 cm is found during screening flexible sigmoidoscopy. The frequency of cancer in adenomas between 1 and 2 cm is more than 10%, whereas those larger than 2 cm have a rate of malignancy of greater than 40%. Most polyps can be satisfactorily treated by endoscopic polypectomy. Laparotomy and partial colectomy are indicated in the presence of invasive adenocarcinoma. The presence of a colonic polyp mandates colonoscopy with polypectomy. Radiographic studies are not indicated to evaluate the progression of growth of a polyp. (*Cecil, Ch. 132; Sleisenger and Fordtran, 2002*)

68. **(A); 69. (E); 70. (C); 71. (D); 72. (A); 73. (B).** *Discussion:* Multiple factors interplay to predispose to cholesterol and pigment gallstones. Obesity and estrogen are associated with increased levels of biliary cholesterol secretion. Crohn's disease is associated with an increased risk of cholesterol gallstones because of bile salt deficiency caused by increased fecal loss. Although these mechanisms lead to supersaturation of bile with cholesterol, this is not sufficient for formation of cholesterol gallstones. One of the best understood risks are conditions associated with defective gallbladder emptying. This occurs in parenteral alimentation, very-low-fat weight reduction diets, and pregnancy, wherein progesterone impairs emptying (as well as lower esophageal sphincter function) and estrogen increases biliary cholesterol. Hemolytic conditions cause increased biliary secretion of unconjugated bilirubin and result in the precipitation of calcium bilirubinate. These are black pigment stones and are typically radiopaque. Brown pigment stones contain calcium bilirubinate as well as calcium soaps of fatty acids and usually form in bile ducts as a result of infection and stasis, which leads to deconjugation of bilirubin in the biliary system. (*Cecil, Ch. 158*)

74. **(B); 75. (E); 76. (D); 77. (C); 78. (A).** *Discussion:* The vast majority of cases of viral hepatitis in the United States are caused by hepatitis viruses A, B, C, and D. Hepatitis E has been identified as a cause of endemic and severe epidemic disease in Asia, Africa, and Mexico. Hepatitis A and E viruses are transmitted by the fecal-oral route. Hepatitis A has been identified as a cause of water-borne point source food handler–related outbreaks in the United States. Hepatitis E infection is uncommon in the United States but has been reported among travelers from endemic areas. It mainly affects adolescents and young adults, and the illness is entirely self-limited with no evidence of chronicity. However, the case-fatality rate for the epidemic form of acute hepatitis E is 1 to 2% and as high as 20% for pregnant women. HBV and HCV are primarily transmitted by the parenteral route. HBV is present in virtually all body fluids and secretions and is readily transmitted by

sexual contact. In contrast, HCV has very low concentration in other body fluids than blood, and transmission by sexual contact is very low. About 50 to 75% of cases of hepatitis C progress to chronicity, and HCV is the most common cause of chronic liver disease in the United States. Hepatitis D is an incomplete RNA virus, which requires simultaneous infection with HBV and has similar risk factors and mode of transmission as HBV. (*Cecil, Chs. 151 and 152; Sjögren, 1996*)

79. **(C); 80. (D); 81. (B); 82. (A).** *Discussion:* The osmolarity of stool is measured by the freezing point depression method. The osmolarity of fecal fluid is also *calculated* by the following formula: $(Na + K) \times 2$. The difference in value between the measured stool osmolarity minus the *calculated* stool osmolarity is called *stool osmolarity gap*. This value is usually around 50 mOsm/kg and never more than 125 mOsm/kg. This "gap" results from the presence of unmeasured osmoles. Because the gastrointestinal tract does not have a diluting mechanism, the osmolarity of fecal fluid is never less than the osmolarity of plasma (i.e., about 280 mOsm/kg). In a patient with osmotic diarrhea caused by a nonmetabolizable substance (e.g., magnesium citrate) (question 79), stool osmolarity will be equal to plasma, but the presence of unmeasured osmoles (e.g., magnesium) will result in a high osmolar gap. Osmotic diarrhea caused by a metabolizable substance (e.g., lactose malabsorption) (question 80), will result in fecal fluid with a stool osmolarity higher than plasma and a significant osmotic gap. The high osmolarity results from the presence of molecules that are the result of bacterial metabolism of larger carbohydrates into smaller molecules, with resultant higher osmotic activity. The presence of large amounts of fecal fluid (i.e., large-volume diarrhea) (question 81) and normal stool fluid osmolarity and no osmotic gap is consistent with a secretory diarrhea such as cholera. Dilution of stool with water, as can be seen in patients with "factitious diarrhea," will result in very low stool osmolarity (question 82). (*Cecil, Ch. 141; Donowitz et al, 1995; Eherer and Fordtran, 1992; Sleisenger and Fordtran, 2002*)

83. **(A); 84. (C); 85. (B); 86. (A).** *Discussion:* Drugs and toxins produce a variety of pathologic lesions in the liver. Diffuse hepatocellular degeneration and necrosis resembling the pathologic lesions of viral hepatitis are produced by many drugs, including halothane, isoniazid (INH), ketoconazole, methyldopa, and phenytoin. Acetaminophen is one of the most important causes of massive liver injury resulting in fulminant hepatic failure. Whereas estrogens, amoxicillin-clavulanate, piroxicam, and trimethoprim-sulfamethoxazole produce predominantly cholestatic injury, fatty liver is most commonly seen with corticosteroid administration. Tetracycline, valproic acid, and didanosine are associated with deposition of small fat droplets in liver. This pattern of liver injury, termed *microvesicular steatosis,* is accompanied by profound lactic acidosis and has been produced by various nucleoside analogues, including didanosine and zidovudine. (*Cecil, Ch. 150*)

87. **(C); 88. (B); 89. (A); 90. (D); 91. (E).** *Discussion:* Large multinucleated cells with Cowdry type A bodies are typically found on biopsy specimens of HSV-infected tissue. The therapy for choice for actinomycosis is penicillin for 6 months to 1 year. Ganciclovir is the treatment of choice for cytomegalovirus esophagitis. Patients with "refractory candidiasis" should be evaluated for aspergillosis. The esophageal damage associated with pills occurs usually in the mid esophagus. (*Cecil, Ch. 136; Monkemuller and Wilcox, 1999; Wilcox and Monkemuller, 1997*)

92. **(A); 93. (C); 94. (E); 95. (D); 96. (B).** *Discussion:* In patients with achalasia, esophageal manometry demonstrates an LES with poor relaxation and esophageal aperistalsis. Nutcracker esophagus is characterized by high-amplitude, long-duration waves that are peristaltic (i.e. normal motility). Diffuse esophageal spasm is characterized by some normal peristaltic waves inter-

spersed with periods of simultaneous esophageal contractions. Scleroderma is characterized by primary muscle failure of the sphincter (low LES pressure) and aperistalsis. Hypertensive LES is characterized by high LES pressures and poor LES relaxation. (*Cecil, Ch. 136*)

97. (C); 98. (B); 99. (D); 100. (A). *Discussion:* Tylenol overdose causes massive hepatocellular necrosis with significant elevations in transaminases. Initially the other liver functions can be within normal limits. Primary biliary cirrhosis causes a cholestatic picture with alkaline phosphatase elevated up to four times normal and GGT elevated up to three times normal. Chronic hepatitis C can present as fluctuating transaminases and mild bilirubin elevations. Up to 30% of patients with hepatitis C will have normal liver function tests. Alcoholic hepatitis frequently presents with AST:ALT ratio of 2 to 3:1. Transaminases are typically under 300 U/L. (*Cecil, Chs. 149 and 150; Sleisenger and Fordtran, 2002*)

101. (D); 102. (E); 103. (B); 104. (A); 105. (C). *Discussion:* HbsAg suggests ongoing hepatitis B disease. Anti-HBc is increased at onset of symptoms and is often the only marker between resolution of HBsAg and the appearance of anti-HBs. HbeAg is the secreted form of HbcAg and is indicative of active viral replication and increased infectivity. Anti-Hbe appears at peak symptoms and, in combination with HBsAg, implies low viral replication and infectivity. (*Cecil, Chs. 151 and 152; Sleisenger and Fordtran, 2002*)

106. (B); 107. (A); 108. (B); 109. (B); 110. (A); 111. (A); 112. (C); 113. (B); 114. (A); 115. (C). *Discussion:* Primary sclerosing cholangitis is characterized by idiopathic inflammation with progressive obliterating fibrosis of the intrahepatic and extrahepatic bile ducts. ERCP reveals multifocal structuring and irregularity of the bile ducts. Patients are at increased risk for cholangiocarcinoma. Eighty percent of cases are associated with inflammatory bowel disease (ulcerative colitis > Crohn's). There is a decreased incidence of disease in smokers. Patients frequently have a positive P-ANCA. Men are more commonly affected than women. Treatment is liver transplantation.

Primary biliary cirrhosis is the most common cholestatic liver disease in the United States. Most affected patients have no cirrhosis. It is associated with a positive ANA test. Women are affected more than men (9:1). Complications of chronic disease include osteopenia, steatorrhea, and hypercholesterolemia. Ursodeoxycholic acid is the only medication with proven benefit. The disease process is characterized by inflammatory destruction of the interlobular and septal bile ducts, resulting in chronic cholestasis. Patients frequently complain of pruritus and fatigue. (*Cecil, Ch. 158; Sleisenger and Fordtran, 2002*)

116. (A) *Discussion:* In a 52-year-old man with liver chemistry abnormalities, hepatosplenomegaly associated with hyperpigmentation of the skin, and peripheral arthritis, one must consider the diagnosis of hereditary hemochromatosis. Ferritin and transferrin saturation should be measured; elevation of transferrin saturation (>62% male; >50% female) and ferritin (twice the normal) are suggestive of hereditary hemochromatosis. In addition, genetic testing is now available and recommended as part of the work-up for hemochromatosis. This test evaluates for 2 major mutations, C282Y and H63D and has significantly decreased the need for liver biopsy to confirm the diagnosis. If the patient is a C282Y homozygote or a C282Y/H63D heterozygote, the iron overload is likely due to the genetic abnormality. (*Sleisenger and Fordtran, 2002*)

117. (B) *Discussion:* This 19-year-old student probably has Wilson's disease. This rare disease is usually asymptomatic when first diagnosed, although cirrhosis, portal hypertension, and splenomegaly are often present. Two useful screening tests are the measurement of serum ceruloplasmin (which is <20 μg/dL in about 85% of patients) and a slit lamp examination to evaluate for Kayser-Fleischer rings. Low ceruloplasmin levels in a patient with Kayser-Fleischer rings confirms the diagnosis of Wilson's disease. Liver biopsy can be obtained to quantify copper, which generally is more than 250 μg/gram of liver tissue in patients with Wilson's disease. (*Cecil, Ch. 224; Sleisenger and Fordtran, 2002*)

118. (C) *Discussion:* This 45-year-old woman probably has primary biliary cirrhosis. The disease typically occurs in middle-aged females. The insidious onset of pruritus is the most characteristic symptom, and many patients have asymptomatic elevation of alkaline phosphatase. As the disease advances, patients become icteric, skin xanthomas are frequently seen, and hepatosplenomegaly becomes evident. Antimitochondrial antibody is present in more than 95% of patients. The presence of antimitochondrial antibody and a compatible liver biopsy confirm the diagnosis. (*Cecil Ch. 156; Sleisenger and Fordtran, 2002*)

119. (E) *Discussion:* This 46-year-old man who has a history of IV drug use is a chronic carrier of hepatitis B. He has recent decompensation of his liver disease. The development of hepatocellular carcinoma is one of the important causes of decline in a patient with stable chronic liver disease. The incidence of hepatocellular carcinoma is much higher in patients with chronic HBV, and the diagnosis is made by an elevated serum concentration of α-fetoprotein; levels of more than 1000 μg/dL in a patient with the appropriate risk factors, such as this patient, are diagnostic of hepatocellular carcinoma. (*Cecil Ch. 202*)

120. (D) *Discussion:* This 28-year-old woman has autoimmune hepatitis. The extrahepatic manifestation of rash, arthritis, amenorrhea, thyroiditis, and vasculitis is seen in more than one third of patients. About half of patients with this disease have a positive ANA test, and about two thirds have a positive anti–smooth muscle antibody test. (*Cecil Ch. 152; Sleisenger and Fordtran, 2002*)

121. (B); 122. (C); 123. (D); 124. (E); 125. (A). *Discussion:* Obstruction caused by a stone is the primary cause of all manifestations of gallstone disease. The mere presence of stones in the gallbladder does not cause symptoms, and between 60 and 80% of patients with gallstones are asymptomatic. When there is transient cystic duct obstruction, biliary pain ("colic") results. If the obstruction is persistent, acute cholecystitis occurs. Because the bile is usually sterile, bacterial infection does not play a primary role in acute cholecystitis. When a stone obstructs the common bile duct, jaundice will result; as with acute cholecystitis, the bile is initially sterile, but with complete biliary obstruction there is greater chance for the bile to become seeded with bacteria (through translocation). When bacterial infection occurs, purulent ascending cholangitis results. Because the infected bile is under high pressure, the bacteria may enter the bloodstream, resulting in severe sepsis. (*Cecil, Ch. 158; Johnston and Kaplan, 1993; Ransohoff and Gracie, 1993*)

126. (A); 127. (D); 128. (B); 129. (C). *Discussion:* Gardner's syndrome differs from familial adenomatous polyposis by the presence of benign extraintestinal tumors, including osteomas and desmoid tumors. Peutz-Jeghers syndrome is characterized by melanotic spots on the lips, buccal mucosa, and skin as well as multiple hamartomatous polyps throughout the gastrointestinal tract. Turcot's syndrome is defined as the presence of hereditary adenomatous polyposis and tumors of the central nervous system. Cronkhite-Canada syndrome is characterized by diffuse gastrointestinal polyposis associated with alopecia, dystrophy of the fingernails, and cutaneous hyperpigmentation. (*Sleisenger and Fordtran, 2002; Rustgi, 1994*)

130. (A); 131. (A); 132. (D); 133. (B); 134. (E). *Discussion:* Long-term sulfasalazine therapy may result in folate deficiency as a result of competitive inhibition of intestinal folate absorption. Supplementation with folic acid (1 mg daily) is indicated in such patients. The sulfapyridine moiety of sulfasalazine is thought to be responsible for the reversible oligospermia and abnormal sperm morphology seen in men taking this medication. Peripheral neuropathy is frequently seen in patients on metronidazole for prolonged periods or at higher doses (>1 g daily). Allergic pancreatitis is seen in up to 15% of patients on azathioprine. Toxic pancreatitis is rarely seen with sulfasalazine therapy. Olsalazine use may be limited by worsening diarrhea in 6% of patients as a result of increased intestinal secretion. (*Cecil, Ch. 142; Das, 1989; Elson, 1996; Kornbluth and Sacchar, 1997*)

135. (B) *Discussion:* Liver disease only occurs in patients homozygous for hemochromatosis. Because the son can get only one allele from his father, the only way he can be homozygous is if he gets a hemochromatosis gene from his mother. Because the gene frequency is 5 to 8%, this is certainly likely enough to recommend screening. The abnormal iron accumulation begins at birth and is cumulative. Normal iron studies at a young age do not necessarily rule out the disorder, and repeated measurements over time may be necessary. This is especially true of women, who accumulate iron at lower rates because of menstrual losses. HLA typing is useful in assessing the risk of disease in siblings; if the sibling shares both haplotypes with the proband, they probably also share the same hemochromatosis genes, because these are very closely linked. However, this screening method is not useful across generations. Although patients with full-blown hemochromatosis may have suggestive abnormalities on CT or MRI, these studies are neither sensitive nor specific. When abnormal screening iron studies are found, a liver biopsy with quantification of total hepatic iron is necessary to confirm the diagnosis. (*Cecil, Ch. 154; Edwards and Kushner, 1993*)

136. (A) *Discussion:* In general, asymptomatic gallstones are not an indication for surgery. Studies have shown no difference in the frequency of symptoms such as vague abdominal pain, bloating, and flatulence between patients with and without gallstones. One attack of biliary colic usually portends future colic in most patients. Although the risk of gallbladder cancer, which is uncommon but seems to occur only in those with gallstones, is not great enough to warrant cholecystectomy in all patients with gallstones, the risk is great enough in the setting of a calcified gallbladder to recommend surgery. Pancreatitis caused by gallstones seems to be related to passage of a stone through the papilla of Vater. When the pancreatitis has resolved, a cholecystectomy is indicated to prevent future attacks. If the pancreatitis is progressive or slow to resolve, it may be necessary to rule out persistent obstruction. (*Cecil, Ch. 158; Johnston and Kaplan, 1993; Ransohoff and Gracie, 1993*)

137. (D) *Discussion:* Approximately 20% of patients with Crohn's disease have similarly affected relatives. However, no clear genetic pattern of inheritance has been defined. (*Cecil, Ch. 142*)

138. (D) *Discussion:* Esophagogastroduodenoscopy should be performed on all patients with nonhealing gastric ulcers to rule out malignancy. Upper endoscopy is useful in the diagnosis of infectious esophagitis, which often presents as odynophagia in immunocompromised individuals. Patients with familial adenomatous polyposis should be screened every 1 to 3 years with upper endoscopy to rule out concurrent gastroduodenal adenomas. Suspected or known perforation is a contraindication to upper endoscopy. (*Cecil, Ch. 132; Rustgi, 1994*)

139. (C) *Discussion:* Patients with A1AT deficiency and cirrhosis have an unusually high incidence of liver cancer. A1AT deficiency is the leading metabolic liver disease for which transplant is performed. (*Cecil, Ch. 154; Sleisenger and Fordtran, 2002*)

140. (D) *Discussion:* A serum-ascites albumin gradient (SAAG) greater than 1.1 suggests portal hypertension as the cause of the ascites. SAAG less than 1.1 suggests alternative causes for ascites, including malignancy, pancreatitis, spontaneous bacterial peritonitis, and tuberculosis. (*Cecil, Ch. 149 ; Sleisenger and Fordtran, 2002*)

141. (D) *Discussion:* E. coli 0157:H7 causes bloody diarrhea in up to 95% of infected patients. It is most commonly associated with ingestion of hamburger. Plain films of the abdomen show mucosal involvement with submucosal edema and thumbprinting in the ascending and transverse colon. Several studies suggest antibiotic use increases the risk of HUS and is therefore not recommended. (*Cecil, Ch. 141; Sleisenger and Fordtran, 2002*)

142. (A) *Discussion:* Celiac sprue is an allergic reaction to wheat gluten that causes small intestinal malabsorption and villous atrophy. Family studies suggest a genetic component. Presenting symptoms typically include diarrhea, steatorrhea, and abdominal bloating. However, a large number of patients are asymptomatic at the time of diagnosis. Serologic markers, given their high specificities, are only helpful when your index of suspicion is low. If it is high, the diagnosis must be confirmed by a small bowel biopsy before committing your patient to a gluten-free diet. (*Cecil, Ch. 141; Sleisenger and Fordtran, 2002*)

143. (D) *Discussion:* An empirical treatment with fluconazole is reasonable given the high frequency of candidal infections when oropharyngeal thrush is documented. If the patient does not symptomatically improve with treatment, then endoscopy with biopsies is indicated. If no thrush had been visible and the patient complained of severe odynophagia, he would have been at increased risk for ulcerative esophagitis. Esophagogastroduodenoscopy with biopsies would have been warranted as the first step. Chest CT and barium swallow can show lesions in the esophagus; however, tissue is required to make the definitive diagnosis. Proton pump inhibitor therapy is indicated for gastroesophageal reflux disease. This is classically described as a substernal burning and/or regurgitation. (*Cecil, Ch. 136; Sleisenger and Fordtran, 2002*)

144. (E) *Discussion:* Current screening recommendations for patients at high risk for liver cancer are serial α-fetoprotein (AFP) measurements every 6 months and annual abdominal ultrasound. Liver function test elevations are nonspecific and can be seen with cirrhosis alone. Only 45% of presymptomatic patients with hepatocellular carcinoma will have elevated AFP levels. The use of AFP levels alone as a screening test can miss smaller tumors. Three-phase CT and MRI are more costly tests and are reserved for doubtful cases or under special circumstances. (*Cecil, Ch. 202; Sleisenger and Fordtran, 2002*)

145. (B) *Discussion:* The patient's history is typical for hemorrhoidal bleeding. Diagnosis of hemorrhoids is made with anoscopy. Flexible sigmoidoscopy and colonoscopy are reserved for cases in which alternative causes of bleeding are suspected (e.g., colitis, malignancy, diverticulosis). Endoscopy would also be indicated if the patient were older than 50 years of age or had a family history of colon cancer. Barium enema plays no role in the diagnosis of hemorrhoids. Stool guaiac cards only tell you blood is present in the stool—which should be apparent from the history. (*Cecil, Ch. 147; Sleisenger and Fordtran, 2002*)

146. (A) Management of liver abscesses begins with broad-spectrum IV antibiotics, including anaerobic coverage. Blood cultures and aspiration of an abscess with cultures help guide antibiotic therapy. Large abscesses often require percutaneous drainage. ERCP is reserved for cases with evidence of biliary stones or obstruction. (*Cecil, Ch. 153, Sleisenger and Fordtran, 2002*)

147. (E) *Discussion:* This patient has cholangiocarcinoma. Patients rarely develop symptoms until the tumor is advanced. In this case, the imaging suggests advanced, metastatic disease. Results of radiation therapy, chemotherapy, and resection are disappointing. Liver transplantation has been successful in select patients with limited disease. ERCP is indicated for this patient to relieve his biliary obstruction and provide some symptomatic relief. (*Cecil, Ch. 158*)

148. **(A)** *Discussion:* Wilson's disease is an autosomal recessive disorder of copper overload. Patients are typically young, with an average age ranging from 6 to 40 years. There is large clinical variability, often making the diagnosis difficult. The disease may present as chronic or fulminant liver disease, often with associated psychiatric illness. The work-up commonly includes *decreased* ceruloplasmin levels (<20 mg/L) and elevated 24-hour urinary copper levels. Kayser-Fleisher rings are caused by copper deposition in Descemet's membrane in the cornea. C282Y mutation and elevated iron indices are associated with hemochromatosis, not Wilson's disease. *(Cecil, Ch. 154; Sleisenger and Fordtran, 2002)*

149. **(A) False; (B) True; (C) True; (D) True; (E) False.**
Discussion: About two thirds of the episodes of variceal hemorrhage will cease spontaneously, but a rapid onset of rebleeding is common without any intervention; thus, endoscopic hemostasis is required. Two endoscopic methods are equally effective in controlling active bleeding in more than 95% of patients. Endoscopic variceal ligation is associated with lower frequency of esophageal ulceration and more rapid obliteration of varices and currently is the method of choice. Pharmacologic therapy with the somatostatin analogue (octreotide) is highly effective in controlling hemorrhage. The Sengstaken-Blakemore tube can be used for controlling hemorrhage after failure of endoscopic techniques or when urgent endoscopic therapy is not available. β-Blockers have been found useful in preventing rebleeding. A transjugular portacaval shunt can be used as salvage therapy in patients who are unresponsive to endoscopic and pharmacologic treatments. *(Cecil, Ch. 133; Sleisenger and Fordtran, 1998)*

BIBLIOGRAPHY

Baron TH, Morgan DE: Acute necrotizing pancreatitis. N Engl J Med 1999;340:1412.

Camilleri M, Prather CM: The irritable bowel syndrome: Mechanisms and a practical approach to management. Ann Intern Med 1992;116:1001.

Das KM: Sulfasalazine therapy in inflammatory bowel disease. Gastroenterol Clin North Am 1989;18:35.

Donowitz M, Kokke FT, Saidi R: Evaluation of patients with chronic diarrhea. N Engl J Med 1995;332:725.

Drossman DA, Thompson WG: The irritable bowel syndrome: Review and a graduated multicomponent treatment approach. Ann Intern Med 1992;116:1009.

Edwards CQ, Kushner JP: Screening for hemochromatosis. N Engl J Med 1993;328:1616.

Eherer AJ, Fordtran JS: Fecal osmotic gap and pH in experimental diarrhea of various causes. Gastroenterology 1992;103:545.

Elson CO: The basis of current and future therapy for inflammatory bowel disease. Am J Med 1996;100:656.

Goldman L, Ausiello D (eds): Cecil Textbook of Medicine, 22nd ed. Philadelphia, WB Saunders, 2004.

Kaplan MM: Primary biliary cirrhosis. N Engl J Med 1996;335:1570.

Kornbluth A, Sacchar DB: UC practice guidelines in adults. Am J Gastroenterol 1997;92:204.

Johnston DE, Kaplan MM: Pathogenesis and treatment of gallstones. N Engl J Med 1993;328:412.

Laine L, Peterson WL: Bleeding peptic ulcer. N Engl J Med 1994;331:717.

Levin B, Lennard-Jones J, Tiddell RH, et al: Surveillance of patients with chronic ulcerative colitis. Bull WHO 1991;69:121.

Lynn RB, Friedman LS: Irritable bowel syndrome. N Engl J Med 1993;329:1940.

Monkemuller KE, Wilcox CM: Diagnosis and treatment of colonic disease in AIDS. Gastrointest Endosc Clin North Am 1998;8:889.

Monkemuller KE, Wilcox CM: Diagnosis and treatment of esophageal ulcers in AIDS. Semin Gastroenterol 1999;10:1.

National Institute of Health Consensus Statement: *Helicobacter pylori* in peptic ulcer disease. JAMA 1994;12:1-22.

Podolsky D: Inflammatory bowel disease. N Engl J Med 1992;325:928, 1008.

Ransohoff DF, Gracie WA: Treatment of gallstones. Ann Intern Med 1993;119:608.

Rustgi A: Hereditary GI polyposis and non-polyposis syndromes. N Engl J Med 1994;331:1694.

Sjögren MH: Serologic diagnosis of viral hepatitis. Med Clin North Am 1996;80:929.

Sleisenger MH, Fordtran JS (eds): GI Disease: Pathophysiology, Diagnosis, Management, 6th ed. Philadelphia, WB Saunders, 2002.

Sontag SJ: The medical management of reflux esophagitis: Role of antacids and acid inhibition. Gastroenterol Clin North Am 1990;19:683.

Steer ML, Waxman I, Friedman S: Chronic pancreatitis. N Engl J Med 1995;332:1580.

Tong MJ, El-Farra NS, Reikes AR, et al: Clinical outcomes after transfusion-associated hepatitis C. N Engl J Med 1995;232:1463.

Walsh JH, Peterson WL: Treatment of *Helicobacter pylori* infection in the management of peptic ulcer disease. N Engl J Med 1995;333:984.

Warshaw AL, Fernandez-Del Castillo C: Pancreatic carcinoma. N Engl J Med 1992;326:455.

Wilcox CM, Monkemuller KE: Review article: The therapy of GI infections associated with AIDS. Aliment Pharmacol Ther 1997;11:425.

Zakim D, Boyer TD (eds): Hepatology, 2nd ed. Philadelphia, WB Saunders, 1990.

Part VIII
Infectious Diseases

Craig J. Hoesley and Peter G. Pappas

MULTIPLE CHOICE

DIRECTIONS: For questions 1–53, choose the *single best* answer to each question.

QUESTIONS 1-3

A 48-year-old male farmer from Arkansas presents with a 6-week history of a slowly enlarging paranasal skin lesion, 10-pound weight loss, low-grade fever, and a nonproductive cough. He has no underlying medical illness. On examination he has a 6 × 4-cm right paranasal verrucous lesion that has a heaped-up, warty appearance with a violaceous hue. There is an area of central healing. A chest radiograph reveals a 5 × 4-cm right parahilar noncavitary mass lesion.

1. What is the most likely diagnosis?

   A. Squamous cell carcinoma
   B. Histoplasmosis
   C. Blastomycosis
   D. Tuberculosis
   E. Nocardiosis

2. A presumptive diagnosis in this patient can best be made through which of the following?

   A. Fungal serology
   B. Blood cultures
   C. Bronchoscopy with bronchoalveolar lavage and transbronchial biopsy
   D. Bacterial, fungal, and mycobacterial cultures of the skin lesion
   E. Skin biopsy with special stains for fungi and acid-fast bacilli

3. Which therapy should be initiated in this patient?

   A. Isoniazid, rifampin, and pyrazinamide
   B. Itraconazole
   C. Amphotericin B
   D. Sulfisoxazole
   E. Radiation therapy to the paranasal and lung lesion

QUESTIONS 4 AND 5

A 30-year-old HIV-infected man presents with a 5-day history of altered mental status and fever of 38.5° C (101.3° F). He has no history of an AIDS-defining opportunistic infection. The patient is currently not on antiretroviral therapy. On physical examination, the patient is obtunded but without focal neurologic findings. There is no meningismus. A CT scan of the brain reveals no mass lesions and no hydrocephalus. A lumbar puncture reveals an opening pressure of 270 cm H_2O, 8 WBCs (100% lymphocytes), 5 RBCs, protein of 85 mg/dL, and glucose of 53 mg/dL. The India ink is positive, and the cryptococcal antigen is 1:512.

4. Initial management of this patient should include:

   A. Immediate ventriculostomy
   B. Flucytosine, 150 mg/kg/day
   C. IV amphotericin B, 0.7 mg/kg/day
   D. Intrathecal amphotericin B, 1 mg/day
   E. Fluconazole, 200 mg/day orally

5. The patient responds to therapy with improved cognitive function and lysis of fever. Long-term management of this patient should include:

   A. Chronic suppression with oral fluconazole
   B. Amphotericin B, 0.6 mg/kg daily for 6 weeks, and then observe off therapy
   C. Repeat lumbar puncture at 4-week intervals, and continue daily amphotericin B until cryptococcal antigen titers are 1:8 or less
   D. Weekly IV amphotericin B, 1 mg/kg
   E. Intermittent amphotericin B or fluconazole for evidence of clinical relapse

QUESTIONS 6 AND 7

A 32-year-old African-American man presents with dysuria and a thick, purulent urethral discharge 3 days after unprotected sexual intercourse with a new female partner. The patient denies any other similar episodes, but he admits to heterosexual promiscuity.

6. What is the most useful initial diagnostic test in this patient?

    A. Venereal Disease Research Laboratories (VDRL)
    B. Urinalysis
    C. Urethral Gram stain
    D. Chlamydial antigen assay
    E. Culture for *Neisseria gonorrhoeae*

7. A urethral Gram stain reveals multiple polymorphonuclear cells and numerous intracellular gram-negative diplococci. What is the most appropriate therapy?

    A. Amoxicillin, 3 g, and probenecid, 1 g PO, followed by doxycycline, 100 mg bid for 7 days
    B. Ceftriaxone, 125 mg IM, followed by doxycycline, 100 mg bid for 7 days
    C. Ciprofloxacin, 500 mg PO, followed by doxycycline, 100 mg bid for 7 days
    D. Procaine penicillin, 4.8 million units IM, followed by doxycycline, 100 mg bid for 7 days
    E. Both B and C are acceptable.

QUESTIONS 8–10

A 44-year-old male engineer from India presents with a 2-week history of fever and right upper quadrant pain. The patient lives in the United States but visits his family in Bombay annually, and he returned from a visit 5 weeks ago. The patient denies illness while in India, but he admits to a recent 7-pound weight loss. Physical examination reveals a chronically ill-appearing man with fever (38.3° C [100.9° F]) in moderate distress. There is moderate right upper quadrant tenderness and moderate hepatomegaly but no splenomegaly. There are no other physical findings. An abdominal ultrasonogram reveals a noncalcified 7 × 6-cm solitary mass in the right hepatic lobe. A plain radiograph of the abdomen is normal.

8. Each of the following are possible causes for his current symptoms and radiologic findings *except:*

    A. Hepatoma
    B. Pyogenic liver abscess
    C. Amebic liver abscess
    D. Echinococcal cyst
    E. Metastatic carcinoma

9. The study that is most likely to be helpful in this patient is:

    A. Serum hepatitis B surface antigen
    B. Stool ova and parasites
    C. Serology of *Echinococcus multilocularis*
    D. Serology of *Entamoeba histolytica*
    E. Needle aspiration of hepatic lesion for Gram stain, culture, and cytology

10. Stool ova and parasites are negative; a serum indirect hemagglutination assay for *E. histolytica* is positive 1:256. Appropriate therapy includes:

    A. Needle aspiration and drainage of the abscess
    B. Metronidazole, 750 mg three times a day for 10 days, then diloxanide furoate
    C. Tetracycline, 250 mg four times a day for 10 days, then diiodohydroxyquin
    D. Clindamycin, 800 mg three times a day for 10 days, then paromomycin
    E. Thiabendazole

QUESTIONS 11 AND 12

A 59-year-old man from rural Louisiana is admitted to the hospital in early September with a 1-day history of a frontal headache, stiff neck, generalized myalgias, and confusion. His past medical history is significant for poorly controlled diabetes mellitus, hypertension, and chronic renal insufficiency. His family reports the patient has spent the summer outdoors, primarily tending to his garden and fishing in local lakes. Physical examination revealed fever (39°C [102.2° F]), meningismus, and altered mental status. A nonenhanced CT of his brain revealed only mild atrophy. A lumbar puncture was performed revealing an opening pressure of 120 cm H_2O, 80 white blood cells (90% lymphocytes), protein of 85 mg/dl, and an elevated cerebrospinal fluid glucose concentration commensurate with an elevated plasma glucose value.

11. What is the most likely diagnosis?

    A. Lyme disease
    B. Rocky Mountain spotted fever
    C. Neurosyphilis
    D. Pneumococcal meningitis
    E. West Nile virus encephalitis

12. What is the most appropriate therapy for this disorder?

    A. Doxycycline, 100 mg twice a day
    B. Penicillin G, 2 million units IV every 4 hours
    C. Ceftriaxone, 2 g IV every day
    D. Acyclovir
    E. Supportive therapy

QUESTIONS 13–15

A 45-year-old man sustained a gunshot wound to the abdomen, leading to a hemicolectomy, partial jejunal resection, and splenectomy. He is placed on ampicillin, gentamicin, and clindamycin preoperatively. He becomes afebrile on postoperative day 2, but fever develops again on day 6 to 39° C (102.2° F) without an apparent source. The patient is clinically stable. Peripheral WBC count is 19,500/μL with a left shift. A subclavian vein central venous catheter has been present since surgery. A chest radiograph is negative. Blood, urine, and abdominal wound drainage cultures are obtained.

13. What is the best approach to anti-infective therapy at this time?

    A. Add vancomycin to current regimen.
    B. Add fluconazole to current regimen.
    C. Add ceftazidime to current regimen.
    D. Stop current regimen, and begin aztreonam and vancomycin.
    E. Stop all antibiotics.

14. The patient remains clinically stable but persistently febrile. There are no new clinical findings, and peripheral leukocytosis persists. Two of four blood cultures drawn 48 hours earlier are positive for yeast. What is the most appropriate intervention?

    A. Replace central venous catheter over a guidewire; do not add antifungal therapy.
    B. Replace central venous catheter at a new site; begin antifungal therapy.
    C. Do not manipulate central venous catheter; begin antifungal therapy.
    D. Begin antifungal therapy; schedule patient for abdominal CT scan.
    E. The blood cultures represent contamination; no intervention is necessary.

15. *Candida glabrata* is isolated from two blood cultures. Which of the following is the best therapy in this clinical situation in a patient with normal renal function?

    A. Fluconazole, 400 mg/day
    B. Amphotericin B, 0.6 mg/kg/day
    C. Amphotericin B, 0.6 mg/kg/day, plus flucytosine, 150 mg/kg/day
    D. Amphotericin B, 0.6 mg/kg/day, plus fluconazole, 400 mg/day
    E. No specific antifungal therapy is necessary.

QUESTIONS 16–18

Five months after exposure to a household case of active pulmonary tuberculosis, a 28-year-old HIV-positive man presents with fever, chills, rash, weight loss, and nonproductive cough for 2 weeks. A CD4 count 3 months ago was 380 cells/mm³. A chest radiograph reveals basilar interstitial infiltrates without cavities, adenopathy, or pleural effusion. A purified protein derivative (PPD) test with controls reveals cutaneous anergy.

16. Which of the following is the most likely explanation for this illness?

    A. *Pneumocystis carinii*
    B. Cytomegalovirus (CMV)
    C. *Toxoplasma gondii*
    D. *Streptococcus pneumoniae*
    E. *Mycobacterium tuberculosis*

17. The patient is placed empirically on parenteral cefotaxime, erythromycin, and trimethoprim/sulfamethoxazole. Five days later, fever and nonproductive cough continue, pulmonary infiltrates have progressed, and the patient is clinically worse. What is the most appropriate intervention?

    A. Begin empirical therapy with IV ganciclovir.
    B. Add IV pentamidine; stop trimethoprim-sulfamethoxazole (TMP-SMX).
    C. Begin empirical amphotericin B.
    D. Begin empirical therapy with an antituberculosis regimen; schedule bronchoscopy.
    E. Schedule open lung biopsy; continue current regimen.

18. A bronchoalveolar lavage specimen reveals numerous acid-fast bacilli. What is the appropriate therapeutic intervention?

    A. Begin clarithromycin, ethambutol, and amikacin.
    B. Begin isoniazid and rifampin.
    C. Begin four-drug antituberculous therapy.
    D. Begin six-drug antituberculous therapy.
    E. Await culture results, and then start specific therapy.

QUESTIONS 19 AND 20

A 20-year-old sexually active female college student presents with vaginal irritation, scant discharge, and odor for 1 week. There is no dysuria. She denies any history of sexually transmitted diseases.

19. Which of the following is the most likely cause of her current complaints?

    A. Primary genital herpes
    B. *Trichomonas* vaginitis
    C. *Candida* vaginitis
    D. Gonococcal cervicitis
    E. Bacterial vaginosis

20. A vaginal examination reveals a thin, grayish discharge with an unpleasant odor, no genital lesions, and minimal cervical friability. Analysis of vaginal secretions reveals the following: pH of 6.5, scant leukocytes, 3+ clue cells, and positive "whiff" test with addition of potassium hydroxide. No trichomonads or yeasts are seen microscopically. What is the likely causative organism(s)?

    A. *Chlamydia trachomatis*
    B. Herpes simplex virus
    C. *Neisseria gonorrhoeae*
    D. Mixed infection with *Gardnerella vaginalis,* anaerobes, and mycoplasmas
    E. *Ureaplasma urealyticum*

QUESTIONS 21 AND 22

A 69-year-old man with mild dementia is noted to have a serum VDRL titer of 1:16 and a positive fluorescent treponemal antibody (FTA) test. The remainder of his evaluation is negative, including cerebrospinal fluid (CSF) analysis, which reveals normal protein and glucose, fewer than five leukocytes, and a negative CSF VDRL. There is no history of prior treatment for syphilis.

21. What is the most appropriate therapy?

    A. Aqueous penicillin G, 20 million units IV for 14 days
    B. Procaine penicillin, 600,000 units IM daily for 14 days
    C. Benzathine penicillin, 2.4 million units IM weekly for three doses
    D. Ceftriaxone, 2 g IV daily for 10 days
    E. No therapy is necessary.

22. If the patient was allergic to β-lactamase antimicrobials, what would be the best alternative therapy?

    A. TMP-SMX, 160/800 mg twice daily for 30 days
    B. Ciprofloxacin, 500 mg twice daily for 30 days
    C. Erythromycin, 500 mg four times a day for 14 days
    D. Doxycycline, 100 mg twice daily for 28 days
    E. Azithromycin, 2 g single dose

QUESTIONS 23–25

An otherwise healthy 33-year-old man plans to join the Peace Corps and will be assigned to Thailand for 2 years. He is leaving in approximately 6 months and has come to your clinic requesting pre-travel advice and recommendations regarding vaccination. On questioning, he states that all of his vaccinations are "up to date" but cannot provide any specifics as to when he received these vaccinations.

23. Which of the following is not a recommended vaccination in this patient?

    A. Hepatitis A
    B. Hepatitis B
    C. Yellow fever
    D. Tetanus
    E. Oral polio vaccine

24. Which would be the most appropriate antimalarial prophylaxis provided he spends the majority of his time in the urban areas of Thailand?

    A. Doxycycline, 100 mg daily
    B. Chloroquine, 300 mg weekly
    C. Fansidar weekly
    D. Mefloquine, 250 mg weekly
    E. No malaria prophylaxis is necessary provided he remains in urban areas of Thailand.

25. Other suggestions for this patient would include each of the following *except:*

A. Avoid undercooked seafood, raw vegetables, and unbottled drinks.
B. Avoid sexual intercourse, especially without the use of a condom.
C. Consider pre-exposure rabies vaccination.
D. Begin ciprofloxacin, 500 mg daily, on entering the country to prevent traveler's diarrhea.
E. If travel to rural areas occurs, use mosquito netting and diethyltoluamide (DEET).

QUESTIONS 26–28

A 63-year-old man with chronic obstructive pulmonary disease (COPD) presents to your office with a temperature as high as 39.2° C (102.5° F) for 3 days, nonproductive cough, headache, abdominal pain, and diarrhea. He has a history of chronic alcoholism but no other underlying medical problems. On examination, he appears toxic; blood pressure is 110/70 mm Hg, heart rate is 95 beats/minute, respiratory rate is 32 breaths/minute, temperature is 38.6° C (101.6° F). Chest examination reveals bilateral rales in the posterior lower lung fields. Chest radiograph demonstrates bilateral patchy lower lobe infiltrates, no effusion, and normal heart size. Laboratory results are as follows:

WBC count	18,600/μL; 90% polymorpho-nuclear leukocytes (PMNs); 10% bands
Hematocrit (Hct)	35%
Arterial blood gases (room air):	
pH	7.49
Po$_2$	52 mm Hg
Pco$_2$	28 mm Hg
Sodium	132 mg/dL
Potassium	4.7 mg/dL
Chloride	110 mg/dL
Bicarbonate	28 mg/dL
Sputum Gram stain (induced)	3+ PMNs, rare mixed organisms

26. What is the most likely cause of this condition?

    A. *Pseudomonas aeruginosa*
    B. *M. tuberculosis*
    C. *Legionella pneumophila*
    D. *Haemophilus influenzae*
    E. Influenzavirus A

27. What is the most appropriate initial therapy for this patient?

    A. Ceftriaxone and azithromycin
    B. Levofloxacin and nafcillin
    C. Isoniazid and rifampin
    D. Vancomycin and gentamicin
    E. Oseltamivir

28. Which of the following is most likely to be diagnostic in this case?

    A. Routine sputum culture
    B. Blood cultures
    C. Urine for *Legionella* antigen
    D. Sputum acid-fast bacillus smear and culture
    E. Nasopharyngeal swab for viral culture

QUESTIONS 29–32

A 28-year-old woman presents with fever for the past 8 weeks. She admits to low back pain and a 10-pound weight loss but has no other complaints. She is otherwise healthy. On physical examination, she has a prominent holosystolic murmur heard best at the apex with radiation to the axilla. No diastolic murmur is heard. There is no rash, and the results of the remainder of the examination are normal. Laboratory results are as follows:

Hct	32%
WBC count	5200/μL; 72 PMNs , 8 bands, 17 lymphocytes, 3 monocytes
Erythrocyte sedimentation rate	81 mm/hour
Electrolytes	Within normal limits
Urinalysis	2+ RBCs, 1+ protein, 0 WBCs, Gram stain negative

29. What is the most appropriate diagnostic test at this time?

    A. Blood cultures
    B. Transthoracic echocardiogram
    C. Transesophageal echocardiogram
    D. Serology for Lyme disease
    E. Abdominal CT scan

30. A diagnosis of endocarditis is established based on clinical findings and positive blood cultures. Which of these organisms is most likely in this patient?

    A. *Staphylococcus aureus*
    B. *Escherichia coli*
    C. Group B *Streptococcus*
    D. Coagulase-negative *Staphylococcus*
    E. *Streptococcus sanguis*

31. There is no history of cardiac disease. What is the most likely underlying valvular disorder?

    A. Atrial septal defect
    B. Mitral valve prolapse with regurgitation
    C. Bicuspid aortic valve
    D. Mitral stenosis
    E. No underlying valvular disorder

32. Which of the following would be most appropriate initial therapy in this patient assuming a fully susceptible organism?

    A. Imipenem and gentamicin
    B. Nafcillin
    C. Vancomycin
    D. Penicillin G
    E. Ceftriaxone and gentamicin

QUESTIONS 33 AND 34

A 65-year-old man is hospitalized for elective surgery. Seven days after discharge, the patient develops fever (38° C [100.4° F]). Physical examination at that time demonstrates a new holosystolic murmur at the cardiac apex, but there are no cutaneous stigmata of infective endocarditis. Blood cultures are positive for S. aureus susceptible only to vancomycin. A transthoracic echocardiogram (TTE) is normal.

33. What is the next step in the management of this patient?

    A. Re-admit the patient to the hospital and administer IV vancomycin alone.
    B. Re-admit the patient to the hospital and administer IV vancomycin and gentamicin.
    C. Re-admit the patient to the hospital, order a transesophageal echocardiogram (TEE), and administer IV vancomycin and gentamicin.
    D. Repeat blood cultures in the outpatient setting and follow clinically.
    E. Placement of long-term intravenous access in outpatient setting and initiate IV linezolid.

34. A TEE was performed and revealed a 1.0-cm vegetation on the mitral valve. Which of the following complications of infective endocarditis would necessitate surgical intervention with valve replacement?

    A. Persistently positive blood cultures after 7 days of appropriate antimicrobial therapy
    B. Congestive heart failure
    C. Recurrent embolic events despite appropriate antimicrobial therapy
    D. Echocardiographic evidence of a large perivalvular abscess
    E. All of the above

35. A 38-year-old man with long-standing HIV infection and an absolute CD4 cell count of 15 cells/mm³ wishes to discontinue all antiretroviral therapy secondary to intolerance and diminishing virologic response. He will continue to comply with certain medications (trimethoprim-sulfamethoxazole and azithromycin) in an effort to prevent opportunistic infections. Which of the following HIV-associated neurologic disorders will be unlikely in this patient?

    A. AIDS dementia complex
    B. Progressive multifocal leukoencephalopathy (PML)
    C. Peripheral sensory polyneuropathy
    D. Primary central nervous system (CNS) B-cell lymphoma
    E. *Toxoplasma gondii* brain abscesses

36. A 17-year-old high school student has recently experienced fever, pharyngitis, and a positive throat culture for *Streptococcus pyogenes*. He was given oral penicillin VK for 10 days and returns without symptoms. He states that he took most of his medication. A repeat throat culture is positive again. What is the most appropriate action?

    A. No intervention is necessary.
    B. Give an additional 10-day course of penicillin VK to the patient because he is clearly noncompliant.
    C. Administer azithromycin, 1 g.
    D. Administer ceftriaxone, 250 mg.
    E. Administer penicillin VK to other family members to prevent secondary cases.

37. The majority of immunocompetent individuals who are acutely infected with cytomegalovirus experience:

    A. Hepatitis
    B. Lymphadenopathy
    C. Heterophil-negative mononucleosis
    D. Fever and debilitating fatigue
    E. No symptoms

38. Hand-foot-and-mouth disease and herpangina are most commonly caused by strains of:

    A. Group A coxsackievirus
    B. Group B coxsackievirus
    C. Echoviruses
    D. Herpes simplex virus
    E. Adenoviruses

39. The gram-negative organism that is the *least* likely cause of infective endocarditis (IE) on a native valve is:

    A. *Cardiobacterium hominis*
    B. *Haemophilus aphrophilus*
    C. *Escherichia coli*
    D. *Eikenella corrodens*
    E. *Actinobacillus actinomycetem comitans*

40. All of the following persons are at increased risk of skin colonization with *S. aureus except*:

    A. Patients on hemodialysis for chronic renal failure
    B. IV drug abusers

C. Insulin-dependent diabetes
D. Patients with atopic dermatitis
E. IgA-deficient patients

41. A 26-year-old male student complains of abdominal cramps, belching, excess flatus, and watery diarrhea for 6 weeks after a 1-month tour of Russia. He describes no fever but has lost 12 pounds. Which of the following organisms likely explains his symptoms?

    A. *Cryptosporidium parvum*
    B. *Giardia lamblia*
    C. Enterotoxigenic *E. coli*
    D. *Salmonella enteritidis*
    E. *Shigella sonnei*

42. Which of the following antimicrobial agents is *not* associated with increased anticoagulation among patients receiving warfarin?

    A. Rifampin
    B. Sulfonamides
    C. Chloramphenicol
    D. Cefotetan
    E. Isoniazid

43. Which of the following statements about pneumococcal pneumonia are *not* true?

    A. Most cases are not bacteremic.
    B. The most important virulence factor is penicillin resistance.
    C. Risk factors include sickle-cell disease, multiple myeloma, and HIV infection.
    D. Untreated mortality may exceed 20%.
    E. The mechanism of penicillin resistance for *S. pneumoniae* is alteration in penicillin binding proteins.

44. Established pathogens among human mycoplasmas include each of the following *except*:

    A. *Mycoplasma hominis*
    B. *M. fermentans*
    C. *M. urealyticum*
    D. *M. lipophilums*
    E. *M. penetrans*

45. What is the most common cause of community-acquired meningitis in adults?

    A. *Haemophilus influenzae*
    B. *Neisseria meningitis*
    C. *Streptococcus pneumoniae*
    D. Group A *Streptococcus*
    E. *Staphylococcus aureus*

46. Which of the following *Salmonella* species is most likely to cause endarteritis?

    A. *S. enteritidis*
    B. *S. typhi*
    C. *S. paratyphi*
    D. *S. cholerae-suis*
    E. *S. hirschfeldii*

47. Which of the following *Bartonella* species is the most common cause of endocarditis?

    A. *B. bacilliformis*
    B. *B. quintana*
    C. *B. henselae*
    D. *B. elizabethae*
    E. *B. vinsoni*

48. Which of the following statements concerning *M. tuberculosis* is *not* true?

    A. Sputum cultures may remain positive for weeks after effective therapy.

B. Among patients with untreated cavitary pulmonary disease, a negative sputum smear for acid-fast bacilli is unusual.

C. Extrapulmonary tuberculosis is rare in HIV-infected individuals.

D. Lifelong risk of clinical tuberculosis is less than 10% in HIV-negative, skin test–positive patients.

E. HIV-infected patients with clinical tuberculosis generally do not require chronic suppressive antimycobacterial therapy after effective treatment.

49. Which statement about Q fever (*Coxiella burnetii*) is *true*?

A. It is a worldwide pathogen.

B. Most patients present with acute pneumonia syndrome.

C. Inhalation of spores leads to infection.

D. Rash is characteristic of Q fever.

E. Endocarditis occurs in men with preexisting valve disease.

50. Which of the following antiviral agents is/are not effective for the treatment of CMV retinitis?

A. Acyclovir

B. Ganciclovir

C. Foscarnet

D. Cidofovir

E. All are effective.

51. Which of the following syndromes is the most common presentation for CMV disease in a recent renal transplant recipient?

A. Mononucleosis-like illness

B. Pneumonia

C. Encephalitis

D. Hepatitis

E. Chorioretinitis

52. Diseases associated with Epstein-Barr virus (EBV) include all of the following *except*

A. Heterophil-positive mononucleosis

B. Nasopharyngeal carcinoma

C. Chronic fatigue syndrome

D. B-cell lymphoma in transplant recipients

E. Burkitt's lymphoma

53. Which is the *least* efficient means of HIV transmission from an HIV-infected patient?

A. Accidental needle exposure

B. Heterosexual intercourse

C. Receptive anal intercourse

D. Deep kissing

E. Active anal intercourse

TRUE OR FALSE

DIRECTIONS: For questions 54–91, decide whether each statement is true or false. Any combination of answers, from all true to all false, may occur.

54. A 38-year-old black man with long-standing sarcoidosis and pulmonary fibrosis presents with a 2-week history of cough, hemoptysis, low-grade fever, and weight loss. He has been on corticosteroids intermittently for the past 10 years but none in the past 2 months. On physical examination, he appears chronically ill and has diffuse inspiratory rales. A chest radiograph reveals apical pulmonary fibrosis with bilateral apical lesions compatible with aspergillomas (mycetomas). Which of the following statements regarding his disease is/are *true*?

A. Life-threatening hemoptysis may occur in the absence of surgical removal of the involved lobes.

B. Systemic amphotericin is warranted to eradicate the mycetomas.

C. Spontaneous regression occurs in 50% of mycetomas.

D. The diagnosis of mycetoma is primarily radiographic.

E. Itraconazole has proven efficacy in the treatment of pulmonary mycetoma.

55. The following are characteristic complications of infection with *Plasmodium falciparum*:

A. Acute renal failure

B. Diarrhea

C. Pulmonary edema

D. Coma

E. Pancreatitis

56. The clinical manifestations of brucellosis include:

A. Subclinical infection, particularly among children living in endemic areas

B. Marked splenomegaly

C. Sacroiliitis

D. Nephrotic syndrome

E. Undulating or intermittent fever pattern

57. The following are characteristic of *Listeria monocytogenes* infection:

A. Ingestion of contaminated food is the source of most human infection.

B. Pregnant women account for 30% of all listeriosis cases.

C. The incubation period for invasive listeriosis averages 30 days.

D. *L. monocytogenes* is the most common cause of bacterial meningitis in persons 60 years of age or older.

E. Serologic testing (antibody to listeriolysin O) is the most effective means of diagnosing listeriosis.

58. Risk factors for the development of reactivation infection with *M. tuberculosis* include:

A. Race

B. Malnutrition

C. Silicosis

D. Chronic renal failure

E. Age

59. Poor prognostic indicators among patients with cryptococcal meningitis include the following:

A. Obtundation

B. High CSF cryptococcal antigen titer

C. Underlying immune deficiency

D. Headache

E. CSF WBC count greater than 20 cells/mm^3

60. Which of the following statements about Hansen's disease (leprosy) are true?

A. Hansen's disease is highly contagious to household contacts.

B. *M. leprae* is easily cultivated in laboratory media.

C. Lepromatous leprosy may result from a selective T-lymphocyte unresponsiveness to *M. leprae* antigen.

D. Palpable peripheral nerves are usually found in patients with lepromatous leprosy.

E. Large numbers of organisms are characteristic in lesions of polar tuberculoid leprosy.

61. The differential diagnosis of pelvic inflammatory disease includes the following:

    A. Appendicitis
    B. Hemorrhagic ovarian cyst
    C. Ectopic pregnancy
    D. Ovarian torsion
    E. Endometriosis

62. Which of the following organisms have been commonly linked to acute and chronic salpingitis?

    A. *Neisseria gonorrhoeae*
    B. *Chlamydia trachomatis*
    C. *Bacteroides* species
    D. Aerobic gram-negative rods
    E. *Staphylococcus aureus*

63. The following are complications associated with salpingitis:

    A. Infertility
    B. Ectopic pregnancy
    C. Ovarian cysts
    D. Chronic pelvic pain
    E. Abnormal uterine bleeding

64. The following are characteristic of disseminated gonococcal infection:

    A. Mostly occurs in females
    B. Diffuse pustular rash, usually with more than 100 lesions
    C. Organisms usually seen in Gram stain of joint fluid
    D. Most patients culture negative
    E. May cause rapidly progressive IE

65. Which of the following statements are true about human ehrlichiosis?

    A. Most cases are tick borne.
    B. There are at least two *Ehrlichia* species that cause human disease.
    C. The disease is at least as severe as Rocky Mountain spotted fever.
    D. The disease is particularly common in the western United States.
    E. Tetracycline or doxycycline is the drug of choice.

66. Combination antimicrobial therapy is warranted under the following circumstances:

    A. Uncomplicated viridans streptococcal endocarditis
    B. Enterococcal endocarditis
    C. Fever in the neutropenic patient
    D. *S. aureus* bacteremia resulting from contaminated central venous catheter
    E. *E. coli* bacteremia complicating pyelonephritis

67. Which of the following statements regarding infection with *Bordetella pertussis* are *true*?

    A. Nonimmune household contacts contract the disease less than 50% of the time.
    B. Vaccination and/or natural infection confer lifelong immunity.
    C. Marked peripheral lymphocytosis is characteristic of acute infection.
    D. Protracted convalescent stage sometimes lasting 3 months is common.
    E. Treatment with erythromycin in the paroxysmal stage clearly ameliorates symptoms and shortens the duration of the disease.

68. Which of the following are *true* regarding human infection with *Francisella tularensis*?

    A. Ticks are a major vector.
    B. Pneumonia may result from skinning or eviscerating an infected rabbit.
    C. Infection may mimic disease caused by *Sporothrix schenckii*.
    D. Diagnosis is usually based on isolates from blood cultures.
    E. Ceftriaxone is the drug of choice for systemic disease.

69. The following are characteristic of nocardiosis:

    A. Underlying host usually has impaired humoral immunity.
    B. Nocardiosis is associated with multiloculated brain abscesses.
    C. Isolation from sputum may occur in the absence of radiographic or clinical disease.
    D. Multiple organ involvement is common, especially in immunocompromised hosts.
    E. Sulfur granules are often seen in clinical specimens from involved sites.

70. The following should receive influenza vaccine routinely:

    A. Persons aged 65 years or older
    B. Physicians, nurses, and other health care workers
    C. Nursing home residents
    D. Solid organ transplant recipients
    E. Anyone wishing to reduce the risk of influenza

71. Which of the following *Plasmodium* species have a chronic intrahepatic stage?

    A. *P. malariae*
    B. *P. ovale*
    C. *P. vivax*
    D. *P. falciparum*

72. A traveler returning from West Africa has fever, severe headache, and anemia. A diagnosis of falciparum malaria is made. The following are appropriate therapies:

    A. Chloroquine
    B. Mefloquine
    C. Quinine
    D. Halofantrine
    E. Pyrimethamine plus sulfadoxine

73. The following cytokines are frequently associated with induction of fever:

    A. Tumor necrosis factor-α
    B. Interleukin-1
    C. Interleukin-6
    D. Interferon-α
    E. Interferon-β

74. The following are increased as an acute-phase response:

    A. C-reactive protein
    B. Ceruloplasmin
    C. α_1-Antitrypsin
    D. Albumin
    E. Ferritin

75. The following conditions are associated with a significantly increased risk of serious bacterial infection:

    A. Splenectomy
    B. IgG deficiency
    C. Hairy cell leukemia
    D. Deficiency of complement factors C1, C2, and C4
    E. Neutropenia (PMNs < 1000 cells/μL)

76. Which of the following statements concerning nosocomial infections are *true*?

    A. *Candida* species are the fourth leading cause of nosocomial bloodstream infections.
    B. Urinary tract infections are the most common nosocomial infections.
    C. Overall, *Pseudomonas aeruginosa* is the most common cause of nosocomial infection.
    D. Wound infections are most commonly caused by *S. aureus*.
    E. The attributable mortality of nosocomial pneumonia exceeds 50%.

77. Which of the following are major criteria in the diagnosis of acute rheumatic fever?

    A. Arthritis
    B. Carditis
    C. Erythema marginatum
    D. Subcutaneous nodules
    E. Fever

78. Ticks are important vectors in the transmission of the following organisms:

    A. *Rickettsia akari*
    B. *Rickettsia rickettsii*
    C. *F. tularensis*
    D. *Coxiella burnetii*
    E. *Rickettsia prowazekii*

79. The following are characteristic of bacterial vaginosis:

    A. pH of 4.5
    B. Clue cells
    C. Odor with potassium chloride
    D. Sheets of PMNs
    E. White curd

80. Which of the following statements are true concerning the acute urethral syndrome?

    A. Pyuria is always present.
    B. Bacterial colony counts are usually less than 104/mL of voided urine.
    C. *C. trachomatis* is a common cause.
    D. Fever and dysuria are common symptoms.
    E. *S. saprophyticus* is a common cause.

81. Which of the following statements regarding gonococcal infections are *true*?

    A. Gonococcal urethritis is the most common form of urethritis in adult males.
    B. Most women with gonococcal cervicitis are symptomatic.
    C. Nucleic acid amplification tests are less sensitive than conventional cervical culture diagnostic methods.
    D. Disseminated gonococcal infection occurs in about 1% of adults with gonorrhea.
    E. A first episode of gonococcal salpingitis leads to infertility in about 50% of women.

82. The following statements concerning Lyme disease are correct:

    A. The disease is transmitted person to person.
    B. Dermatologic findings are the most common.
    C. Cardiac involvement is early and is associated with heart failure.
    D. Amoxicillin or doxycycline for 21 days is an effective regimen for early disease.
    E. An effective vaccination for Lyme disease is available.

83. The following agents are fungistatic:

    A. Amphotericin B
    B. Nystatin
    C. Ketoconazole
    D. Fluconazole
    E. Itraconazole

84. The following individuals are at enhanced risk for disseminated histoplasmosis:

    A. Infants
    B. All HIV-positive individuals
    C. Solid organ transplant recipients
    D. Chronic alcoholics
    E. Individuals with COPD

85. The following statements about coccidioidomycoses are *true*:

    A. Most cases of primary disease are asymptomatic.
    B. The most common pulmonary complication is progressive fibrocavitary disease.
    C. Serology is unhelpful in diagnosis.
    D. Pregnant women are at increased risk of disseminated disease.
    E. Risk of disseminated disease is higher among certain ethnicities.

86. The following statements about cryptococcosis are *true*:

    A. The disease is restricted to North America, Western Europe, and Africa.
    B. All patients with extrapulmonary disease have a measurable immunologic disorder.
    C. It is the most common fungal CNS infection.
    D. Patients with pulmonary disease require surgical resection.
    E. A positive cryptococcal antigen in the CSF is diagnostic for CNS disease.

87. For the following forms of aspergillosis there is good clinical evidence to support the efficacy of systemic antifungal therapy:

    A. Pulmonary aspergillomas
    B. Otitis externa
    C. Chronic necrotizing aspergillosis
    D. Disseminated aspergillosis
    E. Allergic alveolitis

88. Which of the following statements about *Pneumocystis carinii* are *true*?

    A. Only HIV-infected patients with low CD4 lymphocytes (<200 cells/mm^3) are at risk for *Pneumocystis carinii* pneumonia (PCP).
    B. Pneumothorax is a common complication of PCP.
    C. Glucocorticosteroids are warranted in selected patients with PCP.
    D. TMP-SMX is the treatment of choice for acute disease.
    E. Clinicians can consider withdrawing primary prophylaxis against *Pneumocystis carinii* in HIV-infected patients with a sustained response to potent HIV therapy (CD4 > 200 cells/mm^3 with stable low plasma HIV RNA levels).

89. Which of the following neoplasms are associated with an increased incidence among HIV-infected patients?

    A. Anal carcinoma
    B. Hodgkin's disease
    C. Non-Hodgkin's lymphoma
    D. Nasopharyngeal carcinoma
    E. Cervical carcinoma

90. The following characteristics are consistent with the severe acute respiratory syndrome (SARS):
    A. The etiologic agent is a novel coronavirus.
    B. Geographic range of documented outbreaks is limited to Asia.
    C. Suggestive laboratory features include lymphopenia and thrombocytopenia.
    D. Attributable mortality is greater than 50%.
    E. Hospital infection control measures include isolation of patients in negative pressure rooms.

91. The following are potential complications related to highly active antiretroviral therapy:
    A. Cholelithiasis in patients receiving indinavir
    B. Anemia in patients receiving zidovudine
    C. Hyperlactatemia in patients receiving zidovudine
    D. Altered mental status in patients receiving efavirenz
    E. Stevens-Johnson syndrome in patients receiving nevirapine

MATCHING

DIRECTIONS: Questions 92–172 are matching questions. For each numbered item, choose the most likely associated item from those provided. Within each set of questions, each answer may be used once, more than once, or not at all.

Match the organism and the characteristic genital ulceration:

    A. Herpes simplex virus
    B. *Treponema pallidum*
    C. *Haemophilus ducreyi*
    D. *Calymmatobacterium granulomatis*

92. Extensive painless ulceration in the groin with pseudobuboes

93. Painless ulceration with induration

94. Painful shallow ulcerations with associated systemic symptoms, including headache, nausea, vomiting, and fever

95. Painful undermined ulceration with soft edges and associated buboes

Match the retroviruses with the appropriate clinical description.

    A. Human T-cell leukemia virus (HTLV)-1
    B. HTLV-2
    C. HIV-1
    D. HIV-2

96. AIDS-like illness geographically restricted to West Africa, India, and, rarely, Western Europe

97. Tropical spastic paraparesis

98. Adult T-cell leukemia/lymphoma

99. Affects 20 to 40% of childbearing women in certain regions of sub-Saharan Africa

Match the virus with the syndrome described.

    A. Yellow fever
    B. Dengue
    C. Sin nombre
    D. Lassa

100. Adult respiratory distress syndrome and hypotension in a resident of Utah

101. Hemorrhagic complications and severe disease more likely in previously infected persons

102. Person-to-person transmission well documented

103. Fever, jaundice, and gastrointestinal bleeding in a severely ill man returning from the Amazon region.

Match each of the nontuberculous mycobacteria (NTM) with the appropriate description.

    A. *M. avium-intracellulare*
    B. *M. kansasii*
    C. *M. marinum*
    D. *M. abscessus*
    E. *M. gordonae*

104. Most common cause of NTM lymphadenitis

105. Rapidly growing NTM; may cause cutaneous, pulmonary, or disseminated disease

106. Cutaneous ulcer in a fisherman

107. Pulmonary infection resembles *M. tuberculosis,* but therapy is isoniazid, rifampin, and ethambutol for 18 months

108. Rarely a human pathogen, usually indicative of environmental contamination.

Match the following defects in host immunity with the most appropriate infectious complication.

    A. Neutropenia
    B. Decreased cell-mediated immunity
    C. Immunoglobulin A deficiency
    D. Complement deficiency
    E. Asplenia

109. *L. pneumophila* in a renal transplant patient

110. Severe babesiosis

111. Chronic giardiasis

112. Recurrent meningococcal disease

113. Hepatosplenic candidiasis

114. Overwhelming pneumococcal bacteremia

115. *P. aeruginosa* bacteremia

Match the following trypanosomes with the correct clinical description.

    A. *T. brucei brucei*
    B. *T. brucei rhodesiense*
    C. *T. brucei gambiense*
    D. *T. cruzi*

116. Megaesophagus with achalasia, recurrent aspiration pneumonia

117. Winterbottom's sign followed by chronic encephalopathy

118. High temperature, rapid neurologic deterioration, evidence of disseminated intravascular coagulation

119. A nonhuman pathogen that causes wasting illness in cattle and wild animals

Match each arthropod-borne virus with the appropriate clinical description.

    A. Western equine encephalitis
    B. Eastern equine encephalitis
    C. St. Louis encephalitis
    D. California encephalitis

120. Likelihood of apparent disease is greatest in early childhood; overall mortality is 3 to 5%, mostly in children younger than age 5 years.

121. Likelihood of apparent disease increases with age; fatality rare in patients younger than 20 years, approximately 30% in patients 65 or older.

122. Epizootics in horses and exotic birds precede human epidemics; case fatality rate is 35 to 50%.

123. Disease affects younger individuals living in rural areas with close proximity to deciduous hardwood forest; case fatality rate less than 1%.

Match the rickettsial organism with the appropriate clinical or epidemiologic features.

    A. *Rickettsia conorii*
    B. *R. akari*
    C. *R. rickettsii*
    D. *R. typhi*
    E. *R. prowazekii*
    F. *C. burnetii*
    G. *Ehrlichia equi*

124. Humans are infected through body louse feces; symptoms recur years after primary illness.

125. This is associated with tache noire.

126. Rash is uncharacteristic.

127. This is associated with rodent reservoir, truncal rash, and moderate illness.

128. This is associated with mouse reservoir, papulovesicular rash, and self-limited illness.

129. This is associated with severe headache, history of tick exposure, petechial rash, and multisystem involvement.

Match the following organisms and the clinical syndrome.

    A. Enterotoxigenic *E. coli*
    B. *S. enteritidis*
    C. *S. sonnei*
    D. *S. typhi*
    E. *Campylobacter jejuni*
    F. *G. lamblia*

130. A 19-year-old man with crampy abdominal pain and watery diarrhea for 3 weeks after a camping trip.

131. A 42-year-old woman with a 2-day history of abdominal pain, watery diarrhea, and temperature of 100.5° F who just returned from a 7-day tour of Guatemala.

132. An 18-month-old boy with acute-onset bloody diarrhea, seizures, and temperature to 102°F who attends a daycare facility.

133. A 35-year-old woman with fever, abdominal pain, and constipation lasting 10 days who recently visited her family in a small village in Peru.

134. A 70-year-old woman with blood-streaked diarrhea, abdominal pain, hypotension, and positive blood cultures who has had no recent travel and lives alone.

Select the appropriate gram-positive organism for each of the clinical descriptions listed.

    A. *Erysipelothrix rhusiopathiae*
    B. *Actinomyces israelii*
    C. *Nocardia asteroides*

135. A 37-year-old male alcoholic with chronic necrotizing pneumonia involving the left lower lobe experiences erythema and fluctuation over the left lateral chest wall; this spontaneously drains purulent, non–foul-smelling material that contains a yellowish granular substance.

136. A 53-year-old female insulin-requiring diabetic has a recent history of right upper lobe pneumonia, which has resolved; she now presents with altered mental status and fever; CT brain scan reveals a left frontal multiloculated mass with surrounding brain edema.

137. A 63-year-old male butcher acquires a purplish, painful, somewhat indurated ulceration over his left index finger; there is no fever or systemic symptoms.

Select the primary immunodeficiency that is most consistent with each of the cases.

    A. Chronic granulomatous disease
    B. Job's syndrome
    C. Common variable immunodeficiency
    D. Absent C7
    E. IgA deficiency

138. A 23-year-old man with chronic giardiasis and recurrent sinusitis; total serum immunoglobulin levels are normal.

139. A 34-year-old woman with a second episode of meningococcal meningitis; her first episode was 2 years ago.

140. A 45-year-old man with chronic diarrhea and bronchiectasis; he was recently found to be hypogammaglobulinemic.

141. A 5-year-old boy with recurrent staphylococcal skin and pulmonary infections who presents with pain, swelling, and erythema in the left distal femur; radiographs of the femur reveal changes compatible with osteomyelitis.

142. A 30-year-old man with chronic eczema and recurrent staphylococcal abscesses.

For each of the clinical descriptions, select the most likely cause.

    A. *Angiostrongylus cantonensis*
    B. *Strongyloides stercoralis*
    C. *Ascaris lumbricoides*
    D. *Enterobius vermicularis*
    E. *Toxocara canis*

143. Hepatomegaly, fever, and eosinophilia in a 4-year-old

144. Pruritus ani in a 24-year-old mother of three small children

145. Intestinal obstruction in a 5-year-old boy

146. Eosinophilic meningitis after ingestion of undercooked snails

For each antimicrobial agent, select the potential associated toxicity.

    A. Gentamicin
    B. Acyclovir
    C. Imipenem
    D. Levofloxacin
    E. Ceftriaxone
    F. Doxycycline

147. Tendon rupture

148. Biliary sludge

149. Nonoliguric acute tubular necrosis

150. Seizures

151. Crystalline nephropathy

152. Photosensitivity

Match the following malaria parasite with the appropriate characteristic.

    A. *Plasmodium vivax*
    B. *P. falciparum*
    C. *P. malariae*
    D. *P. ovale*

153. High level of parasitemia associated with multiple-organ failure and high mortality

154. Chronic splenomegaly and nephrotic syndrome

155. No known chloroquine resistance

156. Sporadic reports of chloroquine resistance, generally a benign clinical cause

Match the following characteristics of staphylococci with the appropriate clinical condition.

    A. Preformed staphylococcal toxin
    B. Toxin produced after colonization/infection
    C. Coagulase-negative staphylococci
    D. Infection may occur after trauma

157. HIV-infected patient with pain and swelling in anterior thigh

158. Nausea and vomiting 6 hours after a picnic

159. Fever and a new cardiac murmur in a patient with a prosthetic aortic valve placed 1 month ago

160. Fever, hypocalcemia, and diffuse erythematous rash in patient with a wound infection

Match the following organisms with the appropriate description.

    A. *Bacillus anthracis*
    B. *S. schenckii*
    C. *Mycobacterium chelonae*
    D. *Blastomyces dermatitidis*
    E. *Leishmania tropica*
    F. *N. asteroides*

161. A 33-year-old male gardener with nodular lymphangitis involving the right dorsal hand and forearm

162. A 51-year-old female renal transplant recipient with painful erythematous nodules involving the left lower extremity

163. A 57-year-old female diabetic with a right lower lobe pulmonary infiltrate and multiple ring-enhancing lesions on brain CT

164. A 41-year-old male textile worker with 2 × 2-cm painless blade eschar over the left wrist

165. A 76-year-old male retired farmer with a right perihilar mass on chest roentgenogram and five large violaceous plaques on the face and hands

166. A 25-year-old Iranian man with a 3 × 4-cm painful ulceration with heaped-up borders over the left shoulder

Match the following parasites with the appropriate description.

    A. *Leishmania donovani*
    B. *T. gondii*
    C. *Taenia solium*
    D. *Schistosoma mansoni*
    E. *Strongyloides stercoralis*
    F. *T. canis*
    G. *Onchocerca volvulus*

167. Fever, significant eosinophilia, and rash in a 5-year-old boy

168. Massive hepatosplenomegaly and pancytopenia without eosinophilia in a 30-year-old Indian woman

169. Calcified intravascular and intracerebral lesions in an otherwise healthy 25-year-old Mexican man

170. A mononucleosis-like illness in an otherwise healthy 15-year-old girl

171. Abdominal pain, *E. coli* bacteremia, and respiratory failure in a 65-year-old man with steroid-dependent asthma

172. Chronic dermatitis and progressive blindness in a 45-year-old man from West Africa

Part VIII
Infectious Diseases
Answers

1. (C) *Discussion:* The most likely diagnosis is blastomycosis. The demographic features that favor this diagnosis include male gender, occupation, and residence in a high-incidence area. Clinically, the combination of pulmonary and cutaneous disease is consistent with the other diagnoses, but it is most typical of blastomycosis, in which concomitant involvement of lungs and skin occur in up to 60% of patients. Skin lesions may be confused with invasive squamous cell carcinoma, but the lesion described in the case is most characteristic of blastomycosis. Radiographic changes are nonspecific and highly variable, and pulmonary blastomycosis is often confused with primary or metastatic lung neoplasia. *(Cecil, Ch. 381)*

2. (E) *Discussion:* Serology for *Blastomyces dermatitidis* is insensitive and nonspecific and is of limited value in this patient. In addition, blood cultures are almost never positive in patients with blastomycosis. Fungal cultures are necessary for a specific diagnosis, but the 2 to 4 weeks required to isolate and identify the organism could result in a delay in therapy. A presumptive diagnosis can be made by sampling tissue from the skin lesion and demonstrating characteristic fungal organisms in the biopsy. Bronchoscopy might also yield similar results, but it is unnecessarily invasive in this patient. *(Cecil, Ch. 381)*

3. (B) *Discussion:* Both itraconazole and amphotericin B are effective therapy for blastomycosis. Clinical trials demonstrated that itraconazole, 200 to 400 mg daily for at least 6 months, is curative in 95% in patients with non–life-threatening, non–central nervous system disease. Thus, in most ambulatory patients with blastomycosis, itraconazole is the most appropriate initial therapy. *(Cecil, Ch. 381)*

4. (C) *Discussion:* Extrapulmonary cryptococcal disease occurs in about 5% of AIDS patients in the United States. For initial management of AIDS patients with cryptococcal meningitis, most clinicians would initiate IV amphotericin B and treat for 2 weeks before considering an oral alternative such as fluconazole. Flucytosine may be given in combination with amphotericin B but is not given alone. Intrathecal amphotericin B is usually not necessary to control cryptococcal meningitis. *(Cecil, Ch. 383)*

5. (A) *Discussion:* Cryptococcal meningitis in AIDS patients is almost never cured; thus, chronic suppressive therapy is necessary to maintain long-term remission. Oral fluconazole has been shown to be an effective agent for chronic suppression in AIDS patients with cryptococcal meningitis. It appears to have superior efficacy compared with weekly amphotericin B, and it is less toxic and is more easily administered. In 2001, the U.S. Public Health Service (USPHS) guidelines for the treatment of opportunistic infections state discontinuation of secondary prophylaxis (maintenance therapy) can be considered if the HIV-infected patient has successfully completed a course of initial therapy (e.g., IV amphotericin B for 2 weeks), remains clinically asymptomatic, and has a sustained (≥6 months) increase in the absolute CD4 T-cell count (100-200 cells/mm³) on highly active antiretroviral therapy (HAART). *(Cecil, Ch. 383)*

6. (C) *Discussion:* A urethral Gram stain is diagnostic of gonococcal urethritis in more than 90% of culture-positive, symptomatic males. Typical Gram stain findings include the presence of sheets of PMNs and both intracellular and extracellular gram-negative diplococci. *(Cecil, Chs. 345, 346)*

7. (E) *Discussion:* Single-dose ceftriaxone, 125 mg IM, or cefixime, 400 mg PO, are effective agents for the treatment of gonococcal urethritis, including infections caused by penicillinase-producing strains and chromosomally resistant strains of *N. gonorrhoeae*. Single-dose oral therapy with ciprofloxacin, levofloxacin, or ofloxacin are also highly effective against susceptible strains, but it should not be used to treat gonorrhea in Asia, island nations in the Pacific ocean, Hawaii, California, or other geographic areas where resistant gonococci are known to be present. Amoxicillin/probenecid and procaine penicillin are no longer appropriate empirical therapy for gonococcal urethritis because of the increasing prevalence of penicillinase-producing strains and *N. gonorrhoeae*. Doxycycline or another antichlamydial agent must be given in all cases of gonococcal urethritis because of the likelihood of coinfection with *C. trachomatis*. Ofloxacin has potential as a single agent for treatment of gonococcal and nongonococcal urethritis, but it is a very expensive alternative to conventional therapy. *(Cecil, Ch. 346)*

8. (D) *Discussion:* Hepatic echinococcosis is usually associated with a thick, calcified capsule that gradually enlarges over years. The calcified capsule is usually apparent on ultrasonogram and plain radiographs of the abdomen. Acute illness associated with hepatic echinococcosis usually relates to leakage or rupture of the cyst intraperitoneally, leading to acute fever, pain, and hypotension. Hepatoma, amebic abscess, pyogenic abscess, and metastatic carcinoma are more likely possibilities in this patient. *(Cecil, Chs. 300, 399, 401)*

9. (D) *Discussion:* The patient most likely has a hepatic abscess resulting from *E. histolytica*, given his recent history of travel to a hyperendemic area, subacute onset, and focal right upper quadrant findings. Amebic liver abscess usually involves the right hepatic lobe and is usually not associated with coexisting amebic dysentery. Serum antibodies to *E. histolytica* are positive in 99% of cases, and this is the most appropriate diagnostic test. If amebic serology is negative, needle aspiration of the mass for Gram stain, culture, and cytology would be appropriate. *(Cecil, Ch. 399)*

10. (B) *Discussion:* Metronidazole is the drug of choice for extraintestinal amebiasis because of its efficacy and tolerability. It may be given orally or intravenously for 5 to 10 days. Dihydroemetine is an alternative therapy but is more toxic and less efficacious. Intraluminal therapy with diloxanide furoate or paromomycin for 7 days should be given to all patients with extraintestinal disease. *(Cecil, Ch. 399)*

11. (D) *Discussion:* The patient's presentation is most consistent with meningoencephalitis. The West Nile virus, a flavivirus previously confined to the Old World, has become endemic in North America (over 8,000 U.S. cases in 2003). Virus transmission involves mosquitoes (*Culex* species) and wild birds, with mammals, including humans, functioning as incidental end-stage hosts. In endemic areas, there is a high rate of subclinical infection (60%) but older individuals, particularly those with comorbid conditions, are at a higher risk of experiencing the severe manifestations of infection. After being bitten by a mosquito, the incubation period lasts 1 to 6 days, followed by the abrupt onset of fever (38.3-40° C) and the development of drowsiness, frontal headache, ocular pain, myalgia, and pain in the abdomen and back. A rash may occur but is rare. Patients, particularly young children, may present with an undifferentiated febrile illness in the absence of CNS symptoms as well. Diagnosis can be made via the presence of IgM in serum or CSF. Viral RNA is detected in CSF by polymerase chain reaction in less than half of cases. The abrupt onset of symptoms is not consistent with neurosyphilis, and the patient's CSF formula is not consistent with pneumococcal disease. Currently, West Nile virus infection is significantly more common than western equine encephalitis in the United States. (*Cecil, Ch. 377*)

12. (E). *Discussion:* Currently, there is no specific therapy available for West Nile virus meningoencephalitis. Ribavirin has in vitro activity against West Nile virus but has not been clinically efficacious. The administration of immunoglobulin from populations with a high incidence of exposure to West Nile virus (e.g., Israel) is being studied. (*Cecil, Ch. 377*)

13. (A) *Discussion:* Given this patient's history, there is likely an infectious cause of fever and leukocytosis. The most likely possibilities include the development of a wound infection, an intra-abdominal abscess, or a central venous catheter–related infection. Stopping antibiotics is unreasonable at this juncture, and there is little evidence that changing to a different regimen or adding a broad-spectrum cephalosporin is useful. Furthermore, the empirical use of fluconazole in this setting is of no proven value. However, the addition of vancomycin to cover methicillin-resistant *S. aureus* and *S. epidermidis* and multiresistant *Enterococcus* seems reasonable while awaiting further culture and laboratory data. (*Cecil, Ch. 302*)

14. (B) *Discussion:* The patient has candidemia, perhaps related to the central venous catheter. Positive blood cultures for *Candida* species are always considered significant and require some form of antifungal therapy, either systemic amphotericin B or fluconazole. Therapy is usually given for 1 to 2 weeks beyond resolution of clinical findings associated with candidemia. In presumed IV catheter-related candidemia, removal of the catheter is important. If a central venous catheter is essential, then replacement at a different site is important. Guidewire replacement is associated with a higher rate of persistent candidemia. (*Cecil, Ch. 385*)

15. (B) *Discussion:* *C. glabrata* is relatively resistant to fluconazole; therefore, in patients with systemic infections as a result of this organism, amphotericin B is probably the antifungal agent of choice. Lipid-based amphotericin B preparations may be an option in patients with renal insufficiency or in those individuals intolerant of conventional amphotericin B, but they are costly. Caspofungin and voriconazole may be suitable options as well. Combination therapy with flucytosine is warranted for patients with disease unresponsive to amphotericin B alone. Combination therapy with amphotericin B and fluconazole is unproven for systemic fungal infections. (*Cecil, Ch. 385*)

16. (E) *Discussion:* The patient is moderately immunocompromised based on his depressed CD4 lymphocyte count but is not in a range (<200 cells/mm³) that is typical for patients with "classic" opportunistic infections in AIDS. Thus, *P. carinii*, CMV, and *T. gondii* are unlikely pathogens. Furthermore, his illness is rather subacute for pneumococcal pneumonia. His recent exposure to a household contact with pulmonary tuberculosis, the subacute nature of his illness, and the radiographic findings are quite con-

sistent with pulmonary tuberculosis in an HIV-infected patient. (*Cecil, Ch. 341*)

17. (D) *Discussion:* For the reasons given previously, empirical antituberculous therapy is appropriate and probably should have been started at presentation. Empirical antifungal therapy is not warranted at this time nor is empirical therapy for CMV. If the patient is unable to produce sputum, then bronchoscopy is warranted. An open lung biopsy should be reserved for when bronchoscopy has been unhelpful, and the patient's clinical status dictates this aggressive approach. (*Cecil, Ch. 341*)

18. (C) *Discussion:* Given the likelihood of pulmonary tuberculosis, most authorities recommend initial therapy with a four-drug regimen, including isoniazid, rifampin, pyrazinamide, and ethambutol or streptomycin. If a multiresistant organism is suspected based on clinical or epidemiologic data, then a six-drug initial regimen might be appropriate. (*Cecil, Ch. 341*)

19. (E) *Discussion:* The patient's history is most consistent with vaginitis, and the description of foul odor and vaginal irritation are characteristic of bacterial vaginosis. Primary genital herpes presents as painful genital lesions and often as a systemic illness. (*Cecil, Ch. 345*)

20. (D) *Discussion:* Bacterial vaginosis begins with the disappearance of the normal vaginal flora (hydrogen peroxide producing lactobacilli) and their replacement with *Gardnerella vaginalis*, several species of anaerobic bacteria, and mycoplasmas. The inciting event is often inapparent, but the disorder is much more common in sexually active women than in virgins, suggesting it is a sexually associated disorder. To date, bacterial vaginosis has not been proven to be sexually transmitted from one person to another. (*Cecil, Ch. 345*)

21. (C) *Discussion:* This patient appears to have latent syphilis, and standard therapy involves the administration of benzathine penicillin, 2.4 million units IM, in three doses given 1 week apart. Although there is a very small chance that the patient is suffering from neurosyphilis, the normal CSF formula and negative CSF VDRL argue against this. Most authorities would not treat for neurosyphilis. Because the patient has both a positive serum VDRL and FTA, these results cannot be considered as biologic false-positive results; and given no history of therapy, effective therapy for latent syphilis should be given. (*Cecil, Ch. 349*)

22. (D) *Discussion:* Among patients with histories of β-lactam antibiotic intolerance, doxycycline or erythromycin given for 4 weeks is the best alternative. More data support the use of doxycycline in this setting, although neither is an effective therapy for neurosyphilis. (*Cecil, Ch. 349*)

23. (C) *Discussion:* Yellow fever is not endemic to Asia; therefore, pre-travel vaccination is unnecessary. However, hepatitis A and B are hyperendemic in Asia and other developing countries; thus, vaccination is recommended. Oral polio vaccine is given as a "booster" to previously vaccinated adults traveling to developing countries because polio remains endemic in many parts of the world. Revaccination for tetanus is recommended for all adults every 10 years. (*Cecil, Chs. 300 and 375*)

24. (D) *Discussion:* Chloroquine and sulfadoxine-pyrimethamine (Fansidar)-resistant falciparum malaria exists in parts of Thailand, particularly rural areas. There are also mefloquine-resistant strains, but these are less common. Daily doxycycline is given to short-term travelers, but this seems impractical for a 2-year stay. Furthermore, residence in an urban area will significantly decrease the likelihood of malaria. (*Cecil, Ch. 392*)

25. (D) *Discussion:* Traveler's diarrhea occurs in as many as 50% of travelers to foreign countries; however, prophylaxis is generally unwarranted except for unusual circumstances. Therapy with ciprofloxacin is usually started at the onset of symptoms and continued for 3 to 5 days. Sexual intercourse is discouraged among travelers, particularly where the risk of HIV and hepatitis B exposure is significant. Rabies vaccination is also encouraged among travelers to developing countries where rabies among domestic animals remains common. (*Cecil, Chs. 300 and 330*)

26. **(C)** *Discussion:* This patient has classic legionnaires' disease, characterized by toxicity, nonproductive cough, gastrointestinal complaints, and diffuse abnormalities on chest examination and chest radiography. A negative sputum Gram stain and hypoxia are characteristic. COPD, alcoholism, and male gender are strong risk factors for legionellosis. (*Cecil, Ch. 307*)

27. **(A)** *Discussion:* Current guidelines for community-acquired pneumonia support broad coverage for "typical" and "atypical" bacterial pathogens. Thus, ceftriaxone (for "typical" pathogens such as *Streptococcus pneumoniae*) and a macrolide (e.g., erythromycin, azithromycin, or clarithromycin for "atypical" pathogens such as *Legionella pneumophila*) are probably the best selections. (*Cecil, Chs. 307 and 308*)

28. **(C)** *Discussion:* Urine antigen assay for *L. pneumophila* is the most sensitive diagnostic test available, but it is useful only for group 1. Special media and conditions are required for culture of *Legionella* species from sputum, and blood cultures are almost always negative. (*Cecil, Ch. 307*)

29. **(A)** *Discussion:* Persistent fever for 2 months and a significant cardiac murmur together with the laboratory abnormalities are most compatible with a diagnosis of infective endocarditis. Blood cultures are positive in more than 90% of patients without a history of antimicrobial therapy, and a negative culture would cast serious doubt on the diagnosis. Echocardiography should be part of the evaluation, but blood cultures are essential. (*Cecil, Ch. 310*)

30. **(E)** *Discussion:* Without a significant underlying medical illness and no other known risk factors for endocarditis, such as IV drug use or a prosthetic heart valve, the likeliest organisms are the viridans streptococci (*S. sanguis* is one of many viridans streptococci), which cause at least 50% of the cases of native valve endocarditis in nonparenteral drug users. (*Cecil, Ch. 310*)

31. **(B)** *Discussion:* Clinically, the patient has mitral valve endocarditis, and the most common underlying valvular abnormality that predisposes to endocarditis is mitral valve prolapse with an associated regurgitant murmur on examination. Most authorities recommend endocarditis prophylaxis for such patients before dental and other invasive procedures. An atrial septal defect (especially a secundum defect) is not a predisposing factor for endocarditis. (*Cecil, Ch. 310*)

32. **(E)** *Discussion:* Most viridans streptococci are quite susceptible to penicillin G, and 4 weeks of therapy with this alone is effective in most patients. However, newer data suggest that the combination of ceftriaxone and gentamicin for 2 weeks is quite effective in uncomplicated cases of endocarditis caused by penicillin-susceptible viridans streptococci. For viridans streptococci resistant or intermediately susceptible to penicillin, 4 weeks of ceftriaxone alone is also effective. (*Cecil, Ch. 310*)

33. **(C)** *Discussion:* Despite a negative TTE, infective endocarditis remains a serious diagnostic consideration in this scenario (e.g., *S. aureus* bacteremia, fever, and a newly detected heart murmur) and should be evaluated further with a TEE. Both TTE and TEE are highly specific tests (~98%), but the TEE has improved sensitivity (90-95%) when compared with the TTE (48-63%). Despite its antimicrobial resistance, methicillin-resistant *S. aureus* is not more virulent than methicillin-susceptible strains. The combination of vancomycin and gentamicin would allow for synergistic activity in

this bacteremic patient and is an appropriate choice. (*Cecil, Chs. 310 and 311*)

34. **(E)** *Discussion:* Patients with evidence of direct extension of infection to myocardial structures, prosthetic valve dysfunction, or congestive heart failure from infective endocarditis-induced valvular damage should, in most cases, undergo surgery. In addition, many cases of endocarditis caused by fungi or by gram-negative or resistant organisms require surgical management. Progression of disease or persistence of fever and bacteremia for 7 to 10 days in the presence of appropriate antimicrobial therapy may indicate the need for surgery, but other potential foci for infection must be ruled out. Surgical management should also be considered for patients with recurrent (two or more) embolic events or large vegetations (>10 mm) on echocardiography with one embolic event, although the data in these situations are less convincing. (*Cecil, Ch. 310*)

35. **(E)** *Discussion:* HIV is a neurotropic human retrovirus, and the array of neurologic complications with HIV is quite broad, ranging from self-limited aseptic meningitis seen with primary infection to profound dementia and debilitating myelopathy. The majority of patients with advanced HIV disease will have at least one neurologic complication of the disease, most commonly peripheral sensory polyneuropathy. Opportunistic infections involving the CNS may occur with advanced HIV disease (CD4 cells < 75 cells/mm^3), including CMV retinitis or myelitis, reactivation of Epstein-Barr virus infection manifesting as primary B-cell lymphoma involving the brain, PML secondary to JC virus infection, and reactivation of *T. gondii* infection manifesting as ring-enhancing brain lesions. Patients complying with primary or secondary prophylaxis against *Pneumocystis carinii* with trimethoprim-sulfamethoxazole (indicated with CD4 cell counts <200 cells/mm^3) will be at less risk of developing cerebral toxoplasmosis because the sulfa component of this drug is active against this pathogen. This patient's compliance with these preventive measures will not offer protection against the other neurologic disorders listed here. (*Cecil, Chs. 387 and 396*)

36. **(A)** *Discussion:* A repeat throat culture is unnecessary in this patient. Many patients with streptococcal pharyngitis remain culture positive after an adequate course of therapy with oral penicillin. There is no evidence that persistent culture positivity leads to acute rheumatic fever after an adequate course of therapy. (*Cecil, Chs. 308 and 309*)

37. **(E)** *Discussion:* Acute cytomegalovirus (CMV) infection in immunocompetent adults rarely results in clinically apparent disease. Acute CMV infection is the etiology in approximately 8% of persons presenting with an infectious mononucleosis syndrome (heterophil-negative mononucleosis). Symptomatic patients may experience malaise, chemical hepatitis, and low-grade fever. (*Cecil, Ch. 370*)

38. **(A)** *Discussion:* Hand-foot-and-mouth disease is an enteroviral illness causing vesicular stomatitis and exanthem of the extremities. It occurs most commonly in young children and is usually a benign illness, although there are sporadic reports of encephalitis and myocarditis. The disease is usually caused by strains of group A coxsackievirus and less commonly by group B coxsackieviruses and enterovirus 71. Herpangina is a painful enanthem of the posterior pharynx in young children and is characterized by tiny vesicular or ulcerative lesions surrounded by a larger zone of erythema. The disease is usually benign, and group A coxsackieviruses account for the majority of cases of herpangina. (*Cecil, Ch. 373*)

39. **(C)** *Discussion:* Gram-negative infective endocarditis resulting from common aerobic pathogens such as *E. coli, K. pneumoniae,* and *P. aeruginosa* is a rare disease except for two special circumstances: prosthetic valve endocarditis and IV drug use. Endocarditis resulting from fastidious gram-negative bacilli in the

HACEK group (*Haemophilus* species, *A. actinomycetem comitans, Cardiobacterium hominis, Eikenella corrodens,* and *Kingella* species) collectively is an important cause of native valve IE and is responsible for up to 5 to 10% of cases. Each of these organisms may be normal mouth flora. (*Cecil, Ch. 310*)

40. (E) *Discussion:* It is well documented that patients with chronic skin disorders and patients who undergo routine needle-stick injury (dialysis patients, insulin-dependent diabetics, and IV drug users) are at increased risk of skin colonization with *S. aureus.* There are no data to suggest that IgA-deficient patients are at similarly increased risk. (*Cecil, Ch. 311*)

41. (B) *Discussion:* The patient describes chronic diarrhea, weight loss, excessive flatus, belching, but no fever or other signs of systemic illness. These features are classic for chronic intestinal giardiasis. Diarrhea resulting from *E. coli, Salmonella* species, or *Shigella* species is usually acute, self-limited, and associated with fever. Cryptosporidiosis is usually associated with watery diarrhea, vomiting, and low-grade fever and may be difficult to distinguish from giardiasis. (*Cecil, Ch. 398*)

42. (A) *Discussion:* Rifampin is the only compound listed that is associated with decreased anticoagulation resulting from the increased metabolism of warfarin. (*Cecil, Ch. 302*)

43. (B) *Discussion:* The most important virulence factor for *S. pneumoniae* is its polysaccharide capsule. There are no definitive data suggesting that resistant strains are more virulent than penicillin-susceptible organisms, and the mechanism for penicillin resistance is alteration in penicillin binding proteins (as opposed to β-lactamase production). *S. pneumoniae* is the most common etiologic agent of community-acquired pneumonia, and risk factors include many underlying disorders (e.g., myeloma, HIV disease, and sickle-cell disease). (*Cecil, Ch. 308*)

44. (D). *Discussion: M. hominis, M. fermentans,* and *M. urealyticum* are genitourinary pathogens in sexually active persons causing urethritis in males and females and Bartholin's gland infection in women (esp. *M. hominis*). *M. penetrans* is seen in homosexually active men and may be an important immunomodulating infection. *M. lipophilum* is a commensal organism not associated with human disease. (*Cecil, Ch. 304*)

45. (C) *Discussion:* Among adults, *S. pneumoniae* continues to be the most common etiologic agent of meningitis, causing more than 60% of cases. The meningococcus is more common in adolescents and young adults. *H. influenzae* has almost vanished as an invasive pathogen in children where vaccination is available, and group A *Streptococcus* and *S. aureus* are uncommon causes of meningitis in any age. (*Cecil, Ch. 312*)

46. (D) *Discussion:* Worldwide, *S. typhi* and *S. enteritidis* are important forms of salmonellosis, but among non–*S. typhi* strains, *S. choleraesuis* is most commonly associated with bacteremia (about 50% of cases) and together with *S. typhimurium* is the likely cause of metastatic infections. Endothelial sites, especially the aorta, are common sites for extraintestinal involvement. (*Cecil, Ch. 325*)

47. (B) *Discussion: B. quintana,* the agent of trench fever, has been noted to cause endocarditis in homeless alcoholics. *B. elizabethae* and *B. vinsoni* have caused endocarditis rarely. *B. bacilliformis* is the cause of classic bartonellosis. *B. henselae* is most closely limited to cat-scratch disease and to bacillary angiomatosis and peliosis hepatitis in patients with AIDS. (*Cecil, Ch. 340*)

48. (C) *Discussion:* Among non-HIV infected patients with tuberculosis, about 15% will experience extrapulmonary involvement. Among HIV-infected patients, this percentage rises to about 50%. (*Cecil, Ch. 341*)

49. (D) *Discussion: C. burnetii* is a *Rickettsia*-like organism that is transmitted primarily through inhalation of infectious spores. Tick transmission is rare. It is a worldwide zoosis, and acute pneumonia is the most common presentation. Extrapulmonary (chronic Q fever) is manifest by chronic granulomatous hepatitis or chronic endocarditis, the latter occurring primarily in men with preexisting valvular heart disease. Rash may occur but is rare with Q fever. (*Cecil, Ch. 355*)

50. (A) *Discussion:* Ganciclovir, foscarnet, and cidofovir all have activity versus human CMV. Acyclovir has limited CMV activity; CMV does not have virus-specific thymidine kinase, an enzyme required for uptake and phosphorylation of acyclovir. (*Cecil, Chs. 358 and 370*)

51. (A) *Discussion:* CMV causes a variety of syndromes in organ transplant recipients. Most occur within the first 120 days after transplantation and include most commonly a self-limited mononucleosis-like illness. Severe end-organ disease may manifest as pneumonitis, encephalitis, hepatitis, and gastritis and require aggressive therapy. Chorioretinitis is a late and very infrequent complication of CMV infection in organ recipients and may be a more common manifestation in patients with advanced HIV infection (absolute CD4 cell count < 75 cells/mm³). (*Cecil, Ch. 379*)

52. (C) *Discussion:* Chronic fatigue syndrome is mistakenly associated with chronic EBV infection. There are no data to support this association. Classic mononucleosis, nasopharyngeal carcinoma, Burkitt's lymphoma, and post-transplant lymphoproliferative disorder are associated with EBV. (*Cecil, Ch. 371*)

53. (D) *Discussion:* HIV is primarily a sexually, parenterally, and perinatally transmitted virus. All forms of sexual intercourse are potentially risky, but receptive anal or vaginal intercourse are among the highest risk sexual behaviors. Needlestick exposure with a hollow-bore needle carries about a 1 in 300 risk of HIV transmission from an HIV-positive individual. Deep kissing has not been reported as a means of transmission. (*Cecil, Ch. 413*)

54. (A) True; (B) False; (C) False; (D) True; (E) False. *Discussion:* Massive hemoptysis is the most common serious complication of pulmonary mycetomas and may occur in up to 25% of patients. Surgical removal is required in such cases, although the timing of surgery remains controversial, particularly because gross hemoptysis tends to wax and wane. The diagnosis of mycetoma is usually radiologic, with an upper lobe mass occupying a preexisting cavity or bulla. The characteristic "crescent sign" is usually seen. Specific IgG antibodies to *Aspergillus* species are elevated in almost all cases. Spontaneous lysis may occur in up to 10% of cases. Neither parenteral amphotericin B nor itraconazole has proven efficacy in the treatment of pulmonary mycetoma. (*Cecil, Ch. 386*)

55. (A) True; (B) True; (C) True; (D) True; (E) False. *Discussion:* Falciparum malaria is the most severe type of malaria and is associated with a mortality of up to 10% in nonimmune untreated hosts. A number of complications may arise in association with acute infection with *P. falciparum,* the most ominous of which is the development of cerebral malaria. Patients with cerebral malaria may present with altered mental status (including coma), headache, and seizures. Noncardiac pulmonary edema or pulmonary edema resulting from profound anemia may occur. Acute renal failure from massive hemolysis (blackwater fever) may occur independently or concomitant with pulmonary failure. Severe diarrhea is also a common complication of falciparum malaria. Pancreatitis is not a characteristic complication of this disorder. (*Cecil, Ch. 392*)

56. (A) True; (B) False; (C) True; (D) False; (E) True. *Discussion:* More than 500,000 cases of human brucellosis are reported annually to the World Health Organization. *B. melitensis* infection, frequently acquired via the ingestion of goat's milk cheese, has been diagnosed in U.S. travelers to and immigrants from Mexico. Clinically, human brucellosis may be divided into four categories: subclinical illness, acute/subacute disease, relapsing infection, and chronic disease. Detected only by serologic testing, asymptomatic or clinically unrecognized human brucellosis often occurs in high-risk groups (e.g. slaughterhouse workers, farmers, veterinarians) and in children living in endemic areas. Acute brucellosis may occur as a mild transient illness (*B. canis* or *B. abortus*) or as a severe illness with multiple clinical manifestations (*B. melitensis*), including malaise, chills, fatigue, weakness, and a pattern of undulating or intermittent fever. At least 50% of patients will experience myalgias, anorexia, and weight loss. To a lesser extent, patients will experience arthralgias, cough, testicular pain, and blurry vision. Splenomegaly and lymphadenopathy may occur in 10 to 15% of patients. *Brucella* species may localize in almost any organ system but are most commonly localized to bone and joints (particularly the sacroiliac joint), the CNS, heart, lung, spleen, testes, liver, gallbladder, kidney, prostate, and skin. Up to 10% of patients with brucellosis relapse after antimicrobial therapy, usually within months of primary infection, but may occur as long as 2 years after seemingly successful treatment. Disease with duration of greater than 1 year has been termed *chronic brucellosis,* but this diagnosis is controversial and may simply be secondary to persistent or relapsing disease. Patients who carry a diagnosis of chronic brucellosis often complain of persistent fatigue but often do not have clinical, microbiologic, or serologic evidence of active disease, leading some to question the validity of this diagnosis. (*Cecil, Ch. 339*)

57. (A) True; (B) True; (C) True; (D) False; (E) False. *Discussion:* Outbreaks of listeriosis have been documented in association with contaminated coleslaw, milk, soft cheese, deli counter meats, smoked fish, and butter. Neonates and adults older than age 50 years have the highest infection rates. Pregnant women account for 30% of all listeriosis cases, and individuals with impaired cellular immunity (e.g., solid organ transplant recipients) are at increased risk of invasive disease. *L. monocytogenes* is a more common form of bacterial meningitis in patients receiving corticosteroids, transplant recipients, and patients with hematologic malignancies, but *S. pneumoniae* is still the more common etiology in all patients older than 60 years of age. The diagnosis of listeriosis is best made by routine bacterial culture of blood and/or cerebrospinal fluids. Of note, a Gram stain of the CSF in patients with *L. monocytogenes* meningitis will be positive in 40% of cases and is frequently misdiagnosed as "diphtheroids." (*Cecil, Ch. 335*)

58. (All True). *Discussion:* It is well known that advancing age, silicosis, and poor nutrition are significant risk factors in the development of reactivation tuberculosis. Recent observations suggest that patients on chronic hemodialysis and blacks are at higher risk for tuberculosis. (*Cecil, Ch. 341*)

59. (A) True; (B) True; (C) True; (D) False; (E) False. *Discussion:* There are several clearly defined risk factors for a poor outcome in cryptococcal meningitis, among them underlying immune dysfunction (especially HIV infection), absence of headache, altered mental status, high CSF and/or serum cryptococcal antigen titers, and a CSF WBC count of 20 cells/mm³ or less. Thus, in this disease, the absence of inflammation, as evidenced by a low CSF leukocyte count and absent headache, portend a poor outcome. (*Cecil, Ch. 383*)

60. (A) False; (B) False; (C) True; (D) True; (E) False. *Discussion:* In contrast to public perception regarding leprosy, the disease is not highly contagious, afflicting fewer than 5% of household contacts. *M. leprae* is not easily cultivated on artificial media in part because of its very slow growth rate. More severe disease (as

seen with lymphomatous leprosy) may in part be due to selective T cell unresponsiveness to important *M. leprae* antigens. As a neurotropic organism, palpable nerves are found in all stages of the disease but are particularly common in later stages. Polar tuberculoid leprosy is among the milder forms of the disease and is associated with very few organisms on biopsy specimens. (*Cecil, Ch. 343*)

61. (All True). *Discussion:* Pelvic inflammatory disease (PID) is most often a clinical diagnosis, but it is easily confused with other important entities. For this reason, many authorities quip that PID actually stands for "pretty inaccurate diagnosis." A clinical diagnosis of PID is accurate only 65 to 70% of the time based on laparoscopic studies. (*Cecil, Ch. 345*)

62. (A) True; (B) True; (C) True; (D) True; (E) False. *Discussion:* Traditionally, *N. gonorrhoeae* and *C. trachomatis* are linked to acute and chronic salpingitis, respectively. In addition, aerobic gram-negative rods and anaerobes have been isolated from the fallopian tubes of a substantial proportion of women with chronic salpingitis. *S. aureus* is rarely, if ever, associated with salpingitis. (*Cecil, Chs. 345, 346, and 354*)

63. (A) True; (B) True; (C) False; (D) True; (E) False. *Discussion:* The major complications associated with salpingitis include infertility and ectopic pregnancy. Indeed, approximately 15% of women with an episode of salpingitis will become infertile. Chronic pelvic pain is commonly associated with chronic salpingitis and may persist even after effective antimicrobial therapy. (*Cecil, Ch. 345*)

64. (A) True; (B) False; (C) False; (D) True; (E) True. *Discussion:* Disseminated gonococcal infection occurs predominantly in females; the majority have asymptomatic genital infections. The classic presentation is the development of characteristic pustular, necrotic lesions on the extremities. These are usually fewer than 20 in number. Patients may experience tenosynovitis as well. After this phase, many patients will experience monoarticular or pauciarticular arthritis, which is usually culture and Gram stain negative. The diagnosis is usually based on clinical findings. Rarely, an aggressive and rapidly destructive form of endocarditis may occur with fulminant disseminated gonococcal infection. (*Cecil, Ch. 346*)

65. (A) True; (B) True; (C) False; (D) False; (E) True. *Discussion:* Human monocytic ehrlichiosis (HME) has been described in the southern United States and is due to *E. chaffeensis,* an organism transmitted by the vector *A. americanum* (Lone Star tick). Human granulocytic ehrlichiosis (HGE) has been described in the northeastern United State, upper Midwest, and northern California and is caused by *Anaplasma phagocytophilia,* an organism transmitted by the tick vector *Ixodes scapularis.* Another organism, *E. ewingii,* has been the causative agent in immunocompromised patients with HGE in Arkansas. The disease resembles RMSF but is generally milder and is less commonly associated with a rash. The drug of choice for both forms of the disease is tetracycline (doxycycline). (*Cecil, Ch. 355*)

66. (A) True; (B) True; (C) True; (D) False; (E) False. *Discussion:* Combination antimicrobial therapy has proven efficacy in relatively few situations. In uncomplicated viridans streptococcal endocarditis, 2 weeks of therapy with gentamicin and penicillin is equivalent to 4 weeks of therapy with penicillin alone. Enterococcal endocarditis is virtually always treated with two agents: either penicillin or vancomycin plus an aminoglycoside. Fever in the neutropenic patient is empirically treated with two and often three compounds, although monotherapy with a broad-spectrum β-lactam agent is sometimes used. Uncomplicated *S. aureus* and *E. coli* bacteremia cases do not usually warrant combination therapy. (*Cecil, Chs. 302, 310, and 344*)

67. (A) False; (B) False; (C) True; (D) True; (E) False. *Discussion:* Pertussis is one of the more contagious respiratory infections, infecting 80% or more of nonimmune household contacts. Neither infection nor vaccination confer lifelong immunity, so that reinfection in previously vaccinated adults is not uncommon. Acute infection is often associated with marked lymphocytosis. Treatment with erythromycin is effective only in the early stages of infection, and the convalescent stage may last for several months. *(Cecil, Ch. 316)*

68. (A) True; (B) True; (C) True; (D) False; (E) False. *Discussion:* Tularemia may result from ingestion, inhalation, direct inoculation, or tick transmission of the etiologic agent *F. tularensis*. Pneumonia may result from aerosol exposure or bacteremic spread. A sporotrichoid form may result from direct inoculation or tick exposure. The organism is fastidious and hazardous to deal with. Although aminoglycosides remain the drug of choice, tetracycline is a reasonable alternative in milder disease; however, the relapse rate with tetracycline therapy is higher. *(Cecil, Ch. 332)*

69. (A) False; (B) True; (C) True; (D) True; (E) False. *Discussion:* Nocardiosis occurs most commonly in patients with impaired cellular immunity when multiple-organ involvement is common. CNS involvement is usually characterized by focal intracerebral lesions that may be multiloculated. Sulfur granules are typical of actinomycosis, not *Nocardia* infections. Isolation of *Nocardia* species from the sputum of immunocompetent individuals with chronic lung disease but without clinical or radiographic evidence of invasive disease constitutes colonization and may not need to be treated. *(Cecil, Ch. 338)*

70. (All True). *Discussion:* Influenza vaccine is safe, effective, and indicated in older individuals (≥50 years of age), nursing home residents, immunocompromised patients (including HIV-infected individuals), patients with comorbid illnesses (including diabetes mellitus, chronic pulmonary disease, renal insufficiency), all health care providers, and virtually anyone wishing to reduce the risk of influenza and its complications. *(Cecil, Ch. 363)*

71. (A) False; (B) True; (C) True; (D) False. *Discussion:* Among the four human malaria parasites, only *P. vivax* and *P. ovale* have chronic intrahepatic stages that require treatment with primaquine to prevent relapse. *(Cecil, Ch. 392)*

72. (A) False; (B) True; (C) True; (D) True; (E) False. *Discussion:* Chloroquine-resistant *P. falciparum* is now widespread in endemic areas, except for the Middle East and parts of Central America. Thus, a traveler returning from West Africa with falciparum malaria must be assumed to have chloroquine-resistant infection. For patients capable of taking oral medications, options include quinine plus doxycycline, atovaquone plus proguanil (Malarone), mefloquine, and halofantrine. For patients unable to take oral medications, options include IV quinidine or quinine. *(Cecil, Ch. 392)*

73. (All True). *Discussion:* Each of the cytokines listed may function as "endogenous pyrogens," sending signals to the hypothalamus, which may result in the up-regulation of core body temperature. *(Cecil, Ch. 296)*

74. (A) True; (B) True; (C) True; (D) False; (E) True. *Discussion:* The acute-phase response is the nonspecific response in serum proteins that occurs as a result of infection, trauma, acute and chronic inflammation, and neoplasia. There is a wide spectrum of proteins that increase in the acute-phase response, but albumin is usually diminished. *(Cecil, Ch. 297)*

75. (A) True; (B) True; (C) False; (D) False; (E) True. *Discussion:* Multiple conditions may lead to a "compromised host," and each condition may predispose an individual to increased risk of infection based on its effect on PMN number and function, cell-mediated immunity, immunoglobulin synthesis and function, and complement. Splenectomy and IgG deficiency are all associated with serious infections as a result of encapsulated organisms (*S. pneumoniae, N. meningitidis*), whereas neutropenia is associated with increased risk of infection to most bacteria, especially nosocomial organisms. Hairy cell leukemia predisposes to atypical mycobacterial infections, and deficiency of C1, C2, and C4 is usually unassociated with enhanced risk of infection. *(Cecil, Ch. 298)*

76. (A) True; (B) True; (C) False; (D) True; (E) False. *Discussion:* After *S. aureus,* coagulase-negative staphylococci, and enterococci, *Candida* species are the fourth leading cause of bloodstream infections. Urinary tract infections are the most common nosocomial infection (approximately 35%), but pneumonia has the most serious outcome; mortality is up to 30% from all causes. *S. aureus* is both the most common cause of wound infections (approximately 20%) and the most common nosocomial bacterial agent overall (approximately 13% of isolates). *(Cecil, Ch. 299)*

77. (A) True; (B) True; (C) True; (D) True; (E) False. *Discussion:* There are five major criteria for acute rheumatic fever: carditis, arthritis, subcutaneous nodules, erythema marginatum, and chorea. Fever is not a major criteria, but is almost always present at some time during the course of the illness; if untreated, it may continue for weeks. *(Cecil, Ch. 309)*

78. (A) False; (B) True; (C) True; (D) False; (E) False. *Discussion:* The agents of RMSF (*R. rickettsii*) and tularemia (*F. tularensis*) are transmitted by ticks, although not exclusively for *F. tularensis*. *C. burnetii* is an inhaled agent, although there is some evidence of tick transmission. *R. akari*, the agent of rickettsialpox, is transmitted by the mouse mite. *R. prowazekii*, the agent of epidemic typhus, is transmitted by the body louse. *(Cecil, Chs. 332 and 355)*

79. (A) False; (B) True; (C) False; (D) False; (E) False. *Discussion:* Bacterial vaginosis is a polymicrobial process characterized by overgrowth of vaginal anaerobes and *Gardnerella vaginalis*. The characteristic features are a thin, watery discharge, an amine "fishy" odor with potassium chloride, clue cells on microscopic examination, few WBCs, and a pH greater than 5.0. *(Cecil, Ch. 345)*

80. (A) True; (B) True; (C) True; (D) False; (E) True. *Discussion:* Acute urethral syndrome is characterized by frequency, dysuria, and pyuria. Low-colony-count (<104) bacterial infections are common, especially with *S. saprophyticus* and *E. coli*. Other common causes include *C. trachomatis* and herpes simplex virus. The presence of fever, although rare, suggests an upper urinary tract process. *(Cecil, Ch. 361)*

81. (A) False; (B) False; (C) False; (D) True; (E) False. *Discussion: Chlamydia* urethritis is by far more common than gonococcal urethritis in the developed world. At least 50% of women with gonococcal cervicitis are minimally symptomatic or asymptomatic. Cervical Gram stain is only approximately 50% sensitive. Nucleic acid amplification tests (e.g., ligase chain reaction or polymerase chain reaction assays) performed on urine or cervical specimens have enhanced diagnostic sensitivity when compared with standard cervical culture methods but are also more expensive. Disseminated gonococcal infection may be more common in women than men, typically occurs in conjunction with menses, and is estimated to occur in about 1% of infected persons. Infertility associated with a first episode of gonococcal salpingitis is about 15%. After three episodes, the incidence rises to 50% or more. *(Cecil, Ch. 346)*

82. (A) False; (B) True; (C) False; (D) True; (E) True. *Discussion:* Lyme disease is caused by infection with the spirochete *B. burgdorferi* and is transmitted to humans from infected ticks of the *Ixodes* family. The classic finding in early Lyme disease is erythema chromium migrans and is evident in 60 to 70% of patients. Cardiac involvement may occur within 5 to 6 weeks of initial infection but is characterized by conduction abnormalities. Treatment for early disease is either amoxicillin or doxycycline for 21 days and is curative in most patients. A vaccination is currently available and is recommended for those living in or traveling to hyperendemic areas where contact with ticks is likely to occur. (*Cecil, Ch. 352*)

83. **(A) True; (B) True; (C) False; (D) False; (E) False.**
Discussion: The polyenes are fungicidal, although the mechanism of action is unclear. All of the azoles are fungistatic. (*Cecil, Ch. 393*)

84. **(A) True; (B) False; (C) True; (D) False; (E) False.**
Discussion: Disseminated histoplasmosis is seen in infants; in patients with advanced HIV disease (absolute CD4 cell counts typically < 75 cells); in patients taking chronic glucocorticosteroids, including solid organ transplant patients; and in others with cell-mediated immune deficiencies. (*Cecil, Ch. 379*)

85. **(A) True; (B) False; (C) False; (D) True; (E) True.**
Discussion: About 60% of cases of primary coccidioidomycosis are asymptomatic. Among symptomatic cases, most develop as a self-limited atypical pneumonia syndrome or a flulike illness. Progressive fibrocavitary disease occurs in only about 1% of infected individuals. Persons at risk for disseminated disease include those with cell-mediated immune dysfunction (including HIV infection), pregnant women, and members of darker skinned races, especially Filipinos. Serology (complement fixation) is very helpful in establishing diagnosis and assessing response to therapy. (*Cecil, Ch. 380*)

86. **(A) False; (B) False; (C) True; (D) False; (E) True.**
Discussion: C. neoformans is a ubiquitous fungus, and cryptococcosis occurs worldwide. Although the majority of patients with extrapulmonary disease have a discernible immunologic defect, usually in cellular immunity, at least 20% have no underlying disorder. *C. neoformans* is the most common fungal CNS pathogen worldwide. Patients with pulmonary disease may require surgical resection but may also respond to antifungal therapy or observation. A positive cryptococcal antigen from CSF or serum is virtually diagnostic of cryptococcosis. There are very few false-positive assays. (*Cecil, Ch. 383*)

87. **(A) False; (B) False; (C) True; (D) True; (E) False.**
Discussion: Antifungal therapy is warranted for chronic necrotizing and invasive aspergillosis. Historically, systemic amphotericin B has been utilized for these disorders, but newer agents, including liposomal amphotericin B, voriconazole, and caspofungin, may also be efficacious. For aspergillomas and allergic alveolitis, there are no data to suggest routine antifungal therapy is warranted. External otitis is treated with topical antifungals. (*Cecil, Ch. 386*)

88. **(A) False; (B) True; (C) True; (D) True; (E) True.**
Discussion: Potentially, any patient with depressed cell-mediated immunity is at risk for PCP, including transplant recipients. Clinically, patients with AIDS and CD4 counts of less than 200 cells/mm^3 are at greater risk, but PCP occurs in certain patients with higher CD4 counts (200-300 cells/mm^3). Cavitary disease and pneumothorax are commonly seen with PCP. TMP-SMX remains the drug of choice for sulfa-tolerant patents. Glucocorticosteroids have been shown to improve survival and lead to more rapid recovery in patients with Po$_2$ 70 mm Hg or less. Primary or secondary prophylaxis against *Pneumocystis carinii* can be withdrawn in individuals with an appropriate and sustained (>3 months) response to anti-HIV therapy. (*Cecil, Ch. 387*)

89. **(A) True; (B) True; (C) True; (D) False; (E) True.**
Discussion: Anogenital carcinoma associated with oncogenic human papillomavirus types (e.g. HPV type 16) is seen with increased frequency in patients with AIDS. Likewise, the incidences of Hodgkin's disease and of non-Hodgkin's lymphoma are increased severalfold. Nasopharyngeal carcinoma is not known to be more common in AIDS patients. (*Cecil, Ch. 371*)

90. **(A) True; (B) False; (C) True; (D) False; (E) True.**
Discussion: In late 2002, many persons living in or visiting the southern Chinese province of Guangdong developed a severe respiratory illness later termed *severe acute respiratory syndrome* (SARS). The etiologic agent is believed to be a novel coronavirus. Coronaviruses are ubiquitous and cause illness in many animals, including pigs, cattle, dogs, cats, and chickens. Genetic changes occur frequently with these viruses, and it has been suggested that the SARS agent is a recombinant animal coronavirus that crossed species, leading to human infection. Virus transmission occurs via respiratory droplets. The incubation period is estimated to be 2 to 11 days, and typical clinical manifestations include fever greater than 38° C (100.4° F), rigor, dry cough, dyspnea, malaise, headache, and hypoxemia. Laboratory findings associated with the diagnosis include lymphopenia, thrombocytopenia, and an elevated lactate dehydrogenase level. Chest radiographs demonstrate progressive, bilateral air space disease. There is no definitive therapy for patients with SARS, but ribavirin has been suggested as a possible therapeutic option. Through April 2003, there were 3,389 documented SARS cases and 165 deaths (mortality rate of 4.9%) in 27 countries. The largest outbreaks to date have been in China, but smaller outbreaks have also been described in Canada. All patients with confirmed or suspected SARS should be placed in respiratory isolation, with the use of a negative pressure room if possible, along with other infection control measures, including the use of N95 masks, gloves, disposable gowns, and eye protection. (*Drosten, 1967; Kaziazek, 1953; Tsang, 1977*)

91. **(A) False; (B) True; (C) True; (D) True; (E) True.**
Discussion: Indinavir crystalluria occurs in 32 to 67% of patients receiving indinavir and may lead to nephrolithiasis in approximately 9% of patients. Indinavir, a protease inhibitor, also commonly causes an asymptomatic, reversible indirect hyperbilirubinemia but does not cause cholelithiasis. The nucleoside analogue reverse transcriptase inhibitors are capable of causing mitochondrial toxicity, resulting in asymptomatic hyperlactatemia or possibly severe metabolic lactic acidosis. The agents most commonly linked to this toxicity are stavudine, didanosine, and zidovudine. Zidovudine may also induce erythroid hypoplasia in the bone marrow, resulting in anemia in up to 7% of patients. The non-nucleoside reverse transcriptase inhibitors—efavirenz, nevirapine, and delavirdine—are also associated with certain adverse effects. Efavirenz may cause CNS symptoms in up to 53% of patients, including dizziness, insomnia, impaired concentration, somnolence, and hallucinations. These symptoms tend to abate after 2 to 4 weeks of continued use of the medication. Nevirapine-associated rash has been described in up to 7% of patients receiving the drug and, less commonly, Stevens-Johnson syndrome and toxic epidermal necrolysis have been linked to this medication. (*Cecil, Ch.421*)

92. **(D)**; 93. **(B)**; 94. **(A)**; 95. **(C)**. *Discussion:* Granuloma inguinale, caused by *C. granulomatis*, results in extensive local destruction, pseudobuboes, and marching progression. Syphilis, caused by *T. pallidum*, is classically associated with painless, indurated, solitary genital ulceration. Chancroid, caused by *H. ducreyi*, is typically associated with painful, nonindurated ulceration, often with multiple lesions and associated inguinal buboes. Primary genital HSV is associated with not only shallow painful ulcers but also systemic symptoms of headache, nausea, vomiting, and fever. (*Cecil, Chs. 347-349 and 369*)

96. **(D)**; 97. **(A)**; 98. **(A)**; 99. **(C)**. *Discussion:* HIV-2 is endemic in West Africa from whence it has spread to western Europe and India. It generally causes a milder illness than HIV-1

but can be quite virulent, causing full-blown AIDS. Human T-cell leukemia virus type 1 is associated with not only typical spastic paraparesis but also adult T-cell leukemia and lymphoma. HIV-1 is hyperendemic to parts of sub-Saharan Africa and afflicts up to 40% of childbearing women in some cities. HTLV-2 is an "orphan" virus with no true disease association, but it may also be associated with myelopathy. (*Cecil, Ch. 372*)

100. (C); 101. (B); 102. (D); 103. (A). *Discussion:* Hanta virus pulmonary syndrome was described in the Four Corners region of the United States and has been reported in other parts of the country. The virus is called sin nombre, or "without name." Dengue hemorrhagic fever is generally seen in previously infected patients infected with a different dengue strain. Lassa fever can be transmitted by airborne droplets and necessitates strict respiratory isolation. Yellow fever is a severe hemorrhagic fever characterized by hyperbilirubinemia, hemorrhagic complications, and death. (*Cecil, Ch. 376*)

104. (A); 105. (D); 106. (C); 107. (B); 108. (E). *Discussion:* Nontuberculous mycobacteria (NTM) are an increasingly important group of pathogens, particularly among immunocompromised individuals. Each of these organisms can cause disseminated disease or may be localized to one organ system. *M. avium-intracellulare* is the most common cause of NTM lymphadenitis. *M. marinum* exists in aquatic environments and may cause nodular lymphangitis. *M. kansasii* causes pulmonary disease similar to tuberculosis but requires prolonged three-drug therapy. *M. abscessus* is a rapidly growing NTM causing localized or disseminated disease in immunocompromised hosts. *M. gordonae* is usually an environmental contaminant, although occasionally it has been implicated in certain wound infections. (*Cecil, Ch. 342*)

109. (B); 110. (E); 111. (C); 112. (D); 113. (A); 114. (E); 115. (A). *Discussion:* Host immune abnormalities may include defects in cell-mediated immunity, humoral immunity, complement activity, qualitative or quantitative neutrophil dysfunction, and splenic abnormalities. Patients with asplenia (functional or surgical) are at risk for overwhelming sepsis as a result of encapsulated organisms such as the pneumococcus, meningococcus, and *H. influenzae*. Asplenic patients may also experience severe manifestations of babesiosis. Neutropenic patients are at risk for overwhelming sepsis caused by a number of bacteria and fungi, most notably aerobic gram-negative rods, *Staphylococcus* species, and *Candida* species. Patients with IgA deficiency may experience chronic and recurrent sinopulmonary infections but are also at risk for chronic intestinal infections caused by *G. lamblia*. Cell-mediated immune dysfunction is seen in solid-organ transplant recipients who are at risk for invasive protozoan, fungal, mycobacterial, and certain bacterial infections, including legionellosis. The classic presentation of patients with terminal complement deficiency is recurrent systemic infections with *Neisseria meningitidis*. (*Cecil, Ch. 298*)

116. (D); 117. (C); 118. (B); 119. (A). *Discussion:* African trypanosomiasis is divided into two forms: Rhodesian and Gambian sleeping sickness. *T. brucei rhodesiense* (East African trypanosomiasis) causes a much more acute encephalopathy. Surinam is the drug of choice for humans. West African trypanosomiasis (*T. brucei gambiense*) is characterized by a chronic debilitating course with mental deterioration and wasting; approximately 80% of affected persons will have painless supraclavicular and posterior cervical lymphadenopathy (Winterbottom's sign). *T. brucei brucei* is a nonhuman pathogen but causes a chronic wasting illness in African livestock. All three agents are transmitted by the bite of the tsetse fly. American trypanosomiasis (Chagas' disease) is caused by *T. cruzii* and transmitted by the reduviid bug. Chronic manifestations include dilated cardiomyopathy and megaesophagus. (*Cecil, Chs. 393 and 394*)

120. (A); 121. (C); 122. (B); 123. (D). *Discussion:* Arthropod-borne encephalitis viruses occur in summer and early fall. Mortality is unusual in patients with western equine encephalitis and California encephalitis. Mortality is common in eastern equine encephalitis (up to 50%) and increases with age among patients with St. Louis encephalitis (up to 30%). Apparent disease is inversely related to age in western equine encephalitis. (*Cecil, Ch. 377*)

124. (E); 125. (A); 126. (F); 127. (D); 128. (B); 129. (C). *Discussion:* Brill-Zinsser disease is the reactivation form of latent *R. prowazekii* infection characterized by mild typhus-like symptoms, often occurring years after initial infection. Tache noire is the characteristic eschar associated with Mediterranean spotted fever (boutonneuse fever, North African tick typhus), which is caused by *R. conorii*. Rash is not characteristic of Q fever, caused by *C. burnetii*. Murine typhus is a more benign illness than RMSF and is transmitted to humans via the rat flea. The rash of typhus begins in the trunk and face and spreads to the extremities. *R. akari* causes rickettsialpox, a benign illness characterized by a papulovesicular rash on the trunk and abdomen. RMSF, caused by *R. rickettsii*, is the most severe of the rickettsial illnesses and is associated with a 25% mortality in untreated cases. (*Cecil, Ch. 355*)

130. (F); 131. (A); 132. (C); 133. (D); 134. (B). *Discussion:* Giardiasis is frequently associated with outdoor activities and initially with abdominal pain, flatus, and watery diarrhea. Weight loss is common, but fever is almost always absent. Enterotoxigenic strains of *E. coli* are the most common cause of traveler's diarrhea and are usually not associated with severe illness. Fever, bloody diarrhea, and CNS complications are characteristic of shigellosis, especially in infants and toddlers. Several day care outbreaks of shigellosis have been reported. Typhoid is uncommon in the United States, and the majority of cases are imported by visitors from the developing world. Symptoms are severe; untreated mortality approaches 20%. The disease should be suspected in any returning traveler with abdominal pain, fever, diarrhea, or constipation. Salmonellosis is frequently implicated by bacteremia and systemic toxicity in very young and older individuals. (*Cecil, Chs. 324-327, 329, 330, and 398*)

135. (B); 136. (C); 137. (A). *Discussion: Actinomyces* species are a cause of chronic necrotizing pneumonia in debilitated patients. If untreated, this indolent process may spread by direct extension to involve extrapulmonary sites, including the vertebral bodies and ribs, and spontaneous discharge through the chest wall (empyema necessitatis) may occur. The diagnosis is made by isolation of the organism on artificial media in an anaerobic or microaerophilic environment, but a presumptive diagnosis can be made on the basis of clinical findings and the characteristic sulfur granules found at the involved site. *N. asteroides* is a cause of multiloculated brain abscess, and the infection usually occurs in compromised hosts. Cerebral involvement occurs with bacteremic spread from a distant site, usually the lungs. The disease is very uncommon in transplant patients and other immunocompromised individuals who receive chronic prophylaxis with TMP-SMX. The organism is aerobic and slow growing, but it can be isolated on routine, mycobacterial, and fungal media. *E. rhusiopathiae* is a small gram-positive rod that causes chronic cutaneous ulceration in persons exposed to livestock, fish products, shellfish, and uncooked meat. The organism is a ubiquitous zoonotic pathogen that rarely causes systemic disease in humans, although there are occasional reports of septicemia and endocarditis. The typical skin lesion is a violaceous, painful ulcer with surrounding edema but no lymphangitis. (*Cecil, Chs. 336-338*)

138. (E); 139. (D); 140. (C); 141. (A); 142. (B). *Discussion:* Although selective IgA deficiency is fairly common (as many as

1 in 400 persons), most patients remain completely healthy with no demonstrable clinical immunodeficiency. When symptoms develop, they are usually manifest as recurrent sinopulmonary infections. These patients may also experience chronic intestinal parasitosis. Hypersusceptibility to *Neisseria* infections is seen in patients with terminal complement (C7, C8, C9) deficiency. Patients with common variable immunodeficiency have a maturation arrest in globulin synthesis, leading to deficient total IgG serum levels. IgG subclass deficiency and IgA deficiency have been reported in this disorder. Patients experience an array of clinical manifestations, including recurrent sinopulmonary infections, septicemia, and gastrointestinal malabsorption from chronic enteric infections and a spruelike illness. Lymphoma develops in many of those patients who survive long term (years). Children with poor wound healing, recurrent skin and soft tissue staphylococcal infections, and chronic pulmonary infections should be evaluated for possible chronic granulomatous disease. This disorder is a manifestation of a functional polymorphonuclear abnormality in which organisms can be opsonized and ingested, but they are not killed intracellularly because of a defect in the production of superoxide. Job's syndrome is characterized by elevated IgE levels, impaired WBC chemotaxis, and recurrent "cold" staphylococcal abscesses. *(Cecil, Ch. 298)*

143. **(E)**; 144. **(D)**; 145. **(C)**; 146. **(A)**. *Discussion:* Visceral larva migrans is caused by the helminth *Toxocara canis* and occasionally by *Toxocara cati*. Visceral larva migrans occurs most commonly in children younger than age 6 years and is associated with fever, hepatomegaly, and eosinophilia. There is usually a history of pica and exposure to puppies or cats. *E. vermicularis* (pinworm) is worldwide in distribution and is usually seen among families with small children. This nematode infection is largely characterized by perianal and perineal pruritus caused by the migration and ovideposition of adult female worms in the perianal region. *A. lumbricoides* is the largest human nematode, reaching a length of up to 35 cm. It is the most common human helminthic infection, with an estimated worldwide prevalence of 1 billion. The most serious consequence of ascariasis in humans occurs in young children with heavy infections, in whom masses of worms may obstruct the lumen of the small intestine. Eosinophilic meningitis resulting from *A. cantonensis*, the rat lung worm, occurs when humans ingest undercooked snails and other mollusks. Ingested larvae penetrate the gut wall and migrate to the small vessels of the meninges, spinal cord, and eye. *(Cecil, Ch. 404)*

147. **(D)**; 148. **(E)**; 149. **(A)**; 150. **(C)**; 151. **(B)**; 152. **(F)**. *Discussion:* Aminoglycosides are capable of causing reversible acute tubular necrosis and irreversible vestibular toxicity. Precipitation of acyclovir in the kidney may lead to crystalline nephropathy; dehydration and higher doses of acyclovir increase the risk for this reversible adverse effect. Imipenem may cause seizures, particularly in patients with renal insufficiency. Tetracyclines, including doxycycline, may induce photosensitivity, making these agents problematic for individuals who work outdoors or as an agent for

malaria prophylaxis. Ceftriaxone administration may lead to precipitation in the biliary tract, leading to sludging and symptomatic disease. Quinolone administration rarely results in tendon rupture in humans and has been noted to cause arthropathy in animals. Quinolones and tetracyclines are contraindicated in children secondary to the potential for arthropathy and teeth staining, respectively. *(Cecil, Chs. 302 and 358)*

153. **(B)**; 154. **(C)**; 155. **(D)**; 156. **(A)**. *Discussion:* Four *Plasmodia* species are pathogenic in humans. Most deaths are due to *P. falciparum*, which is associated with high levels of parasitemia (>5%) and multiple organ failure. *P. vivax* is a generally benign form of malaria, and chloroquine resistance has been reported. Tropical splenomegaly and nephrotic syndrome have been associated with *P. malariae* (quartan malaria), and relapses are documented years after infection. *P. ovale* is also relatively benign, and there are no reports of chloroquine resistance. *(Cecil, Ch. 392)*

157. **(D)**; 158. **(A)**; 159. **(C)**; 160. **(B)**. *Discussion:* Staphylococcal pyomyositis occurs in the tropics and in HIV-infected individuals. The pathogenesis is unclear but probably relates to prior soft tissue trauma and/or percutaneous inoculation. Staphylococcal food poisoning results from ingesting preformed toxin contaminated from food colonized with *S. aureus*. Symptoms usually occur within 8 hours. Early prosthetic valve endocarditis (≤60 days from surgery) is usually due to coagulase-negative staphylococci, *S. aureus*, gram-negative rods, and diphtheroids. Toxic shock syndrome is caused by toxin-producing *S. aureus*, which elaborate toxic shock syndrome type 1 or related toxins in a colonized individual. Early reports were limited to menstruating women and related to tampon use, but most recent reports are associated with *S. aureus* infections elsewhere. *(Cecil, Ch. 311)*

161. **(B)**; 162. **(C)**; 163. **(F)**; 164. **(A)**; 165. **(D)**; 166. **(E)**. *Discussion:* Each of the organisms listed may cause the cutaneous ulcer syndrome. Because these disorders are similar in their clinical appearance and culture confirmation is often delayed or unavailable, a biopsy with special stains for acid-fast bacilli, fungi, and other likely organisms is appropriate. Finally, a detailed history is important to determine exposure risks. *(Cecil, Chs. 333, 338, 342, 381, 384, and 395)*

167. **(F)**; 168. **(A)**; 169. **(C)**; 170. **(B)**; 171. **(E)**; 172. **(G)**. *Discussion:* Fever eosinophilia and hepatomegaly are characteristic of visceral larva migrans caused by *T. canis*. Kala-azar is the disseminated, visceral form of leishmaniasis, especially *L. donovani*. Cysticercosis occurs in humans who become infected through ingestion of eggs of *T. solium* from contaminated food or water. Toxoplasmosis in a normal healthy person is usually asymptomatic, although a self-limited mononucleosis-like illness may occur. Abdominal pain, gram-negative bacteremia, and acute respiratory distress syndrome are classic complications of hyperinfection syndrome with *S. stercoralis*. One of the leading causes of blindness worldwide, onchocerciasis is usually first manifest as chronic dermatitis. *(Cecil, Chs. 395, 396, 401, 402, and 404)*

BIBLIOGRAPHY

Drosten C, Gunther S, Preiser W, et al: Identification of a novel coronavirus in patients with severe acute respiratory syndrome. N Engl J Med 2003;348:1967-1976.

Goldman L, Ausiello D (eds): Cecil Textbook of Medicine, 22nd ed. Philadelphia, WB Saunders, 2004.

Ksiazek TG, Erdman D, Goldsmith CS, et al: A novel coronavirus associated with severe acute respiratory syndrome. N Engl J Med 2003;348:1953-1966.

Tsang KW, Ho PL, Ooi GC, et al: A cluster of cases of severe acute respiratory syndrome in Hong Kong. N Engl J Med 2003;348:1977-1985.

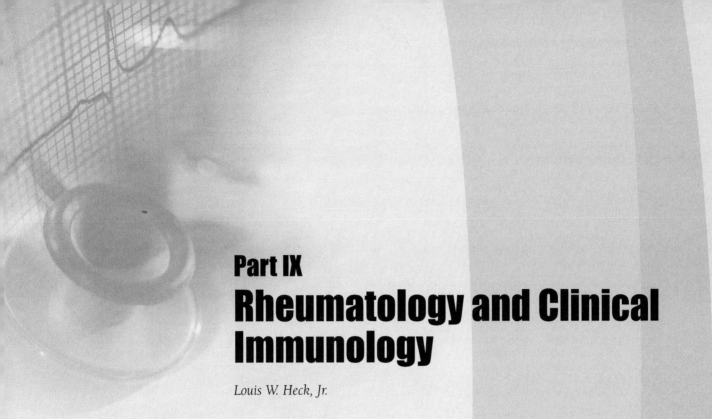

Part IX
Rheumatology and Clinical Immunology

Louis W. Heck, Jr.

MULTIPLE CHOICE

DIRECTIONS: For questions 1 to 26, choose the *single* best answer to each question.

1. A 43-year-old woman presents with a 3-year history of progressive rheumatoid arthritis that has been partially responsive to various nonsteroidal anti-inflammatory drugs (NSAIDs) and to low-dose oral corticosteroids. After the examination, you decide to treat her active arthritis with methotrexate, the most widely used and effective agent currently for rheumatoid arthritis. Some of the facts about methotrexate therapy to tell her include:

   A. Therapeutic effects are delayed so that clinical improvement is not generally seen for 3 to 6 weeks after initiation of treatment.
   B. Adverse effects may include oral ulcers, nausea, vomiting, pneumonitis, bone marrow suppression, and cirrhosis.
   C. Complete blood cell count (CBC), platelet count, alkaline phosphatase level, and aspartate aminotransferase (AST) level should be obtained every 8 to 12 weeks to monitor therapy.
   D. Birth control measures must be in use before methotrexate is started.
   E. All of the above.

2. A 54-year-old woman complains of severe right shoulder pain localized mainly to the mid humerus but also diffusely around the anterolateral shoulder. The onset was sudden and not precipitated by trauma. Physical examination reveals limited abduction with point tenderness over the subacromial bursa and the greater tuberosity of the

humerus. A radiograph reveals a linear calcific density in the supraspinatus tendon. All of the following statements are true *except*:

   A. Treatment consists of cortisone injection into the subacromial bursa, NSAIDs, and physical therapy.
   B. The calcific density is most likely calcium urate.
   C. The diagnosis could not be made by an arthrocentesis.
   D. Local tendon injury may be the major cause.

3. A 74-year-old woman complains of worsening left knee pain with weight bearing and ambulation. Examination of the knee reveals a small effusion without warmth, bony enlargement, and crepitus with flexion and extension of the knee. A diagnostic arthrocentesis is performed. Each of the following characteristics of the synovial fluid would be expected *except*:

   A. Pale yellow color
   B. Good viscosity
   C. Routine culture negative
   D. WBC count of 800/μL
   E. Glucose value of 22 mg/dL

4. A 42-year-old woman with seropositive rheumatoid arthritis has become disabled by pain and tightness behind the right knee. Physical examination reveals cystic swelling over the popliteal fossa and semimembranous tendon. Which of the following is the most appropriate next step?

   A. Arthrogram of the right knee
   B. Synovial biopsy of the right knee
   C. Ultrasound study of the right knee popliteal fossa
   D. Venogram of right lower extremity
   E. None of the above

5. All of the following conditions involve the distal interphalangeal (DIP) joint *except*:

    A. Multicentric reticulohistiocytosis
    B. Erosive osteoarthritis
    C. Psoriasis with nail changes
    D. Juvenile chronic arthritis
    E. Rheumatoid arthritis

6. Rheumatoid factor may be present in each of these conditions *except*:

    A. Adult Still's disease
    B. Subacute bacterial endocarditis
    C. Vasculitis syndromes
    D. Sarcoidosis
    E. Sjögren's syndrome

7. An 82-year-old woman was hospitalized for treatment of congestive heart failure. She experienced a warm, painful right knee on the third hospital day. The most appropriate procedure would be:

    A. Blood cultures followed by IV antibiotics
    B. Arthrocentesis for diagnostic/therapeutic purposes
    C. IV administration of colchicine
    D. Allopurinol
    E. Ultrasound study of right knee, including popliteal fossa

8. A 46-year-old man on hemodialysis for 12 years complains of insidious onset of painful nocturnal dysesthesias involving the thumb and three fingers, relieved by shaking the hand. Physical examination of the hand reveals thenar wasting and numbness over the fingers. Each of the following statements is true *except*:

    A. Deposits of β_2-microglobulin AH (amyloidosis associated with hemodialysis) amyloid compressing the median nerve could produce these findings.
    B. An entrapment neuropathy could explain these findings.
    C. Paresthesias involving the radial side of the thumb, second, third, and fourth fingers suggest compression of the medial nerve.
    D. Carpal tunnel syndrome could explain these findings.
    E. Deposits of amyloid of the primary type AL (amyloidosis associated with light chains) would be typical.

9. Ophthalmologic manifestations of rheumatoid arthritis may include all of the following *except*:

    A. Secondary Sjögren's syndrome with sicca complex
    B. Scleritis
    C. Episcleritis
    D. Corneal melts
    E. Ischemic optic atrophy

10. All of the following are characteristic patterns of joint involvement in rheumatoid arthritis *except*:

    A. Polyarticular involvement
    B. Oligoarticular involvement
    C. Symmetrical involvement
    D. Involvement of the proximal interphalangeal (PIP), metacarpophalangeal (MCP) wrist, and metatarsophalangeal (MTP) joints
    E. Frequent cervical spine involvement

11. A 32-year-old woman presents with left inguinal and groin pain of 1 week's duration that is worse with weight bearing and ambulation. Physical examination reveals full range of motion of the left hip. She walks with a limp. She had previously been treated with mechlorethamine, vincristine, procarbazine, and prednisone therapy for Hodgkin's disease. An anteroposterior film of the pelvis demonstrates no osseous abnormality. Which of the following tests would be most useful in making the diagnosis?

    A. Serum rheumatoid factor
    B. Erythrocyte sedimentation rate
    C. Magnetic resonance imaging (MRI) of the left hip
    D. Arthrogram of the left hip
    E. Blood alcohol level

12. Extra-articular manifestations of rheumatoid arthritis that may be associated with severe morbidity or mortality include:

    A. Rheumatoid vasculitis
    B. Pericarditis
    C. Cachexia
    D. Rheumatoid nodule within the aortic valve
    E. All of the above

13. Each of the following metabolic diseases may be associated with calcium pyrophosphate crystal deposition disease *except*:

    A. Hypothyroidism
    B. Hemochromatosis
    C. Primary hyperoxaluria
    D. Hyperparathyroidism
    E. Gout

14. All of the following statements are true of NSAIDs in general *except*:

    A. They have no major effect on the underlying disease process.
    B. They tend to cause gastric irritation and exacerbate peptic ulcers.
    C. They may suppress vasodilatory functions of renal prostaglandins.
    D. They may increase the pain threshold.
    E. Most are readily absorbed after oral administration.

15. All of the following are consistent with the radiographic manifestation of pyrophosphate arthropathy *except*:

    A. Cystic changes in bones of the wrist with triangular cartilage calcification
    B. Periarticular calcification of the first MTP joint
    C. Severe degenerative changes and subarticular cysts in the knee
    D. Linear subperiosteal resorption most marked in the radial border of the middle phalanx
    E. Linear calcification of the hyaline cartilage of the knee

16. Each of the following is a potential side effect of weekly low-dose (5-15 mg) methotrexate used to treat rheumatoid arthritis *except*:

    A. Leukopenia
    B. Alopecia
    C. Nephropathy
    D. Stomatitis
    E. Thrombocytopenia

17. A 32-year-old homosexual man presents for evaluation and treatment of left ankle pain of 2 weeks' duration. Besides tenderness, swelling, and marked limitation of tibiotalar motion, he has swelling and tenderness over the Achilles tendon insertion on the calcaneus; painful swelling over the left second and third MTP, PIP, and DIP joints; a clear mucoid penile discharge; hyperkeratosis of the soles and palms; and multiple erythematous plaque lesions with scaling over the trunk, arms, and legs. Each of the following would be appropriate diagnostic or treatment possibilities *except*:

A. NSAIDs for 2 weeks to reduce joint pain and swelling
B. Request for patient consent for HIV screening
C. Gram stain and culture of the urethral exudate for gonococcus
D. Strong consideration of adding methotrexate as a disease-modifying agent if there is no improvement within a 2- to 3-week period
E. Arthrocentesis for diagnostic and therapeutic purposes

18. Each of the following statements about immunoglobulin structure and function are true *except*:

A. Among the various classes, the basic structure of all immunoglobulin molecules is similar.
B. Both of the heavy and light chains of an IgG molecule have a variable region.
C. Both of the heavy and light chains of an IgM molecule have a constant region.
D. Complement fixation appears to depend on a structural determinant in the IgG V2 region.
E. The hypervariable regions are in intimate contact with the structural elements of the antigen.

19. Each of the following antibodies have been found in patients with HIV infections *except*:

A. Antinuclear antibodies (ANAs)
B. Anticardiolipin antibodies
C. Cryoglobulins
D. Antilymphocyte antibodies
E. Anti-G protein antibodies

20. A 22-year-old black woman with systemic lupus erythematosus (SLE) experiences worsening arthralgia and is given ibuprofen, 800 mg three times per day. Two days later, she presents to the emergency department with headache, stiff neck, and fever. Cultures of the cerebrospinal fluid are negative for bacteria and fungi. The most appropriate next step would be to:

A. Institute corticosteroids.
B. Give IV cyclophosphamide.
C. Discontinue the ibuprofen.
D. Initiate hydroxychloroquine sulfate (Plaquenil) therapy.
E. Give IV corticosteroids and cyclophosphamide.

21. A 32-year-old white woman presents with a 6-week history of fatigue, lymphadenopathy, and low-grade fever. At age 17, she required splenectomy for thrombocytopenia. In her early 20s, she had three miscarriages, one of which was followed by a deep vein thrombosis. Which laboratory tests would be most helpful in establishing a diagnosis?

A. ANA, anti-Sjögren's syndrome (anti-SS-A and anti-SS-B) antibodies
B. Rheumatoid factor, ANA, antiscleroderma (anti-SCL-70) antibodies
C. Antineutrophilic antibodies, antihistone antibodies
D. ANA, anticardiolipin antibodies, and anti-DNA antibodies
E. ANA, rheumatoid factor, and Lyme disease antibodies

22. A 65-year-old white man is admitted to the hospital for cholecystitis and undergoes cholecystectomy. Postoperatively, he experiences a persistent low-grade fever, intermittent severe crampy abdominal pain, and purpuric lower extremity skin lesions. On the 10th hospital day, he experiences a right footdrop and diplopia. The most appropriate next step in his diagnostic evaluation is to:

A. Obtain a kidney biopsy.
B. Obtain open lung biopsy.
C. Obtain celiac and mesenteric angiography.

D. Obtain a right temporal artery biopsy.
E. Obtain a CT scan of the brain.

23. A 50-year-old white man is transferred to your hospital with a presumptive diagnosis of tuberculosis. His chest radiograph shows nodular cavitary lesions in both lung fields. His urinalysis shows 50 RBCs per high-power field and 3+ proteinuria. He is scheduled for bronchoscopy with transbronchial lung biopsy in the morning. That evening he has a sudden deterioration consisting of massive hemoptysis and progressive renal failure. The most appropriate therapeutic intervention at this point would be supportive management and:

A. IV corticosteroids
B. Antituberculous medications
C. IV cyclophosphamide, 4 mg/kg
D. Oral cyclophosphamide, 2 mg/kg
E. IV corticosteroids and IV cyclophosphamide, 4 mg/kg

24. Each of the following is characteristic of polymyalgia rheumatica *except*:

A. Mild joint inflammation
B. Stiffness of the shoulder and hip girdles
C. Weakness of the shoulder and hip girdles
D. Elevated erythrocyte sedimentation rate
E. Normochromic normocytic anemia

25. A 74-year-old man is noted to have purplish-discolored right third and fourth toes 4 days after coronary angiography and a creatinine level of 2.4 mg/dL (creatinine level was normal on admission). He has a history of adult-onset diabetes mellitus, hypertension, and 50 pack-years of smoking. Cholesterol crystal atheromatous embolization is suspected. Which of the following may be present?

A. Livedo reticularis
B. Elevated erythrocyte sedimentation rate and/or leukocytosis and/or eosinophilia
C. Prominent gastrocnemius pain or claudication
D. Source(s) of the cholesterol emboli are usually the abdominal aorta or iliofemoral arteries rather than the more distal arteries.
E. All of the above

26. An 83-year-old woman presented to the emergency department on a stretcher with severe right hip and thigh pain after falling in the shower. Radiographs revealed generalized osteopenia and a displaced right femoral neck fracture. Each of the following statements about osteoporosis is true *except*:

A. Decreased bone mass is the major risk factor for sustaining a fracture as a result of minor trauma.
B. Lifestyle factors such as calcium intake, cigarette smoking, and ethanol use may modify bone mass.
C. The severity of bone loss is best assessed using plain bone radiographs.
D. There are no symptoms or physical findings in early osteoporosis.
E. The number of osteoporotic fractures in the United States is expected to increase dramatically in the next 40 years.

TRUE OR FALSE

DIRECTIONS: For questions 27-48, decide whether *each* choice is true or false. Any combination of answers, from all true to all false, may occur.

27. Which of the following statements concerning cholesterol (atheromatous) emboli syndrome is/are *true*?

    A. Precipitating factors can always be identified if diligently sought.
    B. Dermal manifestations may include petechiae, hemorrhage, purplish-discolored toes, and digital gangrene.
    C. Transient basophilia is commonly seen.
    D. Cholesterol emboli most commonly arise from atheromatous plaque in the distal lower extremity arteries.
    E. The administration of anticoagulants may be associated with episodes of embolization.

28. Glucocorticoid-induced osteoporosis is currently the most common cause of drug-related osteoporosis in the United States. Which of the following recommendations concerning management of glucocorticoid-induced osteoporosis is/are *true*?

    A. Bone densitometry techniques may detect bone mineral depletion before fractures in patients on chronic glucocorticoid therapy.
    B. Encourage the daily ingestion of 1500 mg of elemental calcium and 400 IU/day of vitamin D.
    C. Decrease or stop all glucocorticoids when osteoporosis is detected.
    D. Encourage weight-bearing activity and exercises.
    E. Give diphosphonate inhibitors if there are no contraindications.

29. Which of the following statements concerning neutrophil/neutrophil-mediated tissue injury is/are *true*?

    A. Proteinases released extracellularly may degrade matrix molecules.
    B. Tissue-bound IgG/immune complexes are the major in vivo signal for degranulation.
    C. The major lipid mediators released extracellularly are leukotriene A_4 and lipoxin B.
    D. The major surface protein-mediating adhesion is IIb/IIIa.
    E. CD11b/CD18 functions as a receptor for iC3b (CR3) and thereby mediates phagocytosis or opsonized particles.

30. Which of the following statements concerning the antiphospholipid antibody syndrome is/are *true*?

    A. It could not be associated with the sudden onset of left paresis in a previously healthy 28-year-old woman.
    B. It could explain recurrent spontaneous abortion in a 24-year-old woman with an ANA 1:40 titer, speckled pattern.
    C. Lupus anticoagulant and anticardiolipin antibody are always identical immunoglobulin molecules.
    D. It could not explain ischemic necrosis of the forefoot in a previously healthy 24-year-old man.

    E. Tests for anticardiolipin antibodies have a low degree of variability and excellent reproducibility and should be done in all hospital laboratories.

31. Which of the following statements concerning rheumatoid factor is/are *true*?

    A. It is present in the blood of approximately 80% of patients with rheumatoid arthritis.
    B. It is clearly implicated as a cause of rheumatoid arthritis.
    C. In most cases it can be demonstrated to be an IgG antibody to autologous IgM.
    D. Its production is restricted to the human leukocyte antigen (HLA) DR4 haplotype.
    E. None of the above

32. Which of the following statements concerning B cells is/are *true*?

    A. They can directly secrete antibodies.
    B. Activation, proliferation, and differentiation require a variety of cytokines.
    C. The binding region of the membrane immunoglobulin of each cell line is unique in its specificity.
    D. They contain immunoglobulin genes located on chromosomes 2, 14, and 22.
    E. Their major receptor is the T3 complex.

33. Which of the following statements concerning hemochromatosis is/are *true*?

    A. Pyrophosphate arthropathy may affect the second and third MCP joints in approximately 50% of patients.
    B. The diagnosis is made by an elevated serum ferritin level.
    C. The diagnosis is made by liver biopsy showing increased iron within parenchymal cells.
    D. Initiating weekly phlebotomies until tissue iron stores are depleted is the usual treatment.
    E. Hepatic cirrhosis, cardiomyopathy, diabetes mellitus, and skin pigmentation may result from increased iron deposition in tissues.

34. Which of the following statements concerning lumbosacral spine films is/are *true*?

    A. Focal or generalized reduction in bone density may be observed in myeloma.
    B. Progression of vertebral body osteomyelitis may lead to involvement of two adjacent vertebrae and the intervening disk space.
    C. Localized rarefaction of the vertebral end-plate is the earliest radiographic change in vertebral osteomyelitis.
    D. Metastatic neoplasms to the vertebral bodies characteristically invade the intervening disk space.
    E. Alternate bands of osteosclerosis and resorption may be seen in renal osteodystrophy.

35. Which of the following statements concerning ankylosing spondylitis is/are *true*?

    A. Monoarthritis or oligoarthritis may precede the onset of back pain.
    B. The earliest recognizable radiographic change in the sacroiliac joints is fusion.
    C. Back pain and morning stiffness may diminish with activity and may recur after periods of inactivity.
    D. Lateral lumbosacral flexion may be assessed with the Schober test.
    E. Aortic insufficiency may be an extra-articular manifestation.

36. Which of the following statements concerning osteoporosis is/are *true*?

    A. Bone mineral and matrix formation rates are always greater than resorption rates.
    B. Bone density in postmenopausal women is the most important determinant for hip and vertebral fractures.
    C. Dual-energy x-ray absorptiometry is the most accurate method for assessing bone density.
    D. Single and dual-photon analysis is the most common technique to assess bone density.
    E. Prevention of symptomatic osteoporosis should be a top public health goal in the United States.

37. Which of the following statements about gonococcal arthritis is/are *true*?

    A. It is a rare problem in healthy, sexually active teenagers and young adults.

B. The diagnosis is easy to make in most cases because of positive synovial fluid Gram stain and culture.

C. Causative organisms are gram-positive diplococci.

D. The arthritis pattern is oligoarticular associated with tenosynovitis and skin lesions.

E. Response to treatment of antibiotics/drainage is slow but definite.

38. Which of the following statements concerning matrix structure and functions is/are *true*?

A. The collagens are the second most abundant class of proteins in the human body.

B. Proteoglycans are the major noncollagenous structural proteins of articular cartilage.

C. The major components of basement membranes are collagen type IV, laminin, entactin, and heparin sulfate proteoglycans.

D. Genetic mutation associated with defects in type I collagen includes Ehlers-Danlos syndrome and osteogenesis imperfecta.

E. Basement membrane alterations are frequently found in diabetes mellitus.

39. Which of the following statements concerning complement is/are *true*?

A. Complement receptor I (CRI) may function to clear circulating immune complexes and enhance phagocytosis.

B. A low CH_{50} (total hemolytic complement) may suggest C2 deficiency.

C. A deficiency of C5, C6, C7, and C8 may be associated with recurrent disseminated staphylococcal infections.

D. The two complement activation pathways (classic and alternative) may lead to the generation of the membrane attack complex.

E. SLE-like syndromes and discoid lupus may be associated with C2 and C4 deficiency.

40. Which of the following statements concerning cytokines is/are *true*?

A. Interleukin (IL)-1α and IL-1β can produce fever, bone and cartilage resorption, and prostaglandin release.

B. Tumor necrosis factor-α can produce fever and macrophage activation and can stimulate bone resorption.

C. IL-2 is produced by T cells and may stimulate proliferation of T cells and natural killer cells.

D. IL-2 has antitumor activity.

E. IL-6 induces antibody secretion.

41. Which of the following statements concerning HLA is/are *true*?

A. More than 100 diseases of diverse manifestations are associated with HLA.

B. The majority of individuals with a given disease associated with HLA haplotype are afflicted with the disease.

C. HLA-A molecules are found on virtually all cells.

D. Certain regions within the DR4 and DR1 class II molecules with the same amino acid sequence may confer predisposition to rheumatoid arthritis.

E. HLA-DR4 occurs in 95% of seropositive individuals with rheumatoid arthritis.

42. Which of the following statements concerning rheumatic manifestations of HIV infection is/are *true*?

A. Fever, myalgias, and arthralgias are distinctly uncommon manifestations of acute HIV seroconversion.

B. A polymyositis-like illness characterized by myalgias, proximal muscle weakness, and wasting has been described as the initial manifestation of HIV infection.

C. An oligoarticular arthritis associated with urethritis, conjunctivitis, painless oral ulcerations, and keratoderma blennorrhagicum are the hallmark of Reiter's syndrome in both HIV-infected and non–HIV-infected individuals.

D. To date, xerophthalmia and xerostomia with abnormal salivary gland biopsies have not been described in HIV-infected individuals.

E. All reported cases of HIV-related periarteritis nodosa have also been hepatitis B surface antigen–positive, suggesting that true vasculitis does not occur with HIV infection.

43. Which of the following statements concerning polyarteritis nodosa is/are *true*?

A. A characteristic pathologic finding in an involved vessel is leukocytoclastic vasculitis with nuclear debris.

B. The lesions tend to involve arteries of medium or small caliber, especially at bifurcations.

C. Eosinophilia with lung involvement is common.

D. Hypocomplementemia is characteristic.

E. Subcutaneous nodules are commonly found in this disease.

44. Which of the following statements regarding the vasculitis syndromes is/are *true*?

A. Wegner's granulomatosis is characterized by infiltration of various organs and vessels with cellular infiltrates consisting of atypical lymphoid and plasmacytoid cells.

B. Hypersensitivity vasculitis is often confined to the skin and often manifested by palpable purpura.

C. Temporal arteritis usually involves small intracranial arterioles and venules.

D. Takayasu's arteritis may involve the subclavian arteries.

E. Henoch-Schönlein purpura is usually progressive, leading to death or renal failure without appropriate therapeutic intervention.

45. Which of the following statements concerning SLE is/are *true*?

A. Although renal glomerular disease is common, renal tubular and interstitial inflammation is rare.

B. Anti-SS-A antibodies (anti-Ro) have been associated with the development of congenital heart block in infants of mothers with SLE.

C. Vasculitic lesions of the skin usually portend CNS vasculitis.

D. Pleural fluid from patients with active SLE is usually exudative, with a low glucose level.

E. The chance that a black woman will acquire SLE in her lifetime is approximately 1:250.

46. Which of the following statement(s) is/are *true*?

A. Idiopathic midline destructive disease is usually treated with a combination of prednisone, cyclophosphamide, and radiation.

B. Elevation of the creatine phosphokinase level and a myopathic pattern in the electromyogram is useful in diagnosing polymyalgia rheumatica.

C. SLE patients with alopecia can be advised that hair will regrow, unless the scalp is involved with discoid lesions.

D. Renal transplantation is contraindicated in patients with end-stage renal failure caused by SLE.

E. A lupus anticoagulant has been identified that prolongs the partial thromboplastin time (PTT) by reacting with phospholipids used in the PTT assay and that is associated with thrombosis rather than bleeding.

47. Which of the following statement(s) is/are *true*?

    A. A neutrophilic leukocytosis and positive rheumatoid factor are often seen in patients with Wegener's granulomatosis.
    B. Anticytoplasmic antibodies are highly specific for Wegener's granulomatosis.
    C. Idiopathic midline destructive disease is a systemic vasculitis.
    D. Lymphomatoid granulomatosis is a systemic vasculitis similar to polyarteritis nodosa.
    E. All patients with Wegener's granulomatosis have lung involvement.

48. Which of the following statements concerning Lyme disease is/are *true*?

    A. Erythema chronicum migrans occurs after an incubation period of 2 months in greater than 95% of affected patients.
    B. Most affected patients experience arthritis, with monoarticular or oligoarticular arthritis in large joints.
    C. Lyme antibody is frequently present early (2-4 weeks) in the disease.
    D. The decision to treat patients with antibiotics in an endemic area should be based on serologic results.
    E. The presence of Lyme disease antibodies may be of most use in the patient with either an atypical manifestation or unexplained recurrent attacks of monoarticular or oligoarthritis over several years.

MATCHING

DIRECTIONS: Questions 49-108 are matching questions. For each numbered item, choose the most likely associated lettered item from those provided. Each numbered item has *only one* answer. Within each set of questions, each answer may be used once, more than once, or not at all.

QUESTIONS 49–52

Match the following histopathologic findings with the most likely associated rheumatic disease.

    A. Calcific masses staining purple with hematoxylin
    B. Dark pigmented hyaline cartilage fragments
    C. Villi infiltrated by lymphocytes with synovial lining cell hyperplasia
    D. Congophilia
    E. Sheets of histiocytes and multinucleated giant cells

49. Ochronosis

50. Pigmented villonodular synovitis

51. Calcium pyrophosphate deposition disease

52. Rheumatoid arthritis

QUESTIONS 53–56

Match the following characteristic ocular manifestations with the rheumatic disease with which they are most likely to be associated.

    A. Corneal melt
    B. Ischemic optic atrophy
    C. Anterior uveitis
    D. Retinal vascular disease

53. Temporal arteritis

54. SLE

55. Rheumatoid arthritis

56. Ankylosing spondylitis

QUESTIONS 57–60

Match the following clinical syndromes with the radiographic description with which they are most likely associated.

    A. Thyroiditis with thyroid acropathy
    B. Synovial osteochondromatosis
    C. Scleroderma
    D. Gout
    E. Acromegaly

57. Hand radiograph showing destruction of the tufts of the terminal phalanges

58. Shoulder radiograph demonstrating marked osteoarthritis with osteophyte formation

59. Punched-out erosion with overhanging bone

60. Lateral knee radiograph demonstrating multiple calcified loose bodies in a popliteal cyst

QUESTIONS 61–64

Match the following sets of clinical problems with the complication in dialysis patients with which they are most likely to be associated.

    A. Bone pain, pathologic fractures, proximal muscle weakness, dementia
    B. Carpal tunnel syndrome, subchondral cysts
    C. Osteolysis of phalangeal tufts, pathologic fractures
    D. Pruritus, periarthritis, acute joint pain
    E. Hypertrophic skin changes, periosteal proliferation

61. Secondary hyperparathyroidism

62. β_2-Microglobulin amyloid arthropathy

63. High serum calcium × phosphorus product

64. Aluminum-related osteomalacia

QUESTIONS 65–68

Match the following cutaneous manifestations with the most likely associated rheumatic disease.

    A. Ring-like erythema that has elevated margins, expands peripherally, and leaves fading centers
    B. Thrombocytopenic purpura
    C. Periorbital swelling with erythema along the lid margins
    D. Nonthrombocytopenic palpable purpura
    E. Hemorrhagic vesicopustules

65. Rheumatic fever

66. Henoch-Schönlein syndrome

67. Disseminated gonococcal arthritis

68. Dermatomyositis

QUESTIONS 69–72

Match the following joint pattern findings with the disease with which they are most likely to be associated.

    A. Inflammatory oligoarthritis in a 21-year-old man

B. Symmetrical polyarthritis in a 32-year-old woman

C. Inflammatory monoarthritis of the first toe interphalangeal joint in a 58-year-old man

D. Monoarticular arthritis in a 6-year-old girl

E. Squaring of the base of the thumb in a 66-year-old woman

69. Gout

70. Reiter's syndrome

71. Rheumatoid arthritis

72. Pauciarticular juvenile chronic arthritis

QUESTIONS 73–76

Match the following characteristic findings with the disease with which they are most likely associated.

A. Digital clubbing, periostitis, and painful swelling of bones and joints

B. Asymptomatic pleural effusions

C. Upper lobe fibrosis

D. Transient arthritis affecting knees, ankles, and wrist

E. Swollen, tender DIP joints

73. Ankylosing spondylitis

74. Bronchogenic carcinoma

75. Sarcoidosis

76. Rheumatoid arthritis

QUESTIONS 77–80

Match the following clinical findings with the most likely associated rheumatic disease.

A. Thenar atrophy, decreased ability to oppose thumb to little finger

B. Fixed facial expression, rigidity of the left arm

C. Acute onset of sagging of the right eyebrow and drooping of the mouth on the right

D. Disturbances of micturition or impotence

E. Sudden, painless loss of vision in the left eye

77. Temporal arteritis

78. Ankylosing spondylitis

79. Lyme disease-related arthritis

80. β_2-Microglobulin hemodialysis arthropathy

QUESTIONS 81–84

Match the following characteristic findings with the most likely associated endocrine disease.

A. Transient Raynaud's phenomenon

B. Vertebral body fractures

C. Finger digit sclerosis with PIP flexion contractures

D. Synovial fluid speckled with dark particles resembling brown pepper

E. Muscle weakness with elevated creatinine kinase level

81. Hyperparathyroidism

82. Hypothyroidism

83. Acromegaly

84. Diabetes mellitus

QUESTIONS 85–88

Match the following characteristic findings with the rheumatic syndromes associated with HIV infection with which they are most likely to be associated.

A. Presents as peripheral sensory or sensorimotor neuropathy

B. Sicca complex symptoms

C. Present in one third of HIV-infected patients

D. Oligoarticular arthritis associated with conjunctivitis, urethritis, painless oral ulcers, and balanitis circinata

E. Presence of nemaline rods

85. Myopathy

86. Arthralgias

87. Reiter's syndrome

88. Vasculitis

QUESTIONS 89–92

Match the following clinical syndromes with the manifestation with which they are most likely to be associated.

A. Rheumatoid arthritis

B. SLE

C. Dermatomyositis

D. Hypersensitivity vasculitis

E. Periarteritis nodosa

89. Palpable purpura

90. Subcutaneous nodules

91. Gottron's papules

92. Hypopigmented skin lesion with central atrophy and telangiectasia

QUESTIONS 93–96

Match the following clinical syndromes with the most likely associated finding.

A. Wegener's granulomatosis

B. Sjögren's syndrome

C. SLE

D. Eosinophilic fasciitis

E. Polyarteritis nodosa

93. C2 deficiency

94. Antibodies against a 29-kD cytoplasmic antigen of neutrophils

95. Renal tubular acidosis

96. Brawny, tender induration of the skin with retraction of subcutaneous tissue

QUESTIONS 97–100

Match the following clinical syndromes with the most likely associated finding.

A. Polyarteritis nodosa

B. SLE

C. Temporal arteritis

D. Behçet's syndrome

E. Scleroderma

97. Cytoid bodies

98. Mononeuritis multiplex

99. Jaw claudication

100. Meningoencephalitis

QUESTIONS 101–104

Match the following laboratory findings with the condition with which they are most likely to be associated.

    A. Anticardiolipin antibodies
    B. Anti-SS-A antibodies
    C. Antihistone antibodies
    D. Anti-Smith antibodies
    E. Anti-SCL-70 antibodies

101. Recurrent abortions

102. Congenital heart block

103. Drug-induced lupus

104. SLE

QUESTIONS 105–108

Match the following clinical syndromes with the most likely associated symptoms.

    A. Eosinophilia-myalgia syndrome
    B. Eosinophilic fasciitis syndrome
    C. Fibromyalgia
    D. Churg-Strauss syndrome
    E. Toxic oil syndrome

105. Pulmonary and systemic vasculitis, eosinophilia, often occurring in patients with a history of allergy or asthma

106. Intense and incapacitating generalized myalgia, fatigue, eosinophilia, and history of ingestion of L-tryptophan

107. Swelling and stiffness of the extremities, eosinophilia, and occurrence in patients after extreme physical exertion

108. Widespread pain in combination with tenderness at specific tender point sites

Part IX
Rheumatology and Clinical Immunology
Answers

1. **(E)** *Discussion:* All of the answers are correct. Methotrexate is currently the best drug used to treat rheumatoid arthritis, with initial improvement seen in 3 to 6 weeks and peak efficacy in 4 to 6 months. Adverse effects such as nausea, abdominal pain, and diarrhea are frequently seen, but serious toxicity is rare. Methotrexate is taken orally (7.5-15 mg/week), and tolerance may be increased by spacing the oral doses over 1 to 2 days, giving a single intramuscular injection each week and daily folic acid (1 mg/day) supplementation. Laboratory tests such as CBC, platelet count, alkaline phosphatase, and AST are done every 4 to 6 weeks. The most toxic drug-related side effects are pancytopenia, neutropenia, thrombocytopenia, pneumonitis, and cirrhosis; all are reasons to stop the medications. Transient or sustained (1.5-2 times normal values) elevations in alkaline phosphatase and AST are common and, in the majority of patients, generally do not portend the development of hepatic fibrosis. Methotrexate is known to be teratogenic and should not be given to women of childbearing potential unless they are using an adequate method of birth control. Because of its potential affect on sperm, men should discontinue methotrexate 3 to 4 months before attempting conception. *(Cecil, Ch. 278)*

2. **(B)** *Discussion:* The clinical features and radiographic pattern are characteristic for calcific tendinitis, an extremely common rheumatic syndrome characterized by deposits of hydroxyapatite crystals within injured rotator cuff muscles near the humeral attachment region. It most commonly involves the supraspinatus tendon, but the infraspinatus and subscapularis tendons may also be involved. Conservative treatment is indicated and is successful in the vast majority of cases. *(Resnick, 2002; Primer 2001)*

3. **(E)** *Discussion:* Clinically, the patient has osteoarthritis of the left knee. Synovial fluid in patients with osteoarthritis is typically "noninflammatory," meaning that the leukocyte count is less than 2000/μL. A low level of glucose in the synovial fluid would not be found in this patient but is suggestive of septic arthritis. *(Cecil, Chs. 274, 286, and 287)*

4. **(C)** *Discussion:* The physical examination is suggestive of a distended Baker's cyst, but physical examination alone is not diagnostic, particularly if there has been a dissection or rupture. Ultrasonography has been found to be very useful in making a diagnosis of popliteal cyst with or without dissection. An arthrogram could also demonstrate a popliteal cyst but is less desirable because it is an invasive procedure. A venogram of the right lower extremity could be performed if a deep vein thrombosis was suspected clinically but would not be indicated in this case. *(Cecil, Ch. 278; Primer, 2001)*

5. **(E)** *Discussion:* Although hand involvement is very common in rheumatoid arthritis and occurs in approximately 95% of patients, DIP joint involvement is distinctly unusual. The most commonly involved joints in the rheumatoid hand are the PIPs, MCPs, and wrist joints in a symmetrical manner. *(Cecil, Ch. 278)*

6. **(A)** *Discussion:* Patients with adult Still's disease are "seronegative" and lack serum rheumatoid factor. Rheumatoid factors are antibodies specific for the region of the Fc portion of human IgG. Although present in 75 to 80% of rheumatoid arthritis patients, primarily those with HLA-DR4 haplotype, they are by no means specific for this disorder and are found in normal individuals as well as patients with a variety of other inflammatory illnesses. *(Cecil, Ch. 278; Primer, 2001)*

7. **(B)** *Discussion:* Clinically, the patient has a monoarthritis that is most likely crystal induced, such as pseudogout or gout. She could also have septic arthritis, although this would be less likely. Gout and pseudogout can be rapidly and definitively diagnosed by proper examination of joint fluid, and infection can also be ruled out in this manner. *(Cecil, Chs. 286 and 287)*

8. **(E)** *Discussion:* Clinically, the patient has carpal tunnel syndrome, an entrapment neuropathy in which the median nerve is compressed within the carpal tunnel area. A new type of amyloid protein identified as β_2-microglobulin has been demonstrated in bone and carpal tunnel tissue of patients undergoing long-term (usually greater than 10 years) hemodialysis. It is hoped that modifications of the dialysis membranes may result in improved β_2-microglobulin clearance with diminished tissue deposition. *(Primer, 2001)*

9. **(E)** *Discussion:* Ischemic optic atrophy is not routinely seen in patients with rheumatoid arthritis but may be a major ophthalmic manifestation of giant cell arteritis, Wegener's granulomatosis, and, less commonly, SLE. *(Cecil, Ch. 278)*

10. **(B)** *Discussion:* Clinically, rheumatoid arthritis is a symmetrical polyarthritis especially involving the PIP, MCP, wrist, and MTP joints. In many of these joints, definite articular deformities will develop over time. Cervical spine involvement is common. Rarely is an oligoarticular pattern observed except in the early course of this illness. *(Cecil, Ch. 278)*

11. **(C)** *Discussion:* Osteonecrosis is one of the most common causes of hip pain and incapacity in patients with a variety of diseases who have been treated with corticosteroids. A major problem in diagnosing osteonecrosis relates to the lag between the onset of symptoms (pain and limp) and defined radiographic changes. MRI has been shown to be extremely valuable in evaluating high-risk patients who are symptomatic but radiographically normal. *(Primer, 2001; Resnick, 2002)*

12. **(E)** *Discussion:* All of the answers are correct. Rheumatoid arthritis may be associated with a number of systemic features that may be associated with severe morbidity or mortality. *(Cecil, Ch. 278)*

13. **(C)** *Discussion:* There is an association of calcium pyrophosphate crystal deposition disease with several metabolic diseases, including primary hyperparathyroidism, hemochromatosis, hypothyroidism, gout, familial hypocalciuric hypercalcemia, hypomagnesemia, and hypophosphatasia, but not with primary hyperoxaluria, which is associated with the tissue deposition of calcium oxalate crystals. The development of premature symptomatic osteoarthritis associated with the features of chondrocalcinosis should initiate a search for underlying associated disorders. In general, treatment of the primary disorder, such as hyperparathyroidism, hemochromatosis, or hypothyroidism, does not lead to resorption of calcium pyrophosphate deposition. Phlebotomy treatment of hemochromatosis may actually exacerbate the arthritis. *(Cecil, Ch. 288; Primer, 2001)*

14. **(D)** *Discussion:* Most NSAIDs are aspirin-like in that they reduce but do not completely eliminate the signs and symptoms of inflammation. A major effect on the underlying disease process has not been demonstrated. They have a broad range of pharmacologic activities, the most well described of which is the inhibition of cyclooxygenase, the enzyme that catalyzes the conversion of arachidonic acid to prostaglandins, prostacyclin, and thromboxanes. Although NSAIDs are well tolerated, they can be associated with a spectrum of adverse reactions, the most notable of which are the gastrointestinal effects, such as the tendency to produce gastritis and antral prepyloric ulcers. *(Primer, 2001)*

15. **(D)** *Discussion:* Linear subperiosteal resorption is seen in primary or secondary hyperparathyroidism. The other manifestations are common radiographic manifestations of calcium pyrophosphate deposition disease. *(Resnick, 2002)*

16. **(C)** *Discussion:* Nephropathy is not an adverse manifestation of oral methotrexate. Methotrexate is usually administered orally, ranging from one to two doses per week separated by 8 to 12 hours. Typically, this protocol results in a reduction in the immunosuppressive and toxic reactions of the drug. Although the mechanism of action may be primarily through inhibition of synovial cell proliferation, its toxicity is primarily associated with effects on rapidly dividing cells such as bone marrow and intestinal epithelium. *(Cecil, Ch. 278; Primer, 2001)*

17. **(D)** *Discussion:* The data presented indicate that the patient has typical Reiter's syndrome, which may or may not be associated with HIV infection. Efforts should be made to screen for HIV, rule out gonorrhea, and refrain from using immunosuppressant drugs such as methotrexate because these are contraindicated in a patient who is HIV positive. *(Cecil, Chs. 279 and 420)*

18. **(D)** *Discussion:* There are five classes of immunoglobulin molecules in humans (IgG, IgA, IgM, IgD, and IgE), which have the same basic four-chain structure, including two heavy (H) and two light (L) chains, but which differ in their chemical and physical properties. Complement activation by the classic pathway appears to be associated with the constant region of IgG, with IgG_1 and IgG_3 subclasses being the most effective. *(Primer, 2001)*

19. **(E)** *Discussion:* A variety of antibodies have been found in patients with HIV infections, but to date no anti–G protein antibodies have been reported. Antinuclear, antilymphocyte, antineutrophil, antiplatelet, and antiphospholipid antibodies, rheumatoid factor, and cryoglobulins have all been demonstrated to occur in patients with HIV infections. The relationship of these antibodies to the rheumatologic diseases associated with the HIV infection is unclear. *(Cecil, Ch. 420)*

20. **(C).** *Discussion:* NSAIDs are commonly used to treat the arthralgias and arthritis in patients with SLE. However, the use of ibuprofen in patients with SLE has been associated with the development of a drug-induced aseptic meningitis. Aseptic meningitis

secondary to sulindac and tolmetin has also been described. *(Cecil, Ch. 280; Boumpas et al, 1995a, 1995b)*

21. **(D)** *Discussion:* The picture of recurrent miscarriages and deep vein thromboses is suggestive of an anticardiolipin antibody syndrome associated with SLE. Thus, it would be important to determine whether anticardiolipin antibodies are present as well as to substantiate a diagnosis of SLE. *(Cecil, Chs. 274 and 280; Boumpas et al, 1995a, 1995b)*

22. **(C)** *Discussion:* This patient has multiorgan manifestations suggesting a systemic necrotizing vasculitis with prominent mesenteric artery involvement. Celiac and mesenteric angiography would be the procedure of choice. Biopsy of other accessible involve tissues, such as the skin and sural nerve, would also be appropriate. *(Cecil, Ch. 284)*

23. **(E)** *Discussion:* The involvement of the lower respiratory tract as well as renal involvement suggests Wegener's granulomatosis. Treatment of Wegener's granulomatosis with cyclophosphamide has resulted in marked improvement in outcome of this condition. Because of the severity and sudden deterioration, administration of IV corticosteroids and IV cyclophosphamide would be indicated. *(Cecil, Ch. 284)*

24. **(C)** *Discussion:* Polymyalgia rheumatica is a common clinical syndrome in patients older than age 55 years and is characterized by stiffness and soreness in the shoulder and hip girdle areas. It is sometimes associated with mild joint swelling. Laboratory findings include normocytic/normochromic anemia and elevated sedimentation rate. Weakness of the proximal upper and lower extremity muscles is distinctly unusual and suggests a proximal myopathy such as polymyositis. *(Cecil, Ch. 285)*

25. **(E)** *Discussion:* All of the answers are correct. Cholesterol crystal (atheromatous) embolization is a common occurrence in patients with advanced atherosclerotic disease but is frequently either not recognized or misdiagnosed as "vasculitis." The exact incidence is currently unknown, but it is associated with significant morbidity and mortality. With a rise in the number of geriatric patients with arthrosclerosis, the recognition of this disorder is critical to prevent unnecessary diagnostic studies and treatment with high-dose corticosteroids/cytotoxic agents, which are of no benefit. The source of most cholesterol emboli is the abdominal aorta or iliofemoral arteries, but cardiac and thoracic aorta sources have been described. Episodes of embolization may occur spontaneously or may be temporally associated with surgery or invasive arterial studies (days) or response to anticoagulant or thrombocytic therapy (weeks). The clinical manifestations may mimic polyarteritis nodosa, with fever, accelerated hypertension, and progressive renal failure; abdominal pain with bleeding or bowel infarction; multiple dermal manifestations such as livedo reticularis, purplish-discolored toes, and digital gangrene; intense thigh and gastrocnemius tenderness; and laboratory findings of elevated erythrocyte sedimentation rate, creatinine, and creatine phosphokinase and leukocytosis, eosinophilia, anemia, and proteinuria. *(Fine et al, 1987)*

26. **(C)** *Discussion:* Osteoporosis is characterized by a reduction of bone mass 2.5 standard deviations below the normal premenopausal mean value. Instead of a single disease, it is heterogeneous and influenced by hereditary, lifestyle, and hormonal factors. It is most treacherous in that the first manifestations may be fractures of the hip and spine, with enormous human and economic costs. Bone mass is inversely related to the risk of hip and spine fractures. Routine bone radiographs do not adequately quantify bone mineral density. *(Cecil, Ch. 258)*

27. **(A) False; (B) True; (C) False; (D) False; (E) True.** *Discussion:* See answer to question 25.

28. **(All True).** *Discussion:* There is no question that glucocorticoid therapy has been beneficial to many patients with a variety of acute and chronic inflammatory disease. However, a common complication of chronic glucocorticoid treatment is severe bone mineral loss and subsequent fracture. Glucocorticoids influence many aspects of calcium and bone metabolism. For example, they may inhibit osteoblast-mediated matrix synthesis; decrease intestinal absorption of calcium and phosphorus; diminish the circulating levels of estrogen, testosterone, follicle-stimulating hormone, and luteinizing hormone; and increase parathyroid hormone secretion, leading indirectly to osteoclast-mediated bone resorption. Some recommendations for management include using the lowest possible dose of glucocorticoids (completely stopping this treatment is not possible in most patients), encouraging ingestion of 1500 mg of elemental calcium (calcium carbonate and calcium citrate contain 40% and 11% elemental calcium, respectively), regular weight-bearing exercise therapy, and measurement of bone mineral density. *(Cecil, Ch. 258; Saag et al, 1998)*

29. **(A) True; (B) True; (C) False; (D) False; (E) True.** *Discussion:* Neutrophils contain within their granules potent proteinases such as elastase and collagenase that can cleave a number of matrix proteins. The major stimulus for the extracellular release of these proteases is by tissue-bound IgG immune complexes binding to the neutrophil Fc receptor. In addition to the release of proteinases, neutrophils may release reactive oxygen species and lipid-derived inflammatory substances such as platelet-activating factor, leukotriene B$_4$, and lipoxin A. CR3 (CDE11/CD18) may demonstrate increased expression with neutrophil activation and binds to iC3b. IIb/IIIa is a major protein complex of platelets, not neutrophils. *(Primer, 2001)*

30. **(A) False; (B) True; (C) False; (D) False; (E) False.** *Discussion:* The presence of antiphospholipid antibodies has been associated with arterial and venous thrombosis, premature stroke syndromes, mesenteric artery insufficiency, and recurrent or multiple spontaneous abortions in patients with lupus or lupus-like illnesses. The lupus anticoagulant (associated with a prolonged PTT) and the anticardiolipin antibody have been shown to be different antibodies but may be present together in approximately 70% of patients. As stressed in the text, measurement of anticardiolipin antibody levels is difficult and should be done only in reference laboratories with multiple controls. *(Cecil, Ch. 274; Boumpas et al, 1995a, 1995b)*

31. **(A) True; (B) False; (C) False; (D) False; (E) False.** *Discussion:* Rheumatoid factor is typically an IgM antibody recognizing Fc determinants of the autologous IgG molecule and is present in the serum of 75 to 80% of patients with rheumatoid arthritis. It is not specific for rheumatoid arthritis and is found in the serum of patients with a variety of inflammatory disorders, such as sarcoidosis and leprosy. It does not cause the disease and is not restricted to the HLA-DR4 haplotype. *(Cecil, Ch. 278; Primer, 2001)*

32. **(A) True; (B) True; (C) True; (D) True; (E) False.** *Discussion:* B cells arise from progenitor cells in the bone marrow. Their activation, proliferation, and differentiation into antibody-secreting plasma cells requires a variety of cytokines. Within their surface membranes, B cells have receptors, allowing them to recognize foreign antigenic determinants. These receptors are membrane immunoglobulins of unique specificity. The T3 complex is part of the T-cell receptor complex. *(Primer, 2001)*

33. **(A) True; (B) False; (C) True; (D) True; (E) True.** *Discussion:* Hemochromatosis is transmitted as an autosomal-recessive disease associated with increased absorption of iron from the gastrointestinal tract, with increased tissue deposition of iron within the liver, heart, pancreas, and skin. Although the serum ferritin level is usually elevated, this is by no means diagnostic and

occurs with a variety of disorders. The diagnosis is made by liver biopsy, which demonstrates increased parenchymal iron by staining as well as by quantitative liver iron measurement. Chondrocalcinosis is a common radiographic manifestation associated with hemochromatosis, primarily involves the second or third MCP joints, and occurs in about 50% of patients. Treatment consists of weekly phlebotomies to decrease the iron content to tissues, but this may aggravate the arthritis. *(Cecil, Chs. 225 and 288)*

34. **(A) True; (B) True; (C) True; (D) False; (E) True.** *Discussion:* Plain radiographs of the lumbosacral spine are indicated primarily in older patients complaining of back pain. These may show patterns of permeative bone destruction such as in myeloma or osteomyelitis. Osteomyelitis of the vertebral body is characterized by localized rarefaction of the vertebral end plate, progressing to destruction of the vertebral body and then to involvement of two adjacent vertebrae and the intervening disk space. Typically, metastatic neoplasms may involve the vertebral body but characteristically spare the intervening disk space. Myeloma may present with either focal, punched-out lesions or generalized reduction in bone density. Patients with renal osteodystrophy may show alternate bands of osteosclerosis and resorption, the so-called rugger jersey sign. *(Resnick, 2002)*

35. **(A) True; (B) False; (C) True; (D) False; (E) True.** *Discussion:* Symptoms of ankylosing spondylitis typically occur in the postpubescent male and consist of back and buttock pain and morning stiffness that diminishes with activity and recurs after periods of rest. Approximately 25% of patients may have an associated peripheral arthritis that is transient or, in a few cases, prolonged. Patients have reduced anterior lumbosacral flexion as measured by Schober's test. The radiographic changes in the adolescent boy are delayed and may not be manifest until the patients are in their early 20s, but they consist of sacroiliac irregularities with areas of sclerosis and/or erosions (widening). Fusion is typically a late radiographic manifestation. Patients may have extra-articular manifestations that include apical lung fibrosis, conduction disturbances, and aortic insufficiency. *(Cecil, Ch. 279; Resnick, 2002)*

36. **(A) False; (B) True; (C) True; (D) True; (E) True.** *Discussion:* Complications of postmenopausal osteoporosis, particularly severe morbidity from hip and vertebral fractures, represent a major health problem in the United States. Typically, bone mineral appears normal but is reduced in amount, suggesting that there is a disorder in which the formation of mineralized bone does not equal the resorption rate. Quantitative assessment of bone density is possible with dual-energy x-ray absorptiometry. *(Cecil, Ch. 258)*

37. **(A) False; (B) False; (C) False; (D) True; (E) False.** *Discussion:* The gonococcus is a gram-negative diplococcus that, when disseminated, may cause arthritis. Disseminated gonococcemia is a common problem in healthy, sexually active teenagers and young adults. Physical presentation is that of an oligoarticular/monarticular arthritis associated with tenosynovitis and skin lesions that vary from small pustules to vesicopustules with central necrotic centers. Diagnosis is frequently presumptive because it is a fastidious organism that is difficult to culture, requiring increased amounts of carbon dioxide and specialized media (Thayer-Martin). Recent advances in diagnosis also include PCR identification of this organism in urine and urethral swabs. Response to treatment with antibiotics is usually dramatic. *(Cecil, Ch. 286)*

38. **(A) False; (B) True; (C) True; (D) True; (E) True.** *Discussion:* Collagens are the most abundant protein in the human body and constitute approximately 30% of the total protein. They serve diverse functions. Defects of type I collagen, the most abundant collagen type, have been associated with genetic syndromes, including Ehlers-Danlos syndrome and osteogenesis imperfecta. In

the formation of specialized collagens, collagen interacts with other components to make functional basement membranes. Type II collagen is the major fibrillar component of hyaline articular cartilage, and proteoglycans are the major noncollagenous structural proteins associated with elastic resistance to compression of this tissue. *(Primer, 2001)*

39. (A) True; (B) True; (C) False; (D) True; (E) True.
Discussion: Phagocytes have on their plasma membrane receptors for C3b (CR1), which may function to clear circulating immune complexes and enhance phagocytosis. Activation of both complement pathways may lead to the generation of terminal components C6, C7, C8, and C9, which attach to the membrane and induce the formation of pores, with ultimate cell lysis. Recurrent sepsis with *Neisseria* species has been demonstrated in patients with deficiencies of the terminal components. C2 deficiency is by far the most common complement deficiency state, and this is usually associated with a low CH_{50}. Several rheumatic diseases, including SLE-like syndrome, vasculitis, and polymyositis, may occur in conjunction with C4 and C2 deficiencies. *(Primer, 2001)*

40. (A) True; (B) True; (C) True; (D) False; (E) True.
Discussion: As noted, cytokines may have diverse or similar physiologic properties. They are all proteins with "hormone-like" properties having profound effects on inflammatory/immune cell function. Reports of treatment of patients with severe rheumatoid arthritis with a soluble recombinant tumor necrosis factor receptor (p75) Fc fusion protein and antibodies to TNF have been published. *(Cecil, Ch. 278).*

41. (A) True; (B) False; (C) True; (D) True; (E) False.
Discussion: Although the relative risk increases in individuals with a given disease associated with an HLA haplotype, a minority are afflicted with the disease. HLA-DR4 occurs in 60 to 70% of seropositive patients with rheumatoid arthritis. *(Cecil, Ch. 278)*

42. (A) False; (B) True; (C) True; (D) False; (E) False.
Discussion: As noted in the text, rheumatic manifestations of HIV disease are being recognized with increased frequency. Musculoskeletal complaints are reported in 33 to 75% of HIV-infected patients and may present as a wide variety of rheumatologic disorders. Manifestations range from arthralgias, myalgias, and fever with acute seroconversion to polymyositis-like illness, Reiter's syndrome (indistinguishable from that in non-HIV-infected patients), Sjögren's syndrome, and a hepatitis B surface antigen–negative periarteritis nodosa syndrome. *(Cecil, Chs. 279 and 420)*

43. (A) False; (B) True; (C) False; (D) False; (E) False.
Discussion: The pathology of polyarteritis consists of fibrinoid necrosis within small- and medium-size vessels with a variable cellular infiltration, primarily neutrophils. Eosinophilia with lung involvement is not seen in patients with polyarteritis. Diminished total serum hemolytic complement with low C3 and C4 levels are seen in a small percentage of the patients. Subcutaneous nodules are infrequently found. *(Cecil, Ch. 284)*

44. (A) False; (B) True; (C) False; (D) True; (E) False.
Discussion: Infiltrates consisting of atypical lymphoid and plasmacytoid cells are characteristic of lymphomatoid granulomatosis, not Wegener's granulomatosis. Hypersensitivity vasculitis is evidenced histologically by a small-vessel leukocytoclastic vasculitis and clinically by palpable purpura. Temporal arteritis usually involves extracranial elastic arteries. Takayasu's arteritis is a giant cell arteritis of the medium and large arteries, primarily of the aorta and vessels adjacent to it. Henoch-Schönlein purpura is usually a self-limited illness with prolonged renal insufficiency; death is an uncommon outcome. *(Cecil, Ch. 284; Primer, 2001)*

45. (A) False; (B) True; (C) False; (D) False; (E) True.
Discussion: Significant renal involvement in SLE occurs in approximately 50% of patients. Although glomerular involvement is marked, renal tubular and interstitial disease is not uncommon. Neonatal lupus syndrome is associated with a placental transfer of maternal anti-Ro IgG antibodies to the fetus, sometimes causing congenital heart block in the fetus. Mothers do not have heart block, and it is thought that there are phase-specific antigens in the fetus that may be targeted by these antibodies. Vasculitic skin lesions are commonly seen in lupus and usually do not portend CNS vasculitis. Pleural fluid from patients with active SLE is usually transudative. *(Cecil, Ch. 274; Boumpas et al, 1995a, 1995b)*

46. (A) True; (B) False; (C) True; (D) False; (E) True.
Discussion: Idiopathic midline granuloma is usually localized to the midline nasopharynx and is most appropriately treated with a combination of prednisone, cyclophosphamide, and radiation. Polymyalgia rheumatica is characterized by proximal upper and lower extremity muscle stiffness and soreness in patients older than 55 years but is not associated with an elevated creatine phosphokinase or myopathic electromyogram. In general, the alopecia associated with active lupus may improve with treatment of the disease, except with discoid lesions, in which there is follicular plugging and scarring that may result in permanent alopecia. A number of patients with end-stage renal disease caused by lupus have successfully received kidney transplants. *(Cecil, Chs. 280 and 285; Primer, 2001)*

47. (A) True; (B) True; (C) False; (D) False; (E) False.
Discussion: Nonspecific laboratory abnormalities such as neutrophilic leukocytosis and positive rheumatoid factor are often seen in patients with active Wegener's granulomatosis. An anticytoplasmic antibody directed to a 29-kD serine protease has been found in patients with active Wegener's granulomatosis. Idiopathic midline destructive disease is not a systemic vasculitis but is confined to the midparanasal sinuses. Lymphomatoid granulomatosis is an angiocentric immunoproliferative lesion with a tissue distribution very similar to that of Wegener's granulomatosis. It can be easily confused with Wegener's granulomatosis, but it is characterized by an angiocentric, inflammatory infiltrate of mononuclear cells with few granulomas that is an Epstein-Barr virus–associated B-cell lymphoproliferative disease. Necrotizing vasculitis involving the lungs and kidney is characteristic of Wegener's granulomatosis. However, limited forms of this disease without clinical renal or pulmonary involvement have been described. *(Cecil, Ch. 284)*

48. (A) False; (B) True; (C) False; (D) False; (E) True.
Discussion: Erythema chronicum migrans is present in 75% of patients with Lyme disease and is manifest after an incubation period of 3 to 32 days. Approximately 60% of the patients experience frank arthritis. Antibodies to the specific IgM antibodies against the Lyme disease spirochete usually peak within 3 to 6 weeks; the specific IgG antibody titers rise more slowly and are present at the time of the arthritis weeks to months after infection. The decision to treat patients with antibiotics in an endemic area should be based on serologic as well as clinical features. *(Cecil, Ch. 352; Primer, 2001)*

49. (B); 50. (E); 51. (A); 52. (C). *Discussion:* The oxidation of homogentisic acid leads to the formation of an ochronotic brown pigment that is preferentially deposited in cartilage and tissue, which eventually leads to a degenerative arthropathy. Pigmented villonodular synovitis is characterized by synovial villous projections with a pleomorphic cellular infiltrate consisting of a variable number of lipid-laden and hemosiderin-laden macrophages, multinucleated giant cells, fibroblasts, and lymphocytes. Calcific deposits associated with calcium pyrophosphate deposition disease may occur not only in the articular and fibrocartilage but also in the joint capsule, ligaments, tendons, and synovial tissues. The calcium salts stain characteristic purple with hematoxylin. The histologic features of rheumatoid arthritis are not specific but characteristically demonstrate synovial cell hyperplasia followed by infiltration of blood-borne lymphocytes and macrophages. (*Primer, 2001*).

53. (B); 54. (D); 55. (A); 56. (C). *Discussion:* Sudden painless loss of vision is a dreaded complication of temporal arteritis and is usually due to ischemic optic atrophy caused by involvement of the short posterior ciliary arteries and pial arterial network, which supply blood to the optic nerve and optic disc. Retinal vascular disease is a hallmark of eye involvement in SLE, usually with cotton-wool spots (cytoid bodies) that are caused by distended and disrupted axons resulting from anoxia. In addition, hemorrhage is commonly observed in the retina. Eye manifestations of rheumatoid arthritis include sicca complex syndrome, with decreased tear formation as a result of secondary Sjögren's syndrome, and "corneal melt" with linear ulcerations usually at the limbus, leading to corneal perforation. Ankylosing spondylitis may be associated with an anterior uveitis, which is usually manifested by a painful red eye that demands attention. Failure to treat may lead to chronic iritis and blindness. (*Primer, 2001*)

57. (C); 58. (E); 59. (D); 60. (B). *Discussion:* Destruction of the tufts of the terminal phalanges is commonly seen in scleroderma, vinyl chloride disease, and secondary hyperparathyroidism. Acromegaly is characterized by premature or exaggerated osteoarthritis, including osteophyte formation. Punched-out erosions with overhanging bone around deposits of monosodium urate are characteristic of gout. Osteochondromatosis is characterized by the formation of multiple foci of metaplastic hyaline cartilage within the synovium. (*Primer, 2001; Resnick, 2002*)

61. (C); 62. (B); 63. (D); 64. (A). *Discussion:* A variety of musculoskeletal syndromes have been observed in patients on long-term (8-10 years) chronic dialysis. Secondary hyperparathyroidism results from a depressed serum calcium level and an elevated serum phosphorus level, which leads to increased release of parathyroid hormone, which in turn results in osteolysis of the pharyngeal tufts, demineralization of the bones of the appendicular and axial skeleton, and pathologic fractures. Deposition of β_2-microglobulin amyloid within the carpal tunnel is associated with carpal tunnel syndrome and deposition in the bone with subchondral cysts. Deposits of calcium salts in the skin and joints may lead to pruritus and periarthritis. Long-term use of aluminum-based antacids to bind phosphate has led to the syndrome of aluminum-related osteomalacia, characterized by muscle weakness and dementia. Some of these patients have been helped with desferrioxamine. (*Primer, 2001*)

65. (A); 66. (D); 67. (E); 68. (C). *Discussion:* Many rheumatic syndromes have cutaneous manifestations. Erythema marginatum is a feature of rheumatic fever, seen in 10 to 20% of afflicted children and rarely in adults. Nonthrombocytopenic purpura, usually involving the lower extremities, is one of the early manifestations of Henoch-Schönlein purpura, which histologically is a leukocytoclastic vasculitis. In addition, IgA may be found in the skin lesions. A variety of skin manifestations are part of the disseminated gonococcal arthritis syndrome, including nonpainful, asymptomatic vesicles and vesiculopustular or hemorrhagic pustular lesions. Heliotrope rash with associated periorbital swelling and erythema is characteristic of dermatomyositis, both the childhood and adult forms. (*Primer, 2001*)

69. (C); 70. (A); 71. (B); 72. (D). *Discussion:* Acute gouty arthritis is the most frequent clinical manifestation of gout and occurs primarily in middle-age and older men. Although the first MTP joint is characteristically involved, the first interphalangeal joint, ankle, and instep area are also commonly involved. The arthritis of Reiter's syndrome has an acute onset and consists of an asymmetrical oligoarthritis primarily affecting the knees, ankles,

and instep and occurs most frequently in young men, presumably as a sexually acquired "reactive" arthritis. Rheumatoid arthritis is typically a symmetrical polyarthritis predominantly involving the wrists, MCPs, PIPs, and MTP joints. The most common presentation pattern in children is a pauciarticular (four joints or less) arthritis. (*Cecil, Chs. 278 and 288*)

73. (C); 74. (A); 75. (D); 76. (B). *Discussion:* One extra-articular manifestation that has been described in patients with ankylosing spondylitis is upper lobe lung fibrosis. Digital clubbing, periostitis, and painful swelling of bones and joints (hypertropic osteoarthropathy) can develop in a wide variety of diseases such as lung malignancies and pulmonary infections. Acute arthritis, which is the common rheumatic manifestation of sarcoidosis, affects the ankles and knees and, less frequently, the PIP joints of the hands, wrists, and elbows. Pleural effusions and pleuritis are often asymptomatic in rheumatoid arthritis patients, and the pleural fluid is typically exudative, with WBC counts rarely exceeding 5000/μL, with characteristically low glucose levels. (*Cecil, Ch. 278; Primer, 2001*)

77. (E); 78. (D); 79. (C); 80. (A). *Discussion:* Sudden painless loss of vision of the left eye associated with optic atrophy caused by occlusion of branches of the posterior ciliary artery is characteristic of temporal arteritis. Cauda equina syndrome can be seen in patients with long-standing ankylosing spondylitis. Bell's palsy, either unilateral or bilateral, may be a neurologic manifestation of Lyme disease–related arthritis. Deposits of β_2-microglobulin in the carpal tunnel area may lead to motor weakness and atrophy of the muscles of the thenar eminence. (*Primer, 2001*)

81. (B); 82. (E); 83. (A); 84. (C). *Discussion:* Elevated levels of circulating parathyroid hormone leading to resorption of bone and vertebral body fractures have been described in primary and secondary hyperparathyroidism. Hypothyroidism can be associated with a proximal myopathy with an elevated creatine kinase level. This condition can easily be confused with polymyositis. Patients with acromegaly may have a transient Raynaud phenomenon–like illness. Patients with both adult and juvenile diabetes experience a painless limitation of joint mobility in the PIP and DIP joints called diabetic cheiropathy. (*Primer, 2001*)

85. (E); 86. (C); 87. (D); 88. (A). *Discussion:* A variety of rheumatic disease syndromes have been described in association with HIV infection. The most common relate to arthralgias and myalgias associated with acute seroconversion. Nemaline rods (thickened Z line seen in congenital myopathy, polymyositis, and secondary myopathies) may also be seen in HIV-related myopathy. Reiter's syndrome indistinguishable from that in non–HIV-infected patients may be seen. Several vasculitis syndromes have been reported; the periarteritis nodosa type is the most common. This usually presents as a peripheral sensory or sensorimotor neuropathy. (*Cecil, Chs. 279 and 420*)

89. (D); 90. (A); 91. (C); 92. (B). *Discussion:* Palpable purpura is a primary skin feature of hypersensitivity vasculitis. Although multisystem involvement may occur in this small-vessel vasculitis, involvement of the skin is the most common manifestation. Subcutaneous nodules occur in 20 to 25% of rheumatoid arthritis cases, may be freely movable or fixed to the periosteum, and occur primarily in the pressure areas but may also be seen in the feet, hands, and scalp. They also occur in SLE and periarteritis nodosa, but this is very unusual. Gottron's papules are a pathognomonic skin finding of dermatomyositis and are seen in one third of afflicted patients. They are manifested by flat-topped papules that overlie the dorsal surface of the MCP or PIP joints of the hands. Discoid lesions typically occur on the face, chest, or arms and may be either independent or associated with SLE and may be associated with permanent scarring. (*Cecil, Chs. 278, 280, and 283*)

93. **(C)**; 94. **(A)**; 95. **(B)**; 96. **(D)**. *Discussion:* C2 deficiency is associated with an SLE-like syndrome as well as vasculitis and polymyositis-like syndromes. Clinically, it is characterized by a low CH_{50} and may be diagnosed by quantitative C2 measurements. Antineutrophil cytoplasmic antibodies are directed against a 29-kD serine protease associated with the azurophil granules and have been found in many patients with Wegener's granulomatosis. The titer is thought to correlate with the severity of disease activity. The most common renal disorder associated with Sjögren's syndrome is renal tubular acidosis. The presence of glomerulonephritis has been described but is distinctly unusual in primary Sjögren's syndrome. Tender induration of the skin with retraction of subcutaneous tissue with eosinophilia is characteristic of diffuse fasciitis with eosinophilia, a syndrome primarily occurring in men, often after unaccustomed strenuous exercise. *(Primer, 2001)*

97. **(B)**; 98. **(A)**; 99. **(C)**; 100. **(D)**. *Discussion:* Cytoid bodies, also called "retinal exudates," are actually degenerating neuronal elements that form as a response to anoxic tissue injury. They are not specific for lupus and may be seen in a variety of disorders, including leukemia and lymphoma. Mononeuritis multiplex, as evidenced by footdrop or wristdrop or cranial nerve abnormalities, is characteristic of patients with polyarteritis nodosa but may also be seen in patients with a vasculitis secondary to SLE or Wegener's granulomatosis. Jaw claudication, a manifestation of ischemia to the lingual arteries, may be seen in patients with temporal arteritis. A variety of neurologic syndromes may occur in patients with Behçet's syndrome. Cerebellar, brain stem, and long tract signs with acute onset of headache and meningitis characterize the meningoencephalitis syndrome. *(Cecil, Chs. 280 and 284)*

101. **(A)**; 102. **(B)**; 103. **(C)**; 104. **(D)**. *Discussion:* Recurrent fetal loss has been described in patients with minimal findings of lupus and has been found to be associated with the presence of anticardiolipin antibodies. Other features associated with the anticardiolipin antibody include premature strokes and recurrent arterial and venous thrombosis. Congenital heart block is one of the features of neonatal lupus and is thought to be mediated by the transplacental passage of IgG anti-SS-A (Ro) antibody during the first trimester of pregnancy. Drug-induced lupus syndrome, most commonly associated with procainamide ingestion, may occur, with the ANAs including antibodies to antihistone components. Although only occurring in 20 to 30% of patients with lupus, the presence of anti-Smith antibodies is quite specific for this disorder. *(Cecil, Ch. 274; Boumpas et al, 1995a, 1995b)*

105. **(D)**; 106. **(A)**; 107. **(B)**; 108. **(C)**. *Discussion:* Churg-Strauss syndrome is a systemic necrotizing vasculitis that has clinical and pathologic manifestations similar to those of polyarteritis but differs with respect to the frequency of pulmonary involvement, eosinophilia, and allergic manifestations. Eosinophilia-myalgia syndrome, a syndrome with protean manifestations, has been causally linked to contaminated preparations of L-tryptophan. Eosinophilic fasciitis is a scleroderma-like disorder characterized by symmetrical sclerosis of the deep fascia, subcutis, and dermis. Fibromyalgia (fibrositis) is an extremely common disorder characterized by generalized pain and the presence of a large number of tender points. *(Cecil, Ch. 284; Primer, 2001)*

BIBLIOGRAPHY

Boumpas DT, Austin HA III, Fessler BA, et al: Systemic lupus erythematosus: Emerging concepts. Ann Intern Med 1995a;122:940.

Boumpas DT, Austin HA III, Fessler BA, et al: Systemic lupus erythematosus: Emerging concepts 1995b;123:42.

Fine MJ, Kapoor W, Falanga V, et al: Cholesterol crystal embolization: A review of 221 cases in the English literature. Angiology 1987;38:769.

Goldman L, Ausiello D (eds): Cecil Textbook of Medicine, 22nd ed. Philadelphia, WB Saunders, 2004.

Klippel JH (ed): Primer on the Rheumatic Diseases, 12th ed. Atlanta, Arthritis Foundation, 2001.

Resnick D: Diagnosis of Bone and Joint Disorders, 4th ed. Philadelphia. WB Saunders, 2002.

Saag KG, Emkey R, Schnitzer TJ, et al: Alendronate for the prevention and treatment of glucocorticoid-induced osteoporosis. N Engl J Med 1998;339:292.

Part X
Endocrinology

Eric S. Albright and Stuart J. Frank

TRUE OR FALSE
QUESTIONS 1-3

1. A cell's concentration of peptide hormone receptors determines the responsiveness of the cell to the hormone.

2. Downregulation of peptide hormone receptors effectively reduces the cellular response even if the peptide hormone level is maintained.

3. A disease state can disrupt peptide hormone receptor binding but cannot interfere with the second messenger system linked to the receptor.

QUESTIONS 4-6

DIRECTIONS: For questions 4-6, decide whether each choice is true or false.

4. Regarding breast development and physiology, which of the following are *true*?

   A. Prepubertal male and female breasts are histologically and functionally the same.
   B. Estradiol and progesterone are the only endocrine factors required for breast development.
   C. Prolactin is the only endocrine factor required for lactogenesis.

5. Premature sexual development (precocious puberty) may be associated with:

   A. Neurofibromatosis
   B. Granulosa-theca tumors of the ovary
   C. McCune-Albright syndrome
   D. Congenital adrenal hyperplasia

6. Which of the following statements are *true* concerning the sick euthyroid syndrome?

   A. It is usually seen in the setting of moderate to severe illness.
   B. Patient outcome can be improved by thyroid hormone supplementation.
   C. Thyroid hormone abnormality occurs as an isolated endocrine disorder.
   D. Thyroid hormone binding is abnormal.

7. You are seeing a 40-year-old black woman with a history of sarcoidosis that has required large doses of glucocorticoids for control of symptoms. One month ago she experienced severe flank pain with hematuria. Work-up revealed calcium-containing kidney stones. She has mild joint pains without swelling, and physical examination is otherwise unremarkable. The following tests were obtained at her most recent visit:

Serum calcium	9.8 mg/dL (normal range, 8.9-10.1 mg/dL)
Albumin	4.0 mg/dL (normal range, 3.5-4.5 mg/dL)
24-Hr urine calcium	450 mg/day (<250 mg/day)

   What additional tests would help determine the cause of this patient's kidney stones (true/false)?

   A. Angiotensin-converting enzyme (ACE) level
   B. 1,25-Hydroxyvitamin D level
   C. Hydroxyproline level
   D. 24-Hour urine sodium

QUESTIONS 8 AND 9

A 30-year-old black woman with a history of hypothyroidism, epilepsy, and iron deficiency anemia comes for renewal of her medications. She underwent gastric bypass 3 years ago for the management of obesity. She feels cold, is constipated, and has a hoarse voice. She is taking levothyroxine, 250 μg/day, ferrous sulfate, 325 mg three times a day, and phenytoin, 100 mg three times a day. She is 5 feet, 4 inches tall and weighs 130 pounds. Her examination is remarkable for a pulse of 58 beats/minute with a blood pressure of 140/90 mm Hg, coarse, dry skin, and hung-up reflexes.

8. Which of the following factors might be responsible for this patient's current symptoms (true/false)?

   A. History of gastrointestinal surgery
   B. Co-administration of ferrous sulfate with thyroid hormone
   C. Noncompliance with medications
   D. Increased clearance of thyroid hormone
   E. None of the above

9. Which of the following abnormalities might this patient have (true/false)?

   A. Impaired hearing
   B. Hyperprolactinemia
   C. Hypernatremia
   D. Osteoporosis
   E. All of the above

QUESTIONS 10 AND 11

A 51-year-old white man comes to see you after a visit to the emergency department 2 days ago. He has noticed progressive swelling of his eyes with pressure-like sensations in the back of his eyes. Two days ago he experienced redness of both eyes followed by double vision. On further questioning, he admits to significant weight loss, heat intolerance, and tremors. He smokes two packs of cigarettes per day and drinks alcohol on weekends. He volunteers a history of thyroid disease in one of his sisters, treated with radioactive iodine (RAI). He takes no medications. The patient is afebrile with a pulse of 110 beats/minute and a blood pressure of 110/70 mm Hg. He has a stare, bilateral exophthalmos with corneal injection, and slight limitation of lateral gaze in the right eye. Thyroid examination reveals a 70-g diffuse goiter with a bruit. He has a smooth shiny skin with pretibial myxedema. The rest of his physical examination is nonrevealing. The following laboratory test results were obtained in the emergency department:

Alkaline phosphatase	Mild elevation
Hemoglobin	12.4 g/dL (normal range, 13.6-17.2 g/dL)
Hematocrit	37% (normal range, 39-49%)
Free T$_4$	3.9 ng/dL (normal range, 0.81-1.76 ng/dL)
Thyroid-stimulating hormone (TSH)	<0.03 mIU/mL (normal range, 0.3-5 mIU/mL)

10. Which of the following medications would you administer immediately (true/false)?

    A. Propylthiouracil (PTU)
    B. Glucocorticoids
    C. β-Blockers
    D. Inorganic iodine
    E. RAI

This patient is rushed back to the emergency department 3 days later after a deterioration of his condition. He did not take his medications properly and, according to his wife, was restless all night and complained of excessive heat and diarrhea. Later he experienced palpitations and shortness of breath and became mentally confused. On examination his temperature is 39.4°C (103°F) and the heart rate is 130 beats/minute. He is in congestive heart failure.

11. Which of the following agents may now be administered immediately (true/false)?

    A. PTU (high dose) after Lugol's solution
    B. Steroids (high dose)
    C. β-Blockers (high dose)
    D. Lugol's solution after high-dose PTU
    E. RAI

12. The following may be associated with diabetes insipidus (DI) (true/false):

    A. Hypokalemia
    B. Hypocalcemia
    C. Lithium treatment
    D. All of the above

QUESTIONS 13–16

You are seeing a 60-year-old black female for the second time. She is being treated for hypertension and has continued to experience episodic headache, palpitations, and diaphoresis. She is taking 240 mg of long-acting verapamil daily. There is no history of hypertension or hypercalcemia in her family. Laboratory test results from the last visit are as follows:

Serum chemistries	Normal
CBC	Normal
Plasma epinephrine	350 pg/mL (normal range, 0-70 pg/mL)
Plasma norepinephrine level	1700 pg/mL (normal range, 65-400 pg/mL)

13. What additional tests would you order now (true/false)?

    A. Clonidine suppression test
    B. 24-Hour urine catecholamine level
    C. Abdominal MRI
    D. 24-Hour urine metanephrine level

14. The correct test is ordered, and the result is abnormal. Which of the following tests would now be appropriate (true/false)?

    A. Clonidine suppression test
    B. Glucagon stimulation test
    C. Abdominal MRI
    D. 24-Hour urine metanephrine

15. Which of the following agents would you prescribe at this point (true/false)?

    A. Phenoxybenzamine
    B. Propranolol
    C. α-Methyltyrosine
    D. All of the above

16. Which of the following disorders may be associated with this patient's disease (true/false)?

    A. Acromegaly
    B. Hypercalcemia
    C. Impaired glucose tolerance
    D. Diarrhea

17. Hormone replacement treatment in a 34-year-old man who has had bilateral adrenalectomy for bilateral pheochromocytoma should include (true/false):

    A. Glucocorticoids
    B. Mineralocorticoids
    C. Catecholamines
    D. Sex steroids

QUESTIONS 18 AND 19

18. The following conditions may be associated with gynecomastia (true/false):

    A. Hyperthyroidism
    B. Hypothyroidism
    C. Refeeding syndrome
    D. Marijuana abuse

19. You are seeing a 47-year-old white man who was recently diagnosed with a human chorionic gonadotropin–secreting tumor of the left testis. He draws your attention to an

enlargement of his breasts, which he noticed 3 months ago. The swellings have not changed in size but have become tender to touch. There is no nipple discharge. The patient also has peptic ulcers and is taking cimetidine, 400 mg twice a day. Physical examination is unremarkable except for bilateral 3-cm gynecomastia, which is mildly tender to touch. What mechanisms are responsible for this patient's gynecomastia (true/false)?

A. Increased testicular estrogen production
B. Increased peripheral estrogen production
C. Impaired testosterone action
D. All of the above

MATCHING

DIRECTIONS: For questions 20-24, match each case described to the most likely diagnosis.

A. Craniopharyngioma
B. Sarcoidosis
C. Suprasellar dysgerminoma
D. Gonadotropin adenoma (pituitary)
E. Langerhans cell histiocytosis
F. Pituitary stalk injury
G. Apoplexy

20. A 25-year-old man was in a motor vehicle accident in which he rear-ended a parked car. He has significant facial trauma and has done well over the past 24 hours after minor surgery. You are called in the middle of the night to evaluate him for severe hypotension. His hematocrit is 44%. He is lethargic and has 3 L of urine output over the past 4 hours.

21. A 35-year-old woman who has complained of shortness of breath for many years presents to your office with galactorrhea. You find an elevated prolactin level (105 ng/mL) and a normal TSH level. A 24-hour urinary cortisol is normal, and the urine volume in the collection was 8 L.

22. A 14-year-old boy is being evaluated for diabetes insipidus and responds to desmopressin (DDAVP) during a water deprivation test. Further work-up with magnetic resonance imaging (MRI) shows a thickened stalk but no masses or lesions.

23. A 68-year-old man presents with recent onset of headaches and a central visual field cut in his right visual field. This patient has been healthy until last year when he was diagnosed with a seizure disorder that is poorly controlled with medications. He also reports loss of his sex drive and impotence for the past 7 months and nocturia × 4 during this same time frame.

24. A 10-year-old boy presents with his parents who are concerned that he is going into puberty. This child over the past year has grown 2 cm in height, developed pubic hair to Tanner stage IV, and had significant enlargement of his phallus. His scrotum contained both testes, which measured 8 to 10 mL with no masses palpated.

MULTIPLE CHOICE
QUESTIONS 25 AND 26

A 30-year-old woman presents for evaluation of depression. The consult is from her obstetrician, who is worried that the patient has not responded to 40 mg of fluoxetine. The patient has no medical history other than the vaginal delivery of her first son 6 months earlier. Her symptoms consist of lack of energy, decreased libido, headache, and morning vomiting. She has not resumed her periods and has galactorrhea even though she chose not to breast feed. Blood work performed 1 month ago revealed a negative urine pregnancy test, normal TSH, and an elevated prolactin level of 80 ng/dL.

25. What tests should be ordered next?

A. Serum human chorionic gonadotropin (hCG), TSH, and adrenocorticotropic hormone (ACTH) stimulation test
B. Urine hCG, free thyroxine (T_4), luteinizing hormone (LH), and follicle-stimulating hormone (FSH)
C. ACTH stimulation test, insulin-like growth factor (IGF)-1, TSH
D. ACTH stimulation test, free T_4, serum hCG

26. You order an MRI of the pituitary to confirm your diagnosis. The report reveals an enlarged pituitary gland with a thick stalk without a post-contrast filling defect. This MRI suggests which of the following diagnosis?

A. Sheehan's syndrome
B. Prolactinoma
C. Lymphocytic hypophysitis
D. Sarcoidosis
E. Hemochromatosis

27. A 45-year-old woman is referred to you for treatment of acromegaly. All of the following are suggestive of the diagnosis *except*:

A. Elevated random IGF-1
B. Thickened heel pad on plain x-ray films
C. Elevated prolactin level
D. Growth hormone less than 2 μg/mL with 75-g glucose suppression test

28. You are asked to see a 30-year-old woman in consultation from her obstetrician. She is 18 weeks' pregnant and has been taking dopamine agonist therapy for a prolactinoma. On examination she is alert with normal vital signs. HEENT examination is unremarkable and visual fields are grossly intact to confrontation. Your history reveals a diagnosis of a prolactinoma 1 year ago after presentation with amenorrhea. The patient has been treated with bromocriptine, 5 mg twice daily, for the past year. Her prolactin level 3 months ago was 20 ng/dL and her MRI showed a 5 × 5-mm right pituitary hypodensity consistent with an adenoma that has not changed from the initial MRI. You are consulted to manage her prolactinoma during the pregnancy and you recommend the following:

A. Measure the prolactin level.
B. Perform formal visual field testing.
C. Order MRI of the pituitary gland.
D. Discontinue the bromocriptine.
E. Switch to cabergoline.

29. All of the following are *true* regarding the evaluation of Cushing's syndrome *except*:

A. Clinical features include facial plethora, hypertension, central obesity, and proximal muscle weakness.
B. A positive 1-mg overnight dexamethasone suppression test (did not suppress) is diagnostic of Cushing's syndrome.
C. Cortisol excess must be diagnosed before determining if the process is ACTH dependent or independent.
D. Cushing's disease is the most common cause of Cushing's syndrome and occurs more commonly in women.

30. A 24-year-old woman presents for a routine physical examination for her medical school admission requirements. She voices no complaints and has a limited medical history that includes appendectomy at age 9 years, fractured radius (skiing accident), and the occasional cold/bronchitis. She has a family history of thyroid disease in her great-grandmother. As part of your work-up you have drawn thyroid function tests that reveal a thyroxine level of 14.0 μg/dL (normal range, 4.5-12.5 μg/dL) and a TSH value of 4.5 μU/mL (normal range, 0.3-6.0 μU/mL). Examination of the thyroid reveals a 20- to 25-g smooth gland without nodularity. The next step to evaluate her abnormal thyroid test should be to:

    A. Order an uptake and scan.
    B. Order reverse T_3.
    C. Order free T_4.
    D. Order thyroid stimulating immunoglobulins (TSI).
    E. Order a thyroid ultrasound.

31. TSH suppression can occur in all of the following situations *except*:

    A. Resistance to thyroid hormone
    B. Pregnancy
    C. Psychiatric illness
    D. Glucocorticoid therapy
    E. Subacute thyroiditis

32. A 66-year-old man is critically ill with urosepsis. The patient has been treated in the intensive care unit (ICU) with IV fluids and antibiotics for the past 24 hours. The admitting physician drew a thyroid function panel because the patient presented with hypothermia. Social history reveals he is a nursing home resident and had been ill for the past week before being found unresponsive in his bed and being admitted. You have been consulted to interpret the thyroid profile and you suspect it represents a nonthyroidial illness. Which of the following profiles listed belongs to this patient?

	TSH (miU/mL) (normal 0.3-6)	T3 (ng/dL) (normal 80-220)	T4 (μg/dL) (normal 4.5-12.5)	rT3 (ng/dL) (normal 20-40)
A.	1.0	70	4.0	40
B.	7.0	200	7.5	35
C.	4.5	170	6.6	22
D.	0.3	60	4.2	100

33. A 43-year-old woman presents with complaints of blurry vision and difficulty with color vision. She has purchased reading glasses that did not help, and she is becoming concerned. Her medical history is positive for Graves' disease, which was treated 10 years ago with radioactive iodine. The only other pertinent finding is that she recently restarted smoking during her divorce. Her examination reveals normal globes, intact ocular movements, and visual acuity of 20/200 in each eye. Funduscopic examination reveals a pale disk and distended veins in both eyes. You suspect that she has the following:

    A. Pituitary macroadenoma with anterior and superior expansion
    B. Graves' ophthalmopathy
    C. Pseudotumor cerebri
    D. Eye strain
    E. Psychogenic visual disturbance

QUESTIONS 34 AND 35

A 39-year-old woman is admitted to your hospital service for RAI treatment for papillary thyroid cancer. On admission the TSH is 66 miU/mL, which is an appropriate elevation to promote radioiodine uptake and thus destruction of any residual thyroid tissue (including the cancer). You order that she resume her home medications on admission except for levothyroxine, which will be restarted by her endocrinologist. You receive a call later that night that the patient is unresponsive and required intubation and transfer to the ICU.

34. Which of the following could explain the respiratory failure?

    A. Iodine allergy
    B. Sepsis
    C. Radiation-induced thyroiditis
    D. Myxedema coma
    E. Acute congestive heart failure from severe hypothyroidism

35. Based on the case described earlier, which one of the following likely contributed to the patient's current condition?

    A. Foley catheter placement
    B. RAI administration
    C. Continuation of her calcium channel blocker
    D. Acute myocardial infarction
    E. Continuation of her benzodiazepine administered at bedtime

36. A 55-year-old man is seen in consultation for evaluation for possible hyperaldosteronism. He is hospitalized for pneumonia and was found to be hypertensive with hypokalemia. He had been in good health until a year ago when he noted weight loss and new-onset hypertension. On review of systems he comments on significant difficulty rising from a chair or from the toilet. He was an avid tennis player up until a year ago when he quit because of fatigue. His social history is otherwise unremarkable. On examination, his blood pressure is 177/100 mm Hg and in general he appears thin. The patient has significant difficulty rising from a chair and multiple bruises on his arms and hands that he reports are from drawing blood. He has mild edema in the lower extremities. The best test to correctly diagnosis this patient is:

    A. 24-Hour urinary aldosterone
    B. Ratio of aldosterone:plasma renin activity
    C. 24-Hour urinary free cortisol
    D. 24-Hour urinary metanephrines and normetanephrines
    E. CT of the adrenal glands to evaluate for adenoma

37. A 45-year-old woman is recovering from an acute myocardial infarction. She received a stent 2 days ago and is thus anticoagulated. You receive a call that the patient has back pain (a common complaint the first 12 hours after catheterization) and you order morphine. Thirty-six hours latter the patient becomes hypotensive, confused, and febrile and complains of abdominal pain. A stat hematocrit is 35%, blood pressure is 70/30 mm Hg, pulse is 110 beats/minute, and an electrocardiogram shows only sinus tachycardia. You administer a fluid bolus and start dopamine but there is only minimal response of her hypotension. What is the next best intervention?

    A. An epinephrine drip
    B. Stat echocardiogram
    C. Stat CT of the head
    D. CT of the abdomen and pelvis

E. Hydrocortisone, 100 mg IV, and CT of abdomen and pelvis

38. A 23-year-old woman presents with complaints of hirsutism. She has significant hair growth on her upper lip, chin, chest, and abdomen which became noticeable around the time of thelarche. She shaves and plucks her facial hair and has waxing to remove unwanted pubic, thigh, and abdominal hair. Further history reveals 9 to 10 periods per year with a wide interval between menstruation and minimal symptoms consistent with ovulation. To diagnosis the patient with polycystic ovarian syndrome you must first rule out congenital adrenal hyperplasia and to do so you order:

A. 21α-Hydroxylase level
B. Plasma renin activity after 4 hours of upright posture
C. Overnight dexamethasone suppression test result of 1 mg
D. 17-Hydroxyprogesterone level before and after ACTH stimulation
E. No further testing is required at this time

QUESTIONS 39 AND 40

A 34-year-old man comes to your office concerned about his 15-year-old son. The patient has had surgery on his thyroid gland for cancer and has also had bilateral removal of adrenaline-releasing tumors. On examination the patient is 5′6″ tall and weighs 160 lbs. Skin examination is remarkable only for the surgical scars, and the rest of the examination is within normal limits. He was told this was genetic and he is concerned that his only son is at risk for the same tumors. The patient was adopted and does not know his family history.

39. Based on the history the patient carries which of the following diagnosis?

A. Multiple endocrine neoplasia type 1
B. Multiple endocrine neoplasia type 2a
C. Multiple endocrine neoplasia type 2b
D. Autoimmune polyglandular syndrome type 1
E. Autoimmune CPE 2

40. Based on the father's diagnosis, what evaluation should you recommend for the patient's son?

A. Measure autoantibodies for the thyroid, adrenal, and pancreas.
B. Measure a thyroid profile and perform a Cortrosyn (ACTH) stimulation test.
C. Measure a gastrin stimulated calcitonin level.
D. Genetic screening for a *RET* proto-oncogene mutation.
E. Genetic screening for a *MENIN* (tumor suppressor gene) mutation.

41. The following statements are true regarding carcinoid syndrome *except*:

A. Carcinoid syndrome is caused by tumors that commonly secrete both serotonin and tachykinins (like substance P).
B. The most common clinical feature is the vasodilator paroxysms, which manifest as cutaneous flushing.
C. Flushing, diarrhea, and tricuspid fibrosis occur as part of the syndrome.
D. Tachycardia and hypertension are a common clinical finding.
E. Exertion, ethanol, and eating may provoke a flushing event.

QUESTIONS 42 AND 43

A 45-year-old British man presents to your clinic with pain in his right femur. On examination he is alert, in mild discomfort from his leg, and is using a cane in his left hand to offset some of the weight bearing on his right leg. He is healthy and on no medications. You evaluate the patient with a full chemistry and liver panel as well as a radiograph of the right femur. Results show a significant elevation of the alkaline phosphatase level, and the radiograph demonstrates mid-shaft increased density with localized hyperlucent foci and mild bowing. On physical examination the bowing is minimal and there is increased temperature over the corresponding area of the thigh.

42. What is your diagnosis?

A. Osteomalacia
B. Osteonecrosis
C. Fibrogenesis imperfecta ossium
D. Osteitis deformans
E. Metastatic prostate cancer involving the femur

43. Based on your diagnosis, which of the following would you recommend?

A. Observation
B. Administration of 1500 mg of elemental calcium and ergocalciferol 2000 IU/day
C. Administration of 1500 mg of elemental calcium and calcitriol, 0.5 μg twice daily
D. Alendronate, 40 mg/day
E. Surgical bone grafting

44. Which of the statements below is *false* regarding peptide hormones?

A. Peptide hormones act by binding to cell surface receptors.
B. Peptide hormones act by triggering rapid conformational changes to existing cell enzymes.
C. Peptide hormones are synthesized from cholesterol precursors.
D. The peptide hormone receptors usually have one of three general structures.

45. A 51-year-old white man was recently diagnosed with a solitary 2.7-cm papillary cancer of the thyroid with no invasion of the capsule, no lymphadenopathy, and no distant metastases. He denies a history of head and neck irradiation, hoarseness, pain, dysphagia, or hemoptysis. His physical examination is otherwise normal, with no laboratory abnormalities. Which of the following measures is most appropriate for his management?

A. Partial thyroidectomy followed by RAI treatment
B. Near-total thyroidectomy followed by RAI treatment
C. Thyroid hormone treatment
D. A and C
E. B and C

46. You saw a 71-year-old white female nursing home resident who was brought in by her daughter for a complete physical examination. Her complaints include a poor appetite, weight loss, cramps, and weakness. She was diagnosed with Crohn's disease 10 years ago but is not taking any medications. Five months ago she had a mammogram and flexible sigmoidoscopy, both of which were normal. Because her examination was normal, she is given a 1-month return appointment and sent for blood work. At the end of the day, the laboratory calls to report a panic value of calcium of

5.6 mg/dL (normal range, 8.5-10.2 mg/dL) with an inorganic phosphate level of 1.8 mg/dL (normal range, 2.7-4.5 mg/dL). She has a creatinine of 0.9 mg/dL (normal range, 0.6-1.4 mg/dL), albumin is 3.5 g/dL (normal range, 3.5-4.5 g/dL), and alkaline phosphatase is 250 U/L (normal range, 42-98 U/L). Which of the following diagnoses is compatible with these laboratory values?

A. Hypoparathyroidism
B. Hypomagnesemia
C. Vitamin D deficiency
D. Renal failure

47. A 38-year-old black woman draws your attention to a swelling in her neck, which she noticed 2 days ago. She denies palpitations, diaphoresis, and weight loss. There is no pain, hoarseness, or dysphagia. Her medical history is notable only for hypertension. Medications include only atenolol, 50 mg once daily. On examination, blood pressure is 150/80 mm Hg; pulse is 70 beats/minute. There is a 2 × 1-cm nontender nodule on the right lobe of the thyroid. No lymphadenopathy is detected. The remainder of the examination is unremarkable. Electrolytes, blood urea nitrogen (BUN), creatinine, liver function tests, calcium, phosphorus, and CBC are normal. What would you do next?

A. Elicit history of head and neck irradiation.
B. Elicit a family history of thyroid cancer.
C. Obtain thyroid function tests.
D. Perform fine-needle aspiration.
E. All of the above

QUESTIONS 48 AND 49

A 60-year-old white man comes to see you for chronic back pain, which worsened 1 week ago. He has been wheelchair bound for 6 months because of severe osteoporosis with multiple lumbosacral spine fractures. He has severe asthma, which has required large doses of glucocorticoids for many years. The patient reports progressive loss of height and kyphosis over the past year. Other medications include albuterol and ipratropium inhalers and long-acting theophylline, 300 mg twice a day. Significant physical findings include bilateral cataracts, multiple ecchymoses, and a prolonged expiratory phase with bilateral wheezes.

48. Which of the following measures may be helpful?

A. Testosterone replacement (only if he is deficient)
B. Physical therapy
C. Vitamin D replacement
D. Calcium supplementation
E. Hydrochlorothiazide
F. All of the above

49. Which of the following underlies his osteoporosis?

A. Decreased bone formation
B. Increased bone loss
C. Decreased calcium absorption from the gastrointestinal tract
D. Increased calcium loss in urine
E. All of the above

50. A 35-year-old black woman comes to see you for a complete physical examination. She has experienced cold intolerance, weakness, and constipation for 3 months. Her menses are regular but scanty. Her history is significant for hypertension and peptic ulcer disease, and her family history includes hypertension and diabetes. The patient is married but has never been pregnant and takes cimetidine, 400 mg at bed-

time, sustained-release nifedipine, 60 mg daily, and docusate sodium, 100 mg three times a day. Her pulse is 58 beats/minute with a blood pressure of 135/90 mm Hg. Her skin is dry and scaly, and she has hung-up reflexes. The rest of her examination is normal, and the following laboratory values are obtained: serum chemistries are normal except for a creatine kinase of 300 U/L (normal range, 26-140 U/L); complete blood cell (CBC) count is normal, free T_4 is 0.5 ng/dL (normal range, 0.7-1.5 ng/dL), and TSH is 1.5 mIU (normal range, 0.3-5.0 mIU). Which of the following tests would you order?

A. Free triiodothyronine (T_3)
B. Thyroid scan
C. Thyroid uptake
D. Pituitary MRI
E. Antithyroid antibodies

51. A 38-year-old black woman presents for renewal of her medications. She has had hypertension since her last pregnancy at age 30 and has been maintained on clonidine, 0.2 mg twice a day. She gets headaches, dyspnea on exertion, swelling of her feet, and orthopnea but denies chest pain. Her father is also being treated for hypertension. She is married and does not smoke. She is 5'7" tall and weighs 257 pounds. Her blood pressure is 180/110 mm Hg; pulse is 92 beats/minute. The rest of her examination is remarkable for hypertensive retinopathy, bibasilar rales, and 1+ pitting edema bilaterally. Initial laboratory results were normal except for a serum potassium level of 3.0 mEq/L (normal range, 3.5-5.0 mEq/L) and serum bicarbonate value of 33 mEq/L (normal range, 22-28 mEq/L). You correct hypokalemia and obtain a random serum aldosterone level of 25 ng/dL (normal range, 5-30 ng/dL) with a plasma renin activity of 0.5 ng/mL/hour (normal range, 1.6-7.4 ng/mL/hour) while the patient is on a normal diet. What additional tests might be appropriate?

A. Adrenal CT scan
B. Adrenal vein sampling
C. 18-Hydroxycorticosterone
D. Saline loading test
E. A, B, and C

52. A 27-year-old white woman was admitted 2 days ago from the emergency department for seizures. She has a history of moderate alcohol use. Two weeks ago she received benzathine penicillin for secondary syphilis. She is complaining of muscle cramps, weakness, and headache. She received 1 g of phenytoin on the day of admission and is now taking 100 mg three times a day. She is also taking acetaminophen, multivitamins, and tapering doses of chlordiazepoxide. There is a history of seizures in her family. She is 5 feet tall and weighs 120 pounds. Her blood pressure is 130/80 mm Hg; pulse is 90 beats/minute. The rest of the physical examination is normal except for a round face, a short neck, short fourth and fifth metacarpals, and bilateral cataracts. Abnormal laboratory results include a calcium value of 6.1 mg/dL (normal range, 8.4-10.2 mg/dL), phosphorus of 5.2 mg/dL (normal range, 2.7-4.5 mg/dL), and an intact parathyroid hormone (PTH) of 200 pg/mL (normal range, 15-65). Which of the following is most likely?

A. Hypothyroidism
B. Hypogonadism
C. Basal ganglia calcification
D. Mental retardation
E. All of the above

53. All of the following thyroid conditions are amenable to RAI treatment *except:*

    A. Papillary cancer
    B. Follicular cancer
    C. Graves' disease
    D. Thyroid lymphoma
    E. Multinodular goiter

54. Which of the following statements is/are *true* regarding PTH?

    A. Secretion is stimulated by hypocalcemia.
    B. Secretion is inhibited by hypercalcemia.
    C. The effect of magnesium on secretion is the same as that of calcium.
    D. Secretion is stimulated by low 1,25-hydroxyvitamin D and inhibited by high levels of 1,25-hydroxyvitamin D.
    E. A, B, and D
    F. All of the above

55. A 30-year-old black woman recently diagnosed with Graves' disease has been on PTU for the past 6 weeks. Today she reports improvement of all of her symptoms. Her thyroid function tests have all normalized except TSH, which is mildly suppressed. The above change can be attributed to:

    A. Inhibition of thyroid hormone 5′-deiodinase type 1
    B. Inhibition of thyroid hormone 5′-deiodinase type 2
    C. Inhibition of the thyroidal peroxidase enzyme
    D. A and C
    E. B and C

56. A 43-year-old white man was admitted 1 week ago for vascular surgery. Three days ago, he experienced atrial fibrillation, which has been very difficult to control. His medical history includes hypertension, diabetes, coronary heart disease, and hypercholesterolemia. Medications include sustained-release verapamil, 180 mg daily, pravastatin, 20 mg daily, and insulin. Family history is positive for diabetes and hypertension. Physical examination reveals a well-developed, well-nourished male in no distress. Blood pressure is 130/80 mm Hg; pulse is 110 beats/minute and irregular. The lungs are clear, and the abdomen is soft and nontender; bowel sounds are normal. Thyroid examination reveals a 20-g gland that is of normal consistency and nontender. The skin is normal; palms are of a normal temperature and are not moist. Significant laboratory test results include a TSH of 0.07 mIU/mL (normal range, 0.35-5.5 mIU/mL) with a free T_4 of 1.0 ng/dL (normal range, 0.81-1.76 ng/dL) and a free T_3 of 2.5 ng/L (normal range, 1.9-5.0 ng/L). What would you recommend?

    A. Starting PTU, 100 mg, three times a day
    B. Thyroid ablation
    C. Measure antithyroid antibody
    D. None of the above

57. A 75-year-old white woman with a history of hypertension was admitted with progressive weakness. She is a widow who lived independently until 2 months ago when, according to her children, she became unable to care for herself and was put in a nursing home. She was noted to be less and less active over 2 to 3 weeks before she became lethargic. Her last bowel movement was 5 days ago, and it consisted of hard stool. She is not taking any medications. Physical examination reveals an elderly woman who is wasted and has dry oral mucosa. She has normal vital signs except for a pulse of 104 beats/minute. Her systemic examination is normal except for slow reflexes. The following laboratory tests are obtained: sodium, 135 mEq/L; potassium, 4.0 mEq/L; chloride, 110 mEq/L; bicarbonate, 18 mEq/L; BUN, 20 mEq/L; creatinine, 1.0 mg/dL; glucose, 98 mg/dL; calcium, 10.1 mg/dL. She has a mild normochromic-normocytic anemia with a normal erythrocyte sedimentation rate. Abdominal x-ray films show fecal impaction with no air-fluid levels. What additional tests would you order?

    A. Thyroid function tests
    B. Serum albumin
    C. Stool occult blood
    D. A, B, and C
    E. A and C only

58. A 55-year-old black man was admitted for management of pharyngeal carcinoma. He underwent radical neck dissection, during which the surgeon removed a 1 × 1-cm lymph node–like structure from the angle of the left jaw; this was pathologically identified as a parathyroid adenoma. The patient has a long-standing history of tobacco abuse and was diagnosed with hypercalcemia 2 years ago. He is taking acetaminophen with codeine for pain. The family history is not significant. Abnormal laboratory values include a calcium level of 11.5 mg/dL (normal range, 8.4-10.2 mg/dL) and an inorganic phosphate level of 2.2 mg/dL (normal range, 2.7-4.5 mg/dL). Albumin is 4.0 g/dL (normal range, 3.5-4.5 mg/dL), and the intact parathyroid hormone level is 110 pg/mL (normal range, 15-65 pg/mL). Which of the following statements is correct?

    A. The gland that was removed was derived from the third brachial pouch.
    B. The gland that was removed was derived from the fourth brachial pouch.
    C. This patient has a 100% chance of having three glands remaining.
    D. A and C
    E. B and C

59. You are seeing a 21-year-old black male college student for a routine physical examination. He has no medical history, has no complaints, and is taking no medications. His family history is unremarkable except for neck exploration in one uncle. Physical examination is remarkable only for a 35-g goiter, which is nontender. Laboratory results are normal except for a calcium concentration of 10.5 mg/dL (normal range, 8.4-10.2 mg/dL), with a normal albumin level. What additional tests would you order?

    A. TSH
    B. Intact PTH
    C. Vitamin D studies
    D. A and B

60. The correct tests are ordered, and the results are within normal limits except for persistence of elevated calcium concentration. What additional tests would you order now?

    A. Obtain a neck ultrasonogram.
    B. Obtain a sestamibi scan.
    C. Obtain a urine calcium/creatinine ratio (calcium clearance ratio).
    D. A and B

61. A 33-year-old white woman comes to see you for a headache, which has been disabling for the past 2 months. It is associated with nausea but no vomiting. Other symptoms include constipation, cold intolerance, and hoarseness. She has been amenorrheic for 4 months and reports mild galactorrhea. She underwent partial thyroidectomy 3 years ago for a solitary thyroid nodule, which was benign. She is not taking any medicines. Her mother was treated for Graves' disease with RAI. Significant physical findings include a well-healed thyroidectomy scar with the left lobe of the thyroid gland being barely palpable, dry and scaly skin, and bilateral nonpitting edema. Visual field testing was normal. Laboratory results are normal except for creatine kinase of 800 U/L (normal range, 26-140 U/L), free T_4 of 0.4 ng/dL (normal range, 0.7-1.5 ng/dL), TSH of 75 mIU/L (normal range, 0.3-5 mIU/L), and a prolactin level of 100 ng/mL (normal range, 0-20 ng/mL). Pregnancy test was negative, and a CT of the head with and without contrast medium enhancement showed diffuse pituitary enlargement. What would you do next?

    A. Recommend pituitary surgery.
    B. Start bromocriptine.
    C. Start thyroid hormone replacement.
    D. B and C
    E. Start estrogen replacement therapy.

62. Which of the following agents are used in the treatment of thyroid storm?

    A. PTU
    B. Corticosteroids
    C. Propranolol
    D. RAI
    E. All of the above
    F. A to C

63. A 31-year-old black woman was admitted with severe headache, visual blurring, nausea, and photophobia, which woke her up at 4:00 AM. The patient is now comatose. She and her husband were involved in a rear-end collision motor vehicle accident 2 days ago, after which she had been complaining of a headache. She has sickle-cell disease and was diagnosed with a prolactinoma 3 years ago. Therapy with bromocriptine led to regularization of her menses and improvement of her headaches. She is now 2 months pregnant and takes prenatal vitamins and acetaminophen as needed for pain. She has been married for 2 years, smokes a half-pack of cigarettes a day, and drinks alcohol on weekends. There is no history of illicit drug use. Which of the following could have led to this patient's condition?

    A. History of smoking
    B. Trauma
    C. Pregnancy
    D. Sickle-cell disease
    E. B, C, and D

64. You are contacted by a nurse practitioner for advice in the management of a 24-year-old white woman who is entering the second trimester of her first pregnancy. She is complaining of excessive thirst and excessive urination. The patient sustained a basilar skull fracture during a head-on motor vehicle collision 1 year ago and experienced increased thirst and urination thereafter; these symptoms worsened significantly after conception. Medications include only prenatal vitamins. The family history is not contributory. She is a married schoolteacher who does not smoke, drink alcohol, or use any illicit drugs. Her review of systems is notable only for mild headaches and excessive thirst without visual dis-

turbance. Her physical examination is unremarkable and the following laboratory results were obtained:

Sodium	143 mEq/L (normal range, 135-143 mEq/L)
Potassium	4.0 mEq/L (normal range, 3.5-5 mEq/L)
Chloride	106 mEq/L (normal range, 97-105 mEq/L)
Bicarbonate	26 mEq/L (normal range, 22-28 mEq/L)
BUN	7 mg/dL (normal range, 7-18 mg/dL)
Creatinine	0.9 mEq/L (normal range, 0.6-1.4 mEq/L)
Serum osmolality	297 mOsm/kg (normal range, 275-295 mOsm/kg)
Urine osmolality	245 mOsm/kg (normal range, 38-1400 mOsm/kg)
24-Hour urine volume	4.5 L

Mechanisms responsible for this patient's disorder include:

    A. Decreased synthesis of arginine vasopressin (AVP)
    B. Increased degradation of AVP
    C. Decreased sensitivity to AVP
    D. All of the above
    E. A and B only

65. The following can be used in the treatment of primary aldosteronism *except*

    A. Spironolactone
    B. Angiotensin-converting enzyme (ACE) inhibitors
    C. Calcium-channel blockers
    D. Thiazide diuretics
    E. None of the above

66. A 20-year-old black woman comes to you for a pre-employment physical examination and is asking for your advice on contraception. She has a 1-year-old infant who was delivered by cesarean section because of toxemia of pregnancy. She has otherwise been in good health since that delivery and is taking no medication. Her mother has diabetes mellitus, and a distant aunt was diagnosed with breast cancer. The patient has smoked a half-pack of cigarettes a day for 3 years. Her physical examination is unremarkable with a blood pressure of 110/70 mm Hg. Preliminary laboratory results are normal, with a negative pregnancy test. Contraindications to combined oral contraceptive pills (OCPs) include:

    A. A history of hypertension during pregnancy
    B. Smoking
    C. A family history of breast cancer
    D. A family history of diabetes mellitus
    E. None of the above

67. A 28-year-old white woman comes to see you after an emergency department visit 2 weeks earlier, during which she was started on phenytoin for seizures. She is taking it faithfully, has been seizure free, and has no specific complaints. She is married and would not like to get pregnant before completion of her master's degree. Other medications include OCPs (containing 35 μg of ethinylestradiol) and acetaminophen as needed. She does not use alcohol or tobacco and has a history of hypertension in her family. What would you recommend?

    A. Do not change medications.
    B. Increase dose of ethinylestradiol to 50 μg/day.
    C. Change to implantable levonorgestrel.
    D. None of the above

QUESTIONS 68 AND 69

A 35-year-old white woman with a history of AIDS and hepatitis B infection was admitted with complaints of abdominal pain, nausea, and vom-

iting for 1 month. She has lost 5 pounds and has lately had severe craving for salt. She reports occasional lightheadedness on rising but has not fainted. She has had diarrhea without hematochezia. She denies cough, fever, difficulty breathing, and chest pain. She is taking inhaled pentamidine every month for Pneumocystis carinii pneumonia prophylaxis. Examination reveals an emaciated woman who is in no distress. Blood pressure is 120/70 mm Hg supine and 100/55 mm Hg standing. The pulse increased from 85 to 100 beats/minute on rising. She has cytomegalovirus retinitis and has hyperpigmentation of the buccal mucosa, knuckles, and elbows. Significant laboratory findings include the following:

Sodium	130 mEq/L (normal range, 135-143 mEq/L)
Potassium	5.7 mEq/L (normal range, 3.5-5.0 mEq/L)
Serum bicarbonate	18 mEq/L (normal range, 22-28 mEq/L)
BUN	30 mg/dL (normal range, 7-18 mg/dL)
Creatinine	1.1 mg/dL (normal range, 0.6-1.4 mg/dL)
Lactate dehydrogenase	400 U/L (normal range, 60-100 U/L)
Albumin	3.8 mg/dL (normal range, 3.5-4.5 mg/dL)
Hemoglobin	9.5 g/dL (normal range, 11.2-15.3 g/dL)
Hematocrit	28.5% (normal range, 33-43%)

68. What additional tests would be appropriate?

    A. Thyroid function tests
    B. Amylase
    C. Stool studies
    D. ACTH stimulation test
    E. All of the above

Appropriate tests were ordered, and the patient was rehydrated with some improvement. She was later started on hydrocortisone, 10 mg in the morning and 5 mg in the afternoon, after a thorough review of her laboratory test results. She continued to improve and was discharged with minimal lightheadedness. Three weeks later she comes to see you in the clinic and is still feeling lightheaded, even though she has been faithful in taking her medications. Her blood pressure is now 120/80 mm Hg with orthostatic changes. The remainder of her examination is unchanged. The following laboratory results are obtained:

Sodium	133 mEq/L
Potassium	5.5 mEq/L
Serum bicarbonate	19 mEq/L

69. What would you do now?

    A. Check serum ACTH.
    B. Add fludrocortisone, 0.1 mg daily.
    C. Increase hydrocortisone to 10 mg bid
    D. None of the above

QUESTIONS 70 AND 71

You are asked to help in the management of a 51-year-old white man who has had progressive lethargy and dizziness for a week. He underwent left upper lobectomy 1 year ago for squamous cell cancer of the lung. Two days ago he had a CT of the brain with contrast medium enhancement, which showed a left parietal mass of 1 cm with surrounding edema. The patient has a pulse of 81 beats/minute with a blood pressure of 110/68 mm Hg. He is afebrile and has no focal neurologic signs. The rest of his physical examination is normal. Abnormal laboratory results include the following:

Sodium	120 mEq/L (normal range, 135-143 mEq/L)
Creatine phosphokinase	1200 U/L (normal range, 26-140 U/L)
Free T_4	0.4 ng/dL (normal range, 0.7-1.5 ng/dL)
TSH	58 mIU (normal range, 0.32-5.0 mIU)
8:00 AM cortisol	32 μg/dL (normal range, 5-25 μg/dL)
Hemoglobin	11.2 g/dL (normal range, 13.6-17.2 g/dL)
Hematocrit	33.5% (normal range, 39-49%)

70. The next step in management should include:

    A. Fluid restriction
    B. Normal saline with IV furosemide
    C. Hypertonic saline
    D. Demeclocycline
    E. None of the above

71. The patient was started on L-thyroxine, 100 μg daily. Which of the following will correct first?

    A. Free T_4
    B. Free T_3
    C. TSH
    D. Total T_3

QUESTIONS 72 AND 73

A 51-year-old black female is admitted with a headache, which started suddenly while she was preparing to go to church. It is associated with nausea, vomiting, and photophobia and is the most severe headache she has ever had. She is being treated for hypertension and hyperlipidemia. The patient gives a history of excessive thirst and excessive urination in the weeks leading up to her admission but denies cold intolerance and galactorrhea. She has had an unexplained weight loss of 5 pounds in the past 2 months. Her mother and an elder sister have been diagnosed with pituitary tumors, and an uncle had neck exploration for reasons unknown to the patient as well as kidney stones. Abnormal physical findings include bitemporal hemianopsia and nuchal rigidity. Significant laboratory results include the following:

Prolactin	417 ng/mL (normal range 0-20 ng/mL)
TSH	1.2 mIU (normal range 0.32-5 mIU)
Serum glucose	305 mg/dL (normal range 65-115 mg/dL)
Free T_4	0.5 ng/dL (normal range 0.8-2.4 ng/dL)
Cortisol	3.3 μg/dL with a peak of 15 μg/dL after ACTH stimulation (normal response > 20 μg/dL).

On review of her fluid balance, you discover that her fluid intake over the past 24 hours was 2 L, with an output of 6 L. Results of FSH and IGF-1 are pending.

72. Management should, among other things, include the following *except*:

    A. Bromocriptine
    B. Desmopressin
    C. Hydrocortisone
    D. Neurosurgery consultation

73. If affected, the offspring of this patient are most likely to have:

    A. Pheochromocytoma
    B. Medullary thyroid carcinoma
    C. Kidney stones
    D. Marfanoid features
    E. None of the above

74. A 28-year-old black woman was diagnosed with Graves' disease 2 years ago and was treated with PTU. Six weeks ago you referred her to an endocrinologist, who treated her with RAI. Her symptoms have improved dramatically, with disappearance of palpitations and diaphoresis. She has gained 2 pounds and has no eye or skin symptoms. All of the following tests will be useful in determining her thyroid status *except*:

    A. Free T_4
    B. Free T_3
    C. TSH
    D. Total T_4

75. You are monitoring a 25-year-old black man who has Klinefelter's syndrome. He is taking testosterone enanthate, 200 mg IM, every 2 weeks, which was started at his last visit 3 months ago. The patient is now having nocturnal erections, and his overall sense of well-being is much improved. He is now shaving more frequently and has no complaints. Examination reveals a tall black male with a well-formed beard and pubic and axillary hair. There is no gynecomastia, and the rest of the examination is normal except for small testes. What would you do at this point?

    A. Check a testosterone level and if low adjust the dose.
    B. Check the LH level and if elevated adjust the testosterone dose.
    C. Check a sperm count.
    D. Observe.

QUESTIONS 76 AND 77

A 70-year-old white woman comes to see you complaining of night sweats, palpitations, and tremors, which she has had for 3 weeks. She has lost 4 pounds despite an excellent appetite. Her medical history is significant for hypertension, an anxiety disorder, and mitral valve prolapse. She takes verapamil slow-release 240 mg daily. On examination she has a pulse of 110 beats/minute and a normal blood pressure. She has warm palms, a fine tremor, a smooth velvety skin, and brisk reflexes. Her thyroid is of normal size, nodular, and nontender. There is no exophthalmos. The following laboratory results are obtained:

Serum chemistries	Normal
CBC	Normal
Free T$_4$	1.4 ng/dL (normal range, 0.7-1.5 ng/dL)
TSH	<0.03 mIU/L (normal range, 0.3-5 mIU/L)

The technetium-99m scan of the thyroid shows patchy inhomogeneous uptake consistent with a multinodular goiter.

76. What additional tests would you order?

    A. Free T$_3$
    B. Thyroid-stimulating immunoglobulin
    C. Thyroglobulin
    D. Antithyroid antibody

77. Long-term management of this patient would include:

    A. β-Blockade
    B. PTU treatment
    C. RAI treatment
    D. Psychiatric referral

78. Which of the following statements regarding pheochromocytoma are correct?

    A. The magnitude of blood pressure elevation is always proportional to serum catecholamine levels.
    B. Complete surgical removal always results in cure of hypertension.
    C. It is never diagnosed in the absence of symptoms.
    D. None of the above.

79. Regarding steroid-induced bone loss, which of the following statements is correct?

    A. It can be prevented by using alternate-day steroid regimens, where applicable.
    B. It can be prevented by the use of inhaled steroids rather than oral steroids, where applicable.
    C. Exercise can be preventive.

    D. It can be minimized if hyperparathyroidism can be prevented.
    E. C and D

80. A 37-year-old white man who has been seeing your partner for the past 6 months presents on a weekend when you are on call. The patient had a prolactinoma removed 3 years ago via a transfrontal approach. At that time he was having visual field defects, which normalized after the procedure. He was lost to follow-up before seeing your partner, who has been evaluating him for abdominal pain and weight loss. Three months ago he was started on omeprazole, 20 mg daily, and levothyroxine, 0.1 mg daily, for secondary hypothyroidism. At his visit 1 month ago he was found to have hyperprolactinemia, for which bromocriptine, 2.5 mg daily, was begun. The patient continues to have abdominal pain with nausea and is now feeling extremely weak. He also reports excessive thirst and excessive urination for the past 3 months. This patient could have:

    A. Anemia
    B. Hypotension
    C. Hypogonadism
    D. Bladder hypertrophy
    E. All of the above

81. A 45-year-old white woman comes to see you because she fears she might have breast cancer just like her mother and sister. She has had galactorrhea for 3 months, which has worsened in the past 4 weeks. She has hot flashes occasionally but denies headaches and visual field problems. She underwent a total abdominal hysterectomy 4 years ago and is not taking any medicines. Physical examination is unremarkable except for the presence of a milky discharge from both breasts. Laboratory results are normal except for a prolactin level of 189 ng/mL (normal range, 0-20 ng/mL). A pituitary MRI showed a 5-mm adenoma. What would you recommend?

    A. Surgery
    B. Bromocriptine
    C. Radiation therapy
    D. Estrogen replacement therapy
    E. Observation

82. Features associated with secondary adrenal failure may include the following *except*:

    A. Eosinophilia
    B. Hypotension
    C. Decreased libido
    D. Hypoglycemia
    E. Hyperkalemia

83. A 71-year-old black woman was brought from a nursing home to your hospital for treatment of pneumonia. In the emergency department she was found to be hypotensive and hypothermic and has received 3 L of saline. A heating blanket has been ordered. Her medical history includes congestive heart failure, peptic ulcers, dementia, and urinary tract infections, and she takes digoxin, ranitidine, and ceftriaxone. Examination reveals an elderly woman who is cachectic and unresponsive, with shallow breathing at a rate of 10 breaths/minute. Her temperature is 35° C (95° F). Blood pressure is 90/50 mm Hg, with a pulse of 80 beats/minute. Neck examination reveals a normal thyroid gland. She has right lower lobe crackles and distant heart sounds, without murmurs or gallops. Her abdomen is slightly distended with

scanty bowel sounds, and there are no masses. Neurologic examination reveals no focal abnormalities. The following laboratory results were obtained:

Arterial blood gases (room air)	
pH	7.29
P_{CO_2}	60 mm Hg
P_{O_2}	50 mm Hg
Oxygen saturation	82%

Serum sodium	145 mEq/L (normal range, 135-143 mEq/L)
Serum potassium	4.1 mEq/L (normal range, 3.5-5.0 mEq/L)
Serum chloride	110 mEq/L (normal range, 97-105 mEq/L)
Serum bicarbonate	26 mEq/L (normal range, 22-28 mEq/L)
BUN	31 mg/dL (normal range, 8-20 mg/dL)
Creatinine	1.5 mg/dL (normal range, 0.6-1.4 mg/dL)
WBC	14.2×10^9/L (normal range, 2.8-10×10^9/L)
Hemoglobin	10 g/dL (normal range, 11.2-15.3 g/dL)
Hematocrit	30% (normal range, 33-43%)
Free T_4	0.3 ng/dL (normal range, 0.7-1.5 ng/dL)
TSH	1.0 mIU/mL (normal range, 0.3-5 mIU/mL)

Chest x-ray film shows a right lower lobe infiltrate. What additional tests would you order?

    A. ACTH stimulation test
    B. LH level
    C. Pituitary MRI
    D. All of the above

84. A 43-year-old white woman comes to see you with a diagnosis of hyperprolactinemia. She has been experiencing galactorrhea, poor vision in both eyes, and headache for more than 6 months. She has taken several courses of steroids for asthma. Her other medications include albuterol and ipratropium inhalers. Her last menstruation was 2 weeks ago, and she has not gained any weight. Examination reveals an obese white woman who has normal blood pressure and pulse. She has bilateral cataracts, but the rest of her examination is normal. Her laboratory results are normal except for a prolactin level of 200 ng/mL. A pituitary MRI showed a 6-mm adenoma. The next step in her management should include the following:

    A. Transsphenoidal surgery
    B. Medical treatment with a dopamine agonist
    C. Radiation therapy
    D. Observation with another MRI in 6 months

85. A 55-year-old white woman sustained a fracture of the left radius after a fall on her outstretched arm. She has had back pain, hot flashes, night sweats, and dyspareunia for several months. Her menarche occurred at 16 years, and she has two grown children. She has smoked two packs of cigarettes a day for 20 years and drinks alcohol on weekends. Her mother suffered from disabling osteoporosis, and she would like to make sure she does not have it. Her vital signs are normal, and physical examination is remarkable only for a slender build and a left forearm encased in a cast. Serum chemistries, CBC, and x-ray films are unremarkable. You order dual-energy x-ray absorptiometry, which confirms osteoporosis of the lumbosacral spine. Which of the following are responsible for this patient's disease?

    A. Positive family history
    B. Low peak bone density

    C. Alcohol and tobacco use
    D. All of the above

86. Regarding the patient in question 85, which of the following is *true*?

    A. Bone loss is faster in trabecular than in cortical bone.
    B. Bone loss is faster in cortical than in trabecular bone.
    C. Bone formation has come to a halt.
    D. A and C
    E. B and C

QUESTIONS 87 AND 88

A 23-year-old college student comes to see you because of a bluish discoloration on her abdomen that she noted 4 months ago. She complains of weakness and finds it extremely difficult to climb stairs. She has gained 10 pounds over the past 3 months despite a meticulous effort at dieting. She has lately developed a ruddy complexion on her face. The patient takes no medication and denies the existence of any significant medical history among her immediate family. Her blood pressure is 150/97 mm Hg; her pulse is 88 beats/minute and regular. Remarkable findings on examination include facial plethora and dorsocervical and supraclavicular fat deposition, along with multiple violaceous abdominal striae. The patient cannot arise from the squatting position without assistance.

87. Which of the following tests would you order?

    A. 24-Hour urine free cortisol
    B. Synthetic ACTH stimulation test
    C. Adrenal CT scan
    D. None of the above

88. The correct tests are obtained and ectopic ACTH secretion is excluded. Which of the following complications can result from delaying treatment?

    A. Hypertension
    B. Diabetes
    C. Infertility
    D. Osteoporosis
    E. All of the above

89. You are seeing a 55-year-old black female for preoperative clearance. Her medical history includes hypothyroidism, multinodular goiter, and degenerative joint disease for which she is now requiring a right knee replacement. The patient reports progressive difficulty breathing, hoarseness, and dysphagia. Her weight is stable, and she denies constipation and cold intolerance. Medications include L-thyroxine, 100 µg daily. Her family history is not significant. Vital signs are normal, and her examination is unremarkable except for a 100-g multinodular goiter with a retrosternal extension and severe right knee arthritis with crepitus and genu valgus deformity. Significant laboratory tests include the following:

Free T_4	1.0 ng/dL (normal range, 0.7-1.5 ng/dL)
TSH	2.1 mIU/L (normal range, 0.3-5 mIU/L)
Calcium	10.6 mg/dL (normal range, 8.5-10.2 mg/dL)
Albumin	4.0 mg/dL (normal range, 3.5-4.5 mg/dL)
Intact parathyroid hormone	70 pg/mL (normal range, 15-65 pg/mL)
24-Hour urine calcium	10.85 mg (normal range, 0-250 mg)
24-Hour urine creatinine	861 mg (normal range, 800-1800 mg)

Which of the following procedures are appropriate for this patient?

A. Knee replacement only
B. Knee replacement and thyroidectomy only
C. Knee replacement and parathyroidectomy only
D. Knee replacement, parathyroidectomy, and thyroidectomy.

MATCHING

DIRECTIONS: For questions 90-107, select the one lettered option that is most clearly associated with it. Each lettered option may be selected once, more than once, or not at all.

QUESTIONS 90–93

For each of the following patients with incidental adrenal tumors, select the most appropriate laboratory tests (A-D).

A. 24-Hour urine for metanephrines and normetanephrines
B. Serum aldosterone level and plasma renin activity
C. 24-Hour free cortisol
D. None

90. A 31-year-old white woman with hypertension and impaired fasting glucose. She has gained 5 pounds in 2 months and has moon facies, a dorsocervical hump, and pink abdominal striae.

91. A 50-year-old black woman recently diagnosed with hypertension. She gets episodes of headaches, palpitations, and diaphoresis.

92. A 42-year-old black man with poorly controlled hypertension on multiple medications. Laboratory testing revealed hypokalemia and metabolic alkalosis.

93. A 35-year-old white man with hydronephrosis. Abdominal MRI showed an adrenal mass with the appearance of myelolipoma.

QUESTIONS 94–98

For each of the following patients seeking referral to a reproductive specialist, decide whether the problem is:

A. An isolated defect of sperm production
B. A defect of both sperm and androgen production
C. None of the above

94. A 28-year-old white man with Klinefelter's syndrome

95. A 42-year-old white man who was treated with the mechlorethamine, vincristine, procarbazine, and prednisone regimen for Hodgkin's disease

96. A 20-year-old black man with Kallmann's syndrome

97. A 32-year-old white man with congenital adrenal hyperplasia

98. A 50-year-old white man who underwent radical prostatectomy 1 year ago for prostate cancer

QUESTIONS 99–102

Match the following medications with the thyroid abnormalities that may occur on exposure.

A. Hypothyroidism
B. Hyperthyroidism
C. Both A and B
D. None of the above

99. Lithium

100. Amiodarone

101. Iodine

102. Corticosteroids

QUESTIONS 103–107

For each of the following patients, select the most appropriate intervention (A-E).

A. Propranolol
B. Counseling
C. PTU
D. RAI
E. Thyroidectomy

103. A 28-year-old black woman presents with anterior neck pain radiating to her right ear. She is biochemically thyrotoxic with a suppressed thyroid uptake.

104. A 34-year-old white woman who has been trying to lose weight presents with palpitations, heat intolerance, and tremors. She is biochemically hyperthyroid, has a low thyroid uptake, and has a suppressed thyroglobulin.

105. A 36-year-old black woman with a history of Graves' disease presents in the second trimester of pregnancy with palpitations and diaphoresis. She is biochemically hyperthyroid.

106. A 45-year-old white woman with a history of Graves' disease was treated with PTU for 2 years. She complains of weight loss, tremors, and palpitations.

107. A 48-year-old black woman with toxic multinodular goiter complains of choking sensations when she swallows.

Select the best one for each of the clinical scenarios below:

A. 21α-Hydroxylase deficiency (classic)
B. 21α-Hydroxylase deficiency (nonclassic)
C. 11β-Hyroxylase deficiency
D. 3β-Hydroxysteroid dehydrogenase deficiency
E. 17α-Hydroxylase/17,20-lyase deficiency
F. Polycystic ovarian syndrome
G. Idiopathic hirsutism
H. 5α-Reductase deficiency
I. Androgen insensitivity
J. Exogenous androgenic steroid use

108. A newborn with incomplete masculinization, elevated pregnenolone, 17-hydroxypregnenolone and dehydroepiandrosterone sulfate (DHEAS) who had sexual reassignment surgery as well as treatment with corticosteroids and mineralocorticoids.

109. A newborn with pseudohermaphroditism with both a penis (severe hypospadias) and a blind vaginal pouch. Ultrasound demonstrates absence of the prostate and uterus but detects normal seminal vesicles and epididymis in the undescended testicles.

110. A 25-year-old woman with moderate hirsutism involving her face, chest, abdomen, and inner thighs with irregular

periods and a 10-times normal 17-hydroxyprogesterone value.

111. A 30-year-old woman with hypertension, enlarged clitoris, hypokalemia with suppressed renin, and low aldosterone levels.

112. An 18-year-old woman currently taking prednisone and mineralocorticoid replacement with history of genital reconstruction surgery as an infant.

113. An 18-year-old female with normal thelarche, minimal adrenarche, and no menarche. Examination reveals testes within the labia, blind vaginal pouch, scant pubic hair, tanner IV breasts. Genetics reveal XY karyotype.

114. A 34-year-old woman with abnormal menstrual cycles, acne, elevated free testosterone levels, normal prolactin level, and a normal Cortrosyn-stimulated 17-hydroxyprogesterone value.

Part X
Endocrinology
Answers

1. (**True**); 2. (**True**); 3. (**False**). *Discussion:* Cell surface receptor concentration regulates the interaction with the hormone and therefore determines the responsiveness of the cells. The feedback system results in upregulation and downregulation of cellular receptors. For example, receptor blockade with receptor antagonists may cause the cell to upregulate receptor numbers. If the antagonist is withdrawn quickly the cell will have an excessive response to the endogenous hormone. Another aspect of the feedback system is the ability of hormone-induced binding to downregulate the number of available receptors, which renders the cell refractory to a given concentration of hormone. If the body senses the need for more hormone effect, an increase in the hormone concentration may result in full biologic response. Many disease states alter the responsiveness of the second messenger system. Some of these diseases are genetic in nature. For example, in pseudohypoparathyroidism, a defect in G protein signaling blunts the response to parathyroid hormone receptor binding. Another example is an autonomous thyroid nodule that is hyperfunctional even in the absence of thyroid-stimulating hormone (thyrotropin) binding. Acquired disorders can also affect post-receptor signaling. Infection with cholera toxin leads to inhibition of certain G-protein–coupled second messenger systems, preventing deactivation or prolonging activation. This results in the massive secretion of sodium, chloride, and water from the intestinal epithelium. (*Cecil, Ch. 234*)

4. (**A**) **True**; (**B**) **False**; (**C**) **True**. *Discussion:* In the prepubertal stage, the male and female breasts are histologically and functionally the same. With the onset of puberty, rising levels of estradiol stimulate the development of the ductal systems and nipples. Action of progesterone (in synergy with estradiol) leads to alveolar development. Cell division and differentiation within the gland are promoted by epidermal growth factor and insulin-like growth factors; transforming growth factor-β plays an inhibitory role. Once breast development is complete, prolactin acts on the breast to bring about milk production. This requires previous priming of the breast by estradiol and progesterone; glucocorticoids, insulin, and thyroxine play a permissive role. (*Wilson, 1998*)

5. (**A**) **True**; (**B**) **True**; (**C**) **True**; (**D**) **True**. *Discussion:* In the female child, precocious puberty refers to the development of breast buds before 8 years of age or the onset of menarche before 9 years of age. In central precocious puberty, there is the premature activation of the gonadotropin-releasing hormone pulse generator, resulting in increase of gonadotropin secretion and an increase in gonadal steroid secretion, as is seen in normal puberty, resulting in ovulatory menstrual cycles. Gonadotropin-independent precocious puberty results from adrenal or ovarian oversecretion of estrogen, leading to feminization without the development of cyclic menses or ovulation. Organic brain lesions like neurofibromatosis have been associated with precocious puberty, but a majority of cases of precocious puberty are due to idiopathic causes. Congenital adrenal hyperplasia resulting from 21-hydroxylase deficiency can lead to gonadotropin-releasing hormone–independent precocious puberty when treatment is started late. In McCune-Albright syndrome (polyostotic fibrous dysplasia), constitutive activation of the gonadotropin receptor is mimicked by activating mutations of a receptor-associated G protein. This leads to estrogen oversecretion with sexual precocity in the absence of gonadotropin secretion. Likewise, granulosa-theca tumors of the ovary cause precocious puberty as a result of excessive secretion of estrogen. (*Carr and Bradshaw, 1998*)

6. (**A**) **True**; (**B**) **False**; (**C**) **False**; (**D**) **True**. *Discussion:* The sick euthyroid syndrome refers to the abnormalities of thyroid function tests that are seen in several acute and chronic illnesses, including myocardial infarction, lung diseases, trauma, infections, and starvation. The most common manifestations of the sick euthyroid syndrome include the low T_3 and low T_4 states; TSH alterations occur less frequently. The cause of the sick euthyroid syndrome is unknown, but it is suggested that defects in peripheral conversion of T_4 to T_3 and thyroid hormone binding might be responsible for the low T_3 and T_4 states, thyroid hormone synthesis being normal. In certain cases, the TSH level may also be abnormal. This may be due to glucocorticoids, dopamine, altered TRH secretion, or endogenous somatostatin. The sick euthyroid syndrome is thought to be part of a broader endocrine response to illness, because insulin-like growth factors, gonadotropins and sex steroids, ACTH, and cortisol are also affected. It is thought to be mediated by cytokines. Some forms of the sick euthyroid syndrome (the low-T_4 form) carry a poor prognosis. In these and other forms of the sick euthyroid syndrome, thyroid hormone replacement has not been shown to improve patient outcome. (*Cecil, Ch. 239*)

7. (**A**) **False**; (**B**) **True**; (**C**) **True**; (**D**) **True**. *Discussion:* A majority (80%) of kidney stones contain calcium complexed with oxalate or phosphate. These calcium-containing complexes form when the concentration of calcium in the urine exceeds the limits of solubility. A majority of patients with calcium-containing stones have hypercalciuria, which can result from increased gastrointestinal absorption of calcium, impairment of renal reabsorption of calcium, or excessive resorption of bone. Hypercalciuria may or may not be accompanied by hypercalcemia. In a minority of patients, calcium-containing stones form in the absence of hypercalciuria. This may be due to a lack of substances that enhance the urinary solubility of calcium. In this patient, hypercalciuria could result from increased formation of 1,25-dihydroxyvitamin D because of sarcoidosis. Elevation of ACE would suggest sarcoidosis; however, this diagnosis is already known and the ACE level does not always correlate with the activity of sarcoidosis. Therefore, it is not indicated in this work-up. If sarcoidosis is the cause of her stones, it would mean that the amount of corticosteroid that she is taking is not sufficient to inhibit the effect of 1,25-dihydroxyvitamin D at the gastrointestinal tract. Excess glucocorticoids, in contrast, can cause hypercalciuria by impairing renal reabsorption of calcium and increasing bone resorption and decreasing bone formation. A high hydroxyproline level will be seen as a result of increased bone resorption. (*Asplin et al, 1998*)

8. **(A) True; (B) True; (C) True; (D) True; (E) False; 9. (A) True; (B) True; (C) False; (D) False; (E) False.** *Discussion:* The treatment of hypothyroidism is aimed at restoring and maintaining the euthyroid state. For most patients with hypothyroidism, thyroid hormone treatment is required for life. They, therefore, need to be educated on the need for lifelong treatment and should be evaluated periodically to determine the adequacy of treatment as well as to reinforce the need for compliance. Thyroid hormone preparations available for the treatment of hypothyroidism include levothyroxine (LT_4), T_3, and T_4/T_3 combinations, as well as thyroid extract. Of these, T_4 is most commonly used. An average adult requires 75 to 125 μg of T_4 for the treatment of hypothyroidism. Higher replacement doses may be required when there is poor absorption or increased clearance of thyroid hormone as well as in obesity. In this patient, higher than average replacement doses will be required to compensate for malabsorption of thyroid hormone because of surgical bypass of the small intestine. Co-administration of ferrous sulfate will add to this requirement because it binds thyroid hormone in the intestine. Moreover, co-administration of phenytoin will lead to increased clearance of thyroid hormone. Finally, noncompliance with the administration of the hormone could also account for apparent inadequacy of an appropriate dose of thyroid hormone. Because thyroid hormone acts on several body tissues, severe hypothyroidism results in dysfunction of several systems. In this patient, impaired hearing can be found. Hyperprolactinemia can be seen as a result of activation of lactotrophs by TRH. Hypothyroidism causes impairment of free water clearance, leading to hyponatremia. There is no association between hypothyroidism and osteoporosis; however, if the short gut syndrome results in vitamin D deficiency and secondary hyperparathyroidism this could result in osteoporosis later in life. Also, untreated primary hypothyroidism may increase the prolactin level, thus inhibiting gonadotrophin release with estrogen deficiency, bone loss, and osteoporosis. Thus the indirect impact of the bowel surgery on long-term hypothyroidism needs to be considered in this patient. *(Cecil, Ch. 239)*

10. **(A) True; (B) True; (C) True; (D) False; (E) False.** *Discussion:* This patient has clinical and biochemical evidence of hyperthyroidism. The presence of a diffuse nontender goiter with bruits makes Graves' disease the most likely cause of hyperthyroidism. Additionally, he has clinical features of ophthalmopathy (proptosis, periorbital edema, chemosis, and diplopia), which is diagnostic for Graves' disease. Clinical evidence of ophthalmopathy is present in 20 to 40% of patients with hyperthyroidism caused by Graves' disease, although measurement of orbital protrusion as well as orbital radiography suggests that a majority of patients are affected. It usually predates or follows hyperthyroidism by 18 months if it does not coincide with its onset and has little, if any, correlation with the severity of hyperthyroidism. A history of smoking tends to put patients at a higher risk for Graves' ophthalmopathy. This patient needs immediate treatment directed at hyperthyroidism as well as ophthalmopathy. PTU should be administered to block thyroid hormone synthesis as well as the conversion of T_4 to T_3. Propranolol should be administered to block peripheral manifestations of thyroid hormone excess. Prednisone should be administered immediately for control of eye symptoms, and an ophthalmology consultation should be arranged to define the precise nature of eye involvement. Additional measures that may be used to control eye involvement include diuretics, eye radiation, and eye surgery. RAI works by reducing the amount of functioning thyroid tissue. Its effect is delayed, and it should be used with caution in patients with severe hyperthyroidism for fear of precipitating a thyroid crisis. Furthermore, it has been suggested that RAI treatment in the presence of ophthalmopathy may lead to exacerbation of eye symptoms. In this situation, patients should be prepared with steroid treatment. Inorganic iodine is used in thyroid storm, for preoperative preparation, and rarely in patients who have received RAI. It would not be appropriate in this patient. *(Cecil, Ch. 239)*

11. **(A) False; (B) True; (C) True; (D) True; (E) False.** *Discussion:* A dreaded complication of uncontrolled hyperthyroidism is the development of thyroid storm, a syndrome of thyrotoxicosis, hyperpyrexia, and neurologic and/or multisystem decline, features of which are apparent in this patient. Although this is a rare complication of hyperthyroidism, it is accompanied by a high mortality. Therefore, a high index of suspicion is required for the diagnosis and treatment of thyroid storm to be made in a timely manner. Thyroid storm can be precipitated by many factors, including infections, surgery, trauma, parturition, cerebrovascular accident, and withdrawal of antithyroid therapy. Treatment of the thyroid storm should be aimed at blocking synthesis and release of thyroid hormone, blocking the peripheral effects of thyroid hormone, and providing supportive care. The precipitating causes should be sought and properly treated. In this patient, high-dose PTU should be instituted immediately to block thyroid hormone synthesis as well as the peripheral conversion of T_4 to T_3, the biologically active form of thyroid hormone. This should be followed (1-2 hours later) by administration of inorganic iodine to block the release of preformed thyroid hormone from the thyroid gland. β-Blockers should be used to control the peripheral manifestations of thyroid hormone excess; however, this should be done with caution in congestive heart failure. Corticosteroids have been used based on their ability to block T_4 to T_3 conversion and thyroid hormone synthesis (in Graves' disease) and because of concerns of impaired adrenocortical reserve in thyroid storm. RAI has no place in the management of thyroid storm. *(Cecil, Ch. 239)*

12. **(A) True; (B) False; (C) True; (D) False.** *Discussion:* DI reflects a reduction of the ability of the body to concentrate urine, resulting in the production of large volumes of dilute urine and excessive thirst. DI can be due to inability to synthesize and secrete adequate amounts of arginine vasopressin (AVP) in response to hyperosmolarity (central DI) or a lack of renal response to AVP (nephrogenic DI). In either case, the renal collecting ducts are incapable of concentrating the filtered fluids, leading to the excretion of excessive volumes of dilute urine. This raises the serum osmolality, which stimulates thirst, leading to polydipsia. Serum AVP level is low in central DI and high in nephrogenic DI. Central DI results from disorders of the hypothalamus in which there is destruction of the supraoptic and paraventricular cells or rarely as an inherited disorder in which there is a single nucleotide substitution (or deletion) in the AVP gene. Congenital forms of nephrogenic DI include disorders of vasopressin V2 receptor (X-linked) and aquaporin-2 water channels (autosomal recessive). Hypercalcemia results in excessive diuresis, but hypocalcemia does not. The acquired forms of DI result from medications (demeclocycline, lithium, fluoride) and electrolyte disorders (hypokalemia and hypercalcemia). *(Cecil, Ch. 238)*

13. **(A) True; (B) True; (C) False; (D) True; 14. (A) False; (B) False; (C) True; (D) False; 15. (A) True; (B) False; (C) True; (D) False; 16. (A) False; (B) True; (C) True; (D) True.** *Discussion:* Pheochromocytoma is a neuroendocrine tumor that causes symptoms by the synthesis, storage, and secretion of excessive amounts of catecholamines. Ninety percent of pheochromocytomas are located in the abdominal cavity and arise from the adrenal gland. Although pheochromocytoma is a rare cause of hypertension, it can be associated with significant morbidity and mortality if diagnosis is delayed or if it is not properly managed. Pheochromocytoma can exist as a sporadic or familial disorder; familial cases can be isolated or exist in association with other endocrine disorders (MEN2a, MEN2b). Thus, it is necessary to consider screening close relatives of the patients in whom it has

been diagnosed. Moreover, pheochromocytomas are sometimes malignant. When pheochromocytoma is suspected, appropriate biochemical studies should be performed to confirm the diagnosis, followed by imaging studies to localize the tumor, which should then be surgically resected after appropriate patient preparation. Biochemical diagnosis of pheochromocytoma relies on the measurement of catecholamines (epinephrine or norepinephrine) and/or catecholamine metabolites (metanephrines or vanillylmandelic acid) in urine or blood. Testing must be performed when the patient is not taking medications or foods that interfere with results. The samples must be properly collected, stored, and processed. Blood samples must be collected under standardized conditions. In this patient, although the catecholamine levels are abnormal, they are not diagnostic of pheochromocytoma (usually epinephrine and norepinephrine levels of 400 pg/mL and 2000 pg/mL, respectively). Thus, additional testing is needed to differentiate physiologic elevations from the pathologic elevation seen in pheochromocytoma. Although urinary catecholamine and catecholamine metabolite levels can be measured, a safe and easy yet sensitive test is the clonidine suppression test. An increase (or no change) in catecholamine level signifies the possible presence of a pheochromocytoma, whereas a decrease in catecholamine makes pheochromocytoma much less likely. After the biochemical confirmation of pheochromocytoma, the next step should be to localize it. Abdominal MRI is appropriate. This should be followed by initiation of treatment aimed at preparing the patient for surgery. Phenoxybenzamine should be initiated to control blood pressure and to restore blood volume. α-Methyltyrosine, a competitive inhibitor of tyrosine hydroxylation (the rate-limiting step in catecholamine synthesis), can also be used to facilitate blood pressure control. β-Blockers should be avoided before complete α-blockade for fear of precipitating unopposed vasoconstriction, which can lead to a hypertensive crisis. Pheochromocytomas may secrete one or more of a number of peptides, including calcitonin, somatostatin, opioid peptides, ACTH, and vasoactive intestinal peptide. Thus, diarrhea and Cushing's syndrome could also be seen in this patient. Hypercalcemia can be seen when pheochromocytoma is diagnosed in the context of MEN 2a and MEN 2b. Although overt diabetes is rare, glucose intolerance is frequently seen in pheochromocytoma because of the anti-insulin effects of catecholamines. (*Cecil, Ch. 241; Keiser, 1995*)

17. **(A) True; (B) True; (C) False; (D) False.** *Discussion:* The adrenal gland is structurally divided into an outer cortex and an inner medulla. The cortex synthesizes, stores, and releases glucocorticoids, mineralocorticoids, and sex steroids. The medulla synthesizes, stores, and releases catecholamines. Glucocorticoids play a central role in intermediary metabolism and immune modulation and a minor role in water regulation. Mineralocorticoids are required for regulation of extracellular fluid volume, potassium, and hydrogen ion concentration. Adrenal androgens are minor regulators of male secondary sexual characteristics. They also have a minor effect on immune and cardiovascular systems. Catecholamines mediate a number of metabolic and cardiovascular effects. They are derived from adrenal glands and nerve terminals. A patient who has had bilateral adrenalectomy will need replacement of glucocorticoids and mineralocorticoids. Sex steroids will not be necessary because a majority of sex steroids are of testicular origin. Catecholamines will not be necessary because the nerve terminals will be an adequate source of catecholamines. (*Cecil, Chs. 240 and 241*)

18. **(A) True; (B) True; (C) True; (D) True; 19. (A) True; (B) True; (C) True; (D) True.** *Discussion:* Gynecomastia refers to the enlargement of the male breast. This can be physiologic or pathologic, is unilateral or bilateral, and may be accompanied by breast tenderness. Bilateral gynecomastia may or may not be symmetrical. The prevalence of gynecomastia is unknown, but it appears to be

more common in the older age groups. Causes of gynecomastia may be congenital or acquired and include those factors that lead to estrogen excess, decreased testosterone secretion (or action), or medications. Estrogen excess may be relative or absolute; it can be due to an exogenous or endogenous source. Likewise, testosterone deficiency may be relative or absolute and can result from testicular, pituitary, or hypothalamic defects. Defective actions of testosterone are due to defects at the receptor level as seen in the androgen insensitivity syndrome. Primary hypothyroidism can lead to gynecomastia by inducing hyperprolactinemia, which may lead to hypogonadotropic hypogonadism. In hyperthyroidism, gynecomastia is sometimes seen as a consequence of increased peripheral conversion of adrenal androgens to estradiol. Gynecomastia of an unknown mechanism is sometimes seen when refeeding is re-established after a period of starvation. Marijuana and several other substances cause gynecomastia by unknown mechanisms. This patient's gynecomastia is the result of excessive testicular production of estrogen due to LH-like action of excessive human chorionic gonadotropin, compounded by the antiandrogenic effect of cimetidine at the receptor level. (*Wilson, 1998*)

20. **(F)** *Discussion:* Head trauma from frontal injuries results in the brain traveling backward with the pituitary remaining fixed within the sella. This can result in stalk injury and frequently presents as pituitary hormone deficiency. Early in the injury the levels of pituitary hormones may be elevated and should always be retested in 72 hours if deficiency is suspected. This patient likely has panhypopituitarism manifesting acutely with adrenal insufficiency and diabetes insipidus. He improved rapidly with corticosteroids, and further work-up 1 week later revealed elevated prolactin, normal TSH with a low normal free thyroxine, low IGF-1, and low testosterone. On discharge from the hospital the patient was given prednisone, thyroxine, and desmopressin with plans to follow up in 2 weeks to discuss hormone replacement therapy, which will depend on his desire for fertility now or in the future. (*Cecil, Ch. 235*)

21. **(B)** *Discussion:* This patient most likely has hypothalamic sarcoidosis causing diabetes insipidus. Her prolactin level is likely elevated because of hypothalamic dysfunction impairing the tonic dopamine inhibition. The patient's age and her current breathing problem can be unified with the diagnosis of sarcoidosis, which can cause interstitial pulmonary fibrosis. Varying degrees of hypopituitarism can occur with or without hyperprolactinemia and diabetes insipidus. This is a difficult diagnosis, and it was made in this case with bronchoscopic biopsy. The normal TSH is helpful to know that the elevation in prolactin is not due to primary hypothyroidism; however, a free T_4 value should be measured to ensure the patient is chemically euthyroid. Corticosteroids will help the breathing and likely the polyuria but are not usually helpful in returning normal pituitary function in those patients with other hormone deficiencies. (*Cecil, Chs. 235, 237, and 238*)

22. **(E)** *Discussion:* Langerhans cell histiocytosis is caused by an eosinophilic granulomatous infiltration of the hypothalamus and commonly causes diabetes insipidus. Pituitary dysfunction and hyperprolactemia may occur in varying degrees. (*Cecil, Ch. 235*)

23. **(A)** *Discussion:* This patient gives a significant number of symptoms that can be caused by a central mass. This patient had a craniopharyngioma that was partially excised, and he recovered his sexual drive and his polyuria and nocturia improved. He was given radiation therapy and therefore has a high risk of developing pituitary deficiency and should be followed closely. This could also represent a gonadotrophic adenoma, which presents as a mass effect. The key is the nocturia × 4, which on closer questioning is of large volume and occurs during the day as well. This suggests diabetes insipidus, which almost never occurs with anterior pitu-

itary adenomas but frequently accompanies a suprasellar cranio-pharyngioma. (Cecil, Chs. 235 and 237)

24. (C) Discussion: This patient has precocious puberty induced by elevated levels of human chorionic gonadotropin (hCG). His testes are the source of testosterone, and the hCG binds the LH receptor to drive production. This patient has a suprasellar dysgerminoma, which is identical to dysgerminomas of the gonads in structure and function. The absences of the "pubertal growth spurt" suggest pituitary dysfunction and merits further endocrinologic evaluation for at least growth hormone and thyroid deficiencies. Commonly, patients will also present with DI, visual field defects, and prolactin elevation. The diagnosis was made by detecting elevated hCG in the CSF, and the patient responded well to radiation therapy. (Cecil, Ch. 235)

25. (D); 26. (C). Discussion: It is critical to evaluate this patient's adrenal function. The ACTH stimulation test yields a general idea of adrenal reserve but must be used with caution in patients suspected of secondary adrenal deficiency. A low-dose ACTH stimulation test may increase the sensitivity of the test, but if secondary adrenal deficiency is suspected, the insulin tolerance test should be performed (unless there is a history of seizure or coronary heart disease) even if an ACTH stimulation test is normal. This patient had a basal serum cortisol of 2 μg/dL and a 1-hour post ACTH cortisol of 8 μg/dL. This demonstrates prolonged ACTH deficiency with adrenal atrophy, and the patient was given 5 mg of prednisone daily. It is important to rule out pregnancy, which could produce many of the described symptoms. One should also screen for central hypothyroidism, by obtaining a free T_4 level. The TSH can be normal in patients with central hypothyroidism. Even though gonadotropin deficiency is suspected, you suspect gonadotrophic deficiency. The prolactin elevation could also diminish FSH and LH release, and it would not be helpful to measure these at this time. (Cecil, Ch. 237)

Each of the just-listed answers should be considered in the differential diagnosis. This patient's history and symptoms make either Sheehan's syndrome or lymphocytic hypophysitis the most likely diagnosis. Prolactinoma would rarely cause adrenal and thyroid deficiency unless it was a macroadenoma. Hemochromatosis can present with the above findings but would not have occurred in an acute fashion. The MRI findings strongly support lymphocytic hypophysitis as the diagnosis. The MRI characteristically demonstrates an enlarged pituitary without a focal lesion. Sheehan's syndrome would likely reveal evidence of bleeding in the acute phase or a hypodensity in the sella that would be consistent with previously infracted tissue. Prolactin levels are typically low in Sheehan's syndrome (Cecil, Ch. 237; Becker)

27. (D) Discussion: Acromegaly is an indolent disease that presents 8 to 10 years after onset of growth hormone (GH) excess. The average age of diagnosis is early in the fifth decade, and the causal adenoma is usually greater than 10 mm in diameter (macroadenoma). GH secretion is pulsatile. Thus, neither high nor low levels can exclude the diagnosis. IGF-1 levels, when matched for age and sex (assuming normal nutritional status) correlate well to daily GH production. It is also common for a GH-producing tumor to present with more than one hormone abnormality and up to 40% co-secrete prolactin with another 10 to 30% of co-secreting glycoproteins. The best test to document GH excess is to perform a 75-g glucose suppression test with measurement of GH levels at 30-minute intervals over 2 hours after glucose administration. GH suppresses in normal patients to less than 2 μg/mL (polyclonal radioimmunoassay) or to less than 0.5 μg/mL (two-site monoclonal assay). A thickened heel pad on a radiograph is suggestive of the diagnosis. (Cecil, Ch. 237)

28. (D) Discussion: This patient has a microprolactinoma and has less than a 2% risk of developing symptoms of tumor enlargement during her pregnancy. The current recommendations for patients with a microprolactinoma are to discontinue the dopamine agonist when the pregnancy is documented and to monitor for clinical symptoms that would suggest enlargement. Measuring a prolactin level will not be helpful because it naturally increases with pregnancy. Thus, the level will not alter clinical management. The patient has no symptoms of mass effect, and visual fields are grossly normal. Therefore, formal visual field testing is not indicated at this time. Visual fields are an essential marker to follow in a patient with a macroprolactinoma. It is important for the physician to evaluate the visual fields grossly in the clinic because gradual progression of visual loss may not be noted by the patient. An MRI is not indicated without symptoms of mass effect (e.g., headache, visual field changes, or cranial nerve palsies). The pituitary naturally increases in size to as much as 12 mm in its greatest dimension during pregnancy, and MRI would not change management unless there is clinical suggestion of a mass effect. The low risk of complications and symptoms from a microprolactinoma during pregnancy allows for cessation of therapy with close observation. If a patient has symptoms or presents with a macroadenoma, bromocriptine should be continued, especially in light of increasing evidence of its safety in pregnancy. (Cecil, Ch. 237)

29. (B) Discussion: A 1-mg overnight dexamethasone suppression test has high specificity. Therefore, patients without the disease will be correctly identified by the test in that normal suppression (a negative test) indicates the absence of Cushing's syndrome. False-positive results (failure to suppress in the absence of disease) can occur up to 30% of the time with this test and can be due to the following: increased metabolism of dexamethasone; depression; recent alcohol withdrawal; or hospitalization. The clinical features of Cushing's syndrome include those listed in A and can be found in Table 237-9 in Chapter 237 of the Cecil textbook. The work-up of Cushing's syndrome is very difficult and must be preformed in a logical manner. It is essential to diagnose hypercortisolism before proceeding with any tests to differentiate the underlying cause. The tests used to determine if the process is ACTH dependent are not designed to diagnose Cushing's syndrome. These tests are only useful for differential diagnosis when performed while the patient is hypercortisolemic. Cushing's disease (hypercortisolism due to an ACTH-secreting pituitary adenoma) is the most common cause (70%) of Cushing's syndrome and occurs eight times more frequently in women compared with men. (Cecil, Ch. 237)

30. (C) Discussion: This patient has no clinical symptoms consistent with hyperthyroidism and the free T_4 value should be measured next. She had a normal free T_4 (1.0 ng/dL), which is consistent with euthyroidism. Abnormalities of the thyroxine-binding globulin (TBG) can alter the total T_4 level because 80% of the bound T_4 level is carried by TBG. Her drug history reveals she had started taking oral contraceptive pills (OCPs) 1 year ago. It is important not to confuse this euthyroid state with hyperthyroidism. The TBG concentration can be elevated by medications including estrogens, tamoxifen, perphenazine, and clofibrate. Physiologic conditions such as pregnancy (increased estrogen) and disease states such as hepatitis, biliary cirrhosis and acute intermittent porphyria can all increase TBG as well. The estrogen content of the OCPs lead to a decrease in TBG clearance and can increase the concentration twofold to threefold. TSI, thyroid scan, and thyroid uptake are not indicated unless thyrotoxicosis has been diagnosed. A reverse T_3 test would not be helpful. However, a T_3 resin uptake that estimates the TBG binding could be used to estimate the free T_4. An ultrasound of the thyroid would not help to determine the function of the gland and should be reserved as

an extension of the physical examination to evaluate palpated or otherwise detected structural abnormalities. (*Cecil, Ch. 239*)

31. (A) *Discussion:* Generalized resistance to thyroid hormone is characterized by normal to minimally elevated TSH and elevated thyroid hormone in the setting of euthyroidism and/or a mixed presentation with findings consistent with both hyperthyroidism and hypothyroidism. Pregnancy leads to an elevation of human chorionic gonadotropin (hCG) during the first trimester and can result in suppression of the TSH, which remits without therapy. Acute psychiatric illness can suppress the TSH and usually resolves soon after presentation once treatment of the psychiatric illness has begun. Moderate doses of glucocorticoids (and dopamine) result in the suppression of TSH release. This is a common combination in the ICU and can further confound thyroid function test abnormalities in the critically ill patient. Any cause of thyrotoxicosis will suppress the TSH unless it is a TRH-or TSH-secreting lesion. The inflammation of the thyroid that occurs with subacute thyroiditis allows leakage of pre-made thyroid hormone into the circulation that results in a transient thyrotoxic episode. This results in suppression of the TSH during the toxic phase and early during the recovery. A small number of patients remain hypothyroid after their thyroiditis resolves, and they will require thyroid hormone replacement. (*Cecil, Ch. 239*)

32. (D) *Discussion:* Nonthyroidal illness syndrome (NTI), sick euthyroid syndrome, and low T_3 syndrome all indicate a thyroid hormone abnormality that has resulted from a disease state that is not thyroid in origin. The key abnormality is a change in the T_3 concentration that is most likely caused by decreased deiodinase activity. The degree of thyroid function test abnormality correlates with the degree of illness. As the severity and duration of the illness progresses, the degree of thyroid dysfunction can increase. In mild to moderate illness the T_3 level falls and the rT_3 level rises with both T_4 and TSH remaining within the normal range. As the illness worsens the T_4 level can fall below normal and the TSH level drifts downward and may dip below the normal values. Additional factors that decrease the level of T_4 include a decrease in thyroid-binding proteins, lowered production of thyroid hormones secondary to declining TSH values, and displacement of T_4 from proteins by free fatty acids. Once the T_4 falls below normal the mortality of the patient is likely greater than 60%, and once the T_4 is less than 2 μg/dL the mortality rate exceeds 80%. Replacement of T_4 has not been shown to affect mortality, which is linked to the severity of the underlying illness. Free T_4 values remain normal when measured by equilibrium dialysis but may become slightly below the normal range in severe illness. (*Cecil, Ch. 239*)

33. (B) *Discussion:* This patient most likely has Graves' ophthalmopathy with optic nerve compression at the posterior apex. The retro-orbital tissues are infiltrated by lymphocytes and other immune mediators, which leads to increased amounts of mucopolysaccharide. This results in muscle edema, which can cause optic nerve compression in the absence of proptosis. Also, Graves' ophthalmopathy can occur at any time, even in patients who have been treated for the hyperthyroidism induced by the underlying autoimmune process. Patients who smoke are more frequently affected by ophthalmopathy, and it likely is triggered by states that may cause flares of autoimmune diseases, such as the postpartum state, severe stress, and withdrawal of corticosteroids. This patient needs immediate evaluation (this is an emergency) by an ophthalmologist, and if one is not locally available, the patient should be treated with glucocorticoids and should travel to the nearest ophthalmologist that day. A pituitary tumor usually causes temporal visual field cuts as a result of optic chiasm compression. Symmetric eye impairment from optic nerve compression would be a *very rare* occurrence from a pituitary lesion. The other choices would not present with the just-listed symptoms. Pseudotumor

cerebri presents as papilledema—swelling of the optic disc that can be seen with ophthalmopathy but does not cause decreased color vision. The patient does not give a history of eye strain that is usually related to excessive reading—including a computer screen. This frequently improves with reading glasses and during weekends when the activity is decreased. No change in color vision occurs. A psychogenic cause would not display the physical findings in this patient. (*Cecil, Ch. 239*)

34. (D); **35. (E)**. *Discussion:* This patient has developed myxedema coma with a depressed respiratory rate, unresponsiveness, and hypotension. This is a rare occurrence in patients admitted for radioiodine therapy, and, like most cases of myxedema coma, an exacerbating event usually must take place. In patients who are profoundly hypothyroid, the development of coma occurs after a myocardial infarction, severe infection, or, in the case of the homeless, cold weather. In a healthy person these events are very unlikely to have occurred. This patient should not have an indwelling urinary catheter for several reasons. Most importantly, it would be a significant radiation safety hazard. Respiratory failure in this case was a result of the patient receiving benzodiazepine, which she takes for sleep. She had been told to discontinue this medication 4 weeks ago with the discontinuation of her levothyroxine, but listed it in her home medications when interviewed for admission. Hypothyroid patients are extremely sensitive to sedative agents and narcotic analgesics, and these should be avoided or given at a greatly reduced dose. Allergy to iodine is not a contraindication to radioiodine therapy because of the very small dose of iodine that is actually given. Sepsis would likely not have developed so rapidly, and myocardial infarction is unlikely in patients who are hypothyroid because of the reduced oxygen demand. One would not expect this patient with no cardiac risk or history to develop a myocardial infarction. Radiation thyroiditis is rarely a complication in thyroid cancer patients because the majority of the thyroid should have been removed and the presentation of radiation thyroiditis is usually limited to neck pain. A calcium channel blocker may accentuate bradycardia if it is a dihydropyridine, however, one would not expect a respiratory collapse. (*Cecil, Ch. 239*)

36. (C) *Discussion:* This patient has catabolic Cushing's syndrome with the symptoms of weight loss, hypertension, hypokalemia, easy bruising, and proximal muscle weakness. This process differs from the classic Cushing's features, which include truncal obesity, dorsicervical fat deposition, and weight gain. The rapid onset of symptoms and the catabolic nature of the process are worrisome for ectopic ACTH production. The best test is to document hypercortisolism. Once that has been documented, the next step is to determine if it is an ACTH-dependent process. The hypertension and hypokalemia seen in this patient is caused by the high level of cortisol that has overwhelmed the enzymatic protection of the mineralocorticoid receptor. 11β-Hydroxysteroid dehydrogenase catalyzes the conversion of cortisol to cortisone. The latter does not bind to the mineralocorticoid receptor. The capacity of this enzyme is overwhelmed and leads to mineralocorticoid independent hypertension. The other laboratory data would not help with the diagnosis, and a CT of the adrenals would not determine if the patient was hypercortisolemic. (*Cecil, Ch. 240*)

37. (E) *Discussion:* This patient has hemorrhaged into her adrenal glands and requires immediate cortisol coverage. The clues in the history include the back pain followed by signs and symptoms of adrenal deficiency 1 to 2 days later. The signs of acute onset of adrenal insufficiency are outlined earlier and one should be very suspicious of adrenal insufficiency in a patient who is unresponsive to volume expansion and pressors. CT is important to document the hemorrhage. The patient has no signs of heart failure, reinfarction, or arrhythmia, and the CT will evaluate for retroperitoneal bleeding, which should always be considered after cardiac arteriography. The patient will also need mineralocorticoid replacement. (*Cecil, Ch. 240*)

38. (D) *Discussion:* 21α-Hydroxylase deficiency can occur in two forms and is the most common cause of congenital adrenal hyperplasia (CAH). The name can be confusing because the adrenal gland hypertrophies as a result of one or more steroid deficiencies. A life-threatening form presents at birth with adrenal crisis. A milder form presents during puberty with irregular menstrual cycles (oligomenorrhea) and signs of androgen excess such as cystic acne and hirsutism. The clinical picture can be difficult to distinguish from polycystic ovarian syndrome (PCOS) and should be ruled out in patients before PCOS is diagnosed. The ACTH stimulation test measuring pre and post 17-hydroxyprogesterone can be used to screen for CAH. Normal subjects rarely exceed the upper limit or normal whereas patients with CAH can achieve plasma levels greater than or equal to four to five times the upper limit of the assay. The deficient enzyme is the 21α-hydroxylase. However, direct measurement to determine the activity is not possible. Plasma renin activity would not likely be helpful in this patient in whom you suspect PCOS but may be helpful in CAH patients if they have the salt-wasting form and you are assessing the adequacy of mineralocorticoid replacement. The dexamethasone suppression test (1 mg overnight) is used to screen for cortisol excess. (*Cecil, Ch. 240*)

39. (B); **40. (D)**. *Discussion:* This patient has multiple endocrine neoplasia type 2a (MEN 2a) based on his history of a thyroid cancer at a very young age and bilateral adrenal tumors that were pheochromocytomas. MEN 2 is the result of a mutation of the *RET* proto-oncogene on chromosome 10. This is an autosomal dominant disease that manifests with medullary thyroid cancer, pheochromocytoma (frequently bilateral), and hyperparathyroidism. MEN 2b has distinctive clinical features that differentiate it from MEN 2a. These include mucosal neuromas and a marfanoid body habitus. This patient had neither of these two physical findings on examination. Therefore, his history and examination support the diagnosis of MEN 2a. MEN 1 is the most common of the multiple endocrine neoplasia syndromes and presents clinically as hyperparathyroidism (four-gland hyperplasia), pancreatic tumors (insulinoma, gastrinoma, somatostatinoma, VIPoma, or glucagonoma), and anterior pituitary adenomas. There is a mutation in the tumor suppressor gene that codes for a protein called MENIN. The mutation is found on chromosome 11. As with MEN 2, this is an autosomal dominant disorder, however, the mutation is in only one copy of the *MENIN* gene and requires a second hit (event that leads to mutation or deactivation of the other copy of the gene) before neoplastic growth. These findings are not consistent with the autoimmune polyglandular syndromes in which endocrine abnormalities result from autoimmune destruction or occasionally stimulation. The only two answers that would be correct for evaluation of MEN 2 would be either the gastrin-stimulated calcitonin level or the genetic analysis for the *RET* proto-oncogene mutation. The genetic screen is much more sensitive and has replaced the stimulated calcitonin. When found early, this knowledge can lead to life-saving thyroidectomy in offspring who have inherited the mutation. There is no role to evaluate for the *MENIN* mutation in MEN 1 because no specific or preventive therapies are available for asymptomatic tumors in this neoplastic disease. (*Cecil, Ch. 245*)

41. (D) *Discussion:* Carcinoid syndrome is the manifestation of neoplastic growth of the enterochromaffin cells and includes vasodilator paroxysms (mainly cutaneous flushing), diarrhea, and cardiac valvular lesions (e.g., tricuspid fibrosis). The presence of tryptophan hydroxylase is a biochemical feature of the carcinoid syndrome and leads to excess formation of 5-hydroxytryptophan (5-HTP), which is decarboxylated to serotonin. Monoamine oxidase and aldehyde dehydrogenase further modify 5-HTP to 5-hydroxyindoleacetic acid (5-HIAA), which can be measured in the urine and used to diagnosis the syndrome. The neurosecretory granules contain both serotonin and tachykinins (likely substance P and neuropeptide K), and these products and their metabolites result in the clinical manifestations of the carcinoid syndrome. The vasodilator paroxysms are most likely the result of the tachykinins and may be associated with tachycardia and a fall or no change in the blood pressure. An elevation of the blood pressure is very rare, and the carcinoid syndrome is not a cause of sustained hypertension. The cutaneous flush can be triggered by excitement, exertion, eating, and ethanol ingestion. (*Cecil, Ch. 245*)

42. (D); **43. (D)**. *Discussion:* Osteitis deformans, also known as Paget's disease, is the second most common abnormality of the bone and affects 5% of the population. The disease involves increased remodeling of the bone, and an affected site may demonstrate a 5-10 fold increase in remodeling activity. This can be detected using both markers of bone formations (alkaline phosphatase) and bone resorption (urinary pyridinoline crosslinks). The radiographic findings described are consistent with Paget's disease with evidence of both patchy osteolysis and sclerosis and thickening of the cortices of the long bones. Skull radiographic findings include a typical "cotton-wool" appearance. It occurs with greater frequency in patients of British descent, and peak presentation is in the sixth decade. Ninety-five percent of patients with Paget's disease are asymptomatic. The underlying increased remodeling leads to excessive bone formation with enlargement and deformity. Despite its increased amount, the bone is less structurally competent and is at risk for fracture. The warmth noted on examination is due to the increased blood flow through the pagetic bone. Because this patient has pain and the bone is weightbearing there is a higher risk of fracture, and treatment with either a bisphosphonate (alendronate, 40 mg/day for 6 months, or pamidronate, 30 to 60 mg for 3 days) or calcitonin (50-100 IU subcutaneous) or both are indicated. Osteomalacia is a diffuse process that leads to defective mineralization of bone. It has numerous causes and usually presents as bone pain and radiographic evidence of decreased mineralization. Osteonecrosis presents as pain in patients with medical problems that places them at risk for impaired blood flow to the affected bone (sickle cell disease, alcoholism, and corticosteroid use). Fibrogenesis imperfecta ossium is a generalized osteopenic disorder with thickening of the residual trabecular bone. It causes intractable skeletal pain in middle aged patients. The bones are tender when palpated. Metastatic prostate cancer would not present with the above clinical or radiologic findings, but the lesions can be either lytic or blastic. All the choices can present with an elevated alkaline phosphatase level, and the diagnosis must be made from the clinical, epidemiologic, and radiographic information. (*Cecil, Chs. 262 and 267*)

44. (C) *Discussion:* Peptide hormones are synthesized and processed as secretory proteins. Peptide hormones must interact with the extracellular domain of a receptor on the cell surface, which imparts a signal, usually through activation of second messenger systems. The end result of this process is to induce a conformational change in, and therefore alter the function of, existing cell enzymes. The receptors for peptide hormones usually are one of three types: (1) a seven membrane-spanning structure (serpentine) that couples to a G-protein–linked second messenger system inside the cell, (2) a membrane-spanning structure with intrinsic enzyme activity in its intracellular domain, and (3) a single membrane-spanning structure that couples to an intracellular second messenger system. Answer C is false because steroid hormones, not peptide hormones, originate from a cholesterol precursor. (*Cecil, Ch. 234*)

45. (E) *Discussion:* Thyroid cancer remains a significant medical problem in the United States; 18,000 new cases are diagnosed and more than 1200 deaths are reported each year. Differentiated thyroid cancer is classified into follicular and papillary (derived from the follicular cells) and medullary thyroid carcinoma (derived from the C cells). Rarely, the thyroid is the site of involvement with lymphoma. Anaplastic cancer arises from the papillary and follicular cancers. The most common type of thyroid cancer is papillary cancer, which accounts for approximately 70% of all thyroid cancers. It is two to three times more common in females and peaks in the third and fourth decades of life. Papillary cancer is usually nonencapsulated and sometimes multifocal and tends to spread by the lymphatic route. Follicular cancer is the second most common form of thyroid cancer, accounting for 15% of all thyroid cancers. It affects a slightly older age group and is more commonly diagnosed in females than in males. Follicular cancer tends to be encapsulated, is usually unifocal, and tends to spread via the hematogenous route; early metastases are seen with small lesions. Thyroid cancer is now diagnosed at an early stage, and its slow rate of growth makes for a favorable outcome in a majority of cases. Sometimes, however, thyroid tumors are encountered that display aggressive features leading to early death despite aggressive treatment. Moreover, the treatment modalities themselves can sometimes be attended by significant complications, making the optimum treatment of thyroid cancer a highly controversial issue. Therefore, an understanding of the factors that affect prognosis should guide selection of treatment modalities. In papillary cancer, prognosis is affected by tumor size, presence or absence of metastases, patient age, and degree of differentiation. Generally, the smaller tumors (<1.5 cm) carry an excellent prognosis in the absence of metastasis, whereas larger tumors (>2.5 cm) tend to carry a poorer prognosis. Patient age greater than 40 years at diagnosis tends to carry a poor prognosis in part because of poor concentration of iodine by most tumors. Poorly differentiated tumors tend to run a more aggressive course. The first line of treatment of thyroid cancer consists of surgical resection. Although the optimum procedure is not known, the more aggressive tumors should be managed with more extensive procedures (near-total or total thyroidectomy with or without lymph node dissection). RAI remnant ablation/therapy should be considered when residual or metastatic disease is present. Finally, thyroid hormone treatment should be used with a goal of keeping the TSH level as low as possible without causing overt hyperthyroidism. RAI ablation and thyroid hormone suppression have been shown to reduce recurrence of thyroid cancer. In this patient, age and tumor size predict a poor outcome. Treatment should, therefore, consist of near-total thyroidectomy, RAI ablation, and thyroid hormone treatment. (*Cecil, Ch. 239; Mazzaferri and Kloos, 2001*)

46. (C) *Discussion:* The causes of hypocalcemia, an abnormal reduction of serum calcium, can quickly be determined by examining the serum phosphorus, creatinine, and calcium levels. In hypoparathyroidism, there is reduced mobilization of calcium from bone, reduced renal reabsorption of calcium relative to the filtered load (along with decreased phosphaturia), and reduced formation of 1,25-hydroxyvitamin D, resulting in reduced intestinal absorption of calcium. Consequently, the hypocalcemia is accompanied by hyperphosphatemia. Hypoparathyroidism can be congenital or acquired; the latter is accounted for by transient or permanent disorders. Hypomagnesemia causes deficient secretion and action of PTH and consequent functional hypoparathyroidism. In vitamin D deficiency, decreased intestinal absorption of calcium leads to secondary hyperparathyroidism, which increases renal tubular loss of phosphate. Vitamin D deficiency can result from inadequate dietary intake, lack of sun exposure, increased catabolism, and malabsorption. Renal failure impairs hydroxylation of 25-hydroxyvitamin D, which results in the malabsorption of calcium. The body compensates by increased secretion of PTH, leading to increased mobilization of calcium from bone. Renal failure is char-

acterized by an abnormal serum creatinine concentration, whereas renal dysfunction is not the critical pathogenetic feature of the other forms of hypocalcemia. (*Cecil, Ch. 264*)

47. (E) *Discussion:* The clinically apparent (>1 cm) thyroid nodule is a common clinical finding; up to 5% of the population is affected. It is more common in women than in men, and a majority (85%) are hypofunctional or cold nodules. The likelihood of malignancy in a solitary thyroid nodule is low (4%); cold nodules carry a higher risk than hot nodules (20% vs. 1%). Evaluation of a solitary nodule should be aimed at detecting potentially malignant lesions so that as many cancers are removed with as few operations as possible. A history of head and neck irradiation raises the likelihood that a thyroid nodule is malignant, as does the presence of a family history of differentiated thyroid cancer or medullary cancer of the thyroid (which can be a component of MEN type 2a or 2b). Fine-needle aspiration of the thyroid gland is a cost-effective procedure with a high sensitivity and specificity for malignancy. Fine-needle aspiration allows the nodule to be characterized cytologically as benign, malignant, suspicious for malignancy, or indeterminate. (*Cecil, Ch. 239*)

48. (F); 49. (E). *Discussion:* Glucocorticoids are used in the treatment of chronic inflammatory diseases of the lungs, connective tissue, and intestines, as well as in transplantation because of their anti-inflammatory effect. When long-term treatment is required, several complications (e.g., cataracts, truncal obesity, skin-thinning, hyperglycemia) may be seen. A particularly disabling complication is bone loss, which can lead to fracture; it can occur with or without the other complications of chronic steroid treatment. The incidence of steroid-induced osteoporosis is unknown, but it appears to be related to the duration of treatment, half-life of the steroid, and its dose. Risk factors associated with increased bone loss include age, body mass index, and duration of use. Steroid-induced osteoporosis proceeds rapidly in the first 6 months of steroid use and slows thereafter. Trabecular bone and the cortical rim of the vertebral body are most susceptible to the effects of steroids. Steroids induce bone loss by several mechanisms. First, they inhibit calcium absorption in the gastrointestinal tract while enhancing calcium loss in the kidneys. These effects induce secondary hyperparathyroidism, which leads to increased bone resorption. Second, they lower sex hormone levels through an effect on the gonadotropin levels and a direct effect at the gonadal level, as well as by decreasing adrenal sex steroid synthesis by inhibiting ACTH release. Third, they have a direct inhibitory effect on osteoblast proliferation, activity, and half-life, leading to decreased bone formation. Fourth, they induce proximal muscle weakness. Short-term studies showed that steroid-induced osteoporosis can be prevented or treated by using measures aimed at minimizing the negative effects of steroids on calcium and bone metabolism. Deficiency of sex steroids should be corrected. Physical therapy should be encouraged to prevent steroid-induced myopathy. Calcium (1000 mg to 1500 mg of elemental) and vitamin D (800 IU) supplementation should be given to all patients receiving long-term corticosteroid therapy. Diuretics have been used to enhance calcium absorption and minimize calcium loss in urine, thereby preventing secondary hyperparathyroidism. Regular monitoring is recommended to prevent hypercalcemia. Treatment with a bisphosphonate is recommended to prevent bone loss in all men and postmenopausal women in whom long-term glucocorticoid treatment at 5 mg/day (prednisone equivalent) or more is being initiated, as well as in men and postmenopausal women receiving long-term glucocorticoids in whom the bone mineral density (BMD) T-score at either the lumbar spine or the hip is below normal. (*Lane and Lukert, 1998; American College of Rheumatology, 2001*)

50. (D) *Discussion:* This patient has central hypothyroidism and should be evaluated for pituitary and end-organ function as well as the presence of a pituitary tumor. The prolactin level should be measured and the pituitary-adrenal, gonadal, and growth hormone axes assessed. The presence of a pituitary tumor can be determined by imaging the pituitary gland with MRI or CT. Where appropriate, this should be followed by evaluation of the visual fields. Measurement of the α subunit, a glycoprotein shared by FSH, LH, and TSH, may also be useful because some pituitary tumors secrete only this peptide. (*Cecil, Ch. 237*)

51. **(E)** *Discussion:* Primary aldosteronism, a disorder characterized by hypertension, hypokalemia, suppressed plasma renin activity, and increased aldosterone secretion, affects 0.05 to 2% of the hypertensive population. This disorder should be suspected in hypertensive patients in whom spontaneous or easily provoked hypokalemia develops that is slow to correct after discontinuation of diuretics. As important as recognizing the presence of primary aldosteronism is the differentiation of lesions that are surgically curable (60-70% of the cases in some series) from those that are best treated medically. In this patient, the presence of hypertension, hypokalemia, and alkalosis appropriately triggered screening for hyperaldosteronism, which led to the findings of an aldosterone-renin ratio of greater than 30, which constitutes a positive screening test if the serum aldosterone level is *greater* than the upper limit of normal. Aldosteronism can be confirmed by the finding of a 24-hour urine aldosterone secretion of 12 μg in the salt-replete state. Adrenal imaging is the next step to differentiate adrenal adenoma from adrenal hyperplasia, although adenomas smaller than 1.5 cm can be missed and thus mistaken for hyperplasia. In confusing cases, adrenal vein sampling for aldosterone measurements is used to localize adenoma with a 95% accuracy. The finding of a lateralizing 10:1 aldosterone ratio in the presence of a symmetrical ACTH-induced cortisol rise diagnoses and localizes an adenoma. Other features suggestive of adenoma include plasma 18-hydroxycorticosterone of 100 ng/dL or more, spontaneous hypokalemia of less than 3 mEq/L, and an anomalous postural decrease of plasma aldosterone concentration. Saline loading is inappropriate in this patient because of heart failure and hypertensive retinopathy. (*Cecil, Ch. 240*)

52. **(E)** *Discussion:* The findings of Albright's hereditary osteodystrophy (short stature, brachydactyly, and soft tissue calcification) along with severe hypocalcemia and elevated PTH are diagnostic of pseudohyperparathyroidism (type IA). This is an autosomal-dominant disorder resulting from a G protein (Gs) defect, which leads to PTH resistance. Hypothyroidism and ovarian failure are also seen because Gs also couples to TSH and gonadotropin receptor signaling, respectively. Mental retardation is seen in 70% of cases. (*Cecil, Ch. 264; Strewler and Rosenblatt, 1995*)

53. **(D)** *Discussion:* Iodine 131 is a radioactive isotope of iodine (RAI) that is selectively concentrated in the thyroid tissue and metabolized by the same pathways as naturally occurring iodine. This, together with its long half-life (8 days), allows it to deliver high doses of radiation to the thyroid gland (β-radiation) sufficient to destroy thyroid follicular cells. Thus, ^{131}I is used in the treatment of Graves' disease, toxic multinodular goiter, and differentiated thyroid cancer. The doses of RAI used in the treatment of Graves' disease and toxic multinodular goiter are relatively low compared with those used in the treatment of thyroid cancer (in which it is used in conjunction with surgery). RAI has no place in the treatment of thyroid lymphoma because lymphoma cells do not concentrate iodine. (*Cecil, Ch. 239; Sarkar and Becker, 1995*)

54. **(E)** *Discussion:* PTH, an 84-amino-acid peptide synthesized and secreted by the parathyroid gland, is a potent regulator of the serum calcium level. Hypocalcemia stimulates the secretion of PTH acutely (with increased PTH synthesis and parathyroid cell hypertrophy and hyperplasia after chronic hypocalcemia), whereas hypercalcemia leads to decreased secretion of PTH. Hypo-

magnesemia inhibits PTH secretion and action. Elevated 1,25-dihydroxyvitamin D affects PTH synthesis and secretion by directly inhibiting the parathyroid gland and indirectly via hypercalcemia. Low levels of 1,25-dihydroxyvitamin D have the opposite effect. (*Cecil, Ch. 261*)

55. **(D)** *Discussion:* Symptoms of thyrotoxicosis caused by Graves' disease usually begin to improve in 1 to 2 weeks after initiation of thionamides (PTU and methimazole), whereas the hyperthyroxinemia takes approximately 3 weeks to normalize, and TSH can take even longer to recover. These changes are due to inhibition of synthesis and secretion of T_4 and T_3 as well as inhibition of T_4 to T_3 conversion (the latter effect occurs with PTU but not with methimazole). Thionamides act by blocking the peroxidase enzymes responsible for organification of iodine and synthesis of thyroid hormones. PTU inhibits 5′-deiodinase (in peripheral tissues—type 1), the enzyme responsible for T_4 to T_3 conversion. (In euthyroid individuals, 80% of circulating T_3 is derived from this peripheral conversion.) The type 2 deiodinase, present in the brain, is resistant to PTU. Once full blockade of thyroid hormone synthesis is accomplished, the degree of normalization of thyroid hormone levels is determined by the magnitude of hyperthyroidism and the half-life of the thyroid hormones (roughly 1 week for T_4, approximately 1 day for T_3). (*Cecil, Ch. 239; Utinger, 1995*)

56. **(D)** *Discussion:* Abnormal thyroid function tests are frequently encountered in severely ill patients in the absence of intrinsic thyroid disease. This sick euthyroid syndrome is thought to be part of a broader endocrine response to illness, with growth hormone, ACTH, cortisol, gonadotropins, and sex hormones all being involved. The low-T_3 state is its most commonly encountered form; T_4 and TSH involvement occurs less frequently. Differentiating sick euthyroid syndrome from hyperthyroidism or hypothyroidism can be a challenge. Signs of preexisting thyroid disease (e.g., goiter, exophthalmos, or preexisting myxedema), when encountered, can point toward a diagnosis of intrinsic thyroid disease. Additional attention should be paid to the magnitude of thyroid hormone abnormality; for example, a TSH greater than 20 μU/mL makes hypothyroidism more likely, whereas a TSH of less than 0.03 μU/mL makes hyperthyroidism more likely. Where the sick euthyroid syndrome is the sole diagnosis, thyroid-directed treatment has not been shown to be beneficial. One should also review medications because TSH suppression can occur with dopamine or higher doses of glucocorticoids. (*Cecil, Ch. 239*)

57. **(D)** *Discussion:* Weakness in an elderly patient is a nonspecific complaint that can result from several causes. In this patient who also has constipation, endocrine causes to be ruled out should include hypothyroidism and hypercalcemia. Hypothyroidism in an adult is most likely to be primary (90%) and may be associated with cold intolerance, a hoarse voice, weight gain, and myxedema with or without a goiter. A normochromic-normocytic anemia may be present. Hypercalcemia can be missed if correction is not made for serum albumin and can be due to PTH or non-PTH related factors. Gastrointestinal malignancy should also be ruled out in this patient with weight loss, abdominal pain, constipation, and anemia. Therefore, a stool occult blood test is important initially. (*Cecil, Ch. 239*)

58. **(A)** *Discussion:* The biochemical and pathologic findings in this patient establish primary hyperparathyroidism as the cause of his hypercalcemia. In non–MEN 1 patients, this disorder is usually due to a solitary adenoma. Normally, there are two superior and two inferior parathyroid glands; the superior glands are located near the upper poles of the thyroid gland, and the inferior glands are located near the inferior poles of the thyroid gland. Each gland measures 2 to 7 mm × 2 to 4 mm × 0.5 to 2 mm. The combined weight of the four glands is approximately 120 mg in males and 145 mg in females. The parathyroid glands are sometimes found at

aberrant locations, leading to difficulty during surgical exploration of the neck for primary hyperparathyroidism, with more extensive neck dissection potentially resulting in surgical complications. In addition, aberrant location may lead to removal of a normal parathyroid gland in nonparathyroid surgery. The superior parathyroid glands develop from the fourth branchial pouches and are typically located at the superior poles of the thyroid glands. Aberrant locations of the superior parathyroids include the tracheoesophageal groove and retroesophageal space. The inferior glands develop from the third branchial pouches and migrate caudad to their final position near the lower poles of the thyroid gland, but they are sometimes aberrantly located at the angle of the jaw or in the anterior mediastinum. The number of parathyroid glands found in a person is variable; up to 5% of people have more than four glands. (*Cecil, Ch. 264*)

59. **(D)** *Discussion:* Mild hypercalcemia in an otherwise asymptomatic patient can be due to a number of factors. Hyperthyroidism can be complicated by hypercalcemia, and further testing should be considered, particularly in this patient with a goiter. Primary hyperparathyroidism is the most common cause of asymptomatic hypercalcemia, and such a diagnosis should be considered in this patient with a family history suggestive of parathyroid surgery. Parathyroid adenomas are not palpable, and the goiter is thyroid tissue. Vitamin D intoxication is unlikely in this patient, who is taking no medications, although granulomatous conditions might exist, in which excessive amounts of 1,25-dihydroxyvitamin D are synthesized. Therefore, vitamin D studies should be ordered only if the patient is euthyroid and PTH is suppressed. (*Cecil, Ch. 264*)

60. **(C)** *Discussion:* A normal PTH level in the face of hypercalcemia is inappropriate and should prompt investigation for abnormal PTH regulation and/or secretion. In this patient, familial hypocalciuric hypercalcemia (FHH) should be ruled in or out by determining a 24-hour calcium-creatinine ratio. This is important in all situations in which parathyroid surgery would otherwise be considered, so that FHH (a disorder resulting from a mutation in the calcium-sensing receptor and not requiring surgery) can be distinguished from primary hyperparathyroidism. Parathyroid imaging is rarely useful in evaluating parathyroid function, and a neck ultrasonogram and sestamibi scan are not appropriate at this stage of this patient's evaluation. Familial hypocalciuric hypercalcemia (FHH) is a rare autosomal-dominant disease that causes a mild hypercalcemia and a low renal excretion of calcium. In most families, the disease is due to a mutation on the long arm of chromosome 3 that encodes an abnormal calcium transport and/or sensing receptor. This results in an exaggerated renal reabsorption of the filtered calcium load, while the parathyroid glands fail to suppress PTH secretion in spite of hypercalcemia. Parathyroid gland mass is usually only mildly increased. The hypercalcemia is usually mild, and evidence of bone and kidney disease is usually lacking. Pancreatitis has been reported, although the association is not certain. Urinary calcium-creatinine ratios less than 0.01 strongly support the diagnosis. For those families in which the disease gene is located on chromosome 3q, genetic diagnosis is possible, but this is not yet widely available. The patient's TSH was normal, no nodules were felt in the goiter, and family history was negative. The goiter size and function should be followed periodically. (*Cecil, Ch. 264*)

61. **(C)** *Discussion:* Hyperprolactinemia in the absence of an obvious pituitary tumor can be a consequence of medications or physiologic or pathologic conditions. In such cases, the hyperprolactinemia is usually mild and may or may not be symptomatic. Primary hypothyroidism sometimes leads to hyperprolactinemia by stimulating hypothalamic output of thyrotropin-releasing hormone (TRH), which in turn stimulates lactotrophs to synthesize

and secrete prolactin. In this patient the initial therapeutic intervention should be directed at correction of the hypothyroidism. Pituitary surgery should not be considered in the absence of a pituitary tumor. Bromocriptine should be considered only if hyperprolactinemia and galactorrhea persist after correction of hypothyroidism. Likewise, estrogen replacement should be considered only if evidence of estrogen deficiency persists after correction of hyperprolactinemia. (*Cecil, Ch. 237*)

62. **(F)** *Discussion:* Treatment of thyroid storm is aimed at blocking thyroidal production of T_3 and T_4, peripheral T_4 to T_3 conversion, and the peripheral actions of thyroid hormones. PTU is useful because it blocks thyroid hormone synthesis and peripheral T_4 to T_3 conversion. The rationale for administering corticosteroids is principally to block T_4 to T_3 conversion (and thyroidal production of T_4 and T_3 in Graves' disease). In addition, administration of corticosteroids provides coverage for adrenal insufficiency that may coexist with the hyperthyroidism. β-Blockers are used to minimize the peripheral effects of thyroid hormone and to decrease T_4 to T_3 conversion (propranolol). Finally, supportive care should be provided as is deemed necessary. RAI treatment is not used in the acute stages of thyroid storm and may indeed worsen the situation by promoting thyroiditis and further release of thyroid hormones. (*Cecil, Ch. 239*)

63. **(E)** *Discussion:* This patient presents with intrapituitary hemorrhage or pituitary apoplexy. The presentation of pituitary apoplexy varies widely depending on the rapidity and extent of the hemorrhage, but when suspected it should be treated as a surgical and medical emergency that requires corticosteroid coverage and possibly surgical decompression. However, it may be asymptomatic in its mildest form or may present as an expanding intrasellar or extrasellar mass. In some cases, it may lead to the spontaneous cure of a hormone-secreting tumor or hypopituitarism, with or without the development of empty sella syndrome. Pituitary apoplexy is most often due to bleeding into a pituitary tumor. Other factors that can lead to intrapituitary hemorrhage include trauma, pregnancy, sickle-cell disease, diabetes mellitus, and anticoagulation. (*Cecil, Ch. 237*)

64. **(E)** *Discussion:* Diabetes insipidus (DI), a disorder characterized by excessive thirst and excessive urination, results from an inability to concentrate urine. It may be due to a lack of arginine-vasopressin (central DI) or a lack of renal response to AVP (nephrogenic DI). This results in serum hyperosmolality and hypernatremia. DI can be diagnosed when urine volumes exceed 30 mL/kg per day with a urine osmolality of less than 250 mOsm/kg. During pregnancy, serum sodium and osmolality are maintained at a lower set point than in the nonpregnant state. This is due to a resetting of the osmostat for thirst and AVP secretion. This makes it easy to miss hypernatremia (and hence DI) during pregnancy. This patient has hypernatremia and serum hyperosmolality with urinary hypo-osmolality. Along with polyuria, this is diagnostic of DI. DI that begins in pregnancy is commonly seen in patients who have preexisting partial neurogenic or nephrogenic DI and fail to compensate for the increased clearance of AVP that is normally seen in pregnancy because of vasopressinase, a placental cystine aminopeptidase. Some of these patients return to their baseline function after the end of pregnancy. In this patient, the beginning of symptoms after head injury suggests hypothalamic damage with development of partial (compensated) DI, which was unmasked by pregnancy. (*Cecil, Ch. 238*)

65. **(E)** *Discussion:* The treatment of primary aldosteronism should be tailored to the source of aldosterone excess. Thus, patients with aldosterone-producing adenoma should be managed surgically if they are young and otherwise healthy. For a majority of these patients, surgery is curative, and for those who are not cured the hypertension and hypokalemia are rendered easier to

control. Response of the blood pressure to surgical resection of an adenoma is not dependent on the severity and duration of hypertension or presence of end-organ damage. The medical management of idiopathic aldosteronism (bilateral adrenal hyperplasia) depends on (1) agents that compete with aldosterone for its intracellular receptor (spironolactone); (2) those that block transmembrane calcium flux, thereby inhibiting aldosterone production resulting from angiotensin II, ACTH, and potassium (calcium-channel inhibitors); and (3) those that inhibit the conversion of angiotensin I to angiotensin II (ACEs) and diuretics. Of these agents, spironolactone most frequently corrects hypertension and hypokalemia. Calcium-channel inhibitors, ACE inhibitors, and diuretics are, therefore, added when spironolactone has failed as a sole agent. (*Bravo, 1994*)

66. (E) *Discussion:* Combination OCPs provide a safe and effective means of preventing unwanted pregnancies. Each combined OCP consists of synthetic estrogens in combination with progestin and is administered for the first 3 weeks of the cycle. The progestin component of the combination pill suppresses ovulation by preventing the LH surge. It also creates a hostile cervical mucus and endometrium to the conceptus. The estradiol component is thought to prevent the development of the graafian follicle by suppressing FSH. Although combined OCPs are safe in a majority of women, there are some in whom alternative methods of contraception should be considered. These include women with a history of thromboembolic disease, active liver disease, known or suspected breast cancer, abnormal vaginal bleeding of unknown cause, or suspected pregnancy and smokers older than age 35 years. OCPs have been shown to cause a mild and insignificant elevation of blood pressure in a majority of users; significant elevations of blood pressure are seen in a minority of patients. Thus, a history of hypertension does not preclude the use of OCPs. Furthermore, a history of toxemia of pregnancy does not predict that a patient will experience hypertension once put on OCPs. A family history of diabetes or breast cancer does not preclude the use of OCPs. (*Sperroff et al, 1994*)

67. (B) *Discussion:* Epilepsy affects 1% of the population, is often diagnosed early in life, and frequently persists into (and often beyond) the childbearing years. It is estimated that 1 in 200 pregnancies occur in women with epilepsy, leading to 20,000 children being born to epileptic mothers each year. Uncontrolled epilepsy during pregnancy can lead to serious complications, including maternal and/or fetal injury, fetal distress, and status epilepticus. Furthermore, unplanned pregnancy while on some antiepileptic drugs can result in fetal exposure to teratogenic drugs, leading to fetal malformations (e.g., spina bifida in fetuses of women taking valproic acid). Therefore, proper contraception is advised for epileptic women of childbearing age. The high efficacy and safety of oral contraceptive pills makes them a valuable means of preventing unnecessary pregnancies in this high-risk group. However, reduced contraceptive protection of the OCPs has been seen in women also taking some antiepileptic medicines, leading to unplanned pregnancy. This contraceptive failure is due to liver enzyme induction by some antiepileptic medicines (phenobarbital, phenytoin, carbamazepine, and paramethadione), although patient noncompliance may also play a role. Thus, if seizures can be controlled only with an agent that is associated with significant enzyme induction, it may be necessary to prescribe OCPs that contain 50 µg of ethinylestradiol rather than 35 µg to compensate for steroid metabolism and maintain contraception. Alternatively, depot medroxyprogesterone acetate may be effective because of its relatively high dose. Moreover, medroxyprogesterone acetate has been shown to reduce seizure frequency. This patient has responded well to phenytoin, and it, therefore, should be continued to maintain seizure control. The dose of ethinylestradiol should be increased to 50 µg to offset the increased steroid clearance caused

by enzyme induction by phenytoin. Implantable levonorgestrel (unlike depot medroxyprogesterone) has not been shown to be protective in the presence of drugs that induce hepatic enzymes. Moreover, some studies reported lower circulatory levels of levonorgestrel during treatment with phenytoin. Women with epilepsy must have close contact with their physicians when considering pregnancy. (*Mattson and Rebar, 1993*)

68. (E); 69. (B). *Discussion:* This patient's history, physical examination, and laboratory findings are highly suggestive of primary adrenal insufficiency, a diagnosis that can be confirmed by the ACTH stimulation test. Although AIDS and related opportunistic infections of the adrenal gland are the most likely cause of adrenal failure in this patient, the polyglandular autoimmune syndrome (particularly type II) should be considered as well. Therefore, autoimmune thyroid disease and diabetes mellitus type I should be ruled out. Pancreatitis is a likely cause of abdominal symptoms in this patient, particularly given that she is on pentamidine. Stool studies need to be done to rule out infections as a cause of her diarrhea.

Primary adrenal failure (unlike secondary adrenal failure) implies a deficiency of both mineralocorticoids and glucocorticoids and is treated by replacing both steroids. Persistence of weakness and lightheadedness along with hyponatremia, hyperkalemia, and metabolic acidosis signals the presence of isolated mineralocorticoid deficiency. This has resulted from not including mineralocorticoids in the treatment regimen. Mineralocorticoid deficiency is treated with fludrocortisone, 0.1 mg per day orally. An adjunct to treatment is adequate salt intake. Patients being treated for adrenal failure should be assessed clinically, and adrenocorticotropin levels should not be relied on in determining adequacy of treatment. (*Cecil, Ch. 240*)

70. (E) *Discussion:* Detection of hyponatremia should prompt a determination of serum osmolality to eliminate factitious causes of a low sodium, such as is seen with hypertriglyceridemia. Once this is done, the patient's volume status should be determined to decide whether fluid restriction and/or diuretic treatment versus rehydration is required (hypervolemic vs. hypovolemic hyponatremia, respectively). Euvolemic causes of hyponatremia include hypothyroidism, hypocortisolism, and the syndrome of inappropriate ADH secretion (SIADH). When specific causes are identified, therapeutic intervention should be directed at the underlying etiologic factors. In SIADH, treatment of hyponatremia should be guided by its degree, its chronicity, and the presence or absence of neurologic manifestations. Hyponatremia of acute onset should be corrected more rapidly, particularly if there are neurologic manifestations; more chronic cases should be corrected slower. In this patient, hypothyroidism should be addressed before any other measures aimed at correcting hyponatremia are instituted. Furthermore, his hyponatremia has been going on for a week, making rapid correction not only unnecessary but perhaps unsafe. Finally, hyponatremia of more than 120 mEq/L is rarely associated with severe symptoms, especially when it has developed slowly.

71. (A) *Discussion:* The goal of treatment of hypothyroidism is to correct the clinical and biochemical abnormalities. This is accomplished by providing thyroid hormone replacement orally or parenterally. Efficacy of treatment is monitored clinically and by measuring levels of thyroid hormones and TSH. The form of thyroid hormone most commonly used in the treatment of hypothyroidism is synthetic T_4. Other forms include T_3, a T_3/T_4 combination, and desiccated animal thyroid. Approximately 80% of an administered dose of thyroid hormone is absorbed in the gastrointestinal tract; the vast majority (>99% of T_3 and T_4) circulates bound to thyroid-binding globulin. Because the half-life of T_4 is longer in hypothyroidism (8-11 days vs. 6 days), it takes 4 to 6 weeks for thyroid hormone levels to reach a steady state on any given dose of thyroid hormone. An adult patient requires

approximately 1.6 μg/kg of T_4 for replacement. Replacement should be started at a lower dose in the elderly and in those who have heart disease. In severe hypothyroidism, both T_4 and T_3 levels are low. Adequate replacement with T_4 restores the levels of both hormones to normal; most T_3 is derived from extrathyroidal deiodination of T_4 if replacement is in the form of T_4. TSH usually corrects last. (*Cecil, Ch. 239*)

72. **(B)** *Discussion:* This patient has a prolactinoma that has bled and is impinging on the optic chiasm. The presence of hypotension raises concern about adrenal insufficiency, and this, along with the presence of secondary hypothyroidism, suggests pituitary failure from compression of pituitary tissue by the tumor. Additionally, she may have diabetes mellitus. Hyperglycemia is a more likely cause of her polyuria than is DI, which is a complication rarely seen with anterior pituitary tumors unless there is compression of the pituitary stalk and/or hypothalamic involvement. Furthermore, she does not have urinary hypo-osmolality. Thus, appropriate initial treatment should include bromocriptine, hydrocortisone, and L-thyroxine. Because of the severity of her symptoms, she needs an immediate neurosurgical consultation.

73. **(C)** *Discussion:* MEN syndromes include groups of endocrine tumors whose cells are of neural crest origin. The syndromes are transmitted via autosomal-dominant mechanisms with a high degree of penetrance and variable expression. Multiple glands may be affected in the same patient or in different members of the family. In MEN 1, the most common manifestation is primary hyperparathyroidism (80-90%) from parathyroid hyperplasia. Pancreatic and pituitary tumors occur less frequently. Pancreatic involvement occurs in the form of benign or malignant gastrinomas or insulinomas and rarely nonfunctioning tumors. Pituitary tumors are most often nonfunctioning. Of the functioning tumors, growth hormone–secreting and prolactin-secreting tumors are most common. Features of MEN 2a include medullary thyroid carcinoma (MTC), pheochromocytoma, and parathyroid neoplasia. Features of MEN 2b include MTC, pheochromocytoma, mucosal and alimentary ganglioneuromatosis, and marfanoid features. In this family, the occurrence of pituitary, parathyroid, and pancreatic tumors defines the presence of the MEN 1 syndrome. (*Cecil, Ch. 265*)

74. **(C)** *Discussion:* In Graves' disease, thyrotoxicosis results from thyroid activation by thyroid-stimulating immunoglobulin (TSI). Correction of the hyperthyroidism can be accomplished by using thionamides or RAI or by thyroidectomy. Thionamides block thyroid hormone synthesis by inhibiting the peroxidase enzyme. This results in clinical improvement within 1 to 2 weeks; maximum effect is seen in 4 to 6 weeks. Many patients may have normal T_3 and T_4 levels by this time; TSH often remains suppressed for longer. Only 50% of the patients treated with thionamides alone experience spontaneous remission from Graves' disease, and over 50% of these patients will relapse over the next 1 to 6 years. Most, like this patient, require definitive treatment with RAI (or surgery) for the long-term management of their disease. RAI is concentrated within the thyroid and delivers a lethal dose of radiation to the follicular cells of the thyroid, which leads to biochemical improvement in 6 weeks to 3 months and likely hypothyroidism requiring replacement therapy. (*Cecil, Ch. 239; Mashio et al, 1997*)

75. **(D)** *Discussion:* Klinefelter's syndrome, a common cause of male hypergonadotropic hypogonadism, is characterized by the presence of one or more supernumerary X chromosomes; classic and variant forms have been identified. Clinical features include small testes, azoospermia, eunuchoid proportions, and gynecomastia. There may be behavioral disorders as well as a low intelligence, and a majority of the patients are infertile. Testosterone replacement is indicated in Klinefelter's syndrome for restoration and maintenance of sexual function and to maintain secondary sexual characteristics. Testosterone is available for intramuscular

injection and transcutaneous administration. Patients receiving testosterone replacement should be monitored closely to determine adequacy of treatment and to avoid systemic side effects of testosterone. When treatment is adequate, patients should experience restoration of sexual function and improvement of body weight, along with appearance of secondary sexual characteristics. Testosterone level can be checked and should be mid normal at mid interval in patients being treated with injectable testosterone. For those receiving transdermal forms, testosterone levels should be at least mid normal 4 hours after application of a scrotal patch and 8 hours after application of a nonscrotal patch. In this patient, who reports restoration of sexual function, the current dose of testosterone should be deemed sufficient. A sperm count will not help in the management of his testosterone replacement. (*Cecil, Ch. 247*)

76. **(A)**; 77. **(C)**. *Discussion:* This patient has the clinical features of thyrotoxicosis, and the findings of the technetium scan suggest that toxic multinodular goiter is the cause of her disease. Some of these nodules have the tendency to selectively hypersecrete T_3, leading to TSH suppression, whereas T_4 levels are normal (T_3 toxicosis). Therefore, free T_3 is the appropriate next test to order in this patient. Unlike in Graves' disease, hyperthyroidism caused by toxic multinodular goiter does not go into spontaneous remission. Therefore, some form of ablative therapy (RAI or surgery) is required for the long-term management of hyperthyroidism. RAI treatment is a convenient way for treating toxic multinodular goiters, particularly in the elderly, who may also have other medical conditions that render surgery unsafe. The dose of RAI used is usually higher than that used for treating Graves' disease because these nodules are generally radioresistant. (*Cecil, Ch. 239*)

78. **(D)** *Discussion:* Pheochromocytoma is a neuroendocrine tumor that causes symptoms by the oversecretion of catecholamines. It affects 0.01% of the hypertensive population, both sexes equally. Pheochromocytoma has been diagnosed in all age groups, but its peak occurrence is in the fourth and fifth decades. It may be sporadic or familial. The familial forms of pheochromocytoma may or may not be associated with endocrine and nonendocrine disorders (e.g., MEN 2a, MEN 2b, von Hippel-Lindau syndrome, and neurofibromatosis). The familial cases of pheochromocytoma tend to be bilateral. Pheochromocytoma is rarely extraabdominal or malignant. The hallmark of pheochromocytoma is hypertension, which may be sustained or sporadic. It is often associated with headache, palpitations, and diaphoresis, which tend to occur in episodes. The relationship between hypertension and the level of catecholamines is not always close; elderly patients manifest an even poorer correlation. Although catecholamine excess is the cause of hypertension in pheochromocytoma, the severity of hypertension does not always correlate with the magnitude of catecholamine excess. This may be due to downregulation of the catecholamine receptors or concurrent release of other vasoactive substances by the pheochromocytoma. Furthermore, autopsy series suggested that up to 50% of pheochromocytomas may be asymptomatic, particularly among elderly patients. Treatment of pheochromocytoma is by surgical removal of the tumor. Because 90% of these tumors are benign, complete surgical removal is possible in a majority of cases. Surgery leads to a cure of hypertension in a majority of cases; those not cured are left with milder forms of hypertension. Those not cured by surgery may also have essential hypertension. (*Cecil, Ch. 241*)

79. **(E)** *Discussion:* Steroid treatment results in several adverse effects on calcium and bone metabolism. In patients who require long-term steroid treatment, these effects can lead to osteoporosis and fractures. Steroid-induced bone loss is most marked in trabecular bone and the cortical rim of the vertebral body. It proceeds most rapidly in the first 6 months of steroid treatment and persists

thereafter at a slower rate. Patients who require long-term treatment with steroids should, therefore, be closely monitored for these effects of steroids on bones and, where indicated, have appropriate measures instituted to minimize or reverse the effect of steroids on bones. Generally, the lowest possible doses of steroids should be used. Steroids with a shorter half-life should be used in preference to those with longer half-lives. When possible, inhaled or topical steroids may be used in place of oral steroids, but both inhaled and topical steroids in high doses may have a negative effect on bone metabolism. The alternate-day schedule of steroid administration, which has been shown to prevent the suppression of the pituitary-adrenal axis, does not prevent the steroid-induced bone loss and, therefore, should not be relied on as a means of preventing osteoporosis. Weight-bearing and isometric exercises should be encouraged to prevent steroid-induced myopathy and muscle weakness, which are thought to lead to the development of osteoporosis by removing the normal forces on bone caused by strong muscle contraction. Additionally, measures to minimize the development of secondary hyperparathyroidism should be instituted early. All patients should receive 1000-1500 mg of elemental calcium and 800 IU of vitamin D and should be considered for bisphosphonate therapy if they are men or postmenopausal women in whom long-term glucocorticoid treatment at 5 mg/day (prednisone equivalent) or more is being initiated, or in any patient receiving long-term corticosteroids in whom the BMD T-score at either the lumbar spine or the hip is below normal. (*Lane and Lukert, 1998; American College of Rheumatology, 2001*)

80. **(E)** *Discussion:* In this patient hypopituitarism has developed from a large pituitary tumor. The surgical procedure performed after the initial diagnosis may have added to the pituitary damage. He now requires treatment for secondary hypothyroidism, and the presence of weakness, weight loss, and chronic abdominal symptoms suggests that he may be developing hypocortisolism (secondary adrenal insufficiency). This deficiency may have presented after the thyroid hormone therapy, which increased the metabolism of any available cortisol. The hypotension may be contributed to by the decreased cortisol. The anemia may be attributable to the combined effects of hypocortisolism and hypothyroidism. This patient can also have hypogonadotropic hypogonadism from gonadotroph cell destruction and/or hyperprolactinemia. The presence of polyuria and polydipsia suggests that DI has developed. This could have been unmasked by thyroid hormone replacement, given the timing of his symptoms. A rare complication of DI is bladder hypertrophy and hydroureter from voluntarily withholding urine. The posterior pituitary damage is almost certainly related to the surgery rather than the initial tumor because anterior pituitary tumors do not typically cause DI. (*Cecil, Chs. 237 and 238*)

81. **(B)** *Discussion:* Like other pituitary tumors, prolactinomas can be classified as microadenomas (<1 cm) versus macroadenomas (>1 cm); clinical features of prolactin excess include galactorrhea, oligomenorrhea, and infertility as well as features of hypoestrogenemia (vaginal dryness, dyspareunia, and loss of libido). Mass effect may be present with larger tumors. Galactorrhea is seen in 50 to 90% of patients with hyperprolactinemia. Oligomenorrhea or amenorrhea occurs in 60 to 90% of the patients and is due to suppression of gonadotropins. Amenorrhea and galactorrhea may precede each other by months to years. Hyperprolactinemia has been associated with bone loss, although it is unclear whether this leads to significant osteoporosis. Studies showed that a majority of prolactin-secreting microadenomas appear not to change in size for up to 5 years. Thus, treatment should not be initiated simply to prevent growth. Patients can be monitored with regular imaging and prolactin measurement. Treatment can be initiated for those tumors that show a growth propensity. Other indications for treatment include control of galactorrhea, amenorrhea, infertility, and concerns about bone loss. Medical treatment is the first line of

management; surgery is reserved for those tumors not responsive to medical treatment. Bromocriptine is a dopaminergic agonist that binds D_2 receptors, thereby decreasing prolactin synthesis, DNA synthesis, cell multiplication, and tumor growth. It normalizes prolactin levels in 80 to 90% of patients. (*Cecil, Ch. 237; Frohman, 1995*)

82. **(E)** *Discussion:* Secondary adrenal failure most commonly results from pituitary suppression by exogenously administered cortisol. Onset depends on the dose and half-life of the steroid used as well as the schedule of administration. Secondary adrenal failure may also result from destructive, inflammatory or infiltrative lesions affecting the pituitary gland or from pituitary surgery. In this case, other pituitary hormones may also be deficient.

Glucocorticoid deficiency is the hallmark of secondary adrenal failure, unlike primary adrenal failure, which is characterized by deficiency of both glucocorticoids and mineralocorticoids. Clinical features include malaise, weight loss, anorexia, and hypotension. Laboratory testing may show anemia (normochromic-normocytic), eosinophilia, prerenal azotemia, and hyponatremia. (*Cecil, Ch. 237*)

83. **(D)** *Discussion:* Myxedema coma is a severe metabolic decompensation seen in hypothyroidism. It is a rare complication seen most commonly in the elderly and during the cold seasons. It is characterized by multisystem decline, often with CNS dysfunction and cardiorespiratory compromise. Seizures may also occur. Although this patient has central hypothyroidism, myxedema coma is seen more commonly in primary hypothyroidism. Myxedema coma can be precipitated by cold, infection, cardiorespiratory disease, narcotics, or analgesics. Because it carries a high mortality, the successful management of myxedema coma depends on a timely diagnosis and institution of treatment. Thyroid hormone should be replaced in the form of intravenously administered LT_4, although some authorities advocate the concomitant use of LT_3 for a rapid onset of action. Appropriate supportive care should be instituted and the precipitating factors addressed. In this patient with central hypothyroidism, appropriate tests would include the ACTH stimulation test and a pituitary MRI. LH level would be useful because it would be expected to be elevated in a postmenopausal woman. Lack of elevation would support the diagnosis of pituitary dysfunction. In the acute setting the patient should be covered with dexamethasone while the Cortrosyn stimulation test is performed and intravenous T_4 should be given shortly after the intravenous dexamethasone. Any imaging of the pituitary should take place only after the patient is stable. Frequently, the evaluation of the gonadal axis can be deferred until the patient follows up as an outpatient. (*Cecil, Chs. 237 and 239*)

84. **(B)** *Discussion:* Although this patient's headache may be related to the prolactinoma, it is unlikely that her visual complaints are attributable to it. The presence of annoying galactorrhea would constitute reason for treatment. A trial of bromocriptine is an appropriate initial treatment; 80 to 90% of prolactinomas respond to bromocriptine not only with normalization of prolactin but also with shrinkage of the adenoma. Of these, 40% decrease by more than 50% in size, 30% show a 25 to 50% decrease in size, and 10% decrease by less than 15%. Some of the tumors respond rapidly; visual field changes are apparent in 1 to 3 days, and radiographic changes can sometimes be seen as early as 2 weeks but most commonly are observed months later. Other tumors respond more slowly. Transsphenoidal surgery may be considered in rapidly expanding tumors or those that fail medical treatment. (*Cecil, Ch. 237*)

85. **(D)**; 86. **(A)**. *Discussion:* Osteoporosis is a disease characterized by loss of bone mass, distortion of the microarchitecture of bone, and increased tendency for bone fracture. Osteoporosis can result from failure to achieve an adequate peak bone density at development, accelerated bone loss, or both. The peak bone density attained in the young adult is due to an interaction of several

factors, including sex steroids, race, gender, genetic factors, exercise, and calcium intake. The postpubertal bone density remains stable for many years before it begins to decline. In women, this begins before cessation of menses and accelerates rapidly with the onset of menopause. During the first 5 to 10 years of menopause, trabecular bone is lost faster than cortical bone. Once the period of rapid postmenopausal bone loss ends, bone loss continues at a more gradual rate throughout life, with a more balanced decrease of both cortical and trabecular bone. Osteoporosis can be diagnosed by measuring bone mineral density in the spine, proximal and distal radius, proximal femur, and heel. Many techniques are available for bone mineral density measurement, including quantitative CT, dual x-ray absorptiometry, and dual-photon absorptiometry. In this patient, factors responsible for osteoporosis include a positive family history, a low peak bone density because of her body habitus, and alcohol and tobacco use. (*Bajaj and Saag, 2003*)

87. (A); 88. (E). *Discussion:* This patient has Cushing's syndrome, a disorder that is due to glucocorticoid excess. It can occur as an isolated entity or in association with hypersecretion of other adrenocortical hormones. A careful medical history and review of the patient's current medications must be done to rule out iatrogenic (or exogenous) Cushing's. Clinical features of the classic syndrome include weight gain, striae, hypertension, plethora, and proximal muscle weakness. An atypical form may manifest few if any of the anabolic features. Glucocorticoid hypersecretion can be sustained or intermittent. When Cushing's syndrome is suspected, glucocorticoid excess should be demonstrated. This can be done using the 24-hour urine free cortisol or overnight dexamethasone suppression test. This should be followed by tests aimed at determining whether the glucocorticoid excess is ACTH dependent (pituitary or ectopic source) or independent (adrenal adenoma, carcinoma, micronodular adrenal disease). This differentiation can be made by assessing whether ACTH is measurable. Pituitary hypersecretion of ACTH can be differentiated from ectopic ACTH hypersecretion by sampling blood from inferior petrosal sinuses (IPSS) after corticotropin-releasing hormone administration. A skilled endocrinologist can use the intact feedback mechanism usually seen in patients with central (Cushing's disease), and a series of biochemical tests can localize the ACTH secreting lesion in the majority of cases when a corresponding lesion within the pituitary is found on MRI. If the IPSS results show a central to peripheral ACTH ratio of more than 3.0 this is compatible with pituitary ACTH hypersecretion (central [or Cushing's] disease). A ratio of 1.8 or less is compatible with ectopic ACTH hypersecretion. Half of ectopic ACTH secreting tumors reside in the lungs and the other half are in various tissues. The most common lung lesions are bronchial carcinoid and small cell carcinoma of the lung. Other tumors that can cause ectopic Cushing's disease include thymic carcinoma, pancreatic carcinoma, islet cell pancreatic tumors, pheochromocytoma, or ovarian tumors. When the ACTH source is localized to the pituitary gland, immediate therapeutic intervention should follow. On the other hand, further testing is required to localize the source of ectopic ACTH hypersecretion. This consists of chest CT and, if necessary, abdominal MRI. Delay of treatment can result in several complications of Cushing's syndrome, including hypertension, infertility, osteoporosis, and diabetes mellitus. (*Cecil, Ch. 240; Becker, 2001*)

89. (B) *Discussion:* This patient with multinodular goiter presents with features of compression of the surrounding structures by the goiter (hoarseness, dysphagia, and difficulty breathing). This requires surgery to relieve compression of the surrounding structures. Surgery should also be considered in patients with toxic multinodular goiter and when there is the threat of cancer. Hypercalcemia in this patient is due to familial hypocalciuric hypercalcemia given a renal calcium-creatinine ratio of less than 1% as determined from the 24-hour urine. This does not require surgery. (*Cecil, Ch. 239*)

90. (C); 91. (A); 92. (B); 93. (D). *Discussion:* Increased use of abdominal imaging studies has resulted in the frequent detection of adrenal tumors in patients who do not have features of adrenal disease. Thus, 1% of people who undergo adrenal imaging may have adrenal tumors, and postmortem studies detected adrenal tumors in up to 9% of cases. Because a majority of these tumors are hormonally inactive, endocrine testing should be guided by the clinical condition of the patient. Because adrenal cancer is rare, a majority of incidentally discovered adrenal tumors can be conservatively managed; surgery is reserved for the larger or hormonally active tumors. Generally, surgery is recommended for tumors that are larger than 4 to 6 cm. The 31-year-old woman has features of Cushing's syndrome and needs to have a 24-hour urine free cortisol test done; the 50-year-old woman should be evaluated for pheochromocytoma with urine studies for metanephrines. The 42-year-old man needs an aldosterone-renin ratio determined to test for primary hyperaldosteronism. The 35-year-old man with myelolipoma needs no further endocrine testing; however a thorough examination by an endocrinologist should be performed to ensure no subtle findings of excess hormone secretion are present. (*Cecil, Chs. 240 and 241*)

94. (B); 95. (B); 96. (B); 97. (A); 98. (C). *Discussion:* Klinefelter's syndrome is the most common cause of primary testicular failure, which leads to failure of spermatogenesis and testosterone production. It is due to chromosomal nondisjunction in meiosis, which leads to more than two X chromosomes with one or more Y chromosome. It is characterized by eunuchoid proportions, small firm testes, azoospermia, gynecomastia, and testosterone deficiency with gonadotropin elevation. More than 90% of patients with Klinefelter's syndrome have azoospermia with low testosterone levels. A common consequence of combination chemotherapy is seminiferous tubule damage, leading to infertility. Treatment with some antineoplastic agents can lead to androgen deficiency as well as failure of spermatogenesis. Kallmann's syndrome is a congenital disorder characterized by hypogonadotropic hypogonadism, which is due to gonadotropin-releasing hormone deficiency. Other features include eunuchoidism, anosmia (or hyposmia), cleft lip or cleft palate, and congenital deafness. The patients have low serum testosterone, LH, FSH, and azoospermia. Untreated congenital adrenal hyperplasia (21-hydroxylase deficiency or 11β-hydroxylase deficiency) leads to excessive production of adrenal androgens. This suppresses gonadotropin secretion, which leads to suppression of sperm production. In the patient who presented with impotence after radical prostatectomy, the problem is due to nerve damage rather than testosterone production or spermatogenesis. (*Cecil, Ch. 247*)

99. (A); 100. (C); 101. (C); 102. (D). *Discussion:* Lithium is concentrated in the thyroid gland, where it inhibits formation and release of thyroid hormones, leading to mild elevations of TSH. Overt hypothyroidism is rare. It is seen in patients with thyroid antibodies who have been on lithium for a long time. Administration of an iodide load can result in hypothyroidism or hyperthyroidism depending on the iodine status of the thyroid gland and whether there is thyroid disease. An iodide load can lead to hypothyroidism in iodine-sufficient patients with chronic autoimmune thyroiditis. It can lead to thyrotoxicosis in patients with autonomously functioning thyroid tissue. Thus iodine exposure to the thyroid will have variable effects based on existence of any thyroid pathology. Amiodarone is 37% iodine and can induce the same thyroidal changes as iodine. Amiodarone can also induce autoimmune disease of the thyroid. Moreover, amiodarone can inhibit both type 1 and type 2 5'-deiodinase as well as the binding of T_3 to its receptor. Glucocorticoid excess inhibits the normal TSH pulse, nocturnal TSH secretion, and the TSH response to TRH. Glucocorticoid excess also blocks the extrathyroidal T_4 to T_3 conversion, leading to a low T_3 and a high reverse T_3. Finally, glucocorticoid excess also alters thyroid hormone binding by decreasing thyroid hormone–binding globulin levels and increasing transthyretin levels. As a result of these actions, glucocorticoid excess results in a low-normal TSH concentration, a low-normal T_4, a normal free T_4, and a low T_3 with a high reverse T_3. (*Utinger, 1995*)

103. **(A)**; 104. **(B)**; 105. **(C)**; 106. **(D)**; 107. **(E)**. *Discussion:* The 28-year-old black woman has thyroiditis and should be managed symptomatically with β-blockade. The 34-year-old, alternatively, is taking exogenous thyroid hormone and needs to be counseled. The best way to manage Graves' disease in pregnancy is to use PTU in doses as low as possible to achieve euthyroidism. Rarely, thyroidectomy may be indicated. When indicated, this should be done in the second trimester. RAI should be avoided in pregnancy because the fetal thyroid is capable of concentrating iodine and could thereby be ablated. The 45-year-old who has had 2 years of thionamides for Graves' disease without remission needs ablative therapy with RAI. The 48-year-old with toxic multinodular goiter is experiencing pressure effect. She needs thyroidectomy. (*Cecil, Ch. 239*)

108. **(D)**; 109. **(H)**; 110. **(B)**; 111. **(C)**; 112. **(A)**; 113. **(I)**; 114. **(F)**. *Discussion:* 3β-Hydroxysteroid dehydrogenase deficiency impairs adrenal steroid production and sex steroid production in both adrenal and gonadal tissue. Adrenal crisis occurs in either sex, and replacement of adrenal steroids is required. Incomplete masculinization leads to ambiguous genitalia in male infants, and female infants develop normally with occasional clitoral enlargement as a result of increased DHEAS. The diagnosis is made by detecting elevated pregnenolone, 17-hydroxypregnenolone, and DHEAS. These patients are treated with glucocorticoid and mineralocorticoids. 5α-Reductase deficiency leads to a decrease in conversion of testosterone into dihydrotestosterone (DHT). This impairs DHT-mediated steps of masculinization and presents as penile and scrotal hypospadias, wolffian duct structures, occasionally a blind vaginal pouch, small or absent prostate, and absence of female internal genital structures. These patients should have surgical correction of the vaginal pouch and cryptorchidism and be reared as males. High doses of testosterone esters can be used in adults. Nonclassic 21α-hydroxylase deficiency is a milder enzyme deficiency and presents around the time of puberty with signs of androgen excess and irregular periods. A random or stimulated elevation of 17-hydroxyprogesterone is required to make the diagnosis, and then appropriate therapy with corticosteroids can be administered. 11β-Hydroxylase deficiency is a rare disorder that results in in-utero virilization in the female fetus and can present as hypertension, hypokalemia, hyporeninism, hypoaldosteronism, and signs of virilization in the female, which include clitoromegaly. The hypertension and suppression of the renin and aldosterone are due to the excess production of 11-deoxycortisol and deoxycorticosterone levels. Corticosteroid treatment can normalize the hypertension. Classic 21α-hydroxylase deficiency presents as adrenal crisis in the newborn and is a medical emergency. Female patients have ambiguous genitalia as a result of the excess androgen production and frequently require surgical correction. Treatment with both corticosteroids and mineralocorticoids is required life long (in both sexes). Androgen insensitivity syndrome has also been called testicular feminization syndrome and is caused by a mutation of or absence of the androgen receptor. The phenotype of an affected male is female with a blind vaginal pouch with or without müllerian derivatives. The testes are abdominal or labial and should be removed because of the risk of neoplasm. Both testosterone and estrogen levels are elevated, and the elevated estrogen leads to breast development. Polycystic ovarian syndrome presents as menstrual irregularity and androgen excess. It is associated with insulin resistance, which likely plays a pathologic role. This is a diagnosis of exclusion, and congenital adrenal hyperplasia should be excluded by an ACTH-stimulated 17-hydroxyprogesterone measurement. (*Cecil, Ch. 246*)

BIBLIOGRAPHY

American College of Rheumatology Ad Hoc Committee on Glucocorticoid-Induced Osteoarthritis: Recommendations for the prevention and treatment of glucocorticoid-induced osteoporosis: 2001 update. Arthritis Rheum 2001;44:1496-1503.

Asplin JR, Coe FL, Favus MJ: Nephrolithiasis. *In* Fauci AS, Braunwald E, Isselbacher KJ, et al (eds): Harrison's Principles of Internal Medicine, 14th ed. New York, McGraw-Hill, 1998, pp 1569-1574.

Bajaj S, Saag KG: Osteoperosis: Evaluation and treatment: Curr Womens Health Rep 2003;3:418-424.

Bravo EL: Primary aldosteronism: Issues in diagnosis and treatment. Endocrinol Metab Clin North Am 1994;23:271.

Carr BR, Bradshaw KD: Disorders of the ovary and female reproductive tract. *In* Fauci AS, Braunwald E, Isselbacher KJ, et al (eds): Harrison's Principles of Internal Medicine, 14th ed. New York, McGraw-Hill, 1998, pp 2097-2115.

Frohman LA: Diseases of the anterior pituitary. *In* Felig P, Baxter JD, Frohman LA (eds): Endocrinology and Metabolism, 3rd ed. New York, McGraw-Hill, 1995, pp 289-383.

Goldman L, Ausiello D (eds): Cecil Textbook of Medicine, 22nd ed. Philadelphia, WB Saunders, 2004.

Keiser HR: Pheochromocytoma and other diseases of the sympathetic nervous system. *In* Becker KL (ed): Principles and Practice of Endocrinology, 2nd ed. Philadelphia, JB Lippincott, 1995, pp 762-772.

Kleerekoper M, Avioli LV: Evaluation and treatment of postmenopausal osteoporosis. *In* Flavus MJ (ed): Primer of Metabolic Bone Diseases and Disorders of Mineral Metabolism, 3rd ed. Philadelphia, New York, Lippincott-Raven, 1996, pp 264-271.

Lane NE, Lukert B: The science and therapy of glucocorticoid-induced osteoporosis. Endocrinol Metab Clin North Am 1998;27:465.

Mashio Y, Beniko M, Matsuda A, et al: Treatment of hyperthyroidism with a small single daily dose of methimazole: A prospective long-term follow-up study. Endocr J 1997;44:553-558.

Mattson RH, Rebar RW: Contraceptive methods for females with neurological disorders. Am J Obstet Gynecol 1993;168:2027.

Mazzaferri EL, Kloos RT: Current Approaches to Primary Therapy for Papillary and Follicular Thyroid Cancer. JCEM 2001;86:1447-1463.

Sarkar SD, Becker DV: Thyroid uptake and imaging. *In* Becker KL (ed): Principles and Practice of Endocrinology, 2nd ed. Philadelphia, JB Lippincott, 1995, pp 307-313.

Sperroff L, Glass RH, Kase NG (eds): Clinical Gynecologic Endocrinology and Infertility, 5th ed. Baltimore, Williams & Wilkins, 1994, pp 715-763.

Strewler GJ, Rosenblatt M: Mineral metabolism. *In* Felig P, Baxter JD, Frohman LA (eds): Endocrinology and Metabolism, 3rd ed. New York, McGraw-Hill, 1995, pp 1407-1516.

Utinger RD: The thyroid. *In* Felig P, Baxter JD, Frohman LA (eds): Endocrinology and Metabolism, 3rd ed. New York, McGraw-Hill, 1995, pp 435-519.

Wilson JD: Endocrine disorders of the breast. *In* Fauci AS, Braunwald E, Isselbacher KJ, et al (eds): Harrison's Principles of Internal Medicine, 14th ed. New York, McGraw-Hill, 1998, pp 2115-2119.

Part XI
Diabetes Mellitus and Metabolism

Eric S. Albright and Fernando Ovalle

MULTIPLE CHOICE

DIRECTIONS: For questions 1-57, choose the one best answer to each question:

QUESTIONS 1–4

A 55-year-old white man comes to your clinic for a routine health screen. He has no complaints other than his weight problem. His past medical history consists of hypertension and gastric reflux disease. A family history reveals a mother with "borderline diabetes" and a father who had a myocardial infarction in his early 50s. Social history reveals inactivity, occasional alcohol use, and 20-pack-year smoking history with cessation 5 years ago. Examination reveals a blood pressure (BP) of 144/88 mm Hg, a pulse of 77 beats/minute, weight of 255 pounds, height of 5'10", and a body mass index (BMI) of 35 kg/m². Remarkable findings on examination include thickened skin with deep, rough creases on the posterior aspect of the neck and obesity with a waist circumference of 46 inches. He currently is taking lisinopril, 10 mg/day, and omeprazole, 20 mg/day.

1. Based on the physical examination and history you suspect the patient has the metabolic syndrome or insulin resistance syndrome and order the following for diagnosis based on the National Cholesterol Education Program—Adult Treatment Panel (ATP) III criteria:

   A. 2-Hour glucose tolerance test
   B. Creatinine clearance
   C. Hemoglobin (Hbg) A1c
   D. Random plasma glucose
   E. Fasting plasma glucose

2. What other interventions should be performed at this visit to assess and treat his risk of atherosclerotic heart disease?

   A. Evaluation of a fasting lipid profile
   B. Therapy with a β-blocker
   C. Evaluation of C-reactive protein
   D. Evaluation of lipoprotein a
   E. Coronary angiography

3. What is the BP target in this individual based on his risk factors?

   A. 140/90 mm Hg
   B. 130/80 mm Hg
   C. 120/75 mm Hg
   D. 110/70 mm Hg
   E. No specific target in this patient

4. You are concerned about the patient's high risk of developing diabetes. Recent clinical evidence has demonstrated a reduction in the development of diabetes with specific intervention therapies. Based on recent clinical trial evidence, the most effective intervention at this time would be to:

   A. Prescribe a thiazolidinedione.
   B. Prescribe a 2500-calorie weight loss diet.
   C. Prescribe metformin.
   D. Prescribe both a weight loss diet and exercise program.
   E. Prescribe a sulfonylurea.

QUESTIONS 5–10

A 55-year-old black woman with diabetes mellitus (DM) type II for 6 years presents to your office for a routine physical examination. She has recently moved to town and has not had consistent medical care for the past few years because of her work travel schedule. She has no microvascular complications of diabetes and reports home fasting AM glucose monitoring values of 140-180 mg/dL. She currently is taking glipizide, 10 mg twice daily, metformin, 1000 mg twice daily, and metoprolol, 25 mg twice daily and has taken these since diagnosis. Her other medical history consists of hypertension, myocardial infarction, hysterectomy with oophorectomy, and sinus surgery. Family history is significant for diabetes type II and coronary disease. She does not smoke and drinks beer occasionally. Examination reveals a healthy woman who weighs 170 lbs with a height of 5′5″, BMI of 28 kg/m², BP of 130/70 mm Hg, and heart rate of 55 beats/minute. Her examination is unremarkable other than the bradycardia. Her blood work is as follows:

Hematocrit (Hct)	33 (normal range 34-44)
Mean corpuscular volume (MCV)	101 (normal range 83-99)
Glucose	140 mg/dL (normal range 70-105 mg/dL)
Creatinine	1.5 mg/dL (normal range 0.4-1.2 mg/dL)
Urinary albumin/ creatinine ratio	18.4 mg/g (normal range 0-13.1)
Hbg A1c	8.8% (normal range < 6.5%)
Total cholesterol	179 mg/dL
Low-density lipoprotein (LDL)	83 mg/dL
High density lipoprotein (HDL)	31 mg/dL
Triglycerides	325 mg/dL

5. Based on the cholesterol profile and her risk factors you recommend the following therapy:

   A. Prescribe step 1 diet with less than 30% fat calories and less than 10% saturated fats.
   B. Prescribe pravastatin.
   C. Prescribe niacin, 1500 mg daily.
   D. Prescribe atorvastatin.
   E. Prescribe gemfibrozil.

6. The patient is estrogen deficient since her hysterectomy 7 years ago and you would recommend hormone replacement for the following reasons:

   A. Cardiovascular protection and lipid profile modifications
   B. Prevention of osteoporosis
   C. Treatment of debilitating vasomotor instability
   D. Increase the metabolic rate
   E. All the above

7. The increased triglycerides is caused by the insufficient activity of:

   A. Hepatic lipoprotein lipase
   B. Lipoprotein lipase
   C. Lecithin:cholesterol acyltransferase
   D. Cholesterol ester transfer protein

8. What modifications should be made to her antidiabetic therapy?

   A. Start insulin therapy.
   B. Increase glipizide to 20 mg twice daily.
   C. Increase metformin to 850 mg three times a day.
   D. Replace metfomin with rosiglitazone, 4 mg/day.
   E. Add pioglitazone, 30 mg/day.
   F. Increase exercise to 30 minutes daily and reduce diet by 500 calories per day.

9. The patient's urinary albumin/creatinine ratio is elevated above normal. What is the best intervention to treat/evaluate this abnormality?

   A. Increase metoprolol to 50 mg twice daily.
   B. Add hydrochlorothiazide, 25 mg/day.
   C. Reorder urinary albumin/creatinine on a different day.
   D. Add an ACE inhibitor and/or an angiotensin II receptor blocker.
   E. Order 24-hour urine test for protein and creatinine.

10. The patient's blood cell count demonstrates anemia and you would start the work by:

    A. Ordering an iron profile
    B. Ordering an erythropoietin level
    C. Ordering a vitamin B_{12} level
    D. Ordering Hemoccult cards with the next three bowel movements
    E. Ordering a vitamin B_{12} level and iron profile

11. Which of the following is not a risk factor for developing diabetes?

    A. BMI > 25 kg/m²
    B. Cousin with DM type II
    C. Gestational diabetes
    D. Polycystic ovarian disease
    E. BP > 140/90 mm Hg

12. The recommended criteria to diagnosis DM is:

    A. Random glucose > 140 mg/dL
    B. 2-Hour glucose tolerance test with glucose value of 140-199 mg/dL
    C. Hbg A1c > 6.5%
    D. Serum glucose ≥ 126 mg/dL
    E. Fasting plasma glucose ≥ 126 mg/dL

13. A 34-year-old woman with type I diabetes wants to become pregnant and wants to know what the chances are for her child to develop type I diabetes. You tell her there is a _____ chance that her child will develop the disease.

    A. 22%
    B. 77%
    C. 51%
    D. 3%
    E. 11%

14. A 70-year-old patient with long-standing diabetes returns for follow-up 2 weeks after your initial visit. Her fasting home glucose monitoring shows elevated blood sugar levels ranging between 200 to 250 mg/dL. Her Hbg A1c was 7.2% from the blood work 2 weeks ago, and the fasting plasma glucose value was 212 mg/dL. You recommend the following to evaluate the discrepancy between the fasting values and the Hbg A1c:

    A. Order a CBC.
    B. Prescribe a new meter.
    C. Order a fructosamine.
    D. Repeat the Hbg A1c.

15. A 33-year-old patient with poorly controlled type I diabetes for 25 years presents with severe pain in his right thigh. The pain was abrupt in onset and has been constant for the last 4 days. Nonsteroidal anti-inflammatory drugs (NSAIDs) do not help with the pain. Examination shows an afebrile alert male with a cool, swollen tender area of the central right thigh with normal distal pulses. What should be ordered next?

    A. Corticosteroids
    B. IV antibiotics
    C. Blood culture
    D. MRI
    E. Creatine kinase

16. The United Kingdom Prospective Diabetes Study demonstrated that diabetic complications can be reduced with lowering of the Hbg A1c. This study found which of the following statements to be *true*?

    A. Significant reduction of any diabetic complication occurred for each 1% reduction of the Hbg A1c.
    B. The greatest benefit was seen when an Hbg A1c of 8.0% was achieved.
    C. No further risk reduction was observed once the Hbg A1c was below 7.0%.
    D. Reduction of the Hbg A1c only demonstrated risk reduction for microvascular complications.

QUESTIONS 17–19

A 55-year-old man with 11 years of diabetes presents with a urinary albumin of 36 mg/day. His blood glucose concentration is 203 mg/dL and he has an Hbg A1c of 9.2% and a plasma creatinine of 1.1 mg/dL.

17. Based on his laboratory work you tell him that he has an increased risk of developing diabetic nephropathy that is the leading cause of end-stage renal disease (ESRD) in the United States. He has a _____ chance of developing end-stage renal disease.

    A. 10%
    B. 30%
    C. 50%
    D. 90%

18. The patient's BP is 144/88 mm Hg on no medications. What BP target should the patient achieve?

    A. 140/90 mm Hg
    B. 130/80 mm Hg
    C. 155/75 mm Hg
    D. 120/55 mm Hg

19. You recommend the following for treatment of his BP:

    A. Lisinopril, 10 mg/day
    B. Hydrochlorothiazide, 50 mg/day
    C. Low sodium diet (< 1 g/day)
    D. Amlodipine, 5 mg/day

QUESTIONS 20–22

A 64-year-old patient with DM type II for 20 years presents to the emergency department with severe chest pain that radiates to the right arm and jaw. An electrocardiogram shows ST wave elevation in the lateral leads, and cardiac markers are elevated. The patient has been taking oral medications for her diabetes: glipizide XL, 10 mg q/day; metformin, 1000 mg twice daily; and pioglitazone, 15 mg/day. You treat her for a myocardial infarction with nitrates, β-blocker, and heparin infusion. The blood glucose concentration is elevated to 239 mg/dL on her admission laboratory tests.

20. How should the elevated blood sugar be managed?

    A. Pattern her blood sugar values and treat with regular sliding scale insulin.
    B. Continue her home medications.
    C. Recheck the blood sugar in 2 hours.
    D. Begin an insulin drip and D₅W.

21. The patient's admission Hbg A1c was 9.8% and home glucose monitoring confirms poor control. After discharge, how should the patient's blood sugar be managed?

    A. Continue previous outpatient therapy.
    B. Discontinue orals and prescribe insulin.

C. Continue metformin and pioglitazone and add multiple daily injections.
D. Change oral agents to acarbose, rosiglitazone, and repaglinide.

22. The patient returns a year later with mild orthopnea and lower extremity edema. Echocardiogram reveals an ejection fraction of 25% with a mildly dilated left ventricle. You should first:

    A. Prescribe Lasix, 60 mg twice daily.
    B. Stop her pioglitazone and metformin therapy.
    C. Order a cardiac angiogram.
    D. Stop her metformin therapy.

23. All of the following are true of insulin action in a fed state *except*:

    A. Accelerates glucose uptake by muscle and fat tissue
    B. Stimulates hepatic glucose uptake
    C. Suppresses hepatic gluconeogenesis
    D. Increases glucagon release

QUESTIONS 24–28

A 48-year-old obese woman presents to her primary physician with complaints of fatigue, weight loss, polyuria, and nocturia of several months' duration. Her fasting plasma glucose concentration is 280 mg/dL (on two different occasions). On review of systems, she denies pain on her lower extremities but refers to an inability to sense the temperature of the water in her bathtub with her feet to the point that she suffered a first-degree burn once in the recent past. Now she tests the water temperature with her hands. On examination her vibratory sensation is normal in all extremities.

24. What is the underlying illness?

    A. Impaired glucose tolerance
    B. DM type II
    C. DM type I
    D. Diabetes insipidus
    E. None of the above

25. What is the most likely cause for her inability to sense the water temperature with her feet?

    A. Diabetic dermopathy
    B. Diabetic neuropathy
    C. Reset thermostat in the hypothalamus
    D. Psychogenic disorder
    E. None of the above

26. Which of the following neurologic findings would you expect?

    A. Diffuse muscle wasting
    B. Decreased pinprick sensation (pain) in both feet
    C. Decreased position sense (proprioception) in both feet
    D. Normal neurologic examination
    E. None of the above

27. Which of the following disorders need to be considered in the differential diagnosis?

    A. Alcohol-induced neuropathy
    B. Uremic neuropathy
    C. Heavy metal intoxication
    D. All of the above
    E. None of the above

28. From which of the following interventions is this patient most likely to benefit?

    A. Blood glucose control
    B. Gabapentin

C. Amitriptyline

D. Carbamazepine

E. Clonazepam

QUESTIONS 29–33

A 23-year-old man is diagnosed with DM after several months of weight loss, fatigue, polyuria, polydipsia, and nocturia. His history is negative for diabetic ketoacidosis. On physical examination, his body mass index (BMI) is 30. The rest of his examination, including ophthalmoscopic, neurologic, and skin, is normal. His fasting blood glucose is 230 mg/dL (on two different occasions), and his urine shows no ketones.

29. At this point, what would be the most likely diagnosis?

A. DM type I

B. DM type II

C. Secondary diabetes

D. Maturity-onset diabetes of the young

E. None of the above

30. Which of the following would make you doubt your diagnosis?

A. A positive history of diabetic ketoacidosis

B. A family history of thyroid disease

C. A family history of DM type I in his father but no one else in the family

D. A family history of DM in his paternal grandfather, father, and two of his five siblings (all of whom are older and in whom diabetes developed in their 20s; they are treated with oral hypoglycemic agents)

E. None of the above

The patient does give you a family history of DM in his paternal grandfather, father, and two of his five siblings (ages 45 and 48). All of them acquired diabetes in their 20s and are treated with oral hypoglycemic agents.

31. Which of the following would be the most likely diagnosis now?

A. DM type I

B. Mitochondrial DM

C. Maturity-onset diabetes of the young

D. Latent autoimmune diabetes of the young

E. None of the above

32. Which of the following statements best describes this diagnosis?

A. X-linked recessive disorder

B. Polygenic disorder

C. Autosomal-recessive disorder

D. Autosomal-dominant disorder

E. None of the above

33. Which of the following statements is correct about this type of diabetes?

A. It is appropriate to defer screening for retinopathy for approximately 5 years.

B. Oral hypoglycemics are appropriate choices for therapy.

C. The chance for his children to develop diabetes is about 25%.

D. This patient's C peptide level is likely to be undetectable.

E. None of the above

QUESTIONS 34–36

A 51-year-old man with DM type I since age 11 comes to your office for routine follow-up. He maintains excellent control of his diabetes and checks his capillary blood glucose four to eight times a day. His blood glu-

cose records show evidence of frequent, almost daily, low blood glucose in the 40- to 50-mg/dL range. The patient denies having had any symptoms when he recorded that low blood glucose value. His Hgb A1c is 6.2%.

34. What is the most likely explanation for this patient's lack of symptoms when his blood glucose is less than 50 mg/dL?

A. Falsification of blood glucose records

B. Malfunction of his blood glucose meter

C. Adrenal insufficiency

D. Hypoglycemia unawareness syndrome

E. None of the above

35. What is the most appropriate next step?

A. Psychiatric counseling

B. Purchase of new blood glucose meter

C. Short cosyntropin (Cortrosyn) stimulation test

D. Strict avoidance of hypoglycemia for at least 2 weeks

E. None of the above

36. Which of the following hormonal responses to hypoglycemia is he most likely to have?

A. Normal glucagon, decreased epinephrine, normal cortisol

B. Decreased glucagon, decreased epinephrine, normal cortisol

C. Decreased cortisol, normal glucagon, normal epinephrine

D. Normal glucagon, normal epinephrine, normal cortisol

E. None of the above

QUESTIONS 37–39

A 21-year-old woman with DM type I since age 14 comes to your office complaining of fatigue and weight loss of several pounds over the last few months. On examination she is a thin white woman in no distress. She has a small diffuse goiter, but the rest of her examination is normal except for mild orthostatic hypotension (supine: BP is 110/70, pulse is 90 beats/minute; standing: BP is 90/50 mm Hg, pulse is 115 beats/minute).

37. Which one of the following diagnoses does *not* need to be initially considered?

A. Hyperthyroidism

B. Adrenal insufficiency

C. Uncontrolled diabetes

D. Psychiatric disorder

On further questioning, she admits increased thirst, and her blood glucose records show evidence of frequent episodes of hypoglycemia. Her Hgb A1c is much better than it had been before these problems without changes in her therapy (now 5.8%).

38. Which of the following tests are indicated?

A. Short Cortrosyn stimulation test

B. Thyroid-stimulating hormone (TSH)

C. Electrolyte profile

D. All of the above

E. None of the above

The results of the appropriate tests confirm your clinical suspicion. A CBC also shows evidence of mild anemia (Hgb = 11 g/dL) with an increased mean corpuscular volume of 110 fL (normal range, 83–89 fL). Her vitamin B_{12} level is found to be low.

39. At this point, which of the following is the most likely diagnosis?

A. Multiple endocrine neoplasia (MEN) type 1

B. MEN 2A

C. Autoimmune polyglandular syndrome type 2

D. Autoimmune polyglandular syndrome type 1

E. None of the above

QUESTIONS 40–43

A 35-year-old white woman with DM type I since age 20 and a history of frequent episodes of diabetic ketoacidosis presents to you for the first time. On ophthalmoscopic examination she has evidence of a few microaneurysms bilaterally. Her skin shows evidence of a few shiny, atrophic, macular areas with hyperpigmentation over her shins. She also has a positive prayer sign. Her fasting blood glucose concentration is 300 mg/dL. Her Hgb A1c is 11%, and her routine urinalysis is normal. Her BP is normal.

40. Which of the following interventions is the most likely to have a significant impact in the long-term prognosis of this patient?
    A. Angiotensin-converting enzyme (ACE) inhibitor therapy
    B. Protein restriction
    C. Birth control pills
    D. Blood glucose control (near-normoglycemia)
    E. None of the above

The patient is 5′ 4″, her weight is 140 pounds, and she is currently being treated with one injection of 20 U of long-acting insulin in the morning.

41. Which of the following regimens would be most appropriate for this patient at this point?
    A. Premixed insulin 70/30 at a dose of 40 U twice a day
    B. 2 units Lispro insulin before each meal and 5 units of NPH at bedtime
    C. 8 units of regular insulin before each meal and 8 units of NPH insulin at bedtime
    D. 15 units Lispro insulin with each meal and 20 units of glargine insulin at bedtime
    E. Sliding scale of regular insulin before each meal and at bedtime

The patient complies with your therapy, and several weeks later this part of her blood glucose record is representative of the rest:

Day	AM	Noon	PM	Bedtime
1	200	120	85	120
2	170	100	88	115
3	190	90	105	120

42. Which of the following would be the most likely appropriate change in her insulin regimen?
    A. Increase her morning regular insulin dose.
    B. Increase her bedtime NPH insulin dose.
    C. Increase her insulin doses at all times.
    D. Add a sliding scale of regular insulin to her morning dose.
    E. Add NPH insulin before breakfast.

After following your advice, her blood glucose levels are now near normal. Now her laboratory test results show normal electrolyte and creatinine values, normal routine urinalysis, but an elevated microalbumin-creatinine ratio on her urine (120 mg albumin per gram of creatinine) on two separate occasions. BP is normal at 120/70 mm Hg.

43. Which of the following would be most appropriate at this point?
    A. Start treatment with an ACE inhibitor.
    B. Watch BP closely and initiate treatment with an ACE inhibitor if BP reaches 130/85 mm Hg or higher.
    C. Start therapy with a calcium-channel blocker.
    D. Extensive search for this patient's cause of microalbuminuria is indicated before any therapy.
    E. No therapy is indicated at this point.

QUESTIONS 44–48

A 32-year-old man is referred to you because of a history of recurrent abdominal pain and DM of several years' duration. On examination his BMI is 24, and he has evidence of lipemia retinalis and eruptive xanthomas on his arms and thighs. There is no family history of diabetes; however, there is premature coronary artery disease. An ultrasonogram of the upper abdomen reveals no cholelithiasis and no biliary duct dilatation. He is not on any medications and drinks only one or two beers a month. His electrolyte profile is normal, including his calcium concentration.

44. Which is the most likely type of diabetes in this man?
    A. Mitochondrial DM
    B. Secondary diabetes
    C. DM type II
    D. Maturity-onset diabetes of the young
    E. Latent autoimmune diabetes of the adult

45. What is the most likely cause of this man's recurrent abdominal pain?
    A. Cholecystolithiasis
    B. Peptic ulcer disease
    C. Pancreatitis secondary to hypertriglyceridemia
    D. Kidney stones
    E. None of the above

46. Which of the following laboratory examination is/are needed?
    A. Fasting lipid profile
    B. Thyroid-stimulating hormone (TSH)
    C. Hgb A1c
    D. Liver function tests, creatinine, and a routine urinalysis
    E. All of the above

47. Which of the following is likely to be this patient's lipid profile?
    A. Total cholesterol, 250; high-density lipoprotein (HDL), 35; triglycerides, 150
    B. Total cholesterol, 260; HDL, 30; triglycerides, 1500
    C. Total cholesterol, 240; HDL, 32; triglycerides, 650
    D. Total cholesterol, 210; HDL, 40; triglycerides, 380

48. Which of the following interventions is indicated?
    A. Glycemic control
    B. Strict avoidance of alcohol
    C. Low-fat diet
    D. Treatment with a fibric acid derivative
    E. All of the above

49. A 54-year-old woman with a history of DM type II diagnosed 2 years ago comes to see you after being lost to follow-up for 1 year. The last time that you saw her you obtained several laboratory tests, which were normal, including electrolytes, creatinine, urinalysis, and a TSH. Her lipid profile showed a total cholesterol of 210 mg/dL and a triglyceride level of 300 mg/dL. Because her Hgb A1c was 8.5% you started her on a glipizide, 10 mg orally every day. You also started her on conjugated estrogens, 0.625 mg orally every day, because she had gone through menopause recently. Now her Hgb A1c is higher at 9.8%; the rest of her tests are again all normal, except her fasting lipid profile, which now shows a triglyceride level of 1300 mg/dL. Which of the following is the most likely cause for her hypertriglyceridemia?
    A. Familial combined dyslipidemia
    B. Sulfonylurea-induced hypertriglyceridemia
    C. Uncontrolled DM
    D. Oral estrogen therapy
    E. None of the above

50. A 58-year-old man with a history of coronary artery disease and dyslipidemia comes to see you for the first time. He has a positive family history of early coronary artery disease. On examination he is approximately 5′ 8″ tall and weighs 200 pounds. His BP is 148/94 mm Hg. There is also evidence of decreased pulses peripherally. His laboratory results show the following: fasting blood glucose, 145 mg/dL; total cholesterol, 210 mg/dL; triglycerides, 375 mg/dL; and uric acid, 10 mg/dL. Which of the following would best describe his problem?

    A. Familial combined hyperlipidemia
    B. Familial hypertriglyceridemia
    C. Impaired glucose tolerance
    D. DM type II
    E. None of the above

51. A 42-year-old businessman comes to see you for the first time. He gives you a history of a myocardial infarction. His examination shows a BP of 110/70 mm Hg; the examination is normal otherwise. He is currently taking atenolol, 50 mg orally twice daily, and one aspirin daily. His fasting lipid profile is as follows: total cholesterol, 210 mg/dL; triglycerides, 100 mg/dL; HDL, 40 mg/dL. He is already following a step II American Heart Association diet. Which of the following would be most appropriate at this point?

    A. Advise him to increase his level of physical activity to raise his HDL.
    B. Discontinue his β-blocker agent.
    C. Check his homocysteine level.
    D. Start therapy with a hydroxymethylglutaryl (HMG)-coenzyme A (CoA) reductase inhibitor to lower his low-density lipoprotein (LDL).
    E. None of the above.

52. By which of the following mechanisms does acarbose exert its therapeutic effect in the glycemic control of diabetics?

    A. Increases insulin production by beta cells
    B. Decreases glucagon production by alpha cells
    C. Inhibits the action of the intestinal enzyme α-glucosidase
    D. Inhibits the aldose reductase enzyme
    E. None of the above

53. In the treatment of diabetic ketoacidosis, which one of the following is *incorrect?*

    A. Hydration is one of the most important aspects of therapy.
    B. It is necessary to monitor the serum potassium levels closely.
    C. The administration of metformin is useful.
    D. The use of insulin is absolutely necessary.
    E. A careful search for a precipitating cause must be performed.

54. Which *one* of the following statements about DM type I is correct?

    A. Insulin resistance is the most important etiopathogenic mechanism.
    B. The presence of anti–glutamic acid decarboxylase (GAD) antibodies, anti–islet cell antibodies, and insulin autoantibodies is quite common.
    C. C peptide levels are most commonly elevated.
    D. Glimepiride is an effective treatment.
    E. The use of glucocorticoids is necessary to avoid ketoacidosis.

55. All of the following statements are appropriate therapeutic measures in painful peripheral diabetic polyneuropathy *except:*

A. Glycemic control
B. HMG-CoA reductase inhibitors
C. Carbamazepine
D. Tricyclic antidepressants
E. Gabapentin

56. All of the following statements about diabetic retinopathy are correct *except:*

    A. Good glycemic control reduces the risk of development and the progression of diabetic retinopathy in both type I and type II diabetics.
    B. Patients with DM type II need to be referred for dilated ophthalmoscopic evaluation yearly starting at the time of diagnosis of their diabetes.
    C. Patients with DM type I need to be referred for dilated ophthalmoscopic evaluation yearly starting at the time of diagnosis of their diabetes.
    D. BP control reduces the risk of and progression of diabetic eye complications.
    E. Diabetic eye disease is the most common cause of blindness in the United States.

57. All of the following are independent risk factors for a myocardial infarction in the diabetic patient *except:*

    A. Glycemic control
    B. Waist-hip ratio
    C. High HDL
    D. Smoking
    E. High LDL

QUESTIONS 58–67

58. All of the following statements are true regarding familial hypercholesterolemia *except:*

    A. Autosomal dominant inherited condition
    B. May cause tendon xanthomas
    C. Frequently associated with early coronary artery disease
    D. Is caused by a defective binding region of apo B
    E. Cholesterol levels 300 to 500 mg/dL are frequently seen in the heterozygous form.

59. A 33-year-old man presents to your clinic stating he has a cholesterol problem. He had a normal cholesterol profile 7 years ago, but last month was found to have both triglyceride and a total cholesterol level in the upper 10%. He is very concerned about his risk of heart disease because of his high cholesterol levels. The patient history is remarkable for a 50-pound weight gain over the past 7 years; otherwise it is unremarkable. Examination was remarkable for obesity, orange tinting in his palm creases, and tuboeruptive xanthomas on the extensor surface of both knees. Which of the following would be inappropriate for this patient?

    A. Order a TSH.
    B. Order liver transaminases.
    C. Recommended a step 2 diet and weight loss.
    D. Reassure the patient that his LDL cholesterol was normal and he has no increased cardiac risk.
    E. Consider treatment with an HMG Co A reductase inhibitor and/or a fibric acid derivative.

60. Which of the following statements is *false* regarding the hypertriglyceridemia seen in alcoholics?

    A. Increased intestinal production of chylomicrons
    B. Increased fatty acid synthesis by the liver
    C. Increased hepatic output of very low density lipoproteins (VLDL)
    D. Inhibition of lipoprotein lipase

61. All of the following statements are *true* regarding galactosemia *except:*

    A. The classic form is an autosomal recessive absence of galactose-1-phosphate uridyl transferase.
    B. It presents in newborns as jaundice, lethargy, and feeding intolerance.
    C. Following a lactose-free diet results in normal development.
    D. Uridine diphosphate-galactose-4-epimerase and galactokinase deficiency can present with less severe elevation of galactose.
    E. All are true.

62. A 22-year-old man presents to your office as a new patient referred by his pediatrician. The patient tells you he has a glycogen storage disease but he cannot remember any specifics. He has been experiencing bad muscle cramps when he walks his dog at night but does not report any symptoms that would be consistent with hypoglycemia. Examination is normal and as you stand to leave the room he tells you he occasionally has tea-colored urine. Based on this information he likely has a deficiency of which enzyme?

    A. Glucose-6-phosphatase
    B. Glycogen synthetase
    C. Acid α-glucosidase
    D. Myophosphorylase

63. A 10-month-old infant presents to your clinic for evaluation of recurrent infections. The parents report recurrent viral infections including chickenpox three times. The infant has missed many milestones and is hypotonic during your examination. When you review the records you notice a uric acid level of 1 mg/dL. You suspect a metabolic deficiency and order the following to confirm your diagnosis:

    A. Erythrocyte purine nucleoside phosphorylase activity
    B. Fat pad biopsy
    C. Varicella antibody titers
    D. Erythrocyte levels of hypoxanthine phosphoribosyltransferase (HPRT)
    E. All the above

64. A 15-year-old boy presents with the chief complaint of severe pain in his arms and legs (acroparesthesias). He describes a burning sensation that occurs after he works out at the gym and states he usually has profound weakness and a low-grade fever as well. He does not recall having this before but states he has been sedentary throughout his life and recently started going to the gym. He attributes these symptoms to overheating because he does not sweat much. On examination you note multiple angiokeratomas on his inner thigh and buttocks that vary in size and do not blanch with pressure. His ophthalmic examination is difficult because of the presence of bilateral corneal opacities. You suspect disease and would expect to find:

    A. An accumulation of sphingomyelin resulting in hepatosplenomegaly
    B. Mild neurologic dysfunction on a detailed neurologic examination
    C. An active urine sediment with red blood cells, casts, and lipid inclusion
    D. An infiltrating lung disease on high-resolution chest CT

65. A 33-year-old man with porphyria cutanea tarda presents to your office complaining of multiple skin lesions. He has been relatively disease free over the past 9 years after phlebotomy after his initial outbreak. Over the past few months he has developed numerous friable vesicles and bullae on his face, forearms, and the dorsa of his hands (identical to his diagnosis 9 years ago). Total plasma porphyrin levels were elevated from a blood sample drawn 1 week ago. Which of the following could have led to this relapse of his condition?

    A. Initiation of a daily multivitamin without iron
    B. Initiation of phenytoin for seizure therapy
    C. Initiation of one to two glasses of red wine daily for cardiac protection
    D. Initiation of a high-protein diet
    E. None of the above

66. A 20-year-old woman is brought to your office because her family feels something is wrong. She has developed a significant change in her personality and has alienated her close friends and sister. She is a sophomore in college and has gone from straight As and president of her freshman class to a D student currently suspended for verbally insulting a teacher. On examination you find an unpleasant woman who resents being in your office. Her examination is remarkable for hepatomegaly, and her eye examination reveals an annular greenish brown discoloration of her blue eyes. All of the following will help confirm your diagnosis *except:*

    A. Coombs-negative hemolytic anemia
    B. Elevated serum ceruloplasmin levels
    C. Low serum copper levels
    D. Increased urinary copper > 100 mg/24 hours
    E. Hepatic copper levels > 200 mg/g on biopsy

67. A 43-year-old man is referred to you for evaluation of fatigue and lower extremity edema. His history is remarkable for fatigue, lethargy, and loss of libido. Examination reveals a healthy blonde-haired blue-eyed, tan individual in no acute distress. His vital signs revealed tachycardia but otherwise were unremarkable. Pertinent findings on examination included scant rales, 2+ pitting edema of the lower extremities, and hepatosplenomegaly. You suspect hemochromatosis and would expect which of the following laboratory data?

	Transferrin Saturation (%)	Ferritin (ng/dL)
A.	35	120
B.	40	200
C.	80	300
D.	80	600

MATCHING

Each answer can be selected more than once or not at all. If more than one answer is correct, select all the correct answers for each question.

    A. Asparte insulin
    B. Regular insulin
    C. NPH insulin
    D. Glargine insulin
    E. All the above
    F. None of the above

68. Has onset of action within 10 to 20 minutes.

69. Should not be mixed (within a syringe) with any other insulin.

70. Has a peak of action within 2 to 4 hours.

71. May require snacking to prevent hypoglycemia.

72. Peakless activity.

73. Works within 5 to 8 minutes when given IV.

Match the triglyceride disorder to the causal defect protein or enzyme.

    A. Hyperlipoproteinemia (type 1)
    B. Mixed hypertriglyceridemia (type V)
    C. Familial dysbetalipoproteinemia (type III)
    D. Familial hypertriglyceridemia (type IV)
    E. None of the above

74. Apolipoprotein C II

75. Apolipoprotein E

76. Lipoprotein lipase deficiency

77. Apolipoprotein B 100

Match the disorder to the predominant plasma lipid.

    A. Hyperlipoproteinemia (type 1)
    B. Mixed hypertriglyceridemia (type V)
    C. Familial dysbetalipoproteinemia (type III)
    D. Familial hypertriglyceridemia (type IV)
    E. None of the above

78. Remnants (β-VLDL)

79. Chylomicrons

80. Chylomicrons and VLDL

81. VLDL

DIRECTIONS: Questions 82-111 are matching questions. For each numbered item, choose the most likely associated lettered item from those provided. Each numbered item has only one answer. Within each set of questions, each answer may be used once, more than once, or not at all.

QUESTIONS 82–86

For each of the following patients, select the most likely diagnosis.

    A. Lipoprotein lipase deficiency
    B. Familial hyperalphalipoproteinemia
    C. Dysbetalipoproteinemia
    D. Familial combined hyperlipidemia
    E. Familial hypercholesterolemia

82. A 90-year-old healthy man. His total cholesterol is 240 mg/dL, triglyceride level is 125 mg/dL, and HDL is 90 mg/dL.

83. A 40-year-old man with premature coronary artery disease. His total cholesterol is 340 mg/dL, and his triglyceride level 400 mg/dL. His examination shows evidence of palmar xanthomas.

84. A 58-year-old woman with premature coronary artery disease. Her total cholesterol is 360 mg/dL, and her triglyceride level is 450 mg/dL.

85. A 15-year-old boy with a triglyceride level of 4000 mg/dL and a total cholesterol level of 340 mg/dL. His examination shows evidence of eruptive xanthomas.

86. A 30-year-old man with a family history of premature coronary artery disease. His total cholesterol is 455 mg/dL, his HDL cholesterol is 40 mg/dL, and his triglyceride level is 325 mg/dL. His examination shows bilateral arcus senilis and tendon xanthomas.

QUESTIONS 87–91

For each of the following patients, select the most likely diagnosis.

    A. Inadvertent sulfonylurea administration
    B. Hypoglycemia unawareness
    C. Insulinoma
    D. Hypoglycemia secondary to renal failure
    E. Factitious hypoglycemia

87. A 26-year-old man has frequent episodes of hypoglycemia when fasting. There is documented venous plasma glucose levels of 35 mg/dL. Two first-degree relatives have been told they have high calcium levels.

88. A 47-year-old female nurse with a history of depression now presents with symptoms consistent with hypoglycemic episodes that happen at random. In your office she has a spell, and you document a venous plasma glucose level of 40 mg/dL, which resolves after drinking a cup of sweetened orange juice.

89. A 72-year-old woman with a history of hypertension but who is otherwise healthy is brought to the emergency department because of altered state of consciousness and is found to have a venous plasma glucose of 30 mg/dL. Her episode resolves after an IV infusion of 50% dextrose. Her other routine laboratory examinations were normal. She returns 2 days later with the same problem. Her husband is a type II diabetic.

90. A 23-year-old female college student has had DM type I since age 10. Her glycemic control is excellent and her last Hgb A1c was 5.8% (normal range, 4-6%). However, she was recently involved in an automobile accident while driving. She does not remember what happened before the accident.

91. A 67-year-old man with a history of poorly controlled DM type II for more than 20 years already has evidence of proliferative diabetic retinopathy and 3+ protein in his urine. Most recently, however, without change in therapy, his blood glucose concentration has been near normal and he has even had two episodes of severe hypoglycemia.

QUESTIONS 92–97

For the following physical examination findings, select the most likely elevated lipoprotein.

    A. HDL
    B. LDL
    C. Chylomicrons
    D. β-VLDL (intermediate-density lipoprotein)
    E. Nonspecific finding

92. Eruptive xanthomas

93. Lipemia retinalis

94. Arcus senilis

95. Tendon xanthomas

96. Palmar xanthomas

97. Xanthelasma

TRUE OR FALSE

DIRECTIONS: For questions 98-111, decide whether each choice is true or false. Any combination of answers, from all true to all false, may occur.

QUESTIONS 98–103

Are the following statements about pregnancy in diabetes true or false?

98. Poor glycemic control at conception is associated with a high incidence of congenital malformations.

99. Macrosomia is the most common neonatal abnormality in diabetic pregnancy.

100. All infants of diabetic mothers need to be carefully monitored for hypoglycemia during the first hours and/or days of life.

101. Gestational DM does not increase the risk of type II diabetes later in life.

102. Gestational DM is more common in whites.

103. Gestational DM occurs in about 20% of all pregnancies.

QUESTIONS 104–111

Are the following statements about diabetic ketoacidosis true or false?

104. Diabetic ketoacidosis is diagnostic of type I diabetes.

105. Abdominal pain may mimic that of surgical emergencies.

106. Death from diabetic ketoacidosis is now only rarely seen.

107. Serum ketones may remain positive after resolution of acidosis.

108. Obtundation and the presence of focal neurologic signs are characteristic features of diabetic ketoacidosis.

109. Resumption of subcutaneous insulin injection therapy should be done at least 1 or 2 hours before stopping IV insulin infusion.

110. Potassium replacement therapy should be started only when a low serum potassium level has been obtained.

111. The most appropriate action when plasma glucose falls below 250 mg/dL, despite persistent acidosis, is to lower the rate of insulin infusion.

Part XI
Diabetes Mellitus and Metabolism
Answers

1. (**E**); 2. (**A**); 3. (**B**); 4. (**D**). *Discussion:* Fasting plasma glucose is the only correct test listed to diagnose the metabolic syndrome by the NCEP ATP III guidelines. To make the diagnosis a patient must have three of the following: abdominal obesity: waist circumference more than 35 inches in females or more than 40 inches in males; triglycerides 150 mg/dL or more, HDL less than 50 mg/dL in females or less than 40 mg/dL in males; BP 130/85 mm Hg or higher; or fasting plasma glucose 110 mg/dL (IFG) or more. This patient has two criteria on his physical examination with both an elevation of his BP and a waist circumference of 46 inches. Either the fasting lipid profile or glucose values should be used for the third criterion. A 2-hour glucose tolerance test can be used to diagnose impaired glucose tolerance (IGT) if the blood glucose concentration is 140-199 mg/dL 2 hours after challenge. This would be part of the World Health Organization criteria for metabolic syndrome, which includes the following: diagnosis of IGT or IFG with at least two of the following: waist-hip ratio greater than 0.85 for females or greater than 0.9 in males and/or a body mass index (BMI) greater than 30 kg/m², triglycerides 150 mg/dL or higher and/or HDL cholesterol less than 35 mg/dL for males or less than 40 mg/dL females, and BP 140/90 mm Hg or higher or microalbuminuria with albumin excretion rate greater than or equal to 20 μg/minute or albumin/creatinine ratio greater than 30 mg/g. A random glucose value has no role to diagnose metabolic syndrome, but is diagnostic of diabetes if greater than 200 mg/dL if symptoms of diabetes are present (i.e., polyuria, polydipsia) (Diabetes Care 2002;25[Suppl 1]:s22). Hbg A1c and creatinine clearance have no role in the diagnosis of the metabolic syndrome.

Clinical trials have clearly shown that treatment of dyslipidemia reduces the risk of atherosclerotic heart disease in patients with average to modestly elevated cholesterol. The ATP III guidelines recommend lipid profile evaluation at age 18 to 20 of all patients with family history of diabetes or obese patients and, if the results are normal, rescreen every 5 years. Treatment is based on a (risk factor weighted) calculated risk of a coronary event over the next 10 years, and treatment targets are stratified over the range from 5-20%. The patient has the following risk factors: age older than 45, hypertension, and family history (event in father before age 55 years old). Using a risk factor calculator without knowing his lipid profile his risk factors attribute a risk between 15 and 20% (www.nhibi.nih.gov/guidelines/cholesterol/atp_iii). A β-blocker will not reduce his cardiac risk of atherosclerosis and is indicated in patients with known coronary disease. Both Lp(a) and C-reactive protein are emerging risk factors for atherosclerotic disease, but it is unclear at this time if these are just markers of disease risk or if targeted intervention will lower cardiac risk. Coronary angiography is clearly not indicated in this patient.

This patient has the metabolic syndrome after laboratory testing was performed. His fasting glucose was 120 mg/dL, and his lipid profile demonstrated an HDL of 33 mg/dL. The JNC VII has very loose recommendations for patients with the metabolic syndrome. The majority of endocrinologist and cardiologist will treat the BP to diabetic targets. There is a direct relationship between BP and risk of cardiovascular disease and the higher the BP, the greater the chance of myocardial infarction, heart failure, stroke, and kidney disease. In patients aged 40 to 70 years, for every 20 mm Hg in systolic BP or 10 mm Hg in diastolic BP above 115/75 mm Hg, the risk of atherosclerotic coronary disease doubles. Treating systolic BP and diastolic BP to target is associated with a reduction of atherosclerotic complications. In diabetic patients the BP target is less than 130/80 mm Hg. The JNC VII recommends intensive lifestyle modification in all individuals with the metabolic syndrome and drug therapy for treatment of any of the abnormalities associated with the diagnosis inferring a blood pressure goal of less than 135/85 mm Hg.

Many studies are underway to evaluate the role of antidiabetic agents to prevent the progression of impaired glucose metabolism into DM type II. For this patient the best evidence is from the Diabetes Prevention Program (DPP), which found a significant risk reduction of developing diabetes among obese individuals with impaired glucose tolerance. The group with intensive lifestyle intervention of both a reduced calorie diet and exercise resulted in a reduction of diabetes progression of 58% compared with controls. Metformin was also used in an intervention arm and only reduced the progression of diabetes by 31%. Thiazolidinediones will likely show impressive results preventing the progression of diabetes based on the outcome of a study with troglitazone (now off the market). This study, the TRIPOD study, demonstrated a reduction of diabetes and beta cell failure in high-risk Hispanic women with a prior history of gestational diabetes. A 2500-calorie diet will not result in weight loss in this individual. Sulfonylurea therapy would place the patient at significant risk of hypoglycemia and would not delay progressive beta cell failure. Until the current trials are complete with the newer thiazolidinediones, the best evidence is for intensive lifestyle intervention. (*Alberti, 1998; American Diabetes Association, 2002; Buchannan, 2002; N Engl J Med 2002; 346:393-403*)

5. (**E**); 6. (**C**); 7 (**B**); 8. (**D**); 9. (**C**); 10. (**E**). *Discussion:* Based on the evidence from the VA Hit Trial (a secondary prevention trial including patients with diabetes, nonelevated LDL cholesterol, and low HDL cholesterol), addition of gemfibrozil reduced coronary heart disease death, nonfatal MI, or stroke by 24% in diabetic patients. The CARE study showed no benefit of lowering the LDL cholesterol below 120 to 125 mg/dL in secondary prevention and therefore a statin medication is not the best choice. Step 1 diet would be beneficial and would improve the cholesterol profile but would not likely decrease the risk of a cardiac events in patients with diabetes (Diabet Med 2000;17:518-523). Niacin would improve the lipid profile; however, the evidence is not as strong as that seen with gemfibrozil regarding cardiovascular outcomes and may worsen glycemic control by increasing insulin resistance.

The only reason to treat a patient with estrogen therapy is for symptoms of vasomotor instability or other symptoms of estrogen deficiency. Based on recent outcome studies, estrogen is not indicated for treatment of abnormal lipid profiles nor as secondary prevention of cardiovascular events. Studies have shown an increase in event rates in the first year that trends down over the next few years and may offer protection after years 5 to 7 of therapy. The role of hormone replacement for primary prevention remains controversial. Estrogen therapy can improve metabolism rates and prevent bone loss (especially if given early in menopause). Hormone replacement must be individualized based on the hormone-deficient symptoms and the patient's risk factors for potential complications of hormone therapy (e.g., thrombotic events, breast cancer).

The triglycerides are elevated because of increased production of VLDL cholesterol by the liver and dietary production of chylomicrons complicated by a decreased clearance by lipoprotein lipase. Lipoprotein lipase mediates hydrolysis of triglycerides carried by VLDL and chylomicrons and produces free fatty acids that are used as fuel and/or stored in adipose and muscle tissue. Lipoprotein lipase activity is decreased in patients with poorly controlled DM, which frequently results in an elevation of triglycerides. Hepatic lipase is a phospholipase and triglyceride hydrolase primarily found on hepatic endothelial cells. It is involved in the final processing of chylomicron remnants, IDL and LDL. It also removes triglyceride and phospholipid from HDL2, which results in the dense, less protective HDL3. Its activity is increased in patients with diabetes. Lecithin:cholestrol acyltransferase circulates in the plasma associated with HDL and functions to esterify free cholesterol; deficiency of this protein results in low levels of both cholesterol esters and HDL and cannot account for the elevated triglycerides. Cholesteryl ester transfer protein facilitates cholesterol ester transfer from HDL to VLDL and IDL. Deficiency results in elevated HDL (not triglycerides) and may be protective against atherosclerotic disease.

Absolute contraindications to metformin therapy include elevated creatinine (Cr > 1.5 mg/mL in males or > 1.4 mg/mL in females), congestive heart failure, metabolic acidosis, intravenous contrast, and hypoxia. Age older than 80 years is not an absolute contraindication to metformin therapy but should be used cautiously with close monitoring and verification of creatinine clearance. The key to this question is to understand the prescription guidelines with metformin. Either rosiglitazone or pioglitazone would be acceptable insulin sensitizers in a patient with renal impairment. The patient should have her antidiabetic regimen increased to reach an Hbg A1c goal of less than 6.5% and fasting blood sugars between 100 and 120 mg/dL. The patient should be followed closely for any change of her creatinine, and if it improves she may resume therapy with metformin. This patient had been hiking in the mountains over the weekend and had a mild degree of dehydration when these laboratory studies were performed. Her follow-up creatinine was 1.2 mg/dL, and she was restarted on metformin therapy. Increasing the glipizide will not result in any improvement of glycemic control.

The patient only has a modest elevation of her albumin/creatinine ratio, which correlates well to excretion of albumin of more than 30 mg/day. The patient's elevation is very mild and should be confirmed on two other occasions (three total) over 3 to 6 months. Other conditions such as hyperglycemia, hypertension, congestive heart failure, urinary tract infections, and exercise can cause transitory microalbuminuria. This patient's albumin/creatinine ratio was 5.5 mg/g 1 month later. She had recently returned from a hiking trip, and the albuminuria was likely caused by the exercise from her trip 16 hours earlier. If the microalbuminuria persisted, an angiotensin-converting enzyme inhibitor (ACE-I) or angiotensin receptor blocker would be indicated. Increasing the patient's β-blocker may improve the albuminuria by lowering the blood pres-

sure but could put the patient at risk of severe bradycardia. The 24-hour urine would likely be negative and would provide useful information but is not the best screening test for microalbuminuria. The patient's blood pressure is at goal and would not merit an additional agent. Strong consideration to switch from a β-blocker to an ACE-I should occur.

Macrocytic anemia can be seen in patients with vitamin B12 deficiency. The elevation of the mean corpuscular volume (MCV) and her history do not suggest iron deficiency. The patient's renal function is normal, and therefore her anemia is unlikely to be caused by renal failure and deficient erythropoietin production. Metformin therapy of long duration and in older patients can result in vitamin B12 deficiency, although it is rarely of clinical relevance. This should be evaluated in addition to an iron profile because deficiency of both could coexist. (*Frank, 1993; Kirpichnikov, 2002; Manley, 2000*)

11. (B) *Discussion:* The risk is highest between first-degree relatives. The American Diabetes Association Committee Report 2002 recommends screening for diabetes in all individuals older than 45 years of age every 3 years. Patients with any of the other risk factors listed earlier or with dyslipidemia with HDL less than 35 mg/dL, triglycerides greater than 250 mg/dL, impaired glucose tolerance or impaired fasting glucose, or of a high-risk racial background (blacks, Hispanics, Native Americans, Asians, and Pacific Islanders) should be screened at a younger age and with greater frequency. (*American Diabetes Association, 2002*)

12. (E) *Discussion:* Fasting plasma glucose concentration greater than or equal to 126 mg/dL is the favored criteria to diagnosis diabetes. Random plasma glucose with symptoms of diabetes including polyuria, polydipsia, and weight loss and a 2-hour glucose tolerance test greater than 200 mg/dL can be used to diagnosis DM. A serum glucose value of 126 mg/dL suggests glucose intolerance and should be followed up with a fasting glucose value. A 2-hour glucose tolerance test value between 140 and 199 mg/dL is impaired glucose tolerance and lifestyle intervention, and modification of other risk factors should occur. (*American Diabetes Association, 2002*)

13. (D) *Discussion:* The risk of type I diabetes in the offspring of a mother with type I is 3% as a lifetime risk. The risk is 8% when the father has type I. The general population risk is 0.4% risk. The patient should be told that her child has a much higher risk than the general population, but the overall lifelong risk is very low and that he has a 97% chance of not having diabetes (NEJM 1994;331:1428-1436).

14. (A) *Discussion:* The patient's plasma glucose and home glucose monitoring correspond and suggest that the Hbg A1c value is artifactually low. The key is to determine if the patient has any underlying medical problems or medications that can lower this value. In this age group, chronic or acute blood loss will decrease the life of the erythrocyte, which will lower the Hbg A1c; therefore, a CBC or hematocrit would be the best initial step. Other conditions that artifactually lower the Hbg A1c are as follows: blood transfusion, pregnancy or childbirth, high doses of vitamin C or E (>1 g/day), hemoglobinopathies (not seen with HPLC analyzer), fetal hemoglobin (seen with immunodetection analyzer), and dapsone. A new meter would help if the laboratory glucose value is different from the home glucose monitoring. A fructosamine could be used to monitor the glucose control over a 2- to 3-week period, but ruling out anemia and determining the cause for the discrepancy should be done first. (*Albright, 2002*)

15. (D) *Discussion:* This patient was found to have a spontaneous diabetic muscle infarct, which is a rare complication of diabetes. The diagnosis can be made with classic clinical presentation, including an abrupt onset of pain in the affected muscle(s) with swelling. Most cases have been reported in the thigh, with the second most reported in the calf muscles. No specific laboratory marker is useful at this time and may delay diagnosis. An increased signal intensity on a T2-weighted MRI is diagnostic and can exclude other conditions within the differential diagnosis. Antibiotics and blood culture are not indicated for this diagnosis because the patient does not have any symptoms consistent with an acute bacterial infection. Most infarcts resolve within 4 weeks, and treatment is based on patient symptoms, but glycemic control is recommended. The prognosis for the muscle infarct is good, but the majority of the patients have microvascular complications of diabetes. Biopsy should be reserved for patients with atypical presentations. (*Trujillo-Santos, 2003*)

16. **(A)** *Discussion:* The UKPDS was the largest longest outcome study ever performed in type II diabetic patients evaluating various end points. All complications of diabetes demonstrated a risk reduction with lowering of the Hbg A1c. Each 1% reduction in Hbg A1c reduced microvascular outcomes 37%, any diabetic complication 21%, death related to diabetes 27%, and myocardial infarction 14%. The greatest benefit was found at or below an Hbg A1c of 7% with no threshold to the risk reduction. (*Stratton, 2000*)

17. **(B)**; 18. **(B)**; 19. **(A)**. *Discussion:* This patient has a 30% chance of progression to end-stage renal disease. Diabetic nephropathy usually occurs 7 to 10 years after the diagnosis of diabetes and elevated blood pressure has a significant role in the progression. Blood pressure targets of less than 130/80 mm Hg will slow the progression of renal insufficiency and the optimal combination of agents should include either an ACE-I or angiotensin receptor blocker. Because microalbuminuria is a cardiovascular risk marker, the patient should be questioned closely for any symptoms and the physician should have a low threshold for cardiac evaluation (*Cecil, Ch. 242; Lasaridis, 2003*)

20. **(D)**; 21. **(C)**; 22. **(B)**. *Discussion:* Insulin drip in the setting of an acute myocardial infarction has shown significant benefits in both DM type I and DM type II patients. The DIGAMI (Diabetes Insulin Glucose Infusion in Acute Myocardial Infarction) demonstrated a 28% mortality reduction when patients were treated initially with an insulin and glucose infusion followed by intensive therapy with insulin over 1 year. Supplying insulin during a myocardial infarction decreases free fatty acid release and increases glucose uptake and ATP generation, which restores calcium hemostasis, which is believed to improve recovery of hibernating or stunned tissue. Oral medication should be discontinued because the glipizide results in unpredictable insulin release and the metformin could accumulate and result in lactic acidosis, especially if the patient has any contrast procedure with underlying renal dysfunction. Sliding scale insulin is dangerous and rarely results in blood glucose control.

The patient's blood sugar is not controlled on triple oral therapy and will likely not be controlled with additional titration or addition of oral medications. Based on the poor glucose control alone the patient should be started on insulin, and with an elevation of the Hbg A1c greater than 9.0%, it has been our clinical experience that multiple daily injections of insulin are required to achieve control. Switching to rosiglitazone will not change blood glucose control, and the addition of acarbose and discontinuation of glipizide XL may worsen control. Continuation of the insulin sensitizers will reduce the amount of insulin required to achieve control as well as provide additional cardiovascular risk reduction benefits. Metformin will also minimize or prevent the weight gain often seen with insulin therapy. Additional support to continue insulin therapy is from the DIGAMI study because mortality reduction was only seen after 1 year of multiple insulin injections.

The best choice is to stop the pioglitazone and metformin. Both drugs are contraindicated in patients with symptomatic congestive heart failure (NYHC III or IV or patients who require medical therapy for CHF). The addition of furosemide (Lasix) would improve the patient's symptoms, but the first intervention is to remove medications that could result in possible harm. An angiogram is indicated to determine the degree of coronary artery disease and if any intervention is required at this time. (*Cecil, Ch. 242; Davies, 2003; Khoury, 2003; Parulkar, 2001; PDR 2002; Yki-Jarvinen, 1999*)

23. **(D)** *Discussion:* Following a glucose load in a fed state, insulin is released to suppress endogenous glucose production (gluconeogenesis), stimulates hepatic glucose uptake, and accelerates glucose uptake by peripheral tissues, predominantly muscle. It does not increase glucagon release. Glucagon counteracts many of the insulin actions and stimulates gluconeogenesis and glycogenolysis. (*Cecil, Ch. 242*)

24. **(B)**; 25. **(B)**; 26. **(B)**; 27. **(D)**; 28. **(A)**. *Discussion:* The diagnosis of DM is usually straightforward when the patient presents with classic symptoms, as this patient did, and a random plasma glucose of 200 mg/dL or greater. The fact that this patient is 40 years old and obese, with an insidious presentation and symptomatic evidence of a chronic complication of diabetes, points to the diagnosis of DM type II rather than DM type I.

Symptomatic, potentially disabling neuropathy affects nearly 50% of diabetic patients. Diabetic neuropathy is commonly present in patients with diabetes at the time of diagnosis of glucose intolerance. The clinical presentation of diabetic neuropathy can be quite varied, depending on the type of neuropathy and the specific nerves affected. It may be completely asymptomatic or may cause dysesthesias, paresthesias, hypoesthesia, or hyperesthesia; allodynia; burning; tingling; "pins and needles"; "electric shock-like sensations"; superficial or deep pain; muscle weakness or cramps; and so on.

Diabetic damage usually affects sensory more than motor fibers and usually encompasses small (pain and temperature) and large (position and touch) sensory fibers. Sometimes small-fiber dysfunction occurs early and may precede objective physical signs or electrophysiologic evidence of large-fiber deficit, as in this case. Sometimes subtle deficits may be detected by testing thermal discrimination or vibratory sense thresholds or by performing nerve conduction studies.

Because the clinical picture of diabetic peripheral neuropathy is not distinguishable from other forms of distal neuropathy (e.g., alcohol, heavy metals, uremia, and amyloidosis), the diagnosis is one of exclusion.

Intensive blood glucose control with achievement of near-normal glycemia has been proved to prevent, delay, and/or stop the progression of peripheral diabetic neuropathy. The other medications listed here are not indicated because this patient has no pain. (*Cecil, Ch. 242; DCCT Research Group, 1993; Dejgaard, 1998*)

29. **(A)**; 30. **(D)**; 31. **(C)**; 32. **(D)**; 33. **(B)**. *Discussion:* With the information provided, stating that this is a young patient, with symptoms of diabetes and a plasma glucose of 230 mg/dL, the most likely diagnosis is DM type I. However, its relatively insidious onset, negative ketonuria, negative history of diabetic ketoacidosis, as well as the patient's BMI of 30 is somewhat unusual.

A history of diabetic ketoacidosis, a family history of thyroid disease, or a family history of DM type I in the father should strengthen suspicion of DM type I. Alternatively, a family history of DM in multiple family members, in an autosomal-dominant pattern, would make one think of some other types of DM that are transmitted in this manner.

Maturity-onset diabetes of the young is a specific type of diabetes in which there is a monogenic defect in beta cell function.

This form of diabetes is frequently characterized by an onset of hyperglycemia at an early age (generally before 25 years). It is also characterized by impaired insulin secretion with minimal or no defects in insulin action. These patients show characteristics similar to those of type II diabetics, although their age at onset may confuse the diagnosis with DM type I.

Maturity-onset diabetes of the young is a specific type of diabetes in which there is a monogenic defect leading to beta cell dysfunction. All of the gene mutations found to date are expressed in the pancreatic beta cell. This type of diabetes is inherited in an autosomal-dominant pattern. Abnormalities on at least six different genes have been found: one encodes for the glycolytic enzyme glucokinase and the others encode for transcription factors. The most common form is associated with mutations on chromosome 12, which codes for a hepatic transcription factor referred to as hepatocyte nuclear factor-1α.

This type of diabetes is characterized by impaired insulin secretion with minimal or no defects in insulin action; thus, oral hypoglycemics are an appropriate choice for therapy. When these agents fail, insulin therapy is indicated. Given the insidious onset of this type of diabetes and the uncertainty of the time of onset, it is appropriate to refer these patients for retinopathy screening at their diagnosis. In contrast, for type I diabetics, in whom the time of onset is well known, referral for retinopathy screening can be deferred for 3 to 5 years. Because this is an autosomal-dominant disorder, the likelihood of diabetes developing in this patient's children is approximately 50%. The C peptide is likely to be detectable in this patient. (*Cecil, Ch. 242; Expert Committee on the Diagnosis and Classification of Diabetes Mellitus, 1999; Wilson and Foster, 1998*)

34. (D); 35. (D); 36. (B). *Discussion:* Patients practicing conventional therapy suffer an average of one episode of symptomatic hypoglycemia per week. Those practicing intensive therapy, like this patient, suffer an average of two such episodes per week. It is also known that about 25% of those practicing intensive therapy suffer at least one episode of severe temporarily disabling hypoglycemia, often with seizure or coma in a given year. Some patients with DM type I, typically those with relatively long-standing disease, lose their neurogenic symptom response to hypoglycemia. In the absence of those warning symptoms, they fail to recognize developing hypoglycemia and, therefore, do not act to prevent development of severe hypoglycemia and its resultant side effects.

There is now considerable evidence in the literature suggesting that the clinical syndrome of hypoglycemia unawareness is reversible. As little as 2 weeks of scrupulous avoidance of iatrogenic hypoglycemia increases symptomatic responses to hypoglycemia.

Although the exact mechanism of hypoglycemia unawareness is not known, it is associated with a reduced plasma epinephrine response to experimental hypoglycemia. It is also associated with the syndrome of defective glucose counter-regulation, especially in those patients with long-standing diabetes. These patients have a decreased glucagon response as well as decreased epinephrine response to hypoglycemia. There is also evidence that strict avoidance of iatrogenic hypoglycemia increases the epinephrine responses to hypoglycemia and perhaps even that of glucagon. (*Cryer, 1997*)

37. (D); 38. (D); 39. (C). *Discussion:* DM type I is an autoimmune disorder. Susceptibility to DM type I appears to be linked to certain human leukocyte antigen alleles. Therefore, type I diabetics have a higher incidence of other autoimmune disorders, including autoimmune thyroid disease, Addison's disease, and others. In the described case, fatigue and weight loss could potentially be due to uncontrolled diabetes but adrenal insufficiency and hyperthyroidism should be considered in the differential diagnosis. The

finding of euthyroid goiter most likely represents Hashimoto's thyroiditis in patients in the United States. The orthostatic hypotension noted in this patient should lead one to consider that the patient might be volume depleted either from uncontrolled diabetes or potentially because of hypoaldosteronism from Addison's disease.

This patient's Hgb A1c and blood glucose records prove that her symptoms are not from hyperglycemia. Given that she is now experiencing frequent episodes of hypoglycemia, without having made changes in her therapy, the diagnosis of adrenal insufficiency should be at the top of the differential. A short Cortrosyn stimulation test would be the most appropriate way to prove or exclude this diagnosis. An electrolyte profile would also help by ruling out the possibility of hyponatremia or hyperkalemia frequently seen with Addison's disease. A TSH is also indicated given that this patient has a goiter and other autoimmune disorders.

This patient's Cortrosyn stimulation test is abnormal (60-minute cortisol < 20 ng/dL) and confirms the clinical suspicion of Addison's disease. Given that she now has two known endocrine autoimmune disorders, the diagnosis of autoimmune polyglandular syndrome can be made. The usual manifestations of this syndrome are Addison's disease, autoimmune thyroid disease, and DM type I. Only two of these three diagnoses need to be present to confirm the diagnosis of this syndrome. Addison's disease and hypothyroidism together are designated Schmidt's syndrome. Many other autoimmune disorders may associate with this autoimmune polyglandular syndrome type 2, including vitiligo, pernicious anemia (which is what this patient most likely has), alopecia, primary hypogonadism, celiac disease, and others. In general, when you discover one autoimmune endocrinopathy, it might be wise to screen for other potentially associated endocrine and nonendocrine organ-specific autoimmunities. (*Wilson and Foster, 1998*)

40. (D); 41. (C); 42. (B); 43. (A). *Discussion:* The Diabetes Control and Complications Trial, published in 1993, proved the value of achieving near-normal glycemia in type I diabetics. It proved that near-normal glycemia does prevent or delay the development of microvascular complications of diabetes, including retinopathy, nephropathy, and neuropathy. ACE inhibitor therapy has also proved to be of benefit in preserving renal function in type I diabetic patients who already have some evidence of renal involvement. However, in the described patient, we do not have evidence of renal impairment.

A single injection of insulin per day is almost never appropriate in the treatment of the type I diabetic patient except in very unusual circumstances. These patients usually require at least two, if not three or four, injections daily to achieve appropriate blood glucose control. The total daily insulin requirements of a type I diabetic are usually between 0.4 and 0.7 U/kg/day. In this case, it would be approximately 32 U of insulin per day (0.5 U/kg/day). The use of a sliding scale of regular insulin without any long-acting insulin usually is not appropriate, especially in a type I diabetic patient. The use of regular insulin at bedtime should also be discouraged.

This patient's blood glucose records are quite good, except in the morning fasting state. The usual target for capillary blood glucose at home is less than 120 mg/dL before meals and less than 140 mg/dL at bedtime. There are three possible explanations for a diabetic patient to show a pattern of fasting hyperglycemia like this patient: (1) the Somogyi phenomenon, (2) the dawn phenomenon, and (3) simple waning of previously injected insulin/inadequate night-time dosing. The Somogyi phenomenon represents a rebound/post-hypoglycemic hyperglycemia that occurs in the morning after an episode of night-time hypoglycemia as a result of activation of the counter-regulatory systems. The dawn phenomenon refers to the frequently observed, early morning increases in plasma glucose concentrations, which are seen without antecedent hypoglycemia in patients with DM. This has been linked to the early-morning rise of growth hormone levels. Clinically, it is important to distinguish between the Somogyi phenomenon, the dawn phenomenon, and simple waning of previously injected insulin as a cause for early-morning hyperglycemia because treatment differs. Management of the dawn phenomenon and insulin waning, as in this case, generally consists of adjusting the evening dose of intermediate-acting insulin or long-acting insulin to provide additional coverage between 4:00 and 7:00 am. Management of the Somogyi phenomenon consists of reducing insulin doses or providing additional late-evening carbohydrate (or both) to avoid hypoglycemia or placing the patient on glargine insulin, which is peakless and has 25% fewer nocturnal hypoglycemic events compared with NPH. The only way to determine the cause of these hyperglycemic episodes is to have the patient check a 3:00 to 4:00 am blood sugar on two to three separate occasions.

Microalbuminuria is known to predict the development of overt nephropathy and ultimately renal failure in diabetic patients. For patients with DM type I and microalbuminuria, even when BP is normal, ACE inhibitors have been clearly shown to slow the progression of nephropathy. (*Cecil, Ch. 242; Cooper, 1998; Cryer and Gerich, 1985; DCCT Research Group, 1993; Isselbacher et al, 1998; Rosenstalk, 2000*)

44. (B); 45. (C); 46. (E); 47. (B); 48. (E). *Discussion:* Although in a patient this young and thin, DM type I should be included in the differential diagnosis, any clues for other less common causes of diabetes need to be carefully considered during history taking. In this case, there are several, including the physical findings reflecting hyperchylomicronemia and recurrent abdominal pain.

This patient's history of recurrent abdominal pain associated with DM and evidence of lipemia retinalis and eruptive xanthomas (which are physical manifestations of severe hypertriglyceridemia) should point to the diagnosis of pancreatitis secondary to hypertriglyceridemia.

The first step in managing a patient with hyperlipidemia is to confirm the diagnosis by a repeat measurement of lipids in the fasting state. It is also important to exclude secondary causes of dyslipidemia, including hypothyroidism, DM, nephrotic syndrome, renal failure, and other less common disorders.

Patients in whom pancreatitis develops secondary to hypertriglyceridemia and those who have evidence of lipemia retinalis or eruptive xanthomas on physical examination usually have triglyceride levels greater than 1000 mg/dL.

Dietary treatment remains the cornerstone treatment in the management of hyperlipidemia because a major cause of hypertriglyceridemia is an accumulation of dietary-induced fat. The treatment is the absolute elimination of fat from the diet until triglyceride levels have fallen to a safe level. In a diabetic, glycemic control always helps as well although by itself usually is not enough when the triglyceride level is greater than 400 mg/dL. The largest reductions in triglyceride concentrations are usually achieved by nicotinic acid or a fibric acid derivative like gemfibrozil. However, nicotinic acid can induce or worsen hyperglycemia, so in this case fibric acid therapy is more appropriate. Alcohol should also be avoided because it increases triglyceride level. (*Cecil, Chs. 191, 206, and 242; Gotto and Pownall, 1992; Wilson and Foster, 1998*)

49. (D) *Discussion:* In this patient in whom there has been a considerable change in triglyceride levels, from mildly elevated to greater than 1000 mg/dL, which can be life threatening, a search for a secondary cause for her dyslipidemia should be performed. Uncontrolled diabetes can be associated in increases of triglyceride concentration but usually to no more than 400 mg/dL. Certain drugs can cause elevations in triglyceride levels, including thi-

azides, β-blockers, and estrogens. In most women receiving estrogen-containing oral contraceptive steroids, some increase in plasma triglycerides and VLDL levels occurs, although usually this increase is mild and the levels remain in the normal range in most instances. However, occasionally massive hypertriglyceridemia can be associated with estrogen therapy when this is given to women with a familial form of hypertriglyceridemia (e.g., familial hypertriglyceridemia or familial combined hyperlipidemia). The mechanism of the estrogen-induced increase in plasma triglyceride levels appears to be related to an enhanced hepatic VLDL triglyceride production rate, perhaps modulated by increased insulin levels. (*Wilson and Foster, 1998*)

50. (D) *Discussion:* This patient's fasting blood is diagnostic for DM type II. The lipid abnormality is the dyslipidemia of diabetes that results in an elevated triglyceride, low HDL, and near-normal LDL. (*Cecil, Ch. 242*)

51. (D) *Discussion:* On the basis of the Friedwald formula [LDL = total cholesterol − (HDL + triglycerides/5)], this patient's calculated LDL is 150 mg/dL. Based on the second report of the National Cholesterol Education Program (NCEP) Expert Panel on detection, elevation, and treatment of high blood cholesterol in adults, drug treatment to lower LDL should be initiated in anyone who has known coronary artery disease and LDL levels of more than 130 mg/dL. The goal should be to bring the LDL level down to less than or equal to 100 mg/dL. (*Cecil, Ch. 206; National Cholesterol Education Program, 1993*)

52. (C) *Discussion:* Acarbose reversibly inhibits α-glucosidases (intestinal enzymes responsible for the breakdown of complex carbohydrate into a monosaccharide), thereby delaying digestion and absorption of carbohydrates. (*Cecil, Ch. 242*)

53. (C) *Discussion:* The goals of therapy for diabetic ketoacidosis are to reverse the metabolic disturbance and replace fluid and electrolyte deficits. These goals thus require prompt delivery of water, electrolytes, and insulin as well as attention to potential complications that might arise during therapy and a search and treatment for any possible underlying precipitating events. Metformin has no role in the treatment of diabetic ketoacidosis. (*Cecil, Ch. 242*)

54. (B) *Discussion:* Patients with DM type I have little or no insulin secretory capacity and depend on exogenous insulin to prevent metabolic decompensation and death. C peptide levels are usually very low or undetectable. Insulin secretagogues like sulfonylureas are of no use in DM type I. Insulin resistance is not involved in the pathophysiology of DM type I. DM type I is an autoimmune disorder and results from an interplay of genetic, environmental, and autoimmune factors that selectively destroy insulin-producing and beta cells. Anti-GAD antibodies, anti-islet cell antibodies, and insulin autoantibodies are commonly present in the blood of patients with DM type I even before the diagnosis has been made. (*Cecil, Ch. 242*)

55. (B) *Discussion:* Glycemic control has been the only proven therapy that might prevent or stop the progression of diabetic peripheral neuropathy. Glycemic control is also an appropriate step in the treatment of pain associated with diabetic peripheral neuropathy; however, usually this will require treatment with certain drugs, including tricyclic antidepressants, carbamazepine, gabapentin, and others. (*Cecil, Ch. 242*)

56. (C) *Discussion:* Proliferative diabetic retinopathy is rare within the first 10 years of DM type I, but its prevalence increases to 50% after 20 years. It is less common in DM type II, appearing in 10 to 15% of patients after 20 years. However, retinopathy affects 15 to 20% of DM type II patients at the time of disease detection, implying that the disease had previously been undetected. Because of this, the current recommendations are to refer DM type II patients for ophthalmologic evaluations annually, but in DM type I patients this referral can be deferred until 3 to 5 years after the diagnosis. The DCCT Trial proved that good glycemic control reduces the risk of and progression of diabetic retinopathy in type I diabetics. The United Kingdom Prospective Diabetes Study showed the same benefits of glycemic control in the type II diabetic population. It also showed that the BP control in diabetics reduces the risk of and progression of diabetic eye disease. Diabetes is the leading cause of blindness in people aged 30 to 65 years. Blindness occurs 20 times more frequently in diabetic patients than in others. (*Cecil, Ch. 242; DCCT Research Group, 1993; United Kingdom PDS Study Group, 1998a, 1998b*)

57. **(C)** *Discussion:* Multiple studies have shown a strong inverse correlation between high HDL concentrations and coronary heart disease events. Alternatively, glycemic control, waist-hip ratio, smoking, and high LDL levels are positively correlated with the rate of coronary heart disease. (*Cecil, Chs. 206 and 242; Gotto and Pownall, 1992*)

58. **(D)** *Discussion:* Familial hypercholesterolemia (FH) is an autosomal dominant disorder that results in a reduction or absence of the LDL receptor. This results in a significant elevation of both cholesterol and LDL, with heterozygotes showing a 2- to 3-fold increase in the LDL and homozygotes showing a 6- to 10-fold increase in the LDL levels. The physical manifestations of this disease can present with tendon xanthomas (only in FH and familial defective apolipoprotein B), xanthelasmas, and corneal arcus. The total cholesterol can reach 300 to 500 mg/dL in the heterozygote patient, and LDL receptor number is decreased by 50%. Homozygotes have absence of LDL receptors and the total cholesterol level reaches 800 to 1000 mg/dL. A similar cholesterol pattern can be seen in patients with familial defective apolipoprotein B, which is an autosomal dominant disorder in which the ligand-binding region of apo B is defective—which is answer D and thus not correct for FH. Patients with the FH defect have a significant increased risk of coronary artery disease and can be seen in the fourth and fifth decades of life. (*Cecil, Ch. 211*)

59. **(D)** *Discussion:* This patient has dysbetalipoproteinemia, which is an autosomal recessive defect in the apolipoprotein E allele. The resulting defect leads to an accumulation of VLDL and chylomicron remnants because the apo E defect decreases binding to the remnant receptors. As in this case, patients can maintain a normal cholesterol level until an aggravating factor increases production. This patient developed obesity, which leads to increased production of the apolipoprotein B–containing lipoproteins. Other potentially aggravating states include hypothyroidism (therefore TSH should be screened for this), diabetes, pregnancy, another genetic abnormality, or some types of liver disease (screen with a liver profile). The planar xanthomas in the palmar creases and the tuboeruptive xanthomas are nearly diagnostic in these patients. Total cholesterol and triglycerides are elevated above the 90th percentile owing to the accumulation of the β-VLDL particles and has been called broad-beta disease. These patients are at greater risk for vascular disease even with the normal or low LDL levels that are commonly seen. Other cardiovascular risk factors should be addressed to lower the patient's risk. Treatment with a combination of medications may be required in severe cases, and one must use great caution because of the rare but serious side effects of myositis and elevation of liver enzymes that is seen with HMG CoA reductase inhibitors and fibric acid derivatives. Fibrates alone may normalize the patient's lipid profile. A step 2 diet, correction of hypothyroidism if present, and weight loss are essential. These rare patients should be seen and treated by a specialist. (*Cecil, Ch. 211*).

60. **(A)** *Discussion:* Alcohol consumption is a very common cause of elevated triglycerides. The elevation of the triglycerides occurs because of an inhibition of the lipoprotein lipase, which decreases disposal. The liver increases the production of both free fatty acids and VLDL, which directly increases the triglyceride level. Alcoholics are frequently malnourished and have decreased food intake and dietary triglycerides in the form of chylomicrons, which do not play a large role in the elevated levels commonly seen. (*Cecil, Ch. 211*)

61. **(C)** *Discussion:* Galactosemia is an autosomal recessive trait that is fatal if not detected within the first few days of life and is part of the newborn screen. If detected, a lactose (galactose) free diet must be followed to prevent or treat jaundice, bleeding, feeding intolerance, lethargy, sepsis, hypotension, or death. The galactose pathway is responsible for development of essential products for cell growth and differentiation, which include glycogen, glycoproteins, and glycolipids. Impairment of either uridine diphosphate-galactose-4-epimerase or galactokinase can result in less severe disease and elevation of blood galactose. Despite therapy for a galactose-free diet, chronic problems emerge later in life and include growth delay, ataxia, tremors, ovarian failure, cerebral dyspraxia, reduced IQ, and cataract formation. The pathology of these late defects is unknown, but the clinician should let the parents know of these possibilities. (*Cecil, Ch. 212*).

62. **(C)** *Discussion:* Glycogen storage diseases (GSD) can present with a spectrum of symptoms, and diagnosis of the deficiency is made with tissue biopsy showing abnormal glycogen concentrations in the tissue or abnormal structure. Type I GSD is a deficiency of glucose-6-phosphatase and presents as an enlarged liver, fasting hypoglycemia, acidosis, and thrombocyte dysfunction. Glycogen synthetase deficiency type 0 results in early death and could not be the defect in this patient. Myophosphorylase deficiency type V GSD (McArdle's disease) presents in the second and third decades of life with muscle cramps and pain after exercise, myoglobinuria in up to 50%, an elevated serum muscle creatine kinase and low lactate levels with exercise. These findings are consistent with our patient and you confirm both an elevated muscle creatine kinase value and myoglobinuria after 10 minutes on a treadmill. Acid α-glucosidase deficiency type II GSD (Pompe's disease) demonstrates glycogen elevation in virtually all tissues and clinically presents as massive cardiomegaly, muscle hypotonia, and rapid respiratory failure a few years after diagnosis. It manifests earlier in life, but a milder adult onset form with a chronic myopathy can occur. (*Cecil, Ch. 213*).

63. **(A)** *Discussion:* This infant has a defect in purine metabolism and has significant T-cell depletion and cellular immune dysfunction. The diagnosis is made by documenting a deficiency of purine nucleoside phosphorylase in the erythrocyte or mononuclear cells. This enzyme catalyzes the cleavage of inosine, 2′-deoxyinosine, guanosine, and 2′-deoxyguanosine to their respective purine bases. In a clinical setting any patient with recurrent viral infections, neurologic abnormalities, autoimmunity, T-cell lymphopenia, and a uric acid level less than 1 mg/dL should be evaluated for purine nucleoside phosphorylase deficiency. Fat pad biopsy is used to diagnose amyloidosis. Varicella titers would be low but would not aid in the diagnosis. HPRT is absent in patients with Lesch-Nyhan syndrome and presents in males as uric acid nephrolithiasis, gout, and severe neurologic/psychologic problems but not immune impairment. These patients have an absent purine salvage pathway, and hypoxanthine and guanine can only be catabolized into uric acid, leading to hyperuricemia. (*Cecil, Ch. 216*)

64. **(C)** *Discussion:* Fabry disease is a lysosomal storage disease that results in the accumulation of globotriaosylceramide in most cells, with particular predilection for vascular endothelial and smooth muscle cells. It is an X-linked disorder and therefore only symptomatic in male patients. This patient had a classic Fabry

crisis that consists of severe burning pain in the extremities followed by fever and fatigue. This commonly occurs after exercise. As these patients age so does their morbidity from this disease—mainly related to the vascular system. The gradual renal deterioration can be detected with the urine sediment described in answer C—RBCs, casts, and lipid inclusions which have a characteristic birefringence—Maltese crosses. Vascular events or uremia result in death by the fifth decade; however, dialysis and transplantation have improved this outcome. Recently, enzyme replacement has become available that has demonstrated both safety and effectiveness in clinical trials. Sphingomyelin accumulation occurs in Niemann-Pick disease, another lysosomal storage disease that results in hepatosplenomegaly (HSM) and progressive neurologic dysfunction. Gaucher's disease is another storage disease that can result in neurologic dysfunction and HSM as a result of glycosylceramide accumulation. Lung disease can occur in Niemann-Pick disease or rarely Gaucher's disease but not in Fabry's disease. *(Cecil, Ch. 217)*

65. (C) *Discussion:* Alcohol ingestion is the most common factor that triggers porphyria cutanea tarda (PCT) by increasing iron absorption and stimulating hepatic heme and porphyrin synthesis and possible by generating free radicals. Estrogen therapy and iron therapy may also trigger or worsen an attack. PCT is caused by a deficiency of uroporphyrinogen decarboxylase in the liver and is both sporadic (type 1) and familial (type 2). Type 1 demonstrates enzyme deficiency only in the liver whereas type 2 has deficiency in all tissues. The risk factors that may be associated with or contribute to the reduced uroporphyrinogen decarboxylase activity (and therefore result in PCT) include normal to increased iron, P450 enzyme oxidation of the porphyrinogen substances, alcohol, hepatitis C, decreased antioxidant levels, and estrogen therapy. None of the other answers has been found to be linked to the worsening of symptoms, and a multivitamin may raise antioxidant levels, which may improve the symptoms. Seizure medication is known to trigger an attack of acute intermittent porphyria, which has a neurologic presentation that is caused by a deficiency of porphobilinogen deaminase *(Cecil, Ch. 223)*

66. (B) *Discussion:* This patient has a classic presentation of Wilson's disease. Wilson's disease is an autosomal recessive disorder of copper metabolism that results in a reduced incorporation of copper into ceruloplasmin and a decreased ability to secrete copper into the bile for excretion. The clinical presentation can vary but includes neurologic abnormalities, psychiatric illness, hemolytic anemia, renal tubular Fanconi's syndrome, and skeletal abnormalities. Commonly, this presentation occurs in patients during their late adolescence and early adulthood, and substance abuse should always be considered. Her examination demonstrated hepatomegaly and Kayser-Fleischer rings, which suggested Wilson's disease over substance abuse. Diagnosis without specific molecular evidence can be made if two of the following symptoms occur: family history, Kayser-Fleischer rings, low copper and ceruloplasmin levels (not elevated), Coombs-negative hemolytic anemia, increased 24-hour urine copper levels (>100 mg/24 hours), elevated hepatic copper levels (biopsy with > 200 mg/g), or a positive penicillamine challenge. *(Cecil, Ch. 224)*

67. (D) *Discussion:* This patient has symptoms suggestive of hereditary hemochromatosis, and these patients have transferring saturation levels of 80 to 100% and ferritin levels of 500 to 6000 ng/dL. Choice C represents levels commonly seen in an asymptomatic patient, and answers A and B are within the normal range. After the abnormal laboratory test results are documented the next step should be genetic analysis to confirm hereditary hemochromatosis and if the *C282Y* gene is positive and the liver transaminase values are within normal limits, therapeutic phlebotomy should occur. *(Cecil, Ch. 225)*

68. (A); **69. (D)**; **70. (B)**; **71. (C)**; **72. (D)**; **73. (E)**. *Discussion:* The new synthetic insulins work within 10 to 15 minutes, with peak activity occurring before 2 hours (both insulin Asparte and insulin Lispro). Insulin glargine has an acidic pH that can be disrupted if mixed with other insulins. This acidic pH is crucial, and when this insulin is injected into the more basic subcutaneous space, a microprecipitate is formed to allow the peakless profile. Regular insulin peak occurs within 2 to 4 hours, and duration of action is between 5 and 8 hours. NPH insulin has a delayed peak action, which may result in hypoglycemia and frequently is prescribed with snacks. All insulins can cause hypoglycemia, which is treated by consuming carbohydrates, but the other insulins are not prescribed with a snack. Glargine has a peakless profile. All insulins when given intravenously have the same action profile. The differences are based on the diffusion from the subcutaneous space into the bloodstream to result in either a rapid or delayed insulin response. *(Cecil, Ch. 242)*

74. (A, B); **75. (C)**; **76. (A, B, D)**; **77. (E)**; **78. (C)**; **79. (A)**; **80. (B)**; **81. (D)**. *Discussion:* Hyperlipoproteinemia (type 1) presents as triglyceride levels in the 99th percentile and consists mainly of chylomicrons resulting from a deficiency of apolipoprotein C II as well as a decreased activity of lipoprotein lipase. Mixed hypertriglyceridemia (type V) also has triglycerides in the 99th percentile consisting of both VLDL and chylomicrons and has the same deficiency of apolipoprotein C II, possibly a deficiency of C III and decrease of activity of the lipoprotein lipase. Familial dysbetalipoproteinemia (type III) has both an elevation of total cholesterol and triglycerides above the 90th percentile and the underlying defect is an abnormal apo E 2/2 phenotype, which increases the remnant (β-VLDL + chylomicrons). Familial hypertriglyceridemia has triglycerides in the 200- to 500-mg/dL range consisting of VLDL particles. This results from a heterozygote inactivation of lipoprotein lipase and may also have a low HDL. *(Williams Textbook of Endocrinology, 2003)*.

82. (B); **83. (C)**; **84. (D)**; **85. (A)**; **86. (E)**. *Discussion:* Individuals with hyperalphalipoproteinemia have an increased HDL cholesterol level, and this condition is associated with increased longevity and decreased risk of coronary artery disease. Dysbetalipoproteinemia, also known as broad-beta or type III hyperlipoproteinemia, is a condition in which there is an abnormal accumulation of cholesterol-rich intermediate-density lipoprotein-type particles, commonly termed β-VLDL. This disorder is due to the interaction of an autosomal defect in apo E that leads to abnormal remnant catabolism and an independent aggravating environmental factor (e.g., obesity, diabetes, pregnancy) or genetic factor (familial combined hypercholesterolemia) resulting in overproduction of apolipoprotein B–containing lipoproteins. The combination of these two factors leads to accumulation of IDL particles and remnants that lead to xanthomas, peripheral vascular disease, and coronary artery disease. Familial combined hyperlipidemia may present as elevations of total and VLDL cholesterol or as elevations of total, LDL, and VLDL cholesterol and triglycerides. Both patterns may be seen within a family. This disorder is quite common in the United States, where it occurs in 1 in 300 persons. Like familial hypercholesterolemia, familial combined hyperlipidemia appears to be inherited as an autosomal trait. The trait carries an increased risk of coronary heart disease. Unlike familial hypercholesterolemia, familial combined hyperlipidemia does not cause xanthomas and does not often occur before age 20 years. The diagnosis is usually one of adulthood. Lipoprotein lipase deficiency is a rare autosomal-recessive trait characterized by the absence of LPL in all tissues, leading to massive hypertriglyceridemia from birth and the clinical consequences of eruptive xanthomas and episodes of pancreatitis. This same clinical syndrome may also occur with a deficiency of apolipoprotein C II, an obligatory activator of lipoprotein lipase, although clinical manifestations in this case tend to occur later in life. Familial hypercholesterolemia (FH) is a common autosomal-dominant disorder caused by absence of or defective LDL receptors, resulting in decreased capacity to remove plasma LDL. In this disorder, the LDL cholesterol levels are strikingly increased and frequently associated with characteristic xanthomas in the Achilles tendon, patella tendon, extensor tendons of the hands, and presence of xanthelasma. It is frequently associated with early coronary artery disease. In heterozygous familial hypercholesterolemia, estimated to be present in 1 in 500 individuals, there is one abnormal allele for the LDL receptor. In this heterozygote state, there is a 50% decrease in the hepatic LDL receptor number with a corresponding decrease in LDL catabolism and an increase of 2- to 3-fold in plasma LDL levels. In the rare homozygous familial hypercholesterolemia patient (only 1 in 1 million people), almost no functional LDL receptors are found, and plasma LDL levels may be increased 6- to 10-fold. In this situation, LDL can be removed from plasma only by low-affinity pathways. If untreated, patients with familial hypercholesterolemia will have premature coronary heart disease as well as other clinical manifestations of atherosclerosis. Risk of peripheral vascular disease and cerebrovascular disease is also increased, although not as much as coronary artery disease. Tendon xanthomas are seen only in familial hypercholesterolemia and in patients with familial defective apo-B. Xanthelasma typically occurs in this setting, and corneal arcus (arcus senilis) is frequently seen as well, although it is seen in other lipoprotein disorders and can be seen in elderly, normal lipidemic patients as well. (Cecil, Ch. 206; Gotto and Pownall, 1992)

87. (C); 88. (E); 89. (A); 90. (B); 91. (D). Discussion: The diagnosis of hypoglycemia is a challenging one. Whipple's triad, which consists of (1) symptoms consistent with the diagnosis, (2) plasma glucose concentration within a range that is compatible with symptoms of hypoglycemia, and (3) prompt relief of symptoms after administration of glucose, needs to be fulfilled before making a diagnosis of hypoglycemia. By far, the most common cause of hypoglycemia is drug-induced hypoglycemia, which, for the most part, is iatrogenic, although it can also be factitious. Insulinoma is a rare disorder that occurs in approximately 1 per 250,000 individuals. The median age at onset is about 50 years, except for those in whom it develops in the context of MEN 1, in which it occurs in the mid 20s. Most insulinomas are small, benign, and single. Tumors are multiple in 7% and malignant in about 5%. Eight percent of patients with insulinoma have MEN 1, and the tumors are much more likely to be multiple. The diagnosis of insulinoma is based on the presence of the Whipple's triad together with inappropriately elevated plasma insulin and C peptide levels in the absence of sulfonylurea in the plasma. The diagnosis is most straightforward when insulin, C peptide, and sulfonylurea determinations are obtained concurrently during an episode of hypoglycemia. In the case presented here, the elevated high calcium levels in two first-degree relatives are likely from primary hyperparathyroidism within the context of MEN 1, which should be a clue for the diagnosis in this case. Hypoglycemia induced by surreptitious administration of insulin or sulfonylureas is probably more common than insulinoma. As a result, the coexistence of hypoglycemia and inappropriate insulin levels does not establish the diagnosis of insulinoma. Most often, factitious hypoglycemia occurs in medical personnel or in family members of patients with diabetes. Insulin has been used for suicide, homicide, and child abuse. The best means for distinguishing insulinoma from surreptitious insulin administration is to measure C peptide along with insulin during hypoglycemia. Drug-induced hypoglycemia is more likely to occur at the extremes of age, in the acutely or chronically undernourished, and in the presence of renal or hepatic dysfunction. In the case of the elderly woman who was

brought to the emergency department with repeated episodes of hypoglycemia, who was otherwise quite healthy, the history of diabetes in her husband should be a clue to the diagnosis because inadvertent administration of sulfonylureas from her husband's medications is quite possible. Those patients practicing intensive insulin therapy suffer an average of two episodes of symptomatic hypoglycemia per week. We also know that about 25% of those practicing intensive therapy suffer at least one episode of severe, temporary disabling hypoglycemia, often with seizure or coma in a given year. In large retrospective series, approximately 4% of deaths of people with DM type I have been attributed to hypoglycemia. After several years of BM type 1 and a history of recurrent hypoglycemia, reflected by an Hgb A1c as low as that noted in the young female college student with type I diabetes presented here, the probability of defective glucose counter-regulation as well as hypoglycemia unawareness is quite high. The hypoglycemia that sometimes accompanies renal failure is often multifactorial and may be due to reduced clearance of hypoglycemic drugs, reduced food intake, and reduced gluconeogenesis, possibly secondary to defective gluconeogenetic substrates. In the last patient presented here, the likelihood of chronic renal insufficiency is quite high, given his history of poorly controlled diabetes for more than 20 years and 3+ protein in the urine. The fact that now his blood sugar levels are relatively normal without changing therapy implies that he probably has reduced clearance of hypoglycemic drugs. (Cecil, Ch. 243; Cryer, 1997a; Service, 1995)

92. (C); 93. (C); 94. (E); 95. (B); 96. (D); 97. (E). Discussion: Eruptive xanthomas are small yellowish papules surrounded by a reddish macular area and result from severe hypertriglyceridemia caused by hyperchylomicronemia, when chylomicrons are taken up by macrophages in the skin. These lesions usually present over the extensor surfaces of the arms and thighs and on the back and buttocks. Lipemia retinalis is also the result of severe hypertriglyceridemia as a consequence of hyperchylomicronemia in which the blood vessels in the fundi appear whitish and overall the retina has a pinkish color. Arcus senilis (also known as corneal arcus) and xanthelasma are frequently seen in patients with hypercholesterolemia or familial defective apolipoprotein B. However, they may be seen in other lipoprotein disorders as well as in the elderly normal lipemic patients. Tendon xanthomas are seen only in familial hypercholesterolemia and patients with familial defective apolipoprotein B. They are bilateral, irregular, firm, and nodular thickenings in the Achilles tendon or extensor tendons of the hands or knees and can be so large as to interfere with normal function, such as wearing shoes. These deposits may also occur elsewhere over the tibial tuberosities and elbows, and in the homozygous state "buttery" xanthomas may be present over the thighs and buttocks. They are related to the impaired LDL clearance from the circulation in both hypercholesterolemia and familial defective apolipoprotein B. Palmar xanthomas are orange discolorations of the creases of the palms. These are typical to the point that they are virtually diagnostic of dysbetalipoproteinemia, also known as broad-beta or type III hyperlipoproteinemia, a condition in which there is abnormal accumulation of cholesterol-rich intermediate-density-lipoprotein type particles, commonly termed β-VLDL. (Cecil, Ch. 206; Gotto and Pownall, 1992; Wilson and Foster, 1998)

98. (True); 99. (True); 100. (True); 101. (False); 102. (False); 103. (False). Discussion: Gestational diabetes is a term used to characterize increased glucose levels that are first detected during pregnancy. It excludes known diabetes before conception. Gestational diabetes occurs in about 2% of pregnancies and usually appears in the second or third trimester at the time of significant elevations of pregnancy-associated insulin antagonistic hormones After delivery glucose tolerance usually reverts to normal. Nevertheless, within 5 to 10 years, DM type II will develop in 30

to 40% of these patients. Occasionally, pregnancy may precipitate DM type I. Although gestational diabetes generally causes only mild asymptomatic hyperglycemia, rigorous treatment, often with insulin, is required to protect against fetal morbidity and mortality. Macrosomia (oversized fetus) is the most common neonatal abnormality in diabetic pregnancy. Because insulin does not cross the placenta, the metabolism of maternal substrates received by the fetus depends entirely on fetal insulin. In a diabetic pregnancy, the fetal nutrient levels, which reflect maternal levels, will exceed the normal range and constitute an important stimulus for the secretion of fetal insulin and other growth factors. If the mother is poorly controlled, the fetus will be hyperinsulinemic and will experience hyperplasia of the beta cells. This hyperinsulinemia will subsequently stimulate fetal growth. Because of this hyperinsulinemia and the possible hyperplasia of the beta cells, all infants of diabetic mothers need to be carefully monitored for hypoglycemia during the first hours and days of life. The incidence of malformations involving many organ systems is increased approximately 2- to 3-fold in infants of diabetic mothers, and such malformations account for 30 to 50% of neonatal mortalities. (*Cecil, Ch. 242; Wilson and Foster, 1998*)

104. (**False**); 105. (**True**); 106. (**False**); 107. (**True**); 108. (**False**); 109. (**True**); 110. (**False**); 111. (**False**). *Discussion:* Diabetic ketoacidosis is an acute, life-threatening complication of DM type I but may occasionally occur in DM type II. Otherwise unexplained abdominal pain occurs frequently in children, less often in adults with diabetic ketoacidosis. The pain is usually periumbilical and constant in nature and can mimic that pain associated with surgical emergencies. The increased circulating levels of prostaglandin I_2 and prostaglandin E_2 present during diabetic ketoacidosis are thought to have a causal relationship with the abdominal pain, nausea, vomiting, and signs of decreased vascular resistance seen during diabetic ketoacidosis. The mortality rate for diabetic ketoacidosis varies between 5 and 10%. For the most part, mortality occurs in elderly patients in whom diabetic ketoacidosis is initiated or complicated by a serious underlying illness. Diabetic ketoacidosis also remains a major cause of death in children with type I diabetes, especially if complicated by cerebral edema. The rapid assessment of serum ketones using dilutions of serum and reagent strips (Ketostix) or tablets (Acetest) depends on nitroprusside reaction with acetoacetate. Acetone, however, reacts weakly with nitroprusside, and β-hydroxybutyrate reacts not at all, making the test results sometimes misleadingly low. Because of the presence of intracellular acidosis, β-hydroxybutyrate levels are often much higher than those of acetoacetate, and the frequent presence of concomitant lactic acidosis further reduces acetoacetate. Conversely, once insulin therapy begins, the nitroprusside reaction often remains positive and gives a false impression of sustained ketosis for many hours or days because some β-hydroxybutyrate is converted to acetoacetate and nonacidic acetone is cleared slowly from the body. Obtundation and the presence of focal neurologic signs are characteristic features of hyperosmolar nonketotic coma. These are rarely seen in diabetic ketoacidosis. In general, the neurologic findings of the hyperosmolar state occur only when the osmolality exceeds 350 mOsm/kg. Of course, when neurologic findings are present, especially at lower osmolality levels, the possibility of an intercurrent neurologic disorder must be considered. Because of the delay in the absorption and onset of action of subcutaneously administered insulin, it is generally appropriate to continue the IV infusion of insulin for at least 1 or 2 hours after the initiation of subcutaneous insulin. The patient should not be treated with a sliding scale of regular insulin. Although most patients in diabetic ketoacidosis have a normal or elevated serum potassium concentration at presentation, virtually every patient in diabetic ketoacidosis has a total body potassium deficit. When therapy is initiated, the serum potassium concentration falls, often rapidly. Consequently, potassium replacement should begin as soon as an adequate urine flow is present and hyperkalemia has been excluded by the determination of the serum potassium concentration and by an electrocardiogram. When the plasma glucose level reaches a value of 250 mg/dL or less, the crystalloid solution being administered should contain 5% glucose to prevent hypoglycemia, allowing the continued administration of insulin to correct the acidosis. (*Cecil, Ch. 242; Axelroad, 1992*)

BIBLIOGRAPHY

Alberti KG, et al: Definition, diagnosis and classification of diabetes mellitus and its complications. Diabet Med 1998;15:535-536.

Albright ES, et al: Artifactually low hemoglobin A1c caused by use of dapsone. Endocr Pract 2002;8:370-372.

American Diabetes Association: Screening for diabetes. Diabetes Care 2002;25(Suppl 1):s22.

Atkinson MA, et al: The pathogenesis of insulin-dependent diabetes mellitus. N Engl J Med 1994;331:1428.

Axelroad L: Diabetic ketoacidosis. Endocrinologist 1992;2:375.

Buchannan T, et al: Preservation of pancreatic beta cell function and prevention of type 2 diabetes by pharmacological treatment of insulin resistance in high-risk Hispanic women. Diabetes 2002;51:2766.

Cooper ME: Pathogenesis, prevention and treatment of diabetic nephropathy. Lancet 1998;352:213.

Cryer PE (ed): Hypoglycemia: Pathophysiology, Diagnosis, and Treatment. New York, Oxford University Press, 1997.

Cryer PE, Gerich JE: Glucose counterregulation, hypoglycemia and intensive insulin therapy in diabetes mellitus. N Engl J Med 1985;313:232.

Dagogo-Jack S, Santiago JV: Pathophysiology of type 2 diabetes mellitus and modes of action of therapeutic interventions. Arch Intern Med 1997;157:1802

Davies MJ, et al: DIGAMI: Theory in practice. Diab Obesity Metab 2002;4:289.

DCCT Research Group: The effect of intensive treatment of diabetes on the development and progression of long term complications in insulin-dependent diabetes mellitus. N Engl J Med 1993;329:977.

Dejgaard A: Pathophysiology and treatment of diabetic neuropathy. Diabet Med 1998;15:97.

Expert Committee on the Diagnosis and Classification of Diabetes Mellitus: Report of the Expert Committee on the Diagnosis and Classification of Diabetes Mellitus. Diabet Care 1999;22(S1):s5.

Expert Committee: Report of the Expert Committee on the Diagnosis and Classification of Diabetes Mellitus. Diabet 2003;25(Suppl 1-47).

Frank B, et al: Postmenopausal hormone therapy and the risk of cardiovascular disease: The epidemiologic evidence. J Lipid Res 1993;34:1255.

Goldman L, Ausiello D (eds): Cecil Textbook of Medicine, 22nd ed. Philadelphia, WB Saunders, 2004.

Gotto AM Jr, Pownall HJ (eds): Manual of Lipid Disorders. Baltimore, MD, Williams & Wilkins, 1992.

Isselbacher KJ, Braunwald E, Wilson JD, et al (eds): Harrison's Principles of Internal Medicine, 14th ed. New York, McGraw-Hill, 1998.

Khoury V, et al: effects of glucose-insulin-potassium infusion on chloric ischaemic left ventricular dysfunction. Heart 2003;89:61.

Kirpichnikov D, et al: Metformin: an update. Ann Intern Med 2002;137:25.

Lasaridis A, et al: Diabetic neuropathy and antihypertensive treatment: What are the lessons from clinical trials? Am J Hypertens 2003;16:689.

Manley SE, et al: Effects of three months' diet after diagnosis of type 2 diabetes on plasma lipids and lipoproteins. Diabet Med 2000;17:518-523.

Parulkar A, et al: Nonhypoglycemic effects of thiazolidinediones. Ann Intern Med 2001;134:61-71.

PDR, 56th ed. 2002.

Service FJ: Hypoglycemic disorders. N Engl J Med 1995;332:1144.

Stratton I, et al: Association of glycemia with macrovascular and microvascular complications of type 2 diabetes (UKPDS 35): Perspective observational study. BMJ 2000;321:405.

Tanwani LK, et al: Minimal change neuropathy and Graves' disease: Report of a case and review of the literature. Endocr Pract 2002;8: 40-43.

Trujillo-Santos AJ: Diabetic muscle infarction. Diabetes Care 2003; 26:211.

United Kingdom PDS Study Group: Tight blood pressure control and risk of macrovascular and microvascular complications in type 2 diabetes: UKPDS 38. BMJ 1998b;317:703.

United Kingdom PDS Study Group: U.K. Prospective Study 33: Intensive blood glucose control with sulfonylureas or insulin compared with conventional treatment and risk of complications in patients with type 2 diabetes. Lancet 1998a;352:837.

Wilson JD, Foster DW (eds): Williams' Textbook of Endocrinology, 9th ed. Philadelphia, WB Saunders, 1998.

Yki-Jarvinen H, et al: Comparison of bedtime insulin regimens in patients with type 2 diabetes mellitus. Ann Intern Med 1999;130:389.

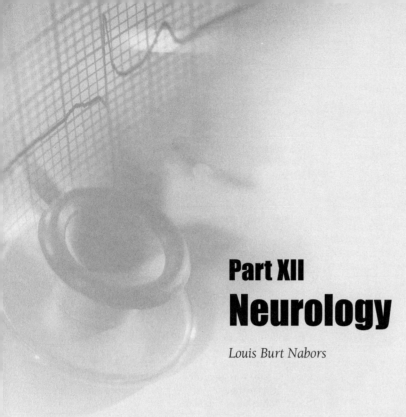

Part XII
Neurology

Louis Burt Nabors

MULTIPLE CHOICE
QUESTIONS 1-68

DIRECTIONS: Select the single best answer for each question.

1. Which of the following is *not* commonly associated with a low cerebrospinal fluid (CSF) glucose level?

   A. Bacterial meningitis
   B. Herpes encephalitis
   C. Fungal meningitis
   D. Carcinomatous meningitis

2. The neuromuscular transmission defect in myasthenia gravis is due to which of the following?

   A. Presynaptic disorder caused by inadequate release of acetylcholine
   B. Presynaptic disorder secondary to an antibody against the voltage-gated calcium channel
   C. Postsynaptic disorder caused by an antibody against the acetylcholine receptor
   D. Nondepolarizing blockade of the acetylcholine receptor
   E. Delayed degradation of acetylcholinesterase

3. In a multiple sclerosis (MS) exacerbation, the CSF is often abnormal. Which one of the following is *specific* to MS?

   A. Increased lymphocytes
   B. Increased total protein
   C. Increased immunoglobulin G (IgG) synthesis rate
   D. Oligoclonal bands
   E. None of the above

4. A 55-year-old man is brought to the emergency department after complaining of a severe headache followed by progressive obtundation. Ocular funduscopic examination reveals subhyaloid hemorrhage. The most likely diagnosis is:

   A. Bacterial meningitis
   B. Brain stem infarction
   C. Intracerebral hematoma
   D. Subarachnoid hemorrhage (SAH)
   E. Glioblastoma multiforme

5. Interferon-β1b is used to decrease relapses and possibly disease progression in MS. Which is *not* an established side effect?

   A. Injection site reactions
   B. Hyponatremia
   C. Depression
   D. Liver function test abnormalities

6. What type of aphasia is characterized by fluent speech with some articulatory deficits and intact comprehension but inability to repeat a phrase?

   A. Wernicke's (sensory)
   B. Broca's (motor)
   C. Transcortical motor
   D. Transcortical sensory
   E. Conductive

7. A patient is self-referred to you for evaluation for memory complaints. He is unaccompanied and answers most of your mental status questions by saying he does not know. He admits to dysphoria. Based on this, what would be the most likely diagnosis?

   A. Pseudodementia secondary to depression
   B. Alzheimer's disease
   C. Pick's disease
   D. Lewy body variant

8. A 70-year-old man is brought to the hospital because of sudden onset of confusion. On examination, he talks with jargon-like phrases. He speaks fluently but selects the wrong words. He is unable to answer your questions but follows visually cued directions well. The examination is otherwise normal. Where is the cerebral lesion most likely located?

   A. Dominant temporal lobe
   B. Dominant frontal lobe
   C. Thalamus
   D. Dominant supramarginal gyrus
   E. Diffuse cortical dysfunction

223

9. Which of the following is *not* a standard part of the routine evaluation for reversible causes in a patient with dementia?

    A. Electroencephalogram (EEG)
    B. Noncontrast computed tomography (CT) of the brain
    C. Vitamin B_{12}
    D. Thyroid function test

10. A 56-year-old woman complains of several weeks of brief, lightning-like pain in the midface area on the left that is brought on by eating. Her neurologic examination is normal. The drug of choice for treatment is:

    A. Lorazepam
    B. Haloperidol
    C. Phenytoin
    D. Carbamazepine
    E. Valproic acid

11. When Parkinson's disease causes a dementia, the dementia usually:

    A. Precedes significant motor impairment
    B. Occurs simultaneously with significant motor impairment
    C. Follows significant motor impairment

12. What is the best treatment for a solitary non–small cell lung metastasis to the brain?

    A. Local irradiation
    B. Whole brain radiation
    C. Chemotherapy with intra-arterial cisplatin
    D. Resection of the tumor
    E. Glucocorticoids alone

13. One of the many types of peripheral neuropathy associated with diabetes is a vascular infarction of the third cranial nerve. The feature that may permit this to be distinguished from other causes of third cranial nerve dysfunction, such as aneurysmal compression, is:

    A. Subacute onset over 1 to 2 weeks
    B. Pupillary sparing
    C. Preservation of lateral eye movements
    D. Being unilateral

14. A state of sustained loss of cognition with intact sleep/wake cycles and autonomic functions is known as:

    A. Stupor
    B. Delirium
    C. Vegetative state
    D. Coma
    E. Locked-in state

15. A 19-year-old woman from the local community college is brought to the emergency department by her roommate for evaluation of headache and confusion. The patient apparently awoke that morning with a headache and stayed home from classes. On her return from class, the roommate found her still in bed and now confused. There is no history of drug or alcohol use. On physical examination her temperature is 39.4° C (103° F) and her neck is stiff. She is oriented only to person. The hospital does not have emergent CT capability. Your next step is:

    A. Transfer the patient to the closest hospital with CT ability.

    B. If her neurologic examination is nonfocal, proceed with lumbar puncture (LP) and antibiotics.
    C. If her neurologic examination has focal findings, proceed with LP and antibiotics.
    D. Perform serial neurologic examinations.

16. A 24-year-old woman is brought to the hospital after being found unresponsive. Examination reveals no withdrawal in response to pain, but all brain stem reflexes are present. An EEG is obtained and is normal. The most likely etiology is:

    A. Phenobarbital overdose
    B. Brain stem stroke
    C. SAH
    D. Psychogenic state
    E. Alpha rhythm coma

17. Which of the following statements concerning migraines and cluster headaches is *correct*?

    A. Cluster headaches are more common in men and migraines more common in women.
    B. Both migraines and cluster headaches are typically bilateral.
    C. Classic migraines have prominent autonomic symptoms such as tearing and rhinorrhea at onset, whereas cluster migraines are preceded by an aura.
    D. The treatment of migraine headaches includes indomethacin and steroids.

18. Temporal arteritis is best treated initially with:

    A. Cyclophosphamide
    B. Prednisone, 20 mg/day
    C. Prednisone, 80 mg/day
    D. Nonsteroidal anti-inflammatory agents
    E. Carbamazepine

19. Which of the following medications is most appropriately used as migraine prophylaxis?

    A. Valproic acid
    B. Sumatriptan
    C. Dihydroergotamine
    D. Ergotamine-caffeine combination (Cafergot)

20. A 60-year-old man with alcohol on his breath is brought to the emergency department and examination reveals ophthalmoplegia, gait difficulties, and confusion. Treatment should include which of the following?

    A. Folate
    B. Phenytoin
    C. Pyridoxine
    D. Thiamine
    E. Benzodiazepine

21. A 75-year-old woman presents for evaluation of several months of worsening tremor, falling, and dizziness. Her medical history is remarkable for hypertension. On examination, you observe an unsteady gait and detect a cogwheel pattern of rigidity. A significant orthostatic blood pressure is noted. The differential diagnosis should include:

    A. Essential tremor
    B. Progressive supranuclear palsy
    C. Shy-Drager syndrome
    D. Diffuse Lewy body disease

22. A 64-year-old man presents with painless weakness in his arms. Examination reveals weakness, atrophy, and fasciculations of multiple muscles in his arms and slight weakness of his right anterior tibialis muscle. Sensation is normal. Deep tendon reflexes are brisk. Electrophysiologic studies reveal

diffuse denervation of multiple muscles with normal sensory nerve conduction studies. The most likely diagnosis is which of the following?

A. Adult-onset spinal muscular atrophy
B. Lambert-Eaton myasthenic syndrome
C. Fascioscapulohumeral muscular dystrophy
D. Amyotrophic lateral sclerosis
E. Multifocal motor neuropathy

23. Tourette's syndrome is associated with which of the following psychiatric diagnoses?

A. Obsessive-compulsive disorder
B. Bipolar disorder
C. Schizophrenia
D. Dysthymia

24. Which of the following is not a neuroleptic-induced movement disorder?

A. Restless leg syndrome
B. Dystonic reaction
C. Akathisia
D. Parkinsonism
E. Tardive dyskinesia

25. Complications related to levodopa therapy for Parkinson's disease include all of the following except:

A. Psychiatric problems
B. Dyskinesias
C. Wearing-off effect
D. Dry mouth

26. A 54-year-old woman reports a 6-month history of difficulty getting out of a chair and difficulty holding her arms overhead. Her serum creatine phosphokinase level is elevated at 350 IU/L. The most likely cause of this acquired myopathy is which one of the following?

A. Inclusion body myopathy
B. Polymyositis
C. Minicore myopathy
D. Mitochondrial myopathy
E. Limb-girdle muscular dystrophy

27. Friedreich's ataxia, a familial progressive ataxia, is characterized by all of the following except:

A. Pes cavus and kyphoscoliosis
B. Dementia
C. Loss of deep tendon reflexes
D. Extensor plantar response

28. A 35-year-old woman reports a 3-week history of left-sided weakness, hyperreflexia, and Babinski's sign. Four years ago she had transient loss of vision in the right eye for several weeks. A cranial MRI is performed that demonstrates multiple areas of white matter signal change in a periventricular distribution, some of which enhance after contrast agent administration. What is the most likely diagnosis?

A. CNS toxoplasmosis
B. Venous thrombosis
C. Multiple sclerosis
D. CNS vasculitis
E. Microangiopathy

29. Which of the following is *not* a congenital myopathy?

A. Central core disease
B. Nemaline rod myopathy
C. Myotubular myopathy
D. Duchenne's muscular dystrophy

30. Which of the following statements concerning inflammatory myopathies is *correct*?

A. Polymyositis is associated with an underlying malignancy.
B. Dermatomyositis is primarily a humoral response resulting in capillary injury and necrosis.
C. Dermatomyositis is responsive to corticosteroids, whereas polymyositis is not.
D. Dermatomyositis is primarily a cellular response directed against muscle fiber antigens.

31. Inclusion body myositis is characterized by which of the following?

A. Patients are older than 50 years.
B. Electromyograph may show a neurogenic component.
C. Muscle biopsy is remarkable for rimmed vacuoles.
D. There is sparing of cervical, facial, and pharyngeal muscles.
E. All of the above

32. The presence of ragged red fibers in a muscle biopsy is indicative of:

A. HIV myopathy
B. Glucocorticoid-induced myopathy
C. Mitochondrial myopathy
D. Carnitine palmityltransferase deficiency

33. While undergoing general anesthesia, a patient experiences tachycardia, rigidity, rising temperature, and cyanosis. Which of the following is *correct*?

A. Condition is inherited in an autosomal-recessive pattern.
B. Mortality is low.
C. Specific therapy includes IV dantrolene.
D. Serum creatine kinase is normal.

34. A 14-year-old patient twisted her ankle during a soccer game. Initial examination and radiographs were normal. Two weeks later, the patient complains of severe burning pain in her foot. The foot is somewhat cold to the touch and discolored, although pedal pulses are intact. Another evaluation, including repeat radiographs, vascular studies, and electrophysiologic studies, is unrevealing. The most likely cause of the pain is which of the following?

A. Vasculitis
B. Small fiber neuropathy
C. Fibromyalgia
D. Reflex sympathetic dystrophy
E. Peroneal neuropathy

35. A 22-year-old man is referred for evaluation of recurrent episodes of myoglobinuria. He gives a history of muscle cramps since childhood and episodes of dark urine after strenuous exercise. There is no family history of neurologic disorders, and otherwise the young man is healthy. He takes no medications and only rarely uses alcohol. An ischemic forearm exercise test is abnormal. Which of the following should be included in the differential diagnosis?

A. Myophosphorylase deficiency
B. Branching enzyme deficiency
C. Kearns-Sayre syndrome
D. Thyrotoxic myopathy

36. Which of the following is/are associated with myotonic dystrophy?

    A. Cardiac arrhythmias
    B. Hypogonadism
    C. Insulin-dependent diabetes
    D. Mental retardation
    E. All of the above

37. All of the following are true of primary central nervous system (CNS) lymphoma *except*:

    A. Increasing incidence in the immunocompromised
    B. Increasing incidence in the immunocompetent
    C. Primarily B cell
    D. Primarily T cell

38. A 65-year-old patient presented initially with focal motor seizures. Cranial MRI with gadolinium enhancement demonstrates a homogeneously enhancing extra-axial mass. What tumor is most likely?

    A. Glioblastoma multiforme
    B. Meningioma
    C. Oligodendroglioma
    D. Primary CNS lymphoma

39. Remote effects of small cell lung cancer on the nervous system include all of the following *except*:

    A. Limbic encephalitis
    B. Eaton-Lambert myasthenic syndrome
    C. Sensory neuronopathy
    D. Stroke

40. Which of the following statements concerning carcinomatous meningitis is *incorrect*?

    A. Protein concentration in CSF is elevated.
    B. Glucose concentration in CSF is elevated.
    C. Cranial neuropathies are common.
    D. CSF cell count is elevated.

41. A 75-year-old man with an 8-year history of chronic lymphocytic leukemia presents to your office complaining of difficulty with his vision over the past 3 weeks. His medical history is otherwise unremarkable. He has been on intermittent chemotherapy for the past 3 years. Physical examination reveals a left homonymous hemianopia. The patient's cranial MRI with contrast medium enhancement demonstrates a nonenhancing lesion in the parieto-occipital white matter. What is the most likely diagnosis?

    A. Multiple sclerosis
    B. Carcinomatous meningitis
    C. Progressive multifocal leukoencephalopathy
    D. Metastatic disease

42. Which of the following is the most common neurotoxicity of methotrexate chemotherapy?

    A. Leukoencephalopathy
    B. Peripheral neuropathy
    C. Myeloradiculopathy
    D. Cerebellar toxicity

43. A 55-year-old woman presents with complaints of midthoracic back pain over the past several months. The pain is constant, dull, and without radiation. Over the past month, she has noticed numbness beginning first in the feet and now extending up to her abdomen. Within the past week, she has experienced difficulty with walking. Her medical history is unremarkable, and her only medication is hormonal replacement. Physical examination reveals a T6 sensory level with increased tone and brisk reflexes in the lower extremities. Babinski signs are present bilaterally. Rectal examination is normal. Which of the following statements is *correct*?

    A. The most likely cause of cord compression is an intramedullary tumor such as an astrocytoma.
    B. Intradural, extramedullary tumors such as meningioma or neurofibroma are the most common cause of cord compression in women of this age group.
    C. Extradural tumors, which may cause cord compression, are typically benign.
    D. Metastatic disease to the cord is typically intramedullary.

44. A 63-year-old man is brought to the hospital by his family, who report that he became confused for 4 hours and was unable to remember where he was. During the episode, he knew who he was and had normal speech and reasoning power. Examination now is normal except the patient is amnestic for the last 12 hours. What is the most likely diagnosis?

    A. Complex partial seizure
    B. Vertebrobasilar insufficiency
    C. Korsakoff's amnesia
    D. Transient global amnesia
    E. Alzheimer's disease

45. Neurologic complications of HIV infection include all of the following *except*:

    A. Dementia
    B. Peripheral neuropathy
    C. Myopathy
    D. Motor neuron disease

46. Which of the following primary tumors is *least* likely to metastasize to the CNS?

    A. Lung
    B. Breast
    C. Melanoma
    D. Prostate

47. Which of the following statements concerning the differentiation of radiation-induced from carcinomatous brachial plexopathy is *correct*?

    A. Radiation-induced brachial plexopathy is typically painful.
    B. Carcinomatous brachial plexopathy is typically painful.
    C. Radiation-induced brachial plexopathy is primarily sensory impairment.
    D. Carcinomatous brachial plexopathy is primarily motor impairment.

48. A 70-year-old man with a history of hypertension and diabetes presents with numbness to the right face, arm, and leg without motor abnormalities. The most likely location for his stroke is:

    A. Left thalamus
    B. Left middle cerebral artery
    C. Left cerebellar hemisphere
    D. Left frontal cortex

49. Hypertensive hemorrhage occurs most commonly in:

    A. Frontal lobe
    B. Cerebellum
    C. Basal ganglia
    D. Pons

50. The North American Symptomatic Carotid Endarterectomy Trial (NASCET) recommends carotid endarterectomy for carotid artery:

A. Symptomatic stenosis greater than 50%
B. Asymptomatic stenosis greater than 66%
C. Symptomatic stenosis greater than 70%
D. Complete occlusion

51. The most likely cause of a lobar hemorrhage in a 86-year-old woman with a history of dementia is:

A. Hypertension
B. Aneurysm
C. Head trauma
D. Amyloid angiopathy

52. A 73-year-old man presents with complaints of headache, malaise, and weight loss over the past 2 months. For the past 3 weeks, he has noted right-sided jaw pain. His medical history is remarkable for hypertension. Physical examination reveals no focal neurologic findings. Laboratory studies are remarkable for an erythrocyte sedimentation rate of 55 mm/hr. Which of the following is indicated?

A. Cranial MRI with magnetic resonance angiography
B. Treatment with corticosteroids
C. Cerebral arteriogram
D. Analgesic medications and antiplatelet therapy

53. Which of the following is not a characteristic typical of narcolepsy?

A. Cataplexy
B. Hypnagogic hallucinations
C. Nocturnal breath cessation
D. Sleep paralysis

54. A 55-year-old woman presents with complaints of double vision over the past 2 days. Her medical history is remarkable for insulin-dependent diabetes. On examination the right eye is looking down and out with a reactive pupil. What is the most likely explanation for her visual deficit?

A. The right third nerve is compressed secondary to an aneurysm.
B. This is a complication of diabetes.
C. The right sixth nerve is compressed secondary to herniation.
D. She has suffered a midbrain stroke.

55. Of the following vascular malformations, which is composed of arteries connecting directly to veins?

A. Venous angioma
B. Telangiectasia
C. Cavernous angioma
D. Arteriovenous malformation (AVM)

56. Which of the following neurons is most vulnerable to ischemia?

A. Hippocampal
B. Cerebellar
C. Striatum
D. Neocortex

57. The following are definite risk factors for stroke except:

A. Hypertension
B. Male gender
C. Smoking
D. Obesity

58. Which of the following antiepileptic drugs is not metabolized by the hepatic system?

A. Phenytoin (Dilantin)
B. Carbamazepine
C. Gabapentin
D. Valproic acid

59. A 60-year-old man is brought to the emergency department by his family for an uncontrolled seizure. They report the onset of generalized tonic-clonic activity about 40 minutes ago. You find the patient in continuous seizure activity. The least appropriate medication would be

A. Lorazepam IV
B. Fosphenytoin intramuscularly
C. Diazepam rectally
D. Valproic acid IV

60. The management of epilepsy in females of reproductive age should include all of the following except:

A. Anticonvulsant appropriate for seizure type
B. Supplementation with folate
C. Birth control
D. Tapering of anticonvulsants before pregnancy

61. A 38-year-old woman with a history of seizures for the past 5 years after head trauma presents with increasing seizure frequency. Her seizures have previously been well controlled. She reports weekly episodes of déjà-vu feelings and a generalized tonic-clonic seizure for each of the past 3 months. Currently, her medication is phenytoin, 300 mg, at bedtime. She is experiencing no side effects. A serum phenytoin level is 16 mcg/mL. The most appropriate intervention is:

A. Change to phenobarbital.
B. Add carbamazepine.
C. Repeat EEG and MRI.
D. Increase phenytoin dose.

62. The drug of choice for primary generalized seizures is:

A. Phenytoin
B. Carbamazepine
C. Valproic acid
D. Gabapentin

63. Which of the following statements concerning febrile seizures of childhood is correct?

A. Seizures typically last longer than 10 minutes.
B. Focal abnormalities during or after the seizure are common.
C. The syndrome is benign, although 5% will experience seizures without fever.
D. An abnormal neurologic examination or mental status change may be a presenting factor.

64. You evaluate a 33-year-old man with a several-year history of tonic-clonic seizures. During the history, the patient's wife reports episodes of blank staring with smacking of his lips and picking at his shirt. These last several minutes and occasionally are followed by a generalized tonic-clonic seizure. After these events, he is unable to speak and appears confused. The patient reports that before these episodes he has a rising feeling in his stomach. As a child, the patient had several seizures with high temperatures. Which of the following best describes this patient?

A. Complex partial seizure with temporal lobe onset
B. Epilepsia partialis continua
C. Rolandic epilepsy
D. Atypical absence

65. Which of the following side effects is associated with carbamazepine use?

A. Hirsutism
B. Alopecia
C. Syndrome of inappropriate antidiuretic hormone
D. Congestive heart failure

66. Which of the following statements concerning the EEG is correct?

    A. A normal study effectively rules out a seizure disorder.
    B. A pattern of slow spike and waves is frequently seen in metabolic encephalopathies.
    C. It is a scalp measure of summated neuronal membrane potentials.
    D. An EEG is required to establish brain death.

67. The most common cause of partial or generalized epilepsy in the elderly is:

    A. Brain tumor
    B. Stroke
    C. Infection
    D. Trauma

68. Tuberculosis meningitis is associated with which of the following?

    A. Serum hyponatremia
    B. Low CSF glucose
    C. Low CSF protein
    D. Albuminocytologic disassociation

TRUE OR FALSE
QUESTIONS 69-85

DIRECTIONS: Answer each question as either true or false. Any combination of answers, from all true to all false, is possible:

69. The CSF abnormalities commonly seen in pseudotumor cerebri include which of the following?

    A. Xanthochromia
    B. Low glucose
    C. 10 to 20 lymphocytes/mm^3
    D. Elevated opening pressure

70. Which of the following administration route(s) of phenytoin is/are contraindicated in a patient in status epilepticus?

    A. Intramuscular
    B. Intravenous in 5% dextrose in water
    C. Oral load of 300 mg
    D. Intravenous in normal saline

71. MRI is a useful adjunct in MS diagnosis and frequently shows:

    A. Hydrocephalus
    B. Increased signal in the white matter on T_2 images *diffusely*
    C. Focal increases in T_2 signal intensity in the periventricular white matter
    D. Petechial hemorrhage surrounding MS "plaques"

72. Clinical symptoms suggestive of the Lewy body variant of Alzheimer's disease include:

    A. Visual hallucinations early in the illness
    B. A classic parkinsonian rest tremor
    C. Rigidity
    D. Pronounced sensitivity to neuroleptics

73. A 34-year-old patient is admitted with acute Guillain-Barré syndrome. Which of the following statements is/are *true* concerning this syndrome?

    A. Autonomic instability is a frequent cause of mortality.
    B. Respiratory failure rarely occurs.
    C. Patients usually are flexic.
    D. Nerve conduction studies typically demonstrate an axonal neuropathy.

74. Mandatory criteria for brain death include which of the following?

    A. Absent pupillary response to light
    B. Absent gag reflex
    C. Absent oculovestibular response to cold water caloric testing
    D. Absent spinal reflexes

75. Features that may help distinguish a frontotemporal dementia from a case of Alzheimer's disease include:

    A. Hyperorality
    B. Early change in personality (more passive)
    C. Increased attention to personal hygiene
    D. Expressive language difficulties

76. Glossopharyngeal neuralgia can be characterized by which of the following?

    A. Lancinating pain in the posterior pharynx
    B. Association with head and neck tumors
    C. Pain triggered by touching posterior auricular area
    D. Can be associated with cardiac arrest
    E. Does not usually respond to carbamazepine

77. The classic symptoms associated with the lower motor neuron dysfunction include which of the following?

    A. Muscle atrophy
    B. Fasciculations
    C. Hypertonia
    D. Weakness

78. A 16-year-old girl presents with a brief spell characterized by a sudden onset of staring and smacking movements of the mouth. Which of the following seizure disorders can be described like this?

    A. Generalized tonic-clonic seizure
    B. Absence seizure
    C. Myoclonic seizure
    D. Complex partial seizure

79. Treatments demonstrated to be effective for some patients with Guillain-Barré syndrome include:

    A. High-dose IV corticosteroids
    B. IV IgG infusions
    C. Plasma exchange cyclophosphamide

80. Concerning treatment of focal brain ischemia, which of the following statements is/are *true*?

    A. A patient with a blood pressure of 190/100 mm Hg who presents with an acute stroke should be treated aggressively with an antihypertensive medication.
    B. Embolic strokes are more likely to become hemorrhagic than thrombotic strokes.
    C. Carotid endarterectomy has been proven more useful than medical therapy in a patient with recent transient ischemic attack and 80% ipsilateral carotid stenosis.

81. Features that should suggest consideration of motor neuron disease (i.e., Lou Gehrig's disease, amyotrophic lateral sclerosis [ALS]) include:

    A. Lower motor neuron findings in the arms with upper motor neuron findings in the legs
    B. Upper and lower motor neuron findings in both the arms and legs
    C. Swallowing difficulties with tongue fasciculations and atrophy
    D. Isolated fasciculations and increased reflexes with normal strength

82. Which of the following can occasionally masquerade as a motor neuron disease?

    A. Lead poisoning
    B. Leprosy
    C. Waldenström's macroglobulinemia
    D. Cervical and lumbar spondylosis

83. Sensory neuropathies, such as those commonly seen with diabetes, are mixed sensory and motor and are associated with dysesthetic feelings that are frequently maximal in the feet. Which of the following are potential therapeutic options?

    A. Amitriptyline
    B. Carbamazepine
    C. Capsaicin
    D. Mexiletine

84. A 58-year-old man presents to the clinic complaining of several months of increasing weakness and fatigue. He denies visual changes or trouble with speech or swallowing. He does report a dry mouth and dizziness on standing. His medical history is unremarkable. The patient has a 50-pack-year history of tobacco abuse but no alcohol use. He takes no medications. Neurologic examination reveals normal mental status and cranial nerve function. Motor examination is remarkable for primarily proximal weakness, which improves with repetition. Sensory examination is normal. Deep tendon reflexes are absent. Which of the following statements is *correct*?

    A. This syndrome is associated with a thymoma.
    B. Electromyography (EMG) would demonstrate a decremental response.
    C. Autoantibodies to calcium channels may be present.
    D. Anticholinesterases are very effective.

85. Which of the following statements is *correct*?

    A. Myopathies typically involve proximal muscles, and neuropathies involve distal muscles.
    B. Muscle atrophy is early and prominent in myopathies and late and mild in neuropathies.
    C. Sensory loss is present in neuropathies and absent in myopathies.
    D. Reflexes are lost early in neuropathies and late in myopathies.

MATCHING

DIRECTIONS: Questions 86-95 are matching questions. For each numbered item, choose the most likely associated lettered item from those provided. Each item has *only one* answer.

QUESTIONS 86-90

Match the following clinical syndrome to a vascular distribution:

    A. Left posterior cerebral artery
    B. Vertebral artery
    C. Lenticulostriate vessels
    D. Right anterior cerebral artery
    E. Left middle cerebral artery

86. Pure motor syndrome

87. Wallenberg's syndrome

88. Right arm/face weak and numb with expressive aphasia

89. Alexia without agraphia

90. Left leg weakness

QUESTIONS 91-95

Match the visual field deficits with the most appropriate anatomic location.

    A. Homonymous hemianopsia with macular sparing
    B. Homonymous hemianopsia without macular sparing
    C. Monocular visual loss
    D. Homonymous superior quadrantanopia
    E. Bitemporal hemianopsia

91. Optic nerve

92. Optic chiasm

93. Lateral geniculate nucleus

94. Unilateral temporal lobe

95. Unilateral occipital lobe

MULTIPLE CHOICE

DIRECTIONS: Select the single best answer for each question.

96. A 50-year-old successful businessman is seen with his extremely anxious spouse. She complains of the acute decline in her husband's cognitive function. This is associated with changes in his sleep pattern and sexual drive. The memory decline has been progressive over the past 6 weeks. Your examination reveals the patient to be demented with myoclonus that is aggravated by auditory startle. He is ataxic and hyperreflexic with bilateral extensor plantar reflexes. Which of the following ancillary tests is most helpful?

    A. MRI of the brain
    B. An EEG that demonstrates periodic complexes.
    C. CSF test for 14-3-3 protein that is negative.
    D. Peripheral muscle biopsy

97. A 75-year-old woman presents with complaints of difficulty with walking and numbness to the extremities. She remarks that symptoms seem worse at night or when she closes her eyes. On examination she has a sensory ataxia, is hyperreflexic, and has marked proprioceptive loss. Your laboratory studies demonstrate a mild megaloblastic anemia. Which of the following would confirm your suspicion of a cobalamin (vitamin B_{12}) deficiency?

    A. Folic acid
    B. Methylmalonic acid
    C. Thiamine
    D. Pyridoxine

98. Patients with Von Hippel-Lindau disease are at increased risk for which malignancies?

    A. Small cell lung cancer
    B. Breast cancer
    C. Renal cell carcinoma
    D. Melanoma

Part XII
Neurology
Answers

1. **(B)** *Discussion:* CSF changes are a major clue to CNS disease. In general, few primary viral infections lower the CSF glucose value, and a low CSF glucose concentration should make one consider other causes. *(Cecil, Ch. 423)*

2. **(C)** *Discussion:* Myasthenia gravis is a disorder of weakness secondary to a defect of neuromuscular transmission that occurs because of autoantibodies that induce acetylcholine receptor depletion at the motor end plate. It presents as fatigable weakness of the voluntary muscles. The eye muscles are the most frequently involved, but the proximal limb and bulbar muscles are also affected in many patients. The diagnosis is confirmed by demonstrating an increased titer of acetylcholine receptor antibody, an abnormal decremental response to repetitive nerve stimulation, and increased strength with anticholinesterase medications (Tensilon test). *(Cecil, Ch. 464)*

3. **(E)** *Discussion:* No laboratory tests (CSF or otherwise) are specific for MS. Suggestive findings include a mild increase in WBCs and protein and a normal glucose value. Oligoclonal bands are often positive, and there is typically increased intrathecal production of IgG. This combination can be seen in other disorders. *(Cecil, Ch. 448)*

4. **(D)** *Discussion:* Subarachnoid hemorrhage frequently presents as severe headache followed by progressive obtundation and neck stiffness. Subhyaloid hemorrhages are retinal hemorrhages that are frequently associated with subarachnoid hemorrhage. Other ocular signs seen include preretinal hemorrhages and papilledema. *(Cecil, Ch. 441)*

5. **(B)** *Discussion:* Interferon-β1b and interferon-β1a have similar side effects and include all those listed except for an altered serum sodium. Copolymer 1 can cause injection site reactions but not depression or liver abnormalities. All three medications are used for treating MS, and none has been proved superior to the others. *(Cecil, Ch. 448)*

6. **(E)** *Discussion:* Conductive aphasia occurs with a lesion in the dominant supramarginal gyrus and is characterized by a deficit in repetition without a loss in fluency or understanding. Wernicke's or sensory aphasia is characterized by fluent speech with deficits in comprehension and repetition. Broca's or motor aphasia is characterized by a loss of fluency and repetition but intact comprehension. Transcortical motor and sensory aphasia are similar to motor and sensory aphasia but repetition is spared. *(Cecil, Ch. 439)*

7. **(A)** *Discussion:* One of the most treatable conditions that can masquerade as a dementia is depression. Frequent clues that depression may be a significant contributor to a dementia are patient's self-referral, an uncooperative mental status examination in which the patient states that he does not know the answers rather than give incorrect responses, and the admission of dysphoria on direct questioning. When in doubt between Alzheimer's disease and depression, a therapeutic trial of an antidepressant may be appropriate. *(Cecil, Ch. 433)*

8. **(A)** *Discussion:* This patient most likely suffers from Wernicke's aphasia, which is a fluent aphasia with loss of comprehension. Although speech is fluent, the patient's well-formed verbal messages are not intelligible. This is frequently interpreted as "confusion." Because of the loss of verbal comprehension, the patient does not realize the deficit. This aphasia occurs with lesions of the posterior and superior temporal lobe. Wernike's aphasia frequently presents without other neurologic signs, unlike Broca's aphasia (dominant frontal lobe), which is frequently associated with contralateral hemiparesis. *(Cecil, Chs. 432 and 439)*

9. **(A)** *Discussion:* The routine evaluation for dementia includes a noncontrast CT scan of the brain, serum chemistries, blood cell count, thyroid test, vitamin B_{12} evaluation, and syphilis serology. Other tests are done in special circumstances. An EEG is not a routine part of an uncomplicated dementia evaluation. If either seizures or a prion disease is suspected, the EEG may prove a useful adjunct. *(Cecil, Ch. 433)*

10. **(D)** *Discussion:* This patient most likely suffers from trigeminal neuralgia, which is a facial pain that is brief, intense, and lancinating. The pain is located in one of the trigeminal nerve branch distributions and can be triggered by touch, talking, or eating. In the idiopathic type, the neurologic examination is normal. Treatment options include carbamazepine (drug of choice), baclofen (Lioresal), phenytoin (less responsive than carbamazepine), and surgery, including gasserian ganglion lesioning. If sensory loss or other abnormality is noted on examination, a search for a structural lesion in the brain stem or along the nerve should be performed. *(Cecil, Ch. 427)*

11. **(C)** *Discussion:* When Parkinson's disease is associated in a causative way with a dementia, it is almost always after the motor symptoms have been present for quite some time and have advanced to a significant degree. *(Cecil, Ch. 443)*

12. **(D)** *Discussion:* Studies have shown that resection of the tumor is the best treatment for most patients with a solitary cerebral metastasis, especially in non–small cell lung cancer. This has resulted in protracted remission for many patients, especially if the lung cancer is resected as well. *(Cecil, Ch. 457)*

13. **(B)** *Discussion:* Diabetic third nerve lesions are frequently pupil sparing. The pupil is almost always involved in a compressive third nerve lesion. Both can be subacute. Lateral eye movements are not supported by the third nerve and would be normal in both circumstances. Both conditions can cause unilateral third nerve palsies. *(Cecil, Ch. 440)*

14. **(C)** *Discussion:* A vegetative state is a condition of altered consciousness in which autonomic function remains intact, including the sleep/wake cycle, but there is complete loss of cognition. This condition can occur with acute, severe bilateral cerebral damage or can develop as the end stage of a dementia. *(Cecil, Chs. 437 and 438)*

15. **(B)** *Discussion:* The combination of headache, fever, and mental status change is a neurologic emergency. The differential diagnosis includes meningitis and subarachnoid hemorrhage. If the neurologic examination is nonfocal and cranial imaging is without mass effect or hydrocephalus, a LP may be performed before the administration of antibiotics. If cranial imaging is not available, a LP may be performed in the presence of a nonfocal neurologic examination and absence of papilledema. If focal findings or papilledema are present, antibiotics should be administered before transport to a facility with cranial imaging capabilities. Under no circumstances should antibiotics be withheld in suspected meningitis to await cranial imaging. *(Cecil, Ch. 423)*

16. **(D)** *Discussion:* A completely normal EEG in an unconscious patient rules out organic causes of unresponsiveness. *(Cecil, Ch. 436)*

17. **(A)** *Discussion:* Cluster headaches are more common in men and migraines more common in women. Cluster headaches are short, intense unilateral headaches that occur in clusters lasting several weeks. Attacks may be associated with rhinorrhea and ipsilateral Horner's syndrome. Migraines are recurrent headaches that are often severe, begin unilaterally, and are associated with malaise, nausea, vomiting, photophobia, and phonophobia. *(Cecil, Ch. 428)*

18. **(C)** *Discussion:* The best initial treatment for biopsy-proven temporal arteritis is high-dose prednisone. Failure to treat can result in blindness secondary to occlusion of the retinal arteries. *(Cecil, Ch. 440)*

19. **(A)** *Discussion:* Migraine prophylaxis may be of benefit in headache patients with a high frequency of migraine headaches. Medications typically used for prophylaxis include tricyclic antidepressants, β-blockers, calcium-channel blockers, and valproic acid. Medications used for abortive therapy include triptans, ergotamines, and combination medications such as Cafergot. *(Cecil, Ch. 428)*

20. **(D)** *Discussion:* Wernicke-Korsakoff syndrome is characterized by the classic triad of ophthalmoplegia, gait disorder, and confusion; it occurs as a result of thiamine (vitamin B_1) deficiency. Thiamine deficiency is frequently found in alcoholics. *(Cecil, Chs. 433 and 458)*

21. **(C)** *Discussion:* Ten to 15% of patients with parkinsonism have more widespread involvement and are considered Parkinson-plus syndromes. Complaints of orthostatic symptoms, incontinence, sexual impotence, and other autonomic symptoms are present in the Shy-Drager variant. *(Cecil, Ch. 443)*

22. **(D)** *Discussion:* Amyotrophic lateral sclerosis is a degenerative disorder characterized by progressive motor neuron loss. Both upper and lower motor neurons are affected, giving a mixed clinical picture of fasciculations and atrophy (lower motor neuron loss) with increased reflexes and Babinski response (upper motor neuron loss). Electrophysiologic studies reveal no abnormalities in the sensory nerves, no significant nerve conduction slowing as seen in neuropathies, and diffuse denervation on needle EMG. *(Cecil, Ch. 447)*

23. **(A)** *Discussion:* Tourette's syndrome is a genetic disorder manifest by tics and a variety of behavioral features. Motor as well as phonic tics are present. Many patients also display features of obsessive-compulsive disorder. *(Cecil, Ch. 459)*

24. **(A)** *Discussion:* Dystonia, parkinsonism, and akathisia are acute movement disorders that may be associated with neuroleptic use. Tardive dyskinesia is a chronic movement disorder seen with neuroleptic use. *(Cecil, Ch. 444)*

25. **(D)** *Discussion:* Management of the side effects of levodopa therapy is a challenging aspect to the treatment of Parkinson's dis-

ease. Common central side effects include psychiatric problems, dyskinesias, and clinical fluctuations. The wearing-off effect is a clinical fluctuation characterized by a return of parkinsonian symptoms resulting from a shorter duration of action of a given dose of levadopa. Anticholinergic side effects such as dry mouth, urinary retention, and constipation are seen with tricyclic antidepressants, which may be used to treat the depression associated with Parkinson's disease. *(Cecil, Ch. 443)*

26. **(B)** *Discussion:* The most common etiology of acquired myopathy during adulthood is inflammatory myopathy (polymyositis, dermatomyositis, inclusion body myopathy). Of these, inclusion body myopathy is extremely rare. It presents as progressive weakness and atrophy with a predilection for the forearm and quadriceps muscles and is poorly responsive to therapy. Polymyositis presents as proximal weakness and in some patients produces myalgias. Dermatomyositis presents like polymyositis but is accompanied by a characteristic rash. Diagnostic evaluation should include electrophysiologic studies, which will reveal small-amplitude and short-duration motor unit potentials as seen in myopathy. Muscle biopsy reveals perivascular and endomysial collections of inflammatory cells and muscle fiber necrosis. *(Cecil, Ch. 463)*

27. **(B)** *Discussion:* Friedreich's ataxia is a familial progressive ataxia inherited in either an autosomal-dominant or an autosomal-recessive pattern. Pes cavus and kyphoscoliosis precede the neurologic symptoms. The initial neurologic symptom is almost always ataxia of gait. Action and intention tremors follow. Mentation is preserved. Tendon reflexes are absent, and plantar responses are extensor. Pathologically, there is degeneration of the dorsal columns, corticospinal tracts, and spinocerebellar tracts. The cause is unknown. *(Cecil, Ch. 446)*

28. **(C)** *Discussion:* Multiple sclerosis is a disorder of central demyelination of unknown etiology but is likely immune mediated. Patients are generally 20 to 45 years old at disease onset and develop relapsing and remitting or chronic progressive focal neurologic signs. Cranial MRI reveals multiple, hyperintense white matter lesions with a predilection for the periventricular regions and corpus callosum. Areas of active inflammation may enhance after the administration of a contrast agent. The MRI findings are not specific for the diagnosis, but, given the age of the patient, the clinical scenario, and the previous history of what was most likely optic neuritis, the most likely diagnosis for this patient is multiple sclerosis. *(Cecil, Ch. 448)*

29. **(D)** *Discussion:* The congenital myopathies are characterized by a nonprogressive course, distinct pattern of inheritance, normal muscle bulk, normal creatine kinase levels, and muscle weakness present from birth or early childhood. Examples include central core disease, nemaline rod myopathy, myotubular myopathy, multicore disease, and fiber-type disproportion. Duchenne's dystrophy is a muscular dystrophy. Muscular dystrophies are characterized by inherited pattern, progressive muscle weakness, destruction and regeneration of muscle, and eventual replacement by fibrous tissue. *(Cecil, Ch. 463)*

30. **(B)** *Discussion:* Dermatomyositis and polymyositis resemble each other clinically as proximal muscle weakness, inflammatory exudates in muscle, myopathic potentials on EMG, and responsiveness to corticosteroids. Dermatomyositis is B-cell mediated against endothelial antigens, resulting in capillary destruction and necrosis. Polymyositis is T-cell mediated against muscle fiber antigens. *(Cecil, Ch. 463)*

31. **(E)** *Discussion:* Inclusion body myositis is one of the inflammatory myopathies. It differs from polymyositis and dermatomyositis in that it does not have an autoimmune cause and does not respond to corticosteroids. Clinically, most patients are older

than 50 years, with a male predominance. Lower limbs are affected first with slow involvement proximally. Cervical, facial, and pharyngeal muscles are not involved. Electrophysiologic studies may also reveal a neurogenic component, and muscle biopsy demonstrates rimmed vacuoles. (*Cecil, Ch. 463*)

32. **(C)** *Discussion:* Ragged red fibers on muscle biopsy indicate mitochondrial myopathy. Ragged red fibers are also seen in azathioprine-related myopathy but not HIV myopathy. (*Cecil, Ch. 463*)

33. **(C)** *Discussion:* Malignant hyperthermia is an autosomal-dominant disorder in which exposure to inhalation anesthetics or succinylcholine triggers an uncontrolled release of calcium from the sarcoplasmic reticulum. Clinical signs include tachycardia, tachypnea, cyanosis, rising temperature, rigidity, and unstable blood pressure. Supportive care includes body cooling, hydration, mechanical ventilation, and diuretics to ensure urine flow. Specific therapy includes dantrolene, 1 to 2 mg/kg IV. (*Cecil, Ch. 463*)

34. **(D)** *Discussion:* Reflex sympathetic dystrophy is a pain disorder characterized by burning, hyperpathic pain associated with autonomic changes, vasomotor instability, and osteoporosis. It frequently follows a trivial trauma and, unless associated with a nerve lesion, the routine electrophysiologic studies are normal. It is believed to be secondary to dysfunction in the autonomic nervous system. It is best treated with sympathetic blockade. (*Cecil, Ch. 427*)

35. **(A)** *Discussion:* Metabolic myopathies such as those caused by glycolytic enzyme defects share common features, including muscle cramps and myoglobinuria after strenuous exertion. A venous lactate level that fails to rise after ischemic exercise is seen in myophosphorylase and phosphofructokinase deficiency. (*Cecil, Ch. 463*)

36. **(E)** *Discussion:* Myotonic dystrophy is transmitted in an autosomal-dominant pattern, with the defective gene residing on the long arm of chromosome 19. The genetic defect is one of trinucleotide repeats. Clinically, patients have weakness, myotonia, and multisystem abnormalities. The systemic abnormalities include cataracts, testicular atrophy, end-organ unresponsiveness to insulin, mental retardation, and cardiac conduction defects. (*Cecil, Ch. 463*)

37. **(D)** *Discussion:* The incidence of primary CNS lymphoma is increasing in both the immunocompromised as well as the competent groups. These tumors are predominantly B-cell phenotype. Radiographically, they have a predilection for the periventricular white matter and may cross the corpus callosum to the opposite hemisphere. (*Cecil, Ch. 457*)

38. **(B)** *Discussion:* Meningiomas are formed from fibroblast-like cells of the dura that are typically attached to the dura of the sphenoidal sinus, sagittal sinus, or cerebral convexities. An enhancing lesion attached to the dura is an extra-axial lesion consistent with meningioma. The tumors are usually benign and slow growing. All the other choices are intra-axial tumors. (*Cecil, Ch. 457*)

39. **(D)** *Discussion:* Paraneoplastic or remote effects of cancer on the CNS are neurologic disorders not caused by local invasion of the CNS by tumor. The cause is believed to be autoimmune, in which the immune system is sensitized to neural antigens presented by the tumor cells. Clinical syndromes include limbic encephalitis, sensory neuronopathy, Eaton-Lambert myasthenic syndrome, and cerebellar ataxia.

40. **(B)** *Discussion:* Carcinomatous meningitis is due to infiltration of the subarachnoid space by neoplastic cells. Malignancies with a tendency to cause meningitis include breast cancer, lymphoma, and melanoma. Clinically, patients often present with cranial neuropathies. CSF examination reveals elevated protein with

depressed glucose. Cell count is typically elevated. Repeated evaluation of CSF with cytology and/or flow cytometry using tumor markers is often diagnostic. (*Cecil, Chs. 423 and 457*)

41. **(C)** *Discussion:* Progressive multifocal leukoencephalopathy (PML) is a white matter disease caused by JC virus infection of oligodendroglia. Progressive multifocal leukoencephalopathy is seen in patients who are chronically immunosuppressed. Clinically, progressive multifocal leukoencephalopathy presents as focal neurologic signs. CSF examination is typically normal. MRI reveals hyperintense T2-weighted signal and hypointense T1-weighted signal. The lesions are nonenhancing, which differentiates PML from other infectious processes (toxoplasmosis) and neoplastic processes seen in the immunosuppressed. The lesions of PML have a tendency to occur in the parieto-occipital white matter. (*Cecil, Ch. 455*)

42. **(A)** *Discussion:* Leukoencephalopathy is the most common and serious neurotoxicity associated with methotrexate. The toxicity develops months to years after administration. The greatest risk is in patients who receive cranial irradiation before chemotherapy. Clinically, patients exhibit cognitive dysfunction and focal neurologic signs, which may progress to dementia, coma, and death. There is no treatment. (*Cecil, Ch. 448*)

43. **(B)** *Discussion:* The patient's clinical syndrome is consistent with a myelopathy. A cause of myelopathy is spinal cord compression from a tumor. The most common tumors to cause cord compression in a patient without known cancer are meningiomas or neurofibromas. These tumors are intradural and extramedullary. Intramedullary tumors, such as astrocytoma and ependymoma, are less common causes of cord compression. Metastatic disease leading to cord compression is typically extradural. Spinal cord compression is a neurologic emergency requiring prompt diagnosis and initiation of treatment. The imaging modality of choice is MRI. Immediate therapy with high-dose dexamethasone (100-mg bolus followed by 24 mg every 6 hours) is recommended pending tissue diagnosis. (*Cecil, Chs. 430 and 457*)

44. **(D)** *Discussion:* Transient global amnesia is a self-limited, isolated memory disorder in which reasoning, attention, and language are unaffected. The patient is disoriented and distressed and frequently asks what is going on. These episodes typically last several hours, leave no impairment, and generally do not recur. The etiology is unclear, but they may be secondary to transient vascular insufficiency. The differential diagnosis includes complex partial seizures, but patients with seizures usually have an alteration of attention. (*Cecil, Ch. 440*)

45. **(C)** *Discussion:* HIV results in many neurologic complications. Risk for neurologic complications is greater with advanced disease and low CD4 counts. The common complications include AIDS dementia complex, peripheral neuropathy, myopathy, and myelopathy. AIDS dementia complex is characterized by cognitive decline, motor dysfunction, and behavioral changes. Peripheral neuropathies common to HIV infection include distal sensory neuropathy, demyelinating motor neuropathy, mononeuritis multiplex, and cytomegalovirus-associated neuropathy. Neuropathies may also be secondary to reverse transcriptase inhibitors such as zidovudine, didanosine, and zalcitabine. Myopathy from either HIV infection itself or from azathioprine-induced mitochondrial myopathy may also be seen. (*Cecil, Ch. 450*)

46. **(D)** *Discussion:* Prostate cancer may metastasize to the skull; however, it is unlikely to spread to brain parenchyma. The most common tumors to metastasize to the brain are the lung in males and the breast in females. Other tumors that may metastasize to the brain include thyroid cancer, melanoma, and gastrointestinal cancer. (*Cecil, Ch. 457*)

47. **(B)** *Discussion:* Clinical signs and symptoms may help in the differentiation of radiation-induced brachial plexopathy from that caused by carcinomatous infiltration. Brachial plexopathy secondary to radiation injury is typically painless and primarily affects motor function. The component of the plexus involved is dependent on the radiation ports. In brachial plexopathy secondary to carcinomatous infiltration, the lower plexus (C8, T1) is primarily affected. The plexopathy is painful and primarily sensory. *(Cecil, Ch. 461)*

48. **(A)** *Discussion:* A pure sensory deficit is a recognized lacunar syndrome typically involving an infarction in the thalamus. Patients at risk for lacunar disease are those with poorly controlled diabetes and/or hypertension. The disease process typically involves lipohyalinization of the media of the small penetrating vessels, which supply much of the diencephalon. *(Cecil, Ch. 440)*

49. **(C)** *Discussion:* The most common location for hypertensive hemorrhage is the basal ganglia (approximately 50%), followed by the pons, cerebellum, and thalamus. Cortical hemorrhages are not due to hypertension but to vascular malformations, amyloid angiopathy, or trauma. *(Cecil, Ch. 441)*

50. **(C)** *Discussion:* Two randomized, controlled trials, the NASCET and the European Carotid Surgery Trial, showed that treatment of symptomatic carotid stenosis of 70% or greater by carotid endarterectomy resulted in a significant reduction in subsequent strokes compared with medical treatment. *(Cecil, Ch. 440)*

51. **(D)** *Discussion:* Amyloid angiopathy is a likely cause of lobar hemorrhage in an elderly demented patient. Less common causes of lobar hemorrhage are vascular malformation, tumor, and infection. *(Cecil, Ch. 441)*

52. **(B)** *Discussion:* Temporal arteritis is characterized by a granulomatous vasculitis of medium-sized arteries. It affects predominantly patients older than 60 years, causing constitutional symptoms such as fever, malaise, weight loss, and headache. Tenderness and pain over the temporal arteries and an elevated erythrocyte sedimentation rate are frequently, but not always, present. Typical features with an elevated sedimentation rate dictate the early initiation of corticosteroid therapy because of the high risk of acute ischemic blindness. *(Cecil, Ch. 440)*

53. **(C)** *Discussion:* Narcolepsy is a disorder characterized by excessive daytime sleepiness with sleep attacks and is associated with cataplexy (sudden loss of muscle tone), sleep paralysis (inability to move on initial awakening), and hypnagogic hallucinations (vivid hallucinations that occur during transition from wakefulness to sleep). Sleep studies reveal sleep-onset rapid eye movement and shortened sleep latency. *(Cecil, Ch. 438)*

54. **(B)** *Discussion:* The third cranial nerve exits the brain stem at the level of the ventral midbrain passing between the posterior communicating artery and superior cerebellar artery before entering the cavernous sinus. Parasympathetic fibers responsible for pupillary constriction are located on the periphery of the nerve; motor fibers to the extraocular muscles are located centrally. This arrangement predisposes the parasympathetic fibers to lesions compressing the nerve from the outside, such as aneurysms and tumors. The vascular supply to the third cranial nerve originates from outside of the nerve and penetrates into the center. With diseases such as diabetes and hypertension, these small penetrating vessels are affected, leading to damage to the center of the nerve that supplies the extraocular muscles and sparing the peripheral parasympathetic fibers. *(Cecil, Ch. 440)*

55. **(D)** *Discussion:* Arteriovenous malformations (AVMs) are composed of tangles of arteries connected directly to veins without intervening capillaries. AVMs can be found anywhere in the brain and may produce headaches, seizures, focal neurologic deficits, or intracranial hemorrhage. *(Cecil, Ch. 441)*

56. **(A)** *Discussion:* Transient arrest of the cerebral circulation for periods of a few minutes causes selective necrosis of neurons that are highly vulnerable to ischemia. For unclear reasons, hippocampal neurons are most vulnerable, followed by cerebellar, striatal, and neocortical neurons. Selective injury to these populations of neurons may be manifest clinically by cognitive impairment and/or movement disorders. *(Cecil, Ch. 440)*

57. **(D)** *Discussion:* Definite genetic and lifestyle risk factors for stroke include hypertension, smoking, age, gender, and race. Possible lifestyle or genetic risk factors include cholesterol, diet, obesity, alcohol, and oral contraceptives. *(Cecil, Ch. 440)*

58. **(C)** *Discussion:* Gabapentin is the only choice of drug that is excreted unchanged by the renal system. The other choices undergo hepatic metabolism. Gabapentin is also the only anticonvulsant that is not protein bound. *(Cecil, Ch. 434)*

59. **(D)** *Discussion:* The definition of status epilepticus is a single seizure lasting longer than 10 minutes or multiple seizures without the return to baseline mental status between seizures. Status epilepticus is a neurologic emergency. The frequency is roughly 100,000 to 150,000 cases per year, with an associated 55,000 deaths. Initial management of status epilepticus includes standard measures applicable to any medical emergency. Pharmacologic intervention with benzodiazepines (lorazepam or diazepam) is recommended as initial therapy because of their potent, fast-acting antiseizure effect. Phenytoin or fosphenytoin is useful for providing a prolonged anticonvulsant effect. Fosphenytoin may be given intramuscularly if IV access is difficult. Valproic acid is available in an IV formulation; however, it is not currently recommended for status epilepticus. *(Cecil, Ch. 434)*

60. **(D)** *Discussion:* The management of epilepsy in females of reproductive age requires active participation by both the clinician and patient. Anticonvulsants have well-known teratogenic potential, and this should be discussed with the patient. However, the effects of a maternal seizure on the developing fetus also carry high risk. Anticonvulsant therapy should be directed toward the seizure type and monotherapy if possible. Supplementation with folate is recommended. *(Cecil, Ch. 434)*

61. **(D)** *Discussion:* The correct management of antiepileptic medications in the patient with increasing seizure frequency without medication side effects would be to increase the dose of the current medication. Anticonvulsant medications should be increased until seizures are controlled or the patient experiences side effects or toxicity from the medication. At that point, a second agent may be added or another agent titrated up for monotherapy. *(Cecil, Ch. 434)*

62. **(C)** *Discussion:* The drug of choice for primary generalized seizures is valproic acid. Carbamazepine may actually worsen absence seizures. *(Cecil, Ch. 434)*

63. **(C)** *Discussion:* One or more febrile convulsions occur in 3 to 4% of children between the ages of 6 months and 5 years and consist of brief tonic-clonic generalized seizures. Although they can be recurrent, the syndrome is benign. Features that would discount the diagnosis of benign febrile convulsions are focal findings on examination, seizure lasting longer than 10 minutes, or focal abnormalities during the seizure. *(Cecil, Ch. 434)*

64. **(A)** *Discussion:* The typical complex partial seizure begins with a stare at the time consciousness is impaired. Purposeless movements called automatisms, which include lip smacking, swallowing, and sucking, are also frequent features of complex partial seizures. Complex partial seizures usually last a few seconds to a

few minutes and may be followed by a generalized convulsion. Postictally, the patient is usually confused and aphasias often occur if the dominant-language hemisphere is involved. (Cecil, Ch. 434)

65. (C) Discussion: The syndrome of inappropriate antidiuretic hormone secretion may be precipitated by carbamazepine use. Other side effects of carbamazepine are hepatotoxic reaction and agranulocytosis. Alopecia and weight gain are side effects of valproate therapy. Hirsutism, gingival hyperplasia, and coarsening of features are seen with phenytoin. (Cecil, Ch. 434)

66. (C) Discussion: The EEG is a scalp measure of summated neuronal membrane potentials during a particular recording interval. A normal EEG does not rule out a seizure disorder. It is not required to establish brain death in the absence of brain stem reflexes, medications that may cause coma (barbiturates), and a normal temperature. Spike and slow waves are seen in epilepsies, not metabolic encephalopathies. The EEG pattern of metabolic encephalopathy is typically of generalized slowing, not spike and slow waves. (Cecil, Ch. 434)

67. (B) Discussion: Stroke is the leading cause of new-onset partial or secondarily generalized seizures in the elderly. Partial seizures are rare during acute stroke unless associated with hemorrhage. Completed strokes may develop scar tissue, which can become epileptogenic months to years later. (Cecil, Ch. 440)

68. (A, B) Discussion: The CSF changes of tuberculosis meningitis include an increase in monocytic leukocytes, an elevation of protein level, and a low glucose value. In addition, tuberculosis meningitis commonly causes the syndrome of inappropriate antidiuretic hormone. (Cecil, Ch. 449)

69. (A) False; (B) False; (C) False; (D) True. Discussion: The only abnormality of the CSF in pseudotumor cerebri is an increased opening pressure. (Cecil, Ch. 457)

70. (A) True; (B) True; (C) True; (D) False. Discussion: In status epilepticus, phenytoin should be given intravenously in normal saline or one-half normal saline. Administration in 5% dextrose in water results in precipitation of the drug, and intramuscular administration results in muscle necrosis. Oral loading can be performed by administering 300 mg every 8 hours for 24 hours, but this should not be performed in status epilepticus because of the inability to obtain adequate drug levels quickly. (Cecil, Ch. 434)

71. (A) False; (B) False; (C) True; (D) False. Discussion: The classic MRI of MS is multiple periventricular hyperintensities, often oriented perpendicular to the long access of the lateral ventricle. This pattern may relate to blood vessels with perivascular inflammation (so-called Dawson's fingers). (Cecil, Ch. 448)

72. (A) True; (B) False; (C) True; (D) True. Discussion: Lewy body disease frequently occurs concomitant with Alzheimer's-type disease, although it may rarely (1 to 2% of dementia) occur in isolation. When seen with Alzheimer's disease, the patient may have many of the same cognitive changes of Alzheimer's disease but in general has an increased incidence of early psychiatric problems, including visual hallucinations and parkinsonian symptoms, excluding a Parkinsonian rest tremor. (Cecil, Ch. 433)

73. (A) True; (B) False; (C) False; (D) False. Discussion: Donepezil is one of the new anticholinesterases available for treatment of the cognitive symptoms of Alzheimer's disease. It is well tolerated and is only taken once a day, typically in the evening, to reduce gastrointestinal intolerance. No blood work is required. (Cecil, Ch. 433)

74. (A) True; (B) True; (C) True; (D) False. Discussion: Brain death requires the absence of all cerebral and brain stem function, including the presence of fixed pupils, absent gag reflex, absent oculovestibular response to cold water calorics, presence of apnea

off the ventilator for 10 minutes, and no behavioral response to noxious stimuli above the foramen magnum. Pure spinal reflexes can be seen. The nature and duration of coma must also be known to exclude a possible reversible cause (i.e., hypothermia, drug intoxication). (Cecil, Ch. 436)

75. (A) True; (B) True; (C) False; (D) True. Discussion: Frontotemporal dementias (which include Pick's disease) are distinct from Alzheimer's disease. The tendency of patients to put things in their mouth is very specific for this subset of dementias but is not very sensitive. These patients often experience personality changes and become less attentive to their personal care and cleanliness. As fits their more anterior disease, expressive language problems are more common in the frontotemporal dementias, whereas comprehension deficits are more frequent in Alzheimer's disease. (Cecil, Ch. 433)

76. (A) True; (B) True; (C) False; (D) True; (E) False. Discussion: Glossopharyngeal neuralgia is characterized by a sharp, lancinating pain in the posterior pharynx with radiation toward the jaw or ear, triggered by eating or swallowing. It can be symptomatic of a tumor or other lesion in the posterior pharynx. Because of vagal involvement, some patients have bradycardia and even cardiac arrest associated with an episode. Many patients respond to carbamazepine and baclofen. Others may require transection of the glossopharyngeal nerve roots. (Cecil, Chs. 423 and 427)

77. (A) True; (B) True; (C) False; (D) True. Discussion: In diagnosing motor system disease, it is important to distinguish between upper and lower motor neuron signs. Lower motor neuron findings include muscle atrophy, muscle fasciculations, decreased muscle tone, and muscle weakness. Often, but invariably, these symptoms are more noticeable distally, but it should be noted that in some types of neuropathy proximal weakness of the legs may be the first symptom. (Cecil, Ch. 461)

78. (A) False; (B) True; (C) False; (D) True. Discussion: Both complex partial and absence seizures can present with staring spells and automatic behaviors such as lip smacking. The typical complex partial seizure of temporal lobe origin consists of a stare associated with an alteration of consciousness followed by automatisms, which are repetitive purposeless complex movements. Typical seizures last 1 to 2 minutes. In absence seizures, there is a sudden lapse of awareness; most seizures last less than 30 seconds. Longer absence seizures are associated with automatisms. Most absence seizures occur in children. Unlike complex partial seizures, patients with absence seizures do not have a postictal state. (Cecil, Ch. 434)

79. (A) True; (B) False; (C) True; (D) False. Discussion: Guillain-Barré syndrome is an acute inflammatory demyelinating polyneuropathy that frequently follows a viral illness. It has been associated with *Campylobacter jejuni* infection. Clinically it is characterized by progressive motor loss and areflexia caused by peripheral nerve demyelination. CSF protein is increased, and nerve conduction studies typically demonstrate demyelination of the peripheral nerves. Cranial nerves can also be affected, leading to severe facial weakness and dysphagia. Dysautonomia is common and is a frequent contributor to morbidity and mortality. Respiratory failure is the other leading cause of morbidity, resulting from involvement of the phrenic nerve. (Cecil, Ch. 462)

80. (A) False; (B) True; (C) True. Discussion: Because cerebral autoregulation is lost in ischemic brain, cerebral blood flow will decrease with aggressive treatment of blood pressure. If hypertension is severe (>200/120 mm Hg), blood pressure should be lowered very slowly and in a stepwise approach. Overaggressive treatment can result in stroke progression. Although all strokes can become hemorrhagic, embolic strokes are more likely to do so than thrombotic events. Many experts advocate anticoagulation for

embolic strokes, but this must be done with caution and is frequently delayed 48 to 72 hours after an embolic stroke to decrease the risk of hemorrhagic conversion. Indications for carotid endarterectomy include recent transient ischemic attack or small stroke, ipsilateral carotid stenosis of 70 to 99%, and low surgical risk. Indications for carotid endarterectomy in asymptomatic patients are still being evaluated. (*Cecil, Ch. 440*)

81. **(A) False; (B) True; (C) True; (D) False.** *Discussion:* The finding of upper motor neuron signs in the legs and lower motor neuron signs in the arm should raise the specter of a cervical level of dysfunction. This is not typical of what is seen in ALS when typically there are upper and motor neuron findings in the same distribution. An alternative form of ALS, progressive bulbar palsy, typically involves the muscles supplied by the lower cranial nerves with wasting, fasciculations, and atrophy. Despite the combination of fasciculations and increased reflexes, one should be hesitant to diagnose ALS in the absence of motor weakness. (*Cecil, Ch. 461*)

82. **(A) True; (B) False; (C) True; (D) True.** *Discussion:* Leprosy is typically associated with a sensory neuropathy and thickening or hypertrophy of the nerves. All the other mentioned items can cause a motor neuropathy and should lead to the evaluation of heavy metals, serum protein electrophoresis, and MRI of the cervical and lumbar spine as part of the evaluation of ALS. (*Cecil, Ch. 449*)

83. **(A) True; (B) False; (C) True; (D) True.** *Discussion:* All the medicines are used to treat some neuropathies, but in general carbamazepine is more effective for neuropathies when there is a brief shocklike or lancinating pain rather than a constant chronic burning pain. (*Cecil, Ch. 462*)

84. **(A) False; (B) True; (C) True; (D) False.** *Discussion:* This clinical description is typical for patients with Eaton-Lambert myasthenic syndrome, which is an acquired autoimmune disease more common in men than women and associated with small cell lung cancer. The clinical signs and symptoms that help to differentiate it from myasthenia gravis are the lack of cranial nerve involvement, association with autonomic symptoms (dry mouth, impotence, orthostatic hypotension), absent deep tendon reflexes, and improvement of motor power with repetition. Electrophysiologically, myasthenia gravis and Eaton-Lambert myasthenic syndrome would demonstrate a decremental response at low rates (2 Hz) and Eaton-Lambert myasthenic syndrome an incremental response at high rates of stimulation (50 to 100 Hz). (*Cecil, Ch. 464*)

85. **(A) True; (B) False; (C) True; (D) True.** *Discussion:* Myopathies are characterized clinically by early proximal muscle involvement, mild muscle atrophy, normal sensation, and preserved reflexes until late in the disease. Neuropathies, alternatively, have a distal pattern of weakness, prominent sensory components, early and prominent muscle atrophy, and early loss of reflexes. (*Cecil, Ch. 463*)

86. **(C);** 87. **(B);** 88. **(E);** 89. **(A);** 90. **(D).** *Discussion:* A pure motor syndrome manifested by face, arm, and leg weakness without sensory disturbance is seen with infarction of the posterior limb of the internal capsule that is supplied by the lenticulostriate vessels. Wallenberg's syndrome is seen with infarction of the lateral medulla. This area is supplied by the posterior inferior cerebellar artery, a branch of the vertebral artery. Infarction in the distribution of the left middle cerebral artery is manifested by expressive aphasia with face and arm weakness with sensory loss. Infarction of the left parieto-occipital region, a distribution of the left posterior cerebral artery, may cause alexia without agraphia (can write but not read). The right anterior cerebral artery supplies the motor region responsible for the left leg. (*Cecil, Chs. 423 and 432*)

91. **(C);** 92. **(E);** 93. **(B);** 94. **(D);** 95. **(A).** *Discussion:* Lesions in front of the chiasm damage the optic nerve from one eye and cause visual loss in that eye alone. The classic cause of visual field defects at the level of the chiasm is a pituitary adenoma. This central pressure impairs the crossing fibers to give a bitemporal hemianopia. The lateral geniculate is a thalamic nucleus that receives optic input and generates the optic radiations. Lesions at this level cause a bilateral hemianopsia only. The fibers from the inferior retina, after synapsing in the thalamus, sweep into the posterior temporal lobe. A lesion at this level thus gives rise to a superior quadrantic field cut. The blood supply to the occipital pole has greater collateral support. Therefore, strokes of the occipital lobe often preserve macular vision despite causing an otherwise typical homonymous hemianopia (so-called macular sparing hemianopia). (*Cecil, Ch. 466*)

96. **(A)** *Discussion:* The patient is exhibiting features of a rapidly progressive dementia such as Creutzfeldt-Jakob disease. This spongiform encephalopathy may present as symptoms of altered sleep patterns, appetite changes, sexual drive changes, and impaired memory and concentration. The examination may be noted for myoclonus provoked by visual, auditory, or tactile stimuli. The EEG is characteristic for periodic complexes. CSF 14-3-3 protein may be elevated; however, this may also be seen in stroke or MS. The gold standard diagnostic test is a brain biopsy and staining for prion protein. (*Cecil, Ch. 456*)

97. **(B)** *Discussion:* Cobalamin deficiency is seen in approximately 15% of the elderly. Patients may present with disturbances of gait and cognition. Serum levels of methylmalonic acid and homocysteine may be used to confirm a clinically significant cobalamin deficiency. (*Cecil, Ch. 458*)

98. **(C)** *Discussion:* Von Hippel-Lindau disease is associated with increase in pheochromocytoma, renal cell carcinoma, and hemangioblastoma. (*Cecil, Ch. 459*)

BIBLIOGRAPHY

Goldman L, Ausiello D (eds): Cecil Textbook of Medicine, 22nd ed. Philadelphia, WB Saunders, 2004.

Part XIII
Dermatology

Julie C. Harper

MULTIPLE CHOICE

DIRECTIONS: For questions 1-23, choose the one best answer to each question.

1. A patient comes to the office with a severe reaction to poison ivy. The cell in the skin responsible for generating this delayed-type hypersensitivity reaction is the:

   A. Melanocyte
   B. Granular cell layer
   C. Langerhans' cell
   D. Mast cell

2. Generalized pruritus without evidence of a rash may be attributed to:

   A. Lymphoma
   B. Uremia
   C. Stress
   D. Obstructive biliary disease
   E. All of the above

3. A patient comes in for a follow-up after a punch biopsy of a generalized rash. All around the biopsy site are erythematous papules, and the patient complains that the site is very itchy. She has been applying Neosporin to the biopsy site as the postbiopsy directions stated. Which of the following is the most appropriate recommendation?

   A. That she switch from Neosporin to Mycitracin
   B. A short course of systemic antibiotics for infection
   C. That she use bacitracin on the site instead of Neosporin
   D. Intralesional steroid injections

4. A patient presents with pruritic, almost vesicular-appearing papules and pustules on the trunk, some of which appear to surround a hair follicle. The previous weekend she had been on a ski trip and was in a swimming pool and a hot tub in the evening. The likely explanation for these findings is:

   A. Intertrigo caused by friction from her ski clothes
   B. Folliculitis caused by *Pseudomonas aeruginosa*
   C. Superficial candidiasis
   D. Multiple *Staphylococcus aureus* carbuncles

5. A 2-month-old girl presents with a rapidly enlarging, bright red, 1.5-cm nodule on the upper trunk. Which of the following is most appropriate?

   A. Recommend immediate excision
   B. Recommend no treatment
   C. Discuss laser therapy with the parents
   D. Recommend hospitalization

6. A patient with a history of ulcerative colitis presents with an enlarging necrotic-appearing ulcer on the lower leg. A surgeon carefully débrides the necrotic tissue and is shocked when the lesion doubles in size. The most likely diagnosis is:

   A. Venous insufficiency
   B. Arterial occlusion
   C. Ecthyma gangrenosum
   D. Pyoderma gangrenosum

7. Mucous membrane erosions and ulcerations are commonly seen in which of the following skin diseases?

   A. Perioral dermatitis
   B. Subacute cutaneous lupus erythematosus
   C. Pemphigus vulgaris
   D. Pemphigus foliaceus
   E. Ecthyma gangrenosum

8. Which of the following diseases is not associated with alopecia areata?

   A. Hashimoto's thyroiditis
   B. Vitiligo
   C. Type II diabetes mellitus
   D. Pernicious anemia

9. The layer of keratinocytes located directly above the basal layer in the epidermis is referred to as the:

   A. Spinous layer
   B. Granular layer
   C. Stratum corneum
   D. Horny layer

10. Which of the following statements regarding melanocytes is *true?*

    A. Differences in skin color are dependent on the number of melanocytes in the epidermis.
    B. Melanocytes reside in the spinous and granular layers of the epidermis.
    C. Melanin may be transferred to keratinocytes from melanocytes via endocytosis of the melanosome.
    D. Individuals with albinism have an absence of melanocytes in the epidermis.

11. The primary type of collagen located in the basement membrane zone lamina densa is:

    A. Collagen I
    B. Collagen III
    C. Collagen IV
    D. Collagen VII

12. A young woman presents to a clinic complaining of hair loss. She has noticed an increased amount of hair loss for about 6 weeks and is concerned that she is going to lose all of her hair. She is otherwise healthy. Her only medication is an oral contraceptive pill. She does not have a family history of hair loss. She recently gave birth to her first child, who also is healthy. What is the most likely explanation for her hair loss?

    A. Her oral contraceptive is causing her hair loss.
    B. She is iron-deficient secondary to recent childbirth.
    C. She is experiencing a telogen effluvium secondary to recent childbirth and her hair will grow back.
    D. She is experiencing an anagen effluvium secondary to recent childbirth and her hair will grow back.

13. All of the following statements are true regarding scabies *except*:

    A. Lindane is an effective treatment but should be avoided in young children.
    B. All household contacts must be treated even if symptoms are absent.
    C. The bedding must be washed in hot water after treatment.
    D. The house and furniture should be fumigated to prevent re-infestation.
    E. All of the above are true.

14. A patient presents to a clinic complaining of thick, dry skin on the feet. There is no sign of redness, and no blistering is evident. There is no scaling or maceration in the toe web spaces and potassium hydroxide (KOH) examination of the dry scale is negative. Which of the following topical medications would be most appropriate?

    A. Ketoconzole
    B. Urea
    C. Terbinafine
    D. Lanolin

15. Which of the following sunscreen ingredients is considered a physical ultraviolet blocker?

    A. Titanium dioxide
    B. Salicylate
    C. Cinnamate
    D. Benzophenone

16. Which of the following clinical features or signs is *not* characteristic of psoriasis?

    A. Koebner's phenomenon
    B. Darier's sign
    C. "Oil drop" sign
    D. Auspitz sign
    E. Fingernail pitting

17. Which of the following statements is *true* regarding infliximab?

    A. Infliximab binds to CD2.
    B. Infliximab is an anti-tumor necrosis factor (TNF)-α mouse-derived monoclonal antibody.
    C. Infliximab is an anti-CD11a humanized monoclonal antibody.
    D. Infliximab is an anti-TNFα humanized monoclonal antibody.

18. A patient presents to a clinic with diffuse skin redness and scaling. He complains of feeling chilled and of the embarrassing amount of scale that is falling from his scalp and skin. On examination there are coalescing red-orange papules with "islands of sparing." The palms and soles are thick and yellow. Which one of the following statements is *true* regarding this patient's diagnosis?

    A. The "islands of sparing" indicate an allergic contact dermatitis and corticosteroids should be administered.
    B. The thick, yellow palms and soles indicate dermatophyte with a diffuse secondary "id" phenomenon.
    C. The patient is erythrodermic, and the scaling on the scalp and skin suggests an underlying cause most likely seborrheic dermatitis.
    D. The patient has pityriasis rubra pilaris and should be treated with systemic retinoids.

19. Which of the following statements is *true* regarding dermatophyte infections?

    A. Tinea cruris affects the inguinal folds but spares the scrotum in men.
    B. Tinea corporis is most commonly observed on the lower extremities.
    C. "One foot–two hand" syndrome is common in the elderly population.
    D. KOH examination will reveal yeast forms under the microscope.

20. A 19-year-old man presents to a clinic with a new, erythematous, finely papular eruption and high fever. He appears ill with injected conjunctiva and bright red, dry, fissured lips. He has marked cervical lymphadenopathy. Review of symptoms is positive for mild arthritis and shortness of breath. He does not take any medications. He denies any recent travel. Which of the following statements is *true* regarding his condition?

    A. He is developing toxic epidermal necrolysis and should be treated with gamma globulin.
    B. He has erythema-multiforme major and his underlying herpes simplex should be treated.
    C. He has Kawasaki disease and should be treated with gamma globulin and aspirin.
    D. He has a viral exanthem and symptoms should be treated as needed.

21. Which of the following human papillomavirus subtypes is associated with malignancy?

   A. 2
   B. 5
   C. 11
   D. 30
   E. All are true.

22. Which of the following statements is *true* regarding leukocytoclastic vasculitis (LCV)?

   A. LCV is characterized clinically by palpable purpura.
   B. Drug reactions are a common cause of LCV.
   C. One example of LCV is seen in Henoch-Schönlein purpura.
   D. Colchicine is an effective treatment for LCV.
   E. All of the above statements are true regarding LCV.

23. A 25-year-old man presents to a clinic complaining of severe itching. He has excoriations and erosions on his elbows and buttocks. He has no other complaints. What organ system other than the skin is most likely involved?

   A. Pulmonary
   B. Cardiovascular
   C. Gastrointestinal
   D. Genitourinary

MATCHING

DIRECTIONS: Questions 24–77 are matching questions. For each numbered item, choose the associated lettered item from those provided. Within each set of questions, each answer may be used once, more than once, or not at all.

QUESTIONS 24–28

Match the following dermatologic terms with the best description.

   A. Raised circumscribed area greater than 1.0 cm
   B. Solid elevation of 1.0 cm or less
   C. Red, raised, edematous area that may change position
   D. Flat lesion
   E. Area of indentation
   F. Fluid-filled lesion 0.5 cm or larger

24. Wheal

25. Macule

26. Plaque

27. Bullae

28. Papule

QUESTIONS 29–34

Specific diagnostic signs can help make a diagnosis for particular disorders. Match the following diseases with their appropriate diagnostic sign.

   A. Darier's sign
   B. Pathergy
   C. Koebner's phenomenon
   D. Nikolsky's sign
   E. Diascopy
   F. Wood's light

29. Psoriasis

30. Toxic epidermal necrolysis

31. Urticaria pigmentosa

32. Lichen planus

33. Pyoderma gangrenosum

34. Sarcoidosis

QUESTIONS 35–39

Microscopic examination of skin conditions may reveal diagnostic findings. Match each disease with the appropriate diagnostic test.

   A. Tzanck smear
   B. Potassium hydroxide (KOH)
   C. Gram's stain
   D. Periodic acid–Schiff (PAS) stain

35. Tinea pedis

36. Cold sore

37. Tinea versicolor

38. Shingles

39. Chickenpox

QUESTIONS 40–44

Eczematous dermatitis is typical of a variety of cutaneous disorders and is characterized by the presence of pruritic erythematous papules and vesicles. Often the distribution or other diagnostic clues may help differentiate between these disorders. Match the following diagnostic clues with the appropriate diagnosis.

   A. Atopic dermatitis
   B. Stasis dermatitis
   C. Nummular dermatitis
   D. Eczema craquelé
   E. Dyshidrotic eczema

40. Involves lower one third of the legs secondary to venous insufficiency, often brown or hyperpigmented

41. Pruritic tiny vesicles on the palms and soles

42. Associated with a family history of allergies, asthma, Dennie-Morgan fold, and flexural distribution

43. Coin-shaped patches, often on extensor surfaces of arms and legs

44. Fissuring of the lower legs, more common in winter time as a result of xerosis

QUESTIONS 45–49

Match each of the following sets of clinical findings with the appropriate disease.

   A. Seborrheic dermatitis
   B. Lichen simplex chronicus
   C. Tinea corporis
   D. Candidiasis
   E. Tinea versicolor

45. Annular, erythematous plaques with peripheral scale on the trunk

46. Yellow greasy scales, often in the central face, nasolabial folds, and eyebrows

47. Bright red erythema of the intertriginous area with satellite pustules

48. Very common hyperpigmented to white scaly patches over central trunk, back, and upper arms

49. Pruritic, lichenified, eczematous eruption often found on the posterior neck folds, legs, or groin as a result of repeated rubbing (often a nervous habit)

QUESTIONS 50–54

Match each of the following skin conditions with the appropriate finding.

A. Autosomal dominant
B. Symmetrical papules or vesicles on elbows, knees, and buttocks
C. Large tense blisters
D. Painful erosions of the oral mucosa are typical
E. Scarring of the conjunctiva that leads to blindness
F. Occurs during pregnancy

50. Pemphigus vulgaris

51. Dermatitis herpetiformis

52. Bullous pemphigoid

53. Herpes gestationis

54. Cicatricial pemphigoid

QUESTIONS 55–58

Match each of the following hair disorders with the appropriate description.

A. Self-induced, with broken hairs of different lengths
B. Transient, diffuse hair loss, often occurring several months after a severe illness or childbirth
C. Round patch of nonscarring hair loss with "exclamation point" hairs
D. Conversion of terminal hairs to vellus hairs
E. Moth-eaten alopecia

55. Alopecia areata

56. Trichotillomania

57. Secondary syphilis

58. Telogen effluvium

QUESTIONS 59–64

Match each item below with the associated gland.

A. Apocrine gland
B. Eccrine gland
C. Sebaceous gland

59. Holocrine secretion

60. Merocrine secretion

61. Moll's gland

62. Ceruminous glands

63. Fordyce spots

64. Meibomian glands

QUESTIONS 65–69

Match the following medications with the appropriate association.

A. Used to treat nodular acne
B. Vitamin D analogue
C. Potential retinopathy
D. Used to treat dermatitis herpetiformis
E. Inhibits TNF-α

65. Dapsone

66. Hydroxychloroquine

67. Thalidomide

68. Isotretinoin

69. Topical calcipotriene

QUESTIONS 70–73

Match the type of ultraviolet light with the appropriate wavelength.

A. 200-290 nm
B. 290-320 nm
C. 320-340 nm
D. 340-400 nm

70. Ultraviolet A-1

71. Ultraviolet A-2

72. Ultraviolet B

73. Ultraviolet C

QUESTIONS 74–77

Match the disease with the appropriate association.

A. Lyme disease
B. Parvovirus B19
C. Lung cancer
D. Hypersensitivity to medication or dermatophyte

74. Erythema annulare centrifugum

75. Erythema gyratum repens

76. Erythema chronicum migrans

77. Erythema infectiosum

MULTIPLE CHOICE

DIRECTIONS: For questions 78-85, choose the one best answer to each question.

78. Which of the following statements is true regarding the use of topical steroids?

   A. Topical steroids penetrate the skin surface most effectively if the skin is first soaked in cool water.
   B. Ointment forms of topical steroids are the least effective because the occlusive nature interferes with permeability through the stratum corneum.
   C. The side effects of topical steroids are least likely to occur in the intertriginous skin and on the face when occluded by dressings or wraps.
   D. Fluorinated steroids can be used on the face to treat perioral dermatitis.
   E. Topical steroids reduce the redness and itchiness of fungal infections of the skin, making them a useful therapeutic agent.

79. A patient with a known history of allergic reaction to poison ivy returns from a trip to Hawaii with a severe pruritic papulovesicular eruption around the mouth. Which of the following is the most likely explanation of her skin findings?

   A. She was re-exposed to poison ivy.
   B. She was eating mangos.
   C. She was eating bananas.
   D. She had a sun-induced "recall" of her poison ivy allergic contact dermatitis.

80. Which of the following is true regarding pityriasis rosea?

    A. Typically involves the palms and soles
    B. May be preceded by a herald patch
    C. Aggressive, early intervention is necessary
    D. Vesicles and bullae develop on the trunk along embryonal lines of cleavage

81. All of the following are true regarding rosacea *except*:

    A. It develops most commonly in middle-aged individuals with a tendency to blush easily.
    B. Spicy foods and hot beverages may worsen the signs and symptoms of rosacea.
    C. Topical steroids will lessen the facial redness of rosacea and are first-line treatment in most cases.
    D. Recurrent chalazion formation may be a sign of ocular rosacea.
    E. Comedones are generally absent.

82. Which is a scarring alopecia?

    A. Traction alopecia
    B. Tinea capitis
    C. Lichen planus
    D. Alopecia areata

83. Guttate psoriasis usually occurs after:

    A. A dermatophyte infection
    B. A streptococcal infection
    C. Surgery (Koebner's phenomenon)
    D. Pregnancy

84. Immunoglobulin A deposits are seen in which disease?

    A. Cicatricial pemphigoid
    B. Epidermolysis bullosa acquisita
    C. Porphyria cutanea tarda
    D. Dermatitis herpetiformis

85. A 50-year-old man with alcoholic liver disease presents to a clinic complaining of sores on the backs of his hands. On further inspection, small milia cysts and vesicles are also observed in the same location. There are no blisters on the face but hypertrichosis is evident under the eyes on both cheeks. What is the most likely diagnosis?

    A. Scurvy
    B. Epidermolysis bullosa acquisita
    C. Lichen planus
    D. Porphyria cutanea tarda

TRUE OR FALSE

DIRECTIONS: Answer questions 86-91 true or false.

86. Intramuscular steroids are recommended for individuals with atopic dermatitis whose disease is not well controlled with topical steroids and emollients.

87. Griseofulvin must be prescribed for 3 months to effectively eradicate onychomycosis.

88. Effective treatment of herpes zoster requires higher doses of antiviral medications than does herpes simplex.

89. Acute exanthematous pustulosis is frequently caused by antibiotics.

90. Polymorphous light eruption flares in the spring and improves toward the end of the summer.

91. Direct fluorescent antibody test can distinguish between herpes simplex virus and varicella-zoster.

MULTIPLE CHOICE

DIRECTIONS: For questions 92-100, choose the one best answer to each question.

92. All of the following statements are true regarding erythema multiforme *except*:

    A. Erythema multiforme minor is commonly associated with underlying herpes simplex virus infection.
    B. NSAIDs are a common cause of both Stevens-Johnson syndrome and toxic epidermal necrolysis.
    C. Toxic epidermal necrolysis exhibits larger targetoid lesions than erythema multiforme minor.
    D. IVIG may be useful in the management of toxic epidermal necrolysis.

93. Pseudoporphyria cutanea tarda may be caused by:

    A. Naproxen
    B. Alcoholic liver disease
    C. Diabetes mellitus
    D. Vitamin A

94. Which of the following statements regarding acne vulgaris is *true*?

    A. Frequent face washing and the use of alcohol-based astringents will help control the excess oil associated with acne vulgaris.
    B. Avoiding chocolate, greasy foods, and carbonated beverages should be recommended for all patients with acne.
    C. Topical retinoids are first-line treatment for acne because they are comedolytic.
    D. Tetracycline antibiotics may be given for 2 weeks in severe acne to manage inflammation.

95. A 23-year-old woman presents to a clinic complaining of premenstrual acne and oily skin. She is healthy and does not take any medications. She does not smoke. She has been thinking about starting an oral contraceptive pill because she heard that it improves acne. What is your response?

    A. Agree that an oral contraceptive pill will improve her acne and oily complexion and write a prescription.
    B. Discourage the use of oral contraceptives because they worsen acne.
    C. Prescribe spironolactone.
    D. Prescribe isotretinoin.

96. Which of the following drugs may cause a phototoxic eruption?

    A. Acetaminophen
    B. Amoxicillin
    C. Captopril
    D. Hydrochlorothiazide

97. Which of the following drugs has been reported to cause drug-induced lupus?

    A. Allopurinol
    B. Ciprofloxacin
    C. Hydralazine
    D. Hydroxychloroquine

98. All of the following statements regarding Kaposi's sarcoma are true *except*:

A. Palatal involvement is common in HIV-associated Kaposi's sarcoma.

B. Elderly patients with endemic Kaposi's sarcoma have a worse prognosis than younger patients.

C. HSV-8 infection is associated with Kaposi's sarcoma.

D. All of the above are true.

99. A 35-year-old woman presents to a clinic complaining of tender, red knots on her shins. They have been present for about 2 weeks. She has two healthy children and is on an oral contraceptive. She denies any recent illnesses or new medications. What do you tell the patient?

A. The diagnosis is erythema nodosum, and the most appropriate treatment is hydroxychloroquine.

B. The diagnosis is erythema nodosum, and the most appropriate treatment is rest, leg elevation, and NSAIDs.

C. The diagnosis is erythema nodosum, and the patient is most likely pregnant.

D. The diagnosis is erythema nodosum, and the patient will need to choose a nonhormonal barrier method of birth control.

100. Which of the following statements is *true* regarding gono-coccemia?

A. Cutaneous involvement is characterized by diffuse erythema followed by necrosis of acral skin.

B. Biopsy of involved skin reveals a leukocytoclastic vasculitis.

C. Skin lesions occur secondary to a circulating exotoxin.

D. Cutaneous lesions are few in number and have the appearance of hemorrhagic pustules.

Part XIII
Dermatology
Answers

1. (C) *Discussion:* The Langerhans' cells are the immunocompetent cells of the skin with surface receptors for immunoglobulins and complement. The *Rhus* antigen (from poison ivy) will be processed and presented by Langerhans' cells in the skin to sensitized T cells, which in turn initiate the delayed-type hypersensitivity response. *(Cecil, Ch. 471)*

2. (E) *Discussion:* Generalized pruritus without primary skin disease may be a sign of internal disease. Lymphoma (Hodgkin's disease), uremia, obstructive biliary disease, myeloproliferative disorders, endocrine disorders, and visceral malignancies may all produce pruritus. Psychiatric disorders, including stress, may also be a cause. *(Cecil, Ch. 471)*

3. (C) *Discussion:* Topical antibiotics are often used on biopsy sites to prevent superficial infection. All topical antibiotics have the potential to sensitize, but neomycin in particular is a frequent cause. Neosporin contains polymyxin and neomycin. Mycitracin also contains neomycin. Polysporin contains polymyxin and bacitracin. A patient who reacts to both Neosporin and Polysporin may be having an allergic reaction to the polymyxin present in both preparations. Bacitracin contains no other active ingredients. Intralesional steroid injections are useful for acne cysts, keloids, or localized areas of alopecia, granuloma annulare, discoid lupus erythematosus, or psoriasis. *(Cecil, Ch. 473)*

4. (B) *Discussion:* Hot tub folliculitis is a pruritic folliculitis caused by *Pseudomonas aeruginosa* from infected hot tubs or swimming pools. It may appear almost vesicular or pustular on the trunk and extremities but spares the head and neck. It may resolve without treatment. Intertrigo usually occurs in areas where the skin becomes macerated, such as under the breasts or in the inguinal folds. Candidiasis is beefy red with peripheral pustules. Carbuncles are multiple, draining, deep-infected follicles that require systemic antibiotics. *(Cecil, Ch. 475)*

5. (B) *Discussion:* Strawberry hemangiomas are benign proliferations of small superficial vessels. Characteristically they develop shortly after birth and rapidly grow during the first 1 or 2 years. No treatment is necessary; hemangiomas generally resolve over time without intervention. An exception occurs when a hemangioma is near the eye or mouth and interferes with normal growth and development. Intervention is certainly warranted in those cases. *(Cecil, Ch. 476)*

6. (D) *Discussion:* Pyoderma gangrenosum is an unusual form of ulceration that presents as an enlarging deep necrotic ulcer with an undermined violaceous border. These lesions demonstrate pathergy, in which trauma, such as surgical débridement, will stimulate their growth. Treatments may include systemic steroids or systemic immunosuppressive medications. Pyoderma gangrenosum is associated with inflammatory bowel disease, rheumatoid arthritis, dysproteinemias, and leukemia or lymphoma. Venous insufficiency usually presents as malleolar ulcers, brawny edema, and hyperpigmentation of the lower legs. Arterial occlusion usually presents as sudden pain, numbness, and the development of an ulcer. Ecthyma gangrenosum typically presents as ulcers of the body folds caused by *Pseudomonas* septicemia. *(Cecil, Ch. 476)*

7. (C) *Discussion:* Mucosal erosions and ulcerations present early in pemphigus vulgaris. Mucosal involvement is absent in pemphigus foliaceus, a more superficial exfoliative type of pemphigus. Perioral dermatitis does not involve the oral mucosa. It is an erythematous, eczematous eruption that develops around the mouth. Perioral dermatitis characteristically spares the skin directly adjacent to the vermillion. Subacute cutaneous lupus erythematosus involves the face, upper trunk, and arms but does not involve the oral mucosa. Ecthyma gangrenosum typically presents as ulcers of the body folds caused by *Pseudomonas* septicemia. *(Cecil, Ch. 475)*

8. (C) *Discussion:* Alopecia areata is an autoimmune disease in which T lymphocytes attack hair bulbs leading to a focal, nonscarring alopecia. It is associated with other lymphocyte-mediated autoimmune diseases such as Hashimoto's thyroiditis, vitiligo, pernicious anemia, and type I diabetes mellitus. *(Cecil, Ch. 477)*

9. (A) *Discussion:* The epidermis is composed of a stratified epithelium of keratinocytes. The basal layer of keratinocytes is the germinative layer of the epithelium and also houses the hemidesmosomes that allow the epidermis to attach to the dermis. Just above the basal layer is the spinous layer. In the spinous layer, the keratinocytes have a "spiny" appearance under the microscope. They are attached to one another and to the basal layer via desmosomes. External to the spinous layer is the granular layer of keratinocytes. Keratohyaline granules are large and well developed in this layer of the epidermis. As the keratinocytes mature and migrate from the basal layer to the granular layer they prepare for apoptosis. Cells in the outermost layer, the stratum corneum or horny layer, have undergone apoptosis and are composed of a hollow shell referred to as the cornified envelope. *(Cecil, Ch. 471)*

10. (C) *Discussion:* Melanocytes reside in the basal layer of the epidermis. They are not normally present in a suprabasilar location. Melanosomes are organelles within melanocytes that contain the enzymatic machinery to produce melanin. Skin color is a factor of the amount of melanin produced not a function of the number of melanocytes. Even in individuals with oculocutaneous albinism, the number of melanocytes is within the normal range. The most common type of oculocutaneous albinism is caused by absence of the enzyme tyrosinase, which is necessary for the production of melanin. Melanin is transferred from melanocytes to keratinocytes via active endocytosis. *(Cecil, Ch. 471)*

11. (C) *Discussion:* Collagen IV is the most prominent type of collagen present in the lamina densa of the basement membrane zone. Collagen type I is the most common type of collagen found in the adult dermis. Collagen III is the most prominent collagen of fetal collagen and remains in the adult dermis but in smaller quantities than seen in the developing fetus. *(Cecil, Ch. 471)*

12. **(C)** *Discussion:* Although medications and iron deficiency can cause hair loss, the most likely explanation is that the woman is experiencing a telogen effluvium. There are three distinct hair growth cycles. Anagen is the phase of the hair cycle when the hair elongates. This phase typically lasts 3 years or longer. After the anagen phase comes the catagen portion of the hair cycle. During the catagen phase, the hairs begin to involute. The telogen phase follows catagen and represents a resting phase that is followed by shedding. Normally, only about 10% of the scalp hair is in telogen at one time. With childbirth, and multiple other medical or psychological events, the hair cycles shift dramatically. Up to 50% of the scalp hair enters the telogen phase, and the end result is a diffuse shedding and thinning. This shedding is usually observed about 3 months after the event because the telogen portion of the cycle lasts for 3 months. *(Cecil, Ch. 477)*

13. **(D)** *Discussion:* Scabies is most commonly treated with topical permethrin (Elimite). Elimite should be applied to the infested patient and to all household contacts. Elimite is applied at bedtime and is washed off the following morning. Laundry and bedding from the previous day should be washed in hot water. It is not necessary to fumigate furniture or homes. Itching may continue even after scabies has been eradicated. Antihistamines will help to alleviate this post-scabetic pruritus. *(Cecil, Ch. 473)*

14. **(B)** *Discussion:* Urea is a keratolytic and will soften and remove thick, dry, calloused skin when used topically. Ketoconazole and terbinafine are topical antiyeast and antifungal medications. KOH examination was negative, eliminating yeast or fungal infection from the differential diagnosis. Other keratolytic agents include salicylic acid and α-hydroxy acids. *(Cecil, Ch. 473)*

15. **(A)** *Discussion:* Titanium dioxide and zinc oxide are considered physical ultraviolet blockers. They reflect light from the skin and offer protection from ultraviolet A and ultraviolet B. Salicylates and cinnamates are chemical ultraviolet blockers. They absorb ultraviolet B wavelengths. Benzophenones are also chemical blockers and absorb both ultraviolet A and B wavelengths. *(Cecil, Ch. 473)*

16. **(B)** *Discussion:* Psoriasis is easily diagnosed in most cases. Distribution on the elbows, knees, and sacral areas is characteristic, as is the clinical appearance of a well-demarcated erythematous plaque with silver scale. When the diagnosis is not certain, there are additional clinical signs that may be helpful if present. The Koebner phenomenon describes the tendency for psoriasis to track into areas of trauma such as surgical scars or skin excoriations. The Auspitz sign refers to the pinpoint bleeding seen when the thick scale of a psoriatic plaque is removed. Microscopically, the epidermis is thin above the dermal papillae in psoriasis and small blood vessels are prominent in these papillae. It is the disruption of these vessels that results in Auspitz's sign. The "oil drop" sign is observed on the fingernails and as a yellow-brown macule that appears to be located under the nail plate. Nail pitting is frequently seen in psoriasis and refers to tiny indentations seen on the nail surface. *(Cecil, Ch. 474)*

17. **(B)** *Discussion:* The biologics are becoming important treatment modalities in dermatology and specifically in psoriasis. The exact cause of psoriasis is not known, but activated T cells and the resulting proinflammatory cytokines are thought to promote the disease process. Several of the biologic therapies target T cells or cytokines that may play a role in the development of psoriasis. Infliximab (Remicade) is a mouse anti-TNFα monoclonal antibody. It is administered intravenously. Etanercept (Enbrel) is an anti-TNF-α fusion protein effective for psoriasis and psoriatic arthritis. It is administered subcutaneously. Alefacept (Amevive) is a fusion protein that binds to CD2 markers and prevents T cell activation. It is administered by IV push or subcutaneously. These biologic agents are all effective treatments for psoriasis. *(Cecil, Ch. 474)*

18. **(D)** *Discussion:* Pityriasis rubra pilaris (PRP) is characterized by an orange-red skin eruption of coalescing papules. Small, coin-shaped areas of uninvolved skin are often observed and are referred to as "islands of sparing." PRP usually starts on the scalp with thick scale and erythema and gradually becomes more diffuse on the skin surface. The face is usually involved, and ectropion formation is very common. PRP is difficult to treat. Systemic retinoids are the most effective treatment available for most patients. *(Cecil, Ch. 474)*

19. **(A)** *Discussion:* Dermatophyte infections are common and may involve the hair, nails, and skin. Tinea corporis refers to dermatophyte infection of the body, and the trunk is the most common location. Tinea corporis is characterized by an erythematous, scaling advancing border. Tinea cruris has a similar appearance but involves the inguinal crease. It does spare the scrotum in men but may involve the intragluteal cleft and buttocks. Two foot–one hand syndrome (not two hand–one foot) is a common presentation. Scaling is seen on one palm and characteristic signs of tinea pedis, including maceration of the web spaces and moccasin distribution of scale, are evident on the feet. A positive KOH examination reveals hyphae; yeast forms are not seen in dermatophyte infections. *(Cecil, Ch. 474)*

20. **(C)** *Discussion:* High fever, cervical lymphadenitis, conjunctival injection, and dry, fissured lips are all features of Kawasaki disease. Although Kawasaki disease more often affects children, adults may be affected as well. Other characteristics of Kawasaki disease include desquamation of the hands and fingers and a strawberry tongue. Myocarditis and coronary artery aneurysms may develop in untreated individuals. Treatment includes gamma globulin and aspirin. Toxic epidermal necrolysis (TEN) usually occurs secondary to a medication, particularly antibiotics and antiepileptics. TEN is characterized by large areas of desquamation with the underlying dermis exposed to the environment. The prognosis of TEN is poor. One potential treatment for TEN is gamma globulin. Erythema multiforme (EM) minor is associated with herpesvirus infection and is characterized by targetoid lesions on the hands and feet. Mild mucosal involvement may be present. Erythema multiforme major is characterized by more widespread atypical targetoid lesions and involvement of two or more mucosal surfaces. EM major is usually triggered by a medication. Viral exanthems are generally maculopapular. Although many of this patient's findings are nonspecific, when taken together they should prompt the observer to strongly consider Kawasaki disease. *(Cecil, Ch. 475)*

21. **(C)** *Discussion:* HPV subtypes 6, 11, 16, 18, 31 and 35 may all be associated with malignancy. HPV infection may cause verruca vulgaris (common warts), flat warts (verruca plana), and genital warts (condyloma acuminata). Most warts remain benign, but genital warts and warts in an immunocompromised patient may, rarely, undergo malignant transformation. *(Cecil, Ch. 475)*

22. **(E)** *Discussion:* Leukocytoclastic vasculitis (LCV) is a small vessel vasculitis characterized clinically by "palpable purpura." Drugs, infections, connective tissue disease, and malignancy are a few of the potential factors that can promote the development of LCV. The diagnosis of idiopathic LCV is given when an underlying stimulus cannot be identified. LCV is an immune-complex–mediated vasculitis with vascular wall necrosis, extravasation of red blood cells, and a neutrophilic infiltrate. Treatments include rest, leg elevation, anti-inflammatory medications such as colchicine, and dapsone. Henoch-Schönlein purpura exhibits a leukocytoclastic vasculitis microscopically and is associated with abdominal pain and renal vasculitis. It most commonly affects children. *(Cecil, Ch. 475)*

23. **(C)** *Discussion:* Dermatitis herpetiformis (DH) is an extremely pruritic disorder. The primary lesions of DH are grouped vesicles but, because of the extreme itching, few of the vesicles remain intact by the time the patient presents to the physician. Erosions and excoriations are more commonly observed on the elbows, knees, buttocks

and occipital scalp. Most patients have a subclinical gluten-sensitive enteropathy, and eliminating gluten from the diet may alleviate skin disease and gastrointestinal symptoms if present. Dapsone is also a very effective treatment for DH, eliminating pruritus within 24 hours in most patients. (*Cecil, Ch. 475*)

24. (C); 25. (D); 26. (A); 27. (F); 28. (B). *Discussion:* Appropriate descriptions of a "rash" will help establish a differential diagnosis. A wheal, typical of urticaria, is usually an erythematous, edematous, annular plaque that typically changes location within 24 hours. A macule is a flat discoloration of the skin, either white as in vitiligo or brown as in a freckle. A plaque is a circumscribed raised area typically greater than 1.0 cm, seen in diseases such as a plaque of psoriasis. Bullae are fluid-filled blisters greater than 0.5 cm, as seen in herpes zoster and with the immunoblistering diseases such as bullous pemphigoid. A papule is a raised area less than 1.0 cm (smaller than a plaque), as seen in eczema or drug eruptions. Atrophy of the skin, as seen in lupus or other scarring processes, will usually leave an area of indentation. (*Cecil, Ch. 472*)

29. (C); 30. (D); 31. (A); 32. (C); 33. (B); 34. (E). *Discussion:* Psoriasis and lichen planus both exhibit the Koebner phenomenon, in which new skin lesions develop in areas that are traumatized. Toxic epidermal necrolysis is a superficial blistering condition of the skin, and pressure on these blisters will make the blister expand, a positive Nikolsky's sign. Urticaria pigmentosa has collections of mast cells in the skin that, when rubbed, will release histamine, making the skin lesion red and raised, a positive Darier's sign. Pyoderma gangrenosum may develop at sites of injury, particularly at needle puncture sites, which is typical of pathergy. Sarcoidosis and other granulomatous diseases will give an apple-jelly color when pressed with a glass slide (diascopy). Wood's light, which is long-wave UVA light, allows appreciation of subtle pigmentary changes in the skin, as in the ash leaf macules of tuberous sclerosis. (*Cecil, Chs. 474 to 476*)

35. (B); 36. (A); 37. (B); 38. (A); 39. (A). *Discussion:* Dermatophyte infections of the skin may be diagnosed by a KOH examination. KOH is added to the scale from the patient on a microscope slide and heated to dissolve the keratin. Dermatophytes, which cause tinea pedis and other tinea infections, may be seen as branching hyphae. Tinea versicolor is caused by the yeast *Malassezia furfur*. On KOH examination, one may see hyphae and spores ("spaghetti and meatballs"). A Tzanck smear is useful for detecting the presence of a herpesvirus, such as HSV or varicella zoster virus. A vesicle base is scraped and allowed to air dry on the slide before staining with Giemsa or Wright's stain, which will demonstrate multinucleated giant cells. Gram's stain may reveal bacteria, and a PAS stain is performed on pathologic sections from skin biopsies to look for fungal and yeast elements. (*Cecil, Ch. 472*)

40. (B); 41. (E); 42. (A); 43. (C); 44. (D). *Discussion:* Stasis dermatitis is an eczematous dermatitis of the lower one third of the legs caused by venous insufficiency. Acutely there would be weeping, and more chronically one may see edema, brawny discoloration, or hyperpigmented plaques with scale. Eczema craquelé often involves the lower legs, although actual fissuring of the skin is seen as a result of excessive dryness. Atopic dermatitis is often familial, occurring in association with asthma and allergic rhinitis. Distribution characteristically involves the antecubital and popliteal fossae and the flexural areas. The Dennie-Morgan fold is a redundant crease below the lower eyelid, present in many atopic individuals. Nummular dermatitis refers to coin-shaped eczematous patches on extensor surfaces. (*Cecil, Ch. 474*)

45. (C); 46. (A); 47. (D); 48. (E); 49. (B). *Discussion:* Tinea corporis can be caused by a variety of species with the similar appearance of an annular, raised, erythematous, scaly edge with central clearing that can occur anywhere on the body. A KOH examination of the scale will reveal hyphae. Seborrheic dermatitis

typically occurs in the areas of skin with a high concentration of sebaceous glands, such as the central face, eyebrows, nasolabial folds, presternal area, and even the groin. Typically, greasy yellow scales are seen with some erythema. Candidiasis often occurs in the intertriginous areas of the groin and inframammary and axillary areas, with bright red erythema with erosions and small satellite pustules. KOH scraping of the scale will reveal pseudohyphae and spores. Tinea versicolor, a superficial infection caused by *Malassezia furfur*, is seen on the upper trunk and may exhibit a lacy appearance with a variety of colors from hypopigmented to brown. KOH reveals hyphae and spores, also known as spaghetti and meatballs. Lichen simplex chronicus, or neurodermatitis, is a result of repeated scratching and itching in one area, often a nervous habit. Typical sites of predilection include the neck, nape, lower legs, or groin. (*Cecil, Ch. 474*)

50. (D); 51. (B); 52. (C); 53. (F); 54. (E). *Discussion:* The vesiculobullous diseases may be differentiated by the level of the blister formation in the skin. Superficial, intraepidermal blisters are characterized by a positive Nikolsky sign, in which the blister spreads easily and the cutaneous lesions may appear only as superficial erosions. The pemphigus family of disorders is a group of autoimmune blistering diseases that have an intraepidermal cleft. Pemphigus vulgaris usually presents as painful oral mucosal erosions and superficial bullae erosions on the skin, especially at sites of pressure or friction. Familial benign pemphigus, also known as Hailey-Hailey disease, is not an autoimmune disorder but is inherited in an autosomal dominant fashion. Superficial blisters and erosions typically occur in the flexural areas of the neck, axillae, and groin. The mouth is spared. Heat and superficial infections will contribute to flares.

The subepidermal blistering diseases typically have tense blisters with a negative Nikolsky sign. Bullous pemphigoid, an autoimmune disorder of the elderly, presents as large tense blisters. Herpes gestationis, which has no association with herpesvirus, is an autoimmune blistering disease that typically occurs during pregnancy and resolves post partum. It may recur with menstrual periods, the use of oral contraceptives, or subsequent pregnancies. There may be an association with fetal mortality and prematurity. Cicatricial pemphigoid typically affects the mucous membranes and conjunctiva and can lead to blindness resulting from scarring. Symmetrical papules and vesicles of the buttocks, elbows, and knees are seen in dermatitis herpetiformis. Dermatitis herpetiformis is very pruritic and may be associated with a gluten-sensitive enteropathy. (*Cecil, Ch. 475*)

55. (C); 56. (A); 57. (E); 58. (B). *Discussion:* Alopecia areata is a well-circumscribed patch of nonscarring alopecia. Typically, the quarter-sized areas will have "exclamation point" hairs, which have tapered hair shafts. Trichotillomania is a self-induced area of alopecia caused by compulsive twisting, or pulling, resulting in broken hairs of different lengths. Secondary syphilis can cause a spotty hair loss described as "moth-eaten." Telogen effluvium is a transient or self-limited phase of diffuse hair loss caused by a change in the hair cycle, usually after extreme stress, severe illness, surgery, childbirth, or by a medication. Male pattern alopecia occurs when terminal hairs are converted to fine, nonpigmented vellus hairs. (*Cecil, Ch. 477*)

59. (C); 60. (B); 61. (A); 62. (A); 63. (C); 64. (C). *Discussion:* Apocrine glands are present in the axilla, around the external genitalia, on the areola and around the nipples and on the perianal skin. Moll's glands are specialized apocrine glands on the eyelid. The ceruminous gland is also a specialized apocrine gland. Sebaceous glands release sebum in a holocrine fashion, meaning that the entire cell disintegrates and is secreted. Sebaceous glands are most numerous on the central face and upper trunk. The meibomian gland on the eyelid margin is a specialized sebaceous

gland, and Fordyce spots are sebaceous glands around the lip margin. Eccrine glands are present diffusely on the body surface. Eccrine glands secrete eccrine sweat via merocrine secretion. (*Cecil, Ch. 471*)

65. (**D**); 66. (**C**); 67. (**E**); 68. (**A**); 69. (**B**). *Discussion:* Dapsone is the treatment of choice for dermatitis herpetiformis. Dapsone inhibits neutrophils, which are prominent in this skin disorder. Hydroxychloroquine is commonly used in dermatology for its sun protective effects. The antimalarials, including hydroxychloroquine, are useful in sun-exacerbated dermatoses such as lupus erythematosus, porphyria cutanea tarda, and polymorphous light eruption. Hydroxychloroquine can cause a retinopathy, and routine eye examinations must be monitored. Thalidomide inhibits TNF-α and is used in dermatology for cutaneous lupus and Behçet's syndrome. Isotretinoin is a systemic retinoid used for the treatment of nodular acne. Both thalidomide and isotretinoin have severe teratogenic capability and must be limited to individuals who will not become pregnant during treatment. Topical calcipotriene is prescribed for psoriasis. It is a topical vitamin D derivative. (*Cecil, Ch. 473*)

70. (**D**); 71. (**C**); 72. (**B**); 73. (**A**). *Discussion:* Ultraviolet (UV) A-1 is in the range of 340 to 400 nm. UVA-1 light penetrates deep into the dermis and may be helpful for morphea and localized scleroderma. UVA-2 consists of wavelengths between 320 and 340 nm. UVB encompasses wavelengths of light between 290 and 320 nm and includes wavelengths that cause sunburn. UVB does not penetrate to the dermis but can cause damage to the germinative basal layer of keratinocytes in the epidermis, promoting the development of skin cancer. UVC light, between 200 and 290 nm, does not reach the Earth's surface. (*Cecil, Ch. 474*)

74. (**D**); 75. (**C**); 76. (**A**); 77. (**B**) *Discussion:* Three of the listed erythematous eruptions are classified as figurate erythemas. They are generally annular or even polycyclic. Erythema annulare centrifugum (EAC), a figurate erythema, is characterized by an annular erythematous eruption with scale on the inner portion of the annulus. This scale is highly characteristic of EAC and is referred to as the "trailing scale" because it trails behind the leading edge of the lesion. EAC may appear as a hypersensitivity response to medications or simple dermatophyte infections. Rarely, it can be a marker of an underlying malignancy, and an age-appropriate cancer screening should be performed in individuals with EAC. An underlying stimulus for the development of EAC may not be found in many cases. Erythema gyratum repens (EGR) has a very characteristic "wood-grain" appearance. This figurate erythema also migrates quickly on the skin and is strongly associated with the presence of an underlying malignancy. A thorough search for underlying malignancy is warranted in those individuals with EGR. Erythema chronicum migrans is seen in Lyme disease. It is a figurate erythema that occurs at the site of the tick bite. Concentric rings radiate from the center, giving an erythematous targetoid appearance. Erythema infectiosum is not a figurate erythema. It is caused by parvovirus B19 virus infection and causes a characteristic "slapped cheek" appearance on the face. (*Cecil, Ch. 475*)

78. (**A**) *Discussion:* Topical steroids are usually applied twice a day. The stratum corneum acts as a reservoir and continues to release the medication throughout the day. Additional applications do not increase absorption. Topical steroids are most effective if applied after the skin has been soaked in cool water. The ointment forms are the most effective because the steroids are more soluble in the ointment vehicles. The ointment vehicle allows greater permeability through the stratum corneum. Side effects of topical steroids are seen most often with the intermediate and high potency preparations when used on the face and intertriginous areas and when occluded. Fluorination of steroids increases their potency and, when used on the face, fluorinated steroids may

cause perioral dermatitis with scale, papules, and pustules. Although topical steroids might initially reduce the erythema and/or pruritus associated with a superficial dermatophyte or candidal infection, they typically worsen or predispose to these infections. Their use may alter the physical characteristics of the infection, causing delay in appropriate diagnosis and therapy. (*Cecil, Ch. 473*)

79. (**B**) *Discussion:* The allergen responsible for allergic contact dermatitis from poison ivy or sumac is pentadecylcatechol. This allergen is also present in mangos, cashews, and gingko trees. The contact dermatitis from mangos and cashews can occur around the mouth when contact with the offending agent occurs. (*Cecil, Ch. 474*)

80. (**B**) *Discussion:* Pityriasis rosea usually begins with a herald patch, a large solitary lesion that precedes the generalized eruption. A generalized rash consists of oval patches with a collarette of scale that follows the skin cleavage lines, creating a Christmas tree–like pattern, especially on the back. Palms and soles are typically spared; however, the differential diagnosis includes secondary syphilis and, if palmar or plantar lesions are noted, a rapid plasma regain test should be performed. Pruritus is a common symptom, but no specific treatment is necessary. Topical steroids, antihistamines, and UVB or sunlight may provide some relief. (*Cecil, Ch. 474*)

81. (**C**) *Discussion:* Rosacea is a common disease of middle-aged people, with the development of papules, pustules, erythema, and telangiectasia of the central face. Flushing is a common complaint and may be triggered by alcohol, caffeine, or spicy foods. Complications of rosacea include rhinophyma, a red bulbous nose, and ocular involvement such as blepharitis, chalazion, conjunctivitis, or keratosis. Treatment includes long-term systemic tetracycline antibiotics and topical antibiotics such as metronidazole. Topical steroids may cause and worsen rosacea. (*Cecil, Ch. 475*)

82. (**C**) *Discussion:* Although there are more causes of scarring than nonscarring alopecia, most of the common forms of alopecia are nonscarring. The two classic scarring alopecias are lupus erythematous and lichen planus. Whereas distribution (localized or diffuse) can sometimes help distinguish these two, biopsy is often necessary. When lichen planus involves the scalp, it is known as lichen planopilaris. (*Cecil, Ch. 477*)

83. (**B**) *Discussion:* Guttate psoriasis frequently presents after a streptococcal infection of the upper respiratory tract. The word "guttate" describes the raindrop-like lesions. These lesions may be very diffuse and may resolve spontaneously or with antistreptococcal antibiotics. UVB and/or topical steroids may also be effective at clearing guttate psoriasis. (*Cecil, Ch. 474*)

84. (**D**) *Discussion:* Dermatitis herpetiformis is a subepidermal bullous disorder typified by small tense blisters on the extensor arms and buttocks. Because of intense pruritus, often only erosions and excoriations remain. For this reason, the distribution is very important. Biopsy helps to confirm the diagnosis with direct immunofluorescence exhibiting granular IgA deposits in the dermal papillae. Dermatitis herpetiformis is commonly associated with an underlying gluten-sensitive enteropathy. (*Cecil, Ch. 475*)

85. (**D**) *Discussion:* Blistering and milia formation on the backs of the hands are seen in both porphyria cutanea tarda (PCT) and in epidermolysis bullosa acquisita (EBA). However, facial hypertrichosis is characteristic of PCT. PCT is characterized by blistering, skin fragility, and milia on the sun-exposed surfaces. The dorsal hands and forearms are the most commonly affected locations. Individuals with PCT have a partial deficiency in uroporphyrinogen decarboxylase. The liver compensates for this enzyme deficiency when possible. However, in individuals with hepatitis or cirrhosis,

this compensation cannot take place and porphyrin biometabolism is interrupted. Porphyrin byproducts proximal to the enzyme deficiency begin to build up and spill into the urine and feces. A urinary analysis of porphyrins will help to confirm the diagnosis. Treatment options include weekly phlebotomy and antimalarials. (*Cecil, Ch. 474*)

86. **False**. *Discussion:* Intramuscular steroids should not be used to treat atopic dermatitis. Although the skin may initially improve, atopic dermatitis will often become even more severe as the steroid dose wanes. Appropriate treatments for atopic dermatitis include emollients, minimizing irritants in the environment, topical steroids, topical tacrolimus or pimecrolimus, and antihistamines. In general, sedating antihistamines are more helpful than nonsedating antihistamines. (*Cecil, Chs. 473 and 474*)

87. **False**. *Discussion:* Griseofulvin is effective against dermatophytes and may be used to treat dermatophyte infections of the skin, scalp, and nails. It does not bind the nail keratin with great affinity and successful treatment of onychomycosis requires 18 months of treatment. Terbinafine is also effective for onychomycosis and must be continued for 3 months to eradicate dermatophyte infection of the toenails. (*Cecil, Ch. 474*)

88. **True**. *Discussion:* Acyclovir and related medications are useful in the treatment of both herpes zoster virus infections and herpes simplex virus infections. Significantly higher doses of these antiviral medications are required to treat herpes zoster virus than herpes simplex. (*Cecil, Ch. 473*)

89. **True**. *Discussion:* Acute generalized exanthematous pustulosis is not infectious. It occurs most often secondary to an antibiotic or other medication. The onset of pustules is within a few days of starting the antibiotic and is associated with high fever. Clinically, the pustules are monomorphous in appearance and are widely disseminated on the skin surface. The fever and pustules will resolve within weeks after the offending agent has been discontinued. (*Cecil, Ch. 475*)

90. **True**. *Discussion:* Polymorphous light eruption (PMLE) presents as erythematous, edematous plaques on sun-exposed skin. It is usually worse in the early spring. It does gradually improve as the summer progresses and the skin becomes less sensitive to sunlight, a phenomenon referred to as skin "hardening." The exact cause is unknown. Treatments include sunscreens, sun protective clothing, and antimalarial agents. (*Cecil, Ch. 474*)

91. **True**. *Discussion:* The direct fluorescent antibody (DFA) test can distinguish between herpes simplex virus and varicella-zoster virus. DFA yields results within 1 day and is quickly becoming a diagnostic standard. (*Cecil, Ch. 475*)

92. **(C)** *Discussion:* Erythema multiforme (EM) is a spectrum of skin diseases ranging from erythema multiforme minor to toxic epidermal necrolysis. EM minor is characterized by erythematous target lesions on the hands and feet. Vesicles may appear in the central portion of the target. EM minor is most commonly triggered by underlying herpes simplex virus infection. EM major is also referred to as Stevens-Johnson syndrome. EM major is characterized by more atypical targets, more widespread skin involvement, and two or more mucosal surfaces with blistering or erosions. EM major usually occurs secondary to a drug. The same is true for toxic epidermal necrolysis. Commonly implicated drugs include NSAIDs, antibiotics, and antiepileptics. Toxic epidermal necrolysis exhibits striking full-thickness desquamation of the epidermis. Diffuse erythema may be present before desquamation, but targetoid lesions are absent. (*Cecil, Ch. 475*)

93. **(A)** *Discussion:* Pseudoporphyria mimics true porphyria cutanea tarda in clinical and histopathologic appearance. However, urinary porphyrins are not abnormal. Pseudoporphyria is usually secondary to a drug, and naproxen is a common offender. Porphyria cutanea tarda and pseudoporphyria are characterized by vesicles and skin fragility on the sun-exposed surfaces of the hands and forearms. Facial hypertrichosis on the cheeks extending to the lower bony orbital rim is also commonly observed. (*Cecil, Ch. 475*)

94. **(C)** *Discussion:* Acne vulgaris is a common skin disorder characterized by comedones (blackheads and whiteheads) and inflammatory papules, pustules, and nodules. Although the exact cause of acne is not known, the first microscopic change is the plugging of the follicle and the development of a microcomedo. The microcomedo is the precursor of all other acne lesions. The only truly comedolytic medications are the retinoids. Therefore, topical retinoids are an important part of any acne treatment regimen in a nonpregnant patient. In more severe acne, topical or systemic antibiotics can be added to the treatment plan. Two to 6 months of treatment is usually required for improvement to be significant. Two weeks of an antibiotic will not be sufficient. Remember that these antibiotics are being utilized for their anti-inflammatory roles at least as much as for their antibiotic roles. Acne is not caused or worsened by chocolate, greasy foods, or carbonated beverages. Frequent face washing and topical alcohols will cause an irritant dermatitis but will not decrease sebum production. Washing with a gentle, nonabrasive cleanser twice a day is sufficient. (*Cecil, Ch. 475*)

95. **(A)** *Discussion:* All combination oral contraceptive pills cause an increase in sex-hormone binding globulin and a resultant decrease in free testosterone. Therefore, they all have at least the potential to decrease sebum production and to improve acne. Production and release of sebum is largely under the control of androgen hormones. Androgen receptors are located in the nucleus of sebocytes. Less free testosterone translates to less androgen receptor binding. Spironolactone is also antiandrogenic and will improve acne and oily skin. Spironolactone can cause dysmenorrhea and feminization of the male fetus. For both of these reasons it is best used in conjunction with an oral contraceptive. Isotretinoin greatly reduces sebum production and is a highly efficacious acne medication. However, it is associated with severe teratogenic effects and a long list of other potential side effects. Its use must be limited to those with severe acne. Women who are prescribed isotretinoin must use two forms of birth control throughout treatment and for 1 month afterward. (*Cecil, Ch. 475*)

96. **(D)** *Discussion:* Thiazide diuretics are notorious for causing sun-sensitivity and phototoxic eruptions. Patients should be warned of this risk and told to avoid sun exposure and to wear sunscreen. Tetracycline antibiotics, particularly doxycycline, are also common photosensitizing medications. (*Cecil, Ch. 476*)

97. **(C)** *Discussion:* Drug-induced lupus has been reported with several medications. Hydralazine, procainamide, and minocycline are a few of the drugs that have been implicated. Allopurinol and amoxicillin certainly can cause skin changes, but they are not lupus-like changes. Hydroxychloroquine is an antimalarial medication commonly used to treat lupus. (*Cecil, Ch. 476*)

98. **(B)** *Discussion:* Kaposi's sarcoma can be classified as endemic or epidemic. Epidemic Kaposi's sarcoma refers to HIV-associated disease. Epidemic Kaposi's sarcoma often presents as violaceous plaques on the hard palate, but lesions can be seen anywhere and may be very widespread. Kaposi's sarcoma can have an aggressive course in individuals infected with HIV and in young patients affected with Kaposi's sarcoma with or without HIV. Treatment of HIV infection may also improve Kaposi's sarcoma in some individuals. Endemic Kaposi's sarcoma refers to Kaposi's sarcoma not associated with HIV infection. It commonly affects Mediterranean males with symmetrical violaceous plaques on the lower extremities. Endemic Kaposi's sarcoma tends to run a more indolent course

than epidemic Kaposi's sarcoma. Both variants are associated with herpes simplex virus (HSV)-8. *(Cecil, Ch. 476)*

99. **(B)** *Discussion:* Tender, red subcutaneous nodules on the shins describes classic erythema nodosum. Potential stimuli for the development of erythema nodosum are myriad. Oral contraceptives and pregnancy can both trigger erythema nodosum in some individuals but so can bacterial, fungal, and viral infections, multiple drugs, inflammatory bowel disease, connective tissue disease, and malignancy. Often a cause for the development of erythema nodosum cannot be identified. In this patient it would be prudent to order a pregnancy test before initiating treatment with NSAIDs, rest, and leg elevation. If the problem persists, substituting the patient's oral contraceptive with a barrier contraceptive would be reasonable. Of course an appropriate history, review of systems and physical examination should be done to eliminate other potential underlying triggers. *(Cecil, Ch. 476)*

100. **(D)** *Discussion:* Gonococcemia may present as acral hemorrhagic pustules that are few in number and associated with fever and joint pain. The skin lesions form secondary to septic emboli. Individuals with acute meningococcemia are critically ill. The skin may be diffusely red early, but petechiae, purpura, and necrosis soon follow as disseminated intravascular coagulation ensues. These skin lesions occur secondary to vasculitis, not septic emboli. *(Cecil, Ch. 477)*

BIBLIOGRAPHY

Goldman L, Ausiello D (eds): Cecil Textbook of Medicine, 22nd ed. Philadelphia, WB Saunders, 2004.